The Evaluation and Treatment
of Mild Traumatic Brain Injury

The Evaluation and Treatment of Mild Traumatic Brain Injury

Edited by

Nils R. Varney

Richard J. Roberts
Veterans' Administration Medical Center
Iowa City, Iowa

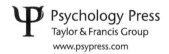 Psychology Press
Taylor & Francis Group
www.psypress.com

Lawrence Erlbaum Associates, Inc., Publishers
10 Industrial Avenue
Mahwah, NJ 07430

Cover design by Kathryn Houghtaling Lacey

Library of Congress Cataloging-in-Publication Data

The evaluation and treatment of mild traumatic brain injury / edited by Nils R. Varney & Richard J. Roberts.
    p. cm.
    Includes bibliographical references and index.
ISBN 0-8058-2393-X (cloth : alk. paper) — ISBN 0-8058-2394-8
(pbk. : alk. paper).
1. Brain damage. I. Varney, Nils R. II. Roberts, Richard J., 1951– .
[DNLM: 1. Brain Injuries. 2. Head Injuries. WL 354 E92 1999]
  RC387.5.E93 1999
  616.8—dc21
  DNLM/DLC
  for Library of Congress   98-33439
                                           CIP

10   9   8   7   6   5   4   3

To Emily Martin

The teacher is faced with the eternal dilemma, whether to present the clear, simple but inaccurate fact or the complex, confusing presumptive truth.

—*Karl Menninger*

When the subject is highly controversial ... one can not hope to tell the truth. One can only show how one came to hold whatever opinion one does hold. One can only give one's audience the chance of drawing their own conclusions as they observe the limitations, the prejudices, the idiosyncrasies of the speaker.

—*Virginia Woolf*

Contents

Preface

This book is concerned with a rather large variety of topics related to minor head injury. It is not intended to be proof that minor head injury is a public health problem, though arguments pro and con are offered in chapters 1 and 13 respectively. Some of the chapters cover aspects of minor head injury about which there is a substantial amount of research already in print. Others, such as Bigler's chapter on imaging or Chwalisz's chapter on collateral stress, while data-driven in content, rely on studies/findings involving more severely injured patients but with results having direct implications for mild head injury. In other words, some chapters deal with what is already known about minor head injury, some address issues that have probable relevance to minor head injury, and some involve a mix of direct proof and inference. This is the state of knowledge about minor head injury. It is anticipated that within the next 5 years, another work (or second edition of this book), will have more facts and less inference. Nevertheless, there has been a need for a work devoted to minor head injury as it is understood to date. The chapters that follow attempt to meet that need.

—*Nils R. Varney*
—*Richard J. Roberts*

1

Mild Head Injury:
Much Ado About Something

B. P. Uzzell
Memorial Neurological Association, Houston, Texas

Mild head injury (MHI) is estimated to occur in the United States at a rate of 1.3 million per year (Malec, chap. 2, this volume). Disorders with this prevalence generally have a scientific base that is clear, precise, and thoroughly understood, but not MHI. Reasons for the chaos of disagreement surrounding MHI have to do with its origins and definition. In this chapter, the set of symptoms associated with MHI is called *MHI syndrome* to avoid some of the negative connotations of some words referring to MHI. Some scientists have claimed MHI is "much ado about nothing," but the aim of this chapter is to provide evidence that MHI is "much ado about something."

One problem with the MHI concept arises from the difficulties in defining MHI. Much of the skepticism stems from an initial inadequate definition of MHI that lacks clarity and generates misunderstanding. Originally, MHI was defined as a posttraumatic amnesia (PTA) period of less than 60 min. But inaccuracies plague this definition due to such factors as suggestibility during the process of obtaining PTA, variation in methods of obtaining PTA, fluctuations in PTA during postinjury measurement times, and excessive alcohol intake (Galbraith, Murray, Patel, & Knill-Jones, 1976). An alternative definition for MHI based on posttraumatic confusion has been offered and used in some situations (Ommaya & Gennarelli, 1974). When the Glasgow Coma Scale (GCS) appeared during the mid-1970s, MHI was defined easily as a GCS score of 13 to 15 (Teasdale & Jennett, 1974). Adding a loss of consciousness of 20 min or less and hospitalization for less than 48 hr further refined the definition (Rimel, Giordani, Barth, Ball, & Jane, 1981). The resulting GCS score with associated time conditions for loss of consciousness and hospitalization provides a more decisive structure, and has become the predominate MHI definition, although the absence of focal findings in the face of GCS scores of 13 to 15 with a loss of consciousness less than 20 min has also defined MHI. A few clinicians still prefer the criterion of the older literature, such as duration of the loss of consciousness in defining MHI.

Another problem with the MHI concept has been the failure of clinical neurology to agree upon neurological origins of MHI syndrome (e.g., headache, anxiety, insomnia, dizziness, irritability, memory losses, concentration losses, etc.; Rutherford, Merrett, & McDonald, 1977, 1979). Some neurologists avoid treatment of MHIs in their clinical practices because of insufficient postgraduate training, and the disorder itself is not intellectually compelling, offering few academic rewards (Alexander, 1995). When the self-reported postconcussive symptoms (e.g., memory losses, difficulties in concentration, dizziness, headache, acoustophobia, vertigo, tinnitus, photophobia, blurred vision, irritability, fatigue, anxiety, depression, hyposexuality, and alcohol intolerance) surface after MHI, they are often discounted because of the symptomatology has not been supported by so-called "hard scientific data." The MHI survivor has often been accused of being a malingerer seeking money and not wanting to return to work. Data more than two decades ago showed 51% of patients have at least one symptom after 6 weeks, whereas 14.5% of patients still had symptoms at 1 year postinjury (Rutherford et al., 1977, 1979). If this percentage is true, then 188,500 MHIs per year (14.5% of 1.3 million MHI per year) have persisting symptoms. Cumulatively, this can amount to large number of patients year after year, although reports a decade later would have us believe symptoms resolve by 3 months (Levin et al., 1987; Hugenholtz, Stuss, Stethem, & Richard, 1988).

The MHI syndrome seems to hinge on the presence or absence of "scientific or objective" data. Few researchers pause long enough to reflect on the fact that observations of "scientific or objective" data are possible only after careful investigation with sensitive or appropriate scientific techniques. One argument is that MHI syndrome exists, but appropriate scientific instruments sufficiently sensitive to reveal it are nonexistent. If that is the case, then the focus should be on establishing careful investigations with adequate or appropriate scientific instruments, rather than rejecting the existence of the MHI syndrome for insufficient evidence.

Despite great strides in uncovering evidence and medical discoveries, scientists do not have sufficient proof for causality or cures for many diseases or disorders, yet this does not mean that any given disease or disorder does not exist. Scientists accept the existence of certain symptoms. For instance, most agree that headaches exist in other individuals besides themselves without experiencing the pain directly. Yet many scientists are unwilling to acknowledge MHI as a genuine disorder with an anatomical and physiological basis. To provide appropriate treatment, it is necessary to determine the cause producing the headache in each clinical case. Similarly, it is necessary to determine the cause or causes of posttraumatic symptoms in each MHI case in order to properly treat the symptoms. Most often, this has not been done. Instead, cynicism rises to such a level that all MHI survivors are presumed to be malingerers, or neurotics looking for excuses not to be gainfully employed, or seeking secondary gain. Certainly there are malingering patients, but not all MHI cases are malingerers. Now is the time to change perspectives and unravel the scientific origins from an array of possibilities in each case of MHI and to decrease easy-to-generate pessimism.

Although much has been written and will continue to be written about MHI, a reflective, analytical examination without rushing into preconceived judgments is necessary. We owe it to those who truly suffer from MHI to raise this syndrome out of the mire of derisiveness and scientific illegitimacy, and to drop the polemics. Chapters in this book addressing MHI from various points of view are designed to provoke thought and reflection, and to engage in the necessary scientific steps in order to arrive at the truth about MHI. The syndrome associated with MHI involves two components: the physical and the neurobehavioral. The question has been, what is the evidence showing which of these two components are responsible for MHI syndrome? To address this question the following review is selective and brief because it is not possible to include the extensive literature in this area in one chapter. To those reading this chapter who believe the symptoms of MHI are mainly psychogenic, suspension of judgment is requested. For those more willing to embrace other conceptions about MHI, attention and understanding are requested.

PHYSICAL EVIDENCE

"Physical evidence must to be present for MHI to be legitimate" is the crux of the matter for many clinicians. Physics surrounding the event of MHI at the time of impact have not been thoroughly explored, although two major mechanisms exist for all types of head injuries: contact phenomena and acceleration. Physical principles are different for each of these mechanisms. Contact phenomena involve an object striking the head and creating local effects at the point of impact, such as skull deformation, as well as far-reaching effects from the impact site. Acceleration of head movement, on the other hand, creates pressure gradients, shear, tensile, and compression strains within the skull and brain (Gennarelli et al., 1982). With sufficient energy or force, death can be instantaneous. With less force, survival may be possible, although primary (intracranial hemorrhage, contusions, etc.) and secondary (raised intracranial pressure, hypoxic, and infection brain damage) complications can occur. The complications may not be clinically apparent until some time after injury. Recently, analyses of physical gravitational forces of acceleration–deceleration have revealed brain damage in 15 MHI human cases during motor vehicle accidents (Varney & Varney, 1995), but more reports at the human level are needed to provide supporting convincing evidence for skeptics.

Because of the mild nature of the injury, humans rarely have routine postmortem analysis. For such evidence, we turn to experimental work. Some time ago, experimental findings showed clear hypoxic damage in Ammon's horn and neocortex of animals with 1- to 3-min loss of consciousness and a 30-sec absence of corneal reflex following acceleration of the head (Adams, Graham, & Gennarelli, 1982). Pathological axonal damage has been documented in MHI experimental preparations (Povlishock, Becker, Cheng, & Vaughan, 1983; Jane, Steward, & Gennarelli, 1985). Evidence suggests the mechanism for MHI damage may be neurochemical (Hayes & Dixon, 1994). Future investigations no doubt will show that neurochemical findings play a greater role in providing physiological underpinnings for MHI, supplementing and/or directing neuroimaging to reveal observable mild brain damage following MHI.

The neuroimaging techniques most often available to provide physical evidence of brain damage have been computed tomography (CT) or magnetic resonance imaging (MRI). When a CT or MRI scan have not shown an abnormality, the conclusion drawn is that no pathology is present. Even with today's technology, absence of a positive finding does not necessarily mean no physiologic or anatomic basis for a MHI. Overlooked, uncontrolled events unrelated to the mildness of the trauma may intercede and negate positive observations of trauma (e.g., poor resolution of neuroimaging techniques and timing of neuroimaging relative to the injury onset).

Computed tomography is the neuroimaging technique initially selected in emergency rooms around the world for all types of head injuries. In the United States, about 14% to 15% of the MHI population have positive CT scans (Livingston, Loder, Koziol, & Hunt, 1991), but the number of MHI cases not receiving CT scans are unknown. The percentage of positive CT scans is the same as the percentage of cases (14%–15%) experiencing symptoms 1 year postinjury (Rutherford et al., 1979). In emergency rooms, CT is the neuroimaging technique of choice because of its accuracy in detecting of life-threatening, intracranial bleeding that necessitates rapid treatment. Although CT may detect intracranial bleeding, it does not seem to be sensitive to detecting smaller lesions laying adjacent to the skull or in other areas. On the other hand, MRI is more sensitive in detecting nonhemorrhagic lesions, such as diffuse axonal injury (DAI), cortical contusions, and brainstem injury. An MRI scan performed in the emergency room with sufficient resolution may be more suitable to demonstrate subtle brain pathology of MHI. Unfortunately, CT, not MRI scans, is generally performed in emergency rooms during initial medical evaluations and treatments of MHIs.

In the climate of recent health care, the radiographic techniques chosen in emergency rooms are evaluated on the basis of cost containment. The cost of identifying the MHI cases with positive CT intracranial abnormalities in the emergency room has revealed a 10% saving when CT is done without the usual combination of CT and skull radiographs, and a 22% saving with skull radiographs alone. These small savings in using skull radiographs rather than CT were reduced by the additional expense related to missed intracranial trauma requiring hospital admissions (Stein, O'Malley, & Ross, 1991). Not addressed was the cost of litigation that may be levied at emergency room physicians or hospitals for not using the usual combination skull radiographs and imaging technique, nor what the cost would be if MRI, rather than CT, were chosen in emergency rooms.

Generally, emergency room physicians are concerned about the "here and now" (i.e., immediate condition and necessary treatment). Consideration is not given to future treatment or rehabilitation where knowledge about the initial documented lesion is beneficial. When MRI scans have been performed in emergency rooms on MHI patients, 10% of the cases have intracranial abnormalities, yet clinical differences between patients with positive MRI scan and those without were not apparent (Doezema, King, Tandberg, Espinosa, & Orrison, 1991). This finding suggests that the brain dysfunction causing clinical symptoms may not be distinctive with a low-magnetic-strength MRI. Many MHI patients with abnormalities and clinical symptoms do not require hospital admission (Pitts, 1991).

So what can be done in emergency rooms? This primarily depends on the clinical judgment of emergency room physicians. CT and MRI are technically available in large medical centers. Some suburban or rural hospitals may only have immediate access to a CT machine. A number of MHI cases may also be discharged from emergency rooms without either a CT or MRI scan. Although missed intracranial lesions are likely in MHI cases, recent developments have produced imaging techniques with greater sensitivity to detect lesions, which will hopefully be available soon in more emergency room settings.

Newer imaging techniques provide anatomic and physiologic explanations for the MHI disorder (Young & Silberstein, 1994). Diffusion-weighted imaging (DWI), which measures diffusion of water through the tissues, may be a technique of choice for MHI patients. As the availability and experience with this technique increase, it is more likely that the technique will be applied to MHI. In white-matter brain tissue, a greater water mobility along myelinated fiber tracts can be observed than along those tracts perpendicular to them. This information is particularly useful in detecting DAI. It can be useful in evaluating patients with minimal impaired consciousness to assess better the patterns of brain injury unrecognized with milder forms of head injury (Ashwal & Holshouser, 1997).

Neuroimaging selection in relation to injury onset and type of pathology are often overlooked factors (Young & Silberstein, 1994). The injury might be observed with CT or MRI only during selected postinjury periods. Certain techniques might not have adequate sensitivity at all time periods to demonstrate physical injury. Perfusion MRI (pMRI) measuring blood volume, blood transit time, and blood flow and functional MRI (fMRI), measuring changes in tissue perfusion based on changes in blood oxygenation, are potentially useful techniques at different type periods. pMRI can demonstrate regions of acute ischemia before MRI lesions can be detected. Evidence now suggests that DWI and pMRI may be more useful in during the acute and subacute phase, while fMRI may be more useful during the later chronic rehabilitation phase when medical and surgical conditions have stabilized (Ashwal & Holshouser, 1997).

Another promising source of identifying a physical basis for MHI has been neurochemical markers. Aberrant neuronal information flow occurring after traumatic brain injury can contribute to acute pathobiologic cascades that produce neurologic deficits in MHI. Loss of calcium homeostasis may mediate this acute excitotoxic cascade. Diffuse reductions in cerebral metabolic activity may occur, although the significance of theses generalized depressions in energy metabolism is not completely understood. MHI can disrupt the blood–brain barrier, allowing excitatory neurotransmitters normally excluded from the brain to gain entry and exacerbate excitatoxic effects (Hayes & Dixon, 1994).

Neurological evidence of organicity has included the presence of anosmia, diplopia, or other positive findings (Rutherford et al., 1977, 1979). Yet these often are ignored. A recent study shows promise in reversing this trend by examining neuroSPECT (single-photon emission computed tomography) images of anosmic MHI patients whose CT and MRI scans show substantial orbital frontal hypoperfusion, the only anatomical region of interest correlating with outcome ratings. Thus, the absence of positive CT and MRI images in anosmic patients does not mean brain damage is not present, as it is detectable with an alternative technique (Varney & Bushnell, 1998). More studies addressing clinical findings in combination with neuroimaging techniques are needed to reveal the physical basis for MHI.

Initial thorough neurological examinations are needed to document the presence or absence of any physical abnormalities, since GCS findings from part of this examination can be misleading. The total GCS score (obtained through observations of eye openings and motor and verbal responses) as part of the clinical neurological examination in most emergency rooms and elsewhere masks important clinical details. Total GCS scores may be the same in MHI patients with different clinical presentations. Although a total GCS of 13 to 15 defines the MHI, a lower score on the verbal part of the GCS may indicate a more serious MHI. A patient who opens his or her eyes to simple questions is different from a patient who opens his or her eyes and answers the simple questions after shouts and shakes, although both will have an eye score of 3 on the GCS. A patient who cannot state the current month on request is different from a patient who can barely give his or her name, although both have a GCS verbal score of 4.

NEUROBEHAVIORAL EVIDENCE

Scarcity of abnormalities on a CT or MRI and persistent postconcussive symptoms (headache, dizziness, memory losses, etc.) lead some professionals to conclude that the sequelae of MHI are strictly psychogenic. The pathogenesis argument for psychogenic versus physiogenic continues unabated without immediate resolution. This argument is analogous to the nature versus nurture argument, where the influence of the two components on human behavior is unclear.

Although a physical component is part of the MHI event, it is not the only part. We are, after all, creatures with feelings and emotions. Looking at the situation from another perspective, it would most likely be considered abnormal if an individual did not react with feelings and emotions after sustaining a MHI. Because the injury is mild, the individual is generally more aware of the circumstances surrounding the injury. Life-threatening events have an impact on most individuals involved. Fearfulness, worry, and interruption of life goals (e.g., education or career threats) have an influence. The emotional response may be heightened by ongoing life events. If a person is in transition at the time of the injury (e.g., has just taken a new job; has started college, trade, or medical school; or has just married or divorced), symptoms may be more intense due to ongoing changes in transition at the time of trauma.

The term *postconcussion syndrome* (PCS) is often used interchangeably with MHI. Heightened sensitivity to light and sound, irritability, headache, dizziness, concentration difficulties, anxiety, sleep disturbances, fatigue, blurred vision, tinnitus, decreased libido, depression, and intolerance to alcohol are some of the PCS symptoms. These are self-reported in varying combinations and severity. Although the symptoms vary inconsistently over time (Rutherford et al., 1977, 1979), they also vary with locale (Levin et al., 1987). Headache and dizziness may dissipate with time, but not anxiety and irritability. In some cases, the PCS can become more intense and persistent. Note that MHI patients are not the only head-injured survivors who have psychological complaints, as these are also found among the severely head injured (Hinkeldey & Corrigan, 1990). Often it is felt that the complaints of the severely injured are more physiogenic and those of the MHI are more psychogenic, but this may not be an accurate assumption. In some cases the PCS may be intense for both mild and severe injuries. Brain damage and psychogenic symptoms can occur together (Binder, 1986).

Because no two MHI cases have exactly the same brain damage, PCS, or preexisting factors (i.e., substance abuse, psychiatric histories, dysfunctional families, and poor interpersonal skills), recovery rates cannot expected to be the same. Clinical experience suggests that not all MHI or severely head-injured patients are alike. Both have subtypes. At least three MHI subgroups have been identified: (a) those with minimal cognitive losses or no complaints, (b) those with transient cognitive losses for a few months, and (c) those with persisting cognitive losses and complaints for several years. Despite evidence to the contrary (Levin et al., 1987), persistent symptoms do not necessarily relate to preexisting neuropsychiatric disorders and/or substance abuse, but can depend on other factors. More studies systematically examining influences of many pre and post variables are needed to understand the MHI subtypes.

Not everyone is going to recover from MHI by 3 months postinjury, as predicted (Hugenholtz et al., 1988; Levin et al., 1987). Efforts need to be made to determine whether participation in studies themselves is therapeutic for the MHI, because studies provide emotional support and information. An invitation to participate in a study can make MHI authentic and attach meaning to the condition. Many MHI individuals feel uncomfortable after having been informed in the past by some professionals that "there is nothing physically wrong with your brain, your complaints are only psychological." They feel comfortable as participants in a study addressing the issues associated with what they are feeling, namely, the MHI syndrome.

The busy, bustling emergency rooms where MHI patients first encounter professionals after injury generally provides no information or misleads intelligent MHI patients by allowing them to draw wrong conclusions about their injuries. Due to the fast pace of emergency rooms and the mildness of the injury relative to other injuries in the emergency rooms, the emergency room staff may, in fact, appear not sympathetic or may not take the reported MHI symptoms seriously. The survivor then is left with little understanding about the disorder and sometimes with disdain for health professionals.

What therapists have known for years—namely, providing patients early with information about MHI reduces symptoms—has been cleverly demonstrated in a recent study (Mittenberg, Tremont, Zielinski, Fichera, & Rayls, 1996). When MHI patients were provided with a printed manual and reviewed the nature and incidence of expected symptoms with a therapist prior to hospital discharge, shorter duration of symptoms, fewer symptoms, and lower mean severity levels at a 6-month follow-up were reported in comparison to untreated controls who received routine hospital treatment and discharge instructions. The implication of this study is clear: More information about the nature and incidence of symptoms needs to be presented to MHI patients prior to discharge from emergency rooms and hospitals, in order to decrease duration, incidence, and severity of symptoms. However, distributing information to MHI patients in emergency rooms and hospitals across the United States is not easily accomplished in terms of cost and personnel time. On the other hand, the cost of not providing information is ethically unforgivable, considering the number of patients experiencing MHI symptoms: the number of work hours lost, the family distress, the medical, psychological, and neuropsychological costs for treatment, and the general loss in productivity in the United States. Postinjury unemployment increases in both mild and severe therapeutically untreated patients (Uzzell, Langfitt, & Dolinskas, 1987) can be reduced in MHI patients with early receipt of information.

Coexistence of posttraumatic stress disorder (PTSD) with MHI has been debated (Bontke, Rattock, & Boake, 1996). Briefly, PTSD has been defined as an anxiety state (Lishman, 1988) with recurrent and intrusive distressing recollections of an event or recurrent distressing dreams of the event with threats of death or serious injury. The theoretical understanding of PTSD is complex (Brewin, Dalgleish, & Joseph, 1996). The risk of PTSD with MHI has generally been relatively low (McMillan, 1996; Middleboe, Andersen, Birket-Smith, & Friis, 1992). The real issue after recognizing a case with PTSD and MHI is planning effective treatment (McGrath, 1997).

Interestingly, neuropsychologists who find no significant changes in functions such as attention, information-processing speed, memory, or other functions after MHI conclude that no cognitive deficits are present. However, this conclusion may be premature. Considering the large number of varied, available neuropsychological assessment techniques, application of a few techniques does not provide conclusive results. For instance, if an examination of visual memory with reproduction of geometric designs after 10-sec exposure reveals no reduction in comparison to norm tables or control subjects, can it be concluded there is no visual memory loss? The simplicity of the geometric designs may not elicit an impaired response. The visual memory function needs to be examined with more complex techniques, or under divided attention conditions. Just as one neuroimaging technique is not sensitive in detecting pathology in MHI, one neuropsychological assessment technique is not always sensitive in detecting dysfunction. On occasion, revealing the predominate dysfunctioning of inattentiveness and loss of concentration after MHI (Gronwall, 1977), which can affect short-term memory and simultaneous processing, can be difficult, but neuropsychologists need to accept the challenge to develop and use instruments to measure dysfunctioning after MHI.

Most neuropsychological studies with MHI do not address functioning ecologically. Answering questions in a quiet laboratory is quite different from the attention required to simultaneously (a) complete an invoice accurately, (b) answer a phone and remember the conversation, and (c) respond to a coworker's questions appropriately. This scenario (or one similar) of multiple simultaneous processing tasks is frequently seen in the workday of an employed MHI survivor. The injured worker can no doubt perform each of these tasks separately well, but not in combination, perhaps due to posttraumatic biochemical disruption. Is it any wonder, the worker complains of headaches, memory losses, or other symptoms after a few work hours? Feelings surge, and the injured worker reminds himself or herself of the preinjury ability to perform all these tasks without problems. In contrast to the severely injured, where a lack of awareness can be a problem, the MHI patient can have too much awareness.

In both clinical practice and scientific investigations selection, neuropsychological instruments need to be sufficiently sensitive to the type of functions affected by MHI, as well as ecologically valid. Conclusions need to be appropriate for the situation, without improper generalizations. Otherwise, the myths and maze of contradictions about MHI will continue. Consistent definitions of PCS, careful patient selection criteria, and follow-up data have been recommended to diminish the controversy surrounding MHI (Bohnen & Jolles, 1992).

Because of the psychogenic features and a dearth of physical evidence with the current imaging techniques, secondary issues of compensation seeking and malingering have been associated with MHI. As a result, far too many malingerers are identified, often reflecting more of clinicians' suspiciousness than the motives of MHI patients. Interestingly, children, who are generally not seeking compensation, have postconcussive symptoms similar to those seen in adults (Mittenberg, Wittner, & Miller, 1997), so the presence of PCS is not sufficient evidence of malingering. When malingerers appear, they can be identified with available techniques (Greiffenstein, Baker, & Gola, 1996; Mittenberg, Rothoic, Russell, & Heilbronner, 1996). In a thorough review of MHI symptoms over a decade ago, Binder (1986) concluded that the effects of compensation claims and preinjury psychopathology were often secondary to organic factors.

CONCLUSIONS

Physical evidence for MHI has been found in pathological, neuroimaging, and biochemical reports, and more evidence will be forthcoming using improved and newly developed imaging techniques. Similarly, old neuropsychological instruments applied in novel ways or newly developed, more sensitive instruments may better disclose MHI dysfunctioning in the future. The trick for both neuroimaging and neuropsychological techniques is to apply them appropriately at selected times. Behaviors associated with physical changes may be long- or short-lived, and may be related to one or more factors (e.g., preinjury health status, life circumstances, coping ability, emergency room experiences, and timing of post-traumatic treatment). PTSD conceivably is a natural development of a life-threatening event, with a low incidence associated with MHI. With provisions for early information and treatment in emergency rooms, PCS and PTSD can be minimized. Focusing exclusively on PCS or PTSD symptoms ignores the physical basis for MHI. No doubt, malingering can occur after MHI (as well as in other disorders), but not every MHI survivor is a malingerer. Scientific energy needs to be directed toward developing newer technical and clinical methods to increase knowledge about the disorder, rather than promoting suspiciousness and cynicism. The premise of this chapter is that MHI syndrome is a legitimate entity supported by physical and neurobehavioral evidence. Although the controversy will not end soon, the future holds a promise of finding further evidence that MHI is "much ado about something."

REFERENCES

Adams, J. H., Graham, D. I., & Gennarelli, T. A. (1982). Neuropathology of acceleration-induced head injury in the subhuman primate. In R. G. Grossman & P. L. Gildenberg (Eds.), *Head injury: Basic and clinical aspects* (pp. 141–150). New York: Raven Press.

Alexander, M. P. (1995). Mild traumatic brain injury: Pathophysiology, natural history and clinical management. *Neurology, 45,* 1253–1260.

Ashwal, S., & Holshouser, B. A. (1997). New neuroimaging techniques and their potential role in patients with acute brain injury. *Journal of Head Trauma Rehabilitation, 12,* 13–35.

Binder, L. M. (1986). Persisting symptoms after mild head injury: A review of the postconcussive syndrome. *Journal of Clinical and Experimental Neuropsychology, 8,* 323–346.

Bohnen, N., & Jolles, J. (1992). Neurobehavioral aspects of postconcussive symptoms after mild head injury. *Journal of Nervous and Mental Disease, 180,* 683–692.

Bontke, C. F., Rattok, J., & Boake, C. (1996). Do patients with mild brain injuries have posttraumatic stress disorder, too? *Journal of Head Injury Rehabilitation, 11,* 95–102.

Brewin, C. R., Dalgleish, T., & Joseph, S. (1996). A dual representation theory of posttraumatic stress disorder. *Psychological Review, 103,* 670–686.

Doezema, D., King, J. N., Tandberg, D., Espinosa, M. C., & Orrison, W. W. (1991). Magnetic resonance imaging in minor head injury. *Annals of Emergency Medicine, 20,* 1281-1285.

Galbraith, S., Murray, W. R., Patel, A. R., & Knill-Jones R. (1976). The relationship between alcohol and injury and its effect on the conscious level. *British Journal of Surgery, 63,* 128–130.

Gennarelli, T. A., Segawa, H., Wald, U., Czernicki, A., Marsh, K., & Thompson, C. (1982). Physiological response to angular acceleration of the head. In R. G. Grossman & P. L. Gildenberg (Eds.), *Head injury: Basic clinical aspects* (pp. 129–140). New York: Raven Press.

Greiffenstein, M. F., Baker, W. J., & Gola, T. (1996). Comparison of multiple scoring methods for Rey's malingered amnesia measures. *Archives of Clinical Neuropsychology, 11,* 283–293.

Gronwall, D. (1977). Paced auditory serial addition task: A measure of recovery from concussion. *Perceptual Motor Skills, 44,* 367–373.

Hayes, R. L., & Dixon, E. (1994). Neurochemical changes in mild head injury. *Seminars in Neurology, 14,* 25–31.

Hinkeldey, N. S., & Corrigan, J. D. (1990). The structure of head-injured patients' neurobehavioral complaints. *Brain Injury, 4,* 115–133.

Hugenholtz, H., Stuss, D. T., Stethem, B. A., & Richard, M. T. (1988). How long does it take to recover from a mild concussion? *Neurosurgery, 22,* 853–858.

Jane, J. A., Steward, O., & Gennarelli, T. A. (1985). Axonal degeneration induced by experimental noninvasive minor head injury. *Journal of Neurosurgery, 62,* 96–100.

Levin, H. S., Mattis, S., Ruff, R. M., Eisenberg, H. M., Marshall, L. F., Tabaddor, K., High, W. M., Jr., & Frankowski, R. F. (1987). Neurobehavioral outcome following minor head injury: A three-center study. *Journal of Neurosurgery, 66,* 234–243.

Lishman, W. A. (1988). Physiogenesis and psychogenesis in the "postconcussive syndrome." *British Journal of Psychiatry, 153,* 460–469.

Livingston, D. H., Loder, P. A., Koziol, J., & Hunt, C. D. (1991). The use of CT scanning to triage patients requiring admission following minimal head injury. *Journal of Trauma, 31,* 483–489.

McGrath, J. (1997). Cognitive impairment associated with post-traumatic stress disorder and minor head injury: A case report. *Neuropsychological Rehabilitation, 7,* 231–239.

McMillan, T. M. (1996). Post-traumatic stress disorder following minor and severe closed head injury: 10 Single cases. *Brain Injury, 10,* 749–758.

Middelboe, T., Andersen, H. S., Birket-Smith, M., & Friis, M. L. (1992). Minor head injury: Impact on general health after 1 year. A prospective follow-up study. *Acta Neurologica Scandinavica, 85,* 5–9.

Mittenberg, W., Rothoic, A., Russell, E., & Heilbronner, R. (1996). Identification of malingered head injury on the Halstead-Reitan Battery. *Archives of Clinical Neuropsychology, 11,* 271–281.

Mittenberg, W., Tremont, G., Zielinski, R. E., Fichera, S., & Rayls, K. R. (1996). Cognitive-behavioral prevention of postconcussion syndrome. *Archives of Clinical Neuropsychology, 11,* 139–145.

Mittenberg, W., Wittner, M. S., & Miller, L. J. (1997). Postconcussion syndrome occurs in children. *Neuropsychology, 11,* 447–452.

Ommaya, A. K., & Gennarelli, T. A. (1974). Cerebral concussion and traumatic unconsciousness. *Brain, 97,* 633–654.

Pitts, L. H. (1991).The role of neuroimaging in mild head injury. *Annals of Emergency Medicine, 20,* 1387–1388.

Povlishock, J. T., Becker, D. P., Cheng, C. L. Y., & Vaughan, G. W. (1983). Axonal change in minor head injury. *Journal of Neuropathology and Experimental Neurology, 42,* 225–242.

Rimel, R. W., Giordani, B., Barth, J. T., Ball, J. T., & Jane, J. (1981). Disability caused by minor head injury. *Neurosurgery, 9,* 221–228.

Rutherford, W. H., Merrett, J. D., & McDonald, J. R. (1977). Sequelae of concussion caused by minor head injuries. *Lancet, 1,* 1–4.

Rutherford, W. D., Merrett, J. D., & McDonald, J. (1979). Symptoms at one year following concussion from minor head injuries. *Injury, 10,* 225–230.

Stein, S. C., O'Malley, K. F., & Ross, S. E. (1991). Is routine computed tomography scanning too expensive for mild head injury? *Annals of Emergency Medicine, 20,* 1286–1289.

Teasdale, G., & Jennett, B. (1974). Assessment of coma and impaired consciousness: A practical scale. *Lancet, 2,* 81–84.

Uzzell, B. P., Langfitt, T. W., & Dolinskas, C. A. (1987). Influence of injury severity on quality of survival after head injury. *Surgical Neurology, 27,* 419–429.

Varney, N. R., & Bushnell, D. (1998). NeuroSPECT findings in patients with post-traumatic anosmia: A quantitative analysis. *Journal of Head Trauma Rehabilitation, 13,* 63–72.

Varney, N. R., & Varney, R. N. (1995). Brain injury without head injury: Some physics of automobile collisions with particular reference to brain injuries occurring without physical trauma. *Applied Neuropsychology, 2,* 47–62.

Young, W. B., & Silberstein, S. D. (1994). Imaging and electrophysiologic testing in mild head injury. *Seminars in Neurology, 14,* 46–52.

2

Mild Traumatic Brain Injury: Scope of the Problem

James F. Malec
Mayo Medical Center and Medical School

Estimates of the occurrence of mild traumatic brain injury (MTBI) have ranged greatly, from 131 per 100,000 (Kraus et al., 1984) to 149 per 100,000 (Annegers et al., 1980)—or approximately 325,000 to 375,000 occurrences per year—to over 2 million occurrences per year (National Head Injury Foundation, 1993). In part because many cases of MTBI do not result in hospital admission, inclusive surveillance systems for MTBI are nonexistent and incidence estimates are often not based on reliable data. One of the best studies of incidence (Sosin, Sniezek, & Thurman, 1996) was based on a household survey of a national sample conducted through the U.S. Census Bureau. This study resulted in an estimate of 618 cases per 100,000 of mild to moderate TBI in 1991 that resulted in loss of consciousness (LOC) but not death or institutionalization. Of these, 59 per 100,000 resulted in only an overnight stay in the hospital, with an additional 460 per 100,000 resulting in no hospitalization. These data can be interpreted to indicate an annual incidence of MTBI of 519 per 100,000 or—based on a national population of 250 million—approximately 1.3 million mild brain injuries per year. This is a conservative estimate because MTBI may occur without LOC.

In a sample of 1,345 high school and 2,321 university students, Segalowitz and Lawson (1995) reported a prevalence of 30%–37% for mild head injury, 12%–15% for MTBI with LOC, and 11.8%–12.6% for multiple head injuries. In this sample, a self-reported history of head injury was correlated with sleep disturbance, with social problems, and with diagnoses of attention deficit, depression, and speech, language, and reading disorders.

These studies indicate that MTBI is a relatively common health problem that brings with it the risk of significant sequelae, including persistent impairment and disability. Nonetheless, many aspects of emergent, acute, and chronic diagnosis and management following MTBI remain controversial. This chapter explores controversies in the diagnosis and management of MTBI and postconcussive symptoms (PCS).

CONTROVERSIES IN DIAGNOSIS

Diagnostic criteria for MTBI continue to be debated. It is generally accepted that an initial Glasgow Coma Scale (GCS) score above 12 following head trauma indicates a milder injury. However, a GCS score of 15 after head trauma provides no evidence of brain injury because persons with normal brain functioning will obtain a normal GCS score of 15.

Some clinicians require the occurrence of LOC to substantiate the occurrence of brain trauma. However, both animal and human models have identified mechanisms by which axonal brain injury can occur without LOC (Hayes, Povlishock, & Singha, 1992). There is also clinical evidence that significant brain trauma can occur without a clearly defined period of posttraumatic amnesia (PTA). Kelly and colleagues (1991), for example, reported a case in which a high school football player died from cerebrovascular congestion after the second of two MTBIs, neither of which resulted in LOC or clear PTA. In a series of 1,448 cases evaluated in the emergency room after MTBI, Borczuk (1995) reported 27 positive CT scans and 2 cases requiring emergent neurosurgical interventions among patients with no reported LOC or amnesia.

The now familiar definition of MTBI developed by the American Congress of Rehabilitation Medicine (ACRM) Brain Injury Interdisciplinary Special Interest Group Mild Traumatic Brain Injury Committee (ACRM BI-ISIG MTBI Committee) indicates that not only LOC or interruption of continuous memory but any disruption of mental state (e.g., feeling stunned or "foggy") associated with head injury is evidence that mild brain trauma has occurred (Kay et al., 1993). According to this definition, focal neurologic deficit after head trauma may also be evidence of brain trauma. The application of the ACRM definition of MTBI, however, requires clinical judgment to verify that the change in mental state is due to head injury and not to psychological causes or other physical injuries. For instance, a person who has sustained no brain trauma may report feeling "stunned" after witnessing a catastrophic event or in response to severe pain associated with nonbrain injuries.

Criteria for distinguishing mild from moderate TBI also lack consensus. The ACRM definition classifies as *moderate* those cases in which the GCS score is less than 13, LOC is greater than approximately 30 min, or PTA extends beyond 24 hr. A small percentage of individuals with MTBI may develop life-threatening sequelae (i.e., subdural hematoma, cerebrovascular congestion) or demonstrate structural brain damage on neuroimaging studies. Williams, Levin, and Eisenberg (1990) found poorer outcomes for cases of MTBI in which intracranial lesions were apparent on CT scan. Such cases may be more appropriately classified as *moderate TBI*. The ACRM definition does not exclude patients with intracranial lesions from the mild category and may merit revision in this regard.

Grading MTBI

Efforts have been made to identify finer grades of MTBI (Esselman & Uomoto, 1995), particularly in the assessment of sports-related injuries. The *second impact syndrome* represents the occurrence of more severe sequelae following a second MTBI sustained shortly after an initial MTBI that resulted in no or minimal sequelae. The case described by Kelly and colleagues (1991) is a dramatic example of the severe consequences that may occur following a second impact. Recent recommendations from the American Academy of Neurology (AAN) for the diagnosis and management of MTBI in sports specified three grades of MTBI (Quality Standards Committee, 1997; see Table 2.1). These grades of MTBI may have application in other clinical settings. For instance, the grade of MTBI might determine emergency room management of the patient or the potential for persistent PCS. At present, however, research supporting the application of AAN recommendations in various practice settings is lacking.

Injury Severity Versus Severity of Sequelae

MTBI may result in one or more symptoms that persist for a month or two after injury. The most common PCS are increased headache frequency, fatigue, dizziness, impaired concentration, impaired memory, anxiety, depression, irritability, tinnitus, and hypersensitivity to light or sound. In some cases, PCS may become chronic, resulting in a *postconcussional disorder*.

The most recent edition of the American Psychiatric Association *Diagnostic and Statistical Manual* (*DSM–IV*) includes research criteria for *postconcussional disorder* (American Psychiatric Association, 1994). A number of issues about the validity of the *DSM–IV* definition of postconcussional disorder have been raised by the ACRM BI-ISIG MTBI Committee (Malec, 1996). These are summarized in Table 2.2. For instance, the development of persistent PCS is not related to LOC or PTA as the *DSM–IV* criteria suggest,

AAN System for Grading Concussion in Sports

Grade	Recommendations for Return to Play After First Injury	Recommendations for Return to Play After Second Injury
Grade 1 Transient confusion No LOC Concussion symptoms or mental status abnormalities on examination resolve in less than 15 min	Remove from contest Examine immediately and every 5 min for mental status abnormalities or PCS at rest and with exertion Return to contest if mental status abnormalities or PCS clear within 15 min	After a second Grade 1 concussion in same contest, remove from play for that day Return to play after asymptomatic for 1 week at rest and with exertion
Grade 2 Transient confusion No LOC Concussion symptoms or mental status abnormalities on examination last more than 15 min	Remove from contest and disallow return to play that day Examine on-site for signs of evolving intracranial pathology Reexamination by a trained person the next day Neurologic exam to clear for return to play after 1 full week without symptoms at rest and with exertion CT or MRI recommended if headache or other symptoms worsen or persist longer than 1 week	After a second Grade 2 concussion, return to play only after at least 2 weeks without symptoms at rest and with exertion Terminate season if any abnormality on CT or MRI consistent with brain swelling, contusion, or other intracranial pathology
Grade 3 LOC (a) Brief (seconds) (b) Prolonged (minutes)	Transport athlete to the nearest hospital emergency department by ambulance if the athlete is still unconscious or if worrisome signs are detected (with cervical spine immobilization if indicated) for neurologic exam with neuroimaging, hospital admission, and transfer to a Trauma Center with persistent or worsening symptoms If initial medical evaluation is normal, send home with written instructions; follow up with daily assessment of neurologic status until symptoms have stabilized or resolved After brief LOC: return to play after 1 week without symptoms at rest and with exertion After prolonged LOC: return to play after 2 weeks without symptoms at rest and with exertion	After a second Grade 3 concussion, withhold from play for a minimum of 1 month without symptoms If any abnormality on CT or MRI consistent with brain swelling, contusion, or other intracranial pathology: terminate season, seriously discourage return to play in the future

Note. From Quality Standards Committee (1997). Reprinted with permission.

TABLE 2.2
DSM–IV Research Criteria for Postconcussional
Disorder and ACRM BI-ISIG Response

DSM–IV Research Criteria Requirements	*ACRM BI-ISIG Response*
A history of head trauma that has caused significant cerebral concussion. LOC, PTA, or seizures are evidence of concussion.	MTBI can occur without LOC, PTA, or seizures.
Evidence from neuropsychological testing or quantified cognitive assessment of impaired attention or memory.	Cognitive symptoms may not be present. Impairment of executive cognitive functions should be included.
Three (or more) of the symptoms listed below should be present and persistent for at least 3 months:	Only two symptoms should be required for diagnosis. Tinnitus and hypersensitivity to light or sound should be included in the symptom list.
(1) becoming fatigued easily	Three-month criteria may prevent early intervention. A diagnosis of
(2) disordered sleep	*postconcussional disorder prodrome* is
(3) headache	recommended to describe a post-
(4) vertigo or dizziness	concussional disorder that has been
(5) irritability or aggression on little or no provocation	present for less than 3 months.
(6) anxiety, depression, or affective lability	
(7) changes in personality (e.g., social or sexual inappropriateness)	
(8) apathy or lack of spontaneity	
Significant impairment in social or occupational functioning and significant decline from a previous level of functioning.	The determination of "significant" impairment may be overly subjective. It is unclear whether the significance is determined from the viewpoint of the evaluating professional, the patient, family or significant others, or some other source (e.g., legal system, society).
Rule out: dementia due to head trauma, amnestic disorder due to head trauma, personality change due to head trauma.	Also rule out: adjustment disorder, posttraumatic stress disorder, somatoform disorder, pain disorder, other anxiety or depressive disorder, substance abuse or dependency, conversion disorder, factitious disorder, malingering.

and the emergence of seizure disorder after MTBI is no greater than in the normal population. Not all patients report cognitive impairment, and many patients report less than three persistent symptoms. Persistent symptoms may include impairment of executive cognitive abilities (complex attention, initiation, reasoning, problem solving), tinnitus, and hypersensitivity to light or sound. Requiring a 3-month duration of symptoms before establishing a diagnosis may prevent early intervention. The ACRM BI-ISIG MTBI Committee suggested that a preliminary diagnosis of *postconcussional disorder prodrome* might be utilized to initiate early treatment.

PCS do not in themselves provide evidence of MTBI because PCS may also occur on a psychological or motivational basis. Furthermore, PCS do not correlate consistently with indicators of initial injury severity. The occurrence of PCS is related to CT abnormalities, but not to LOC or PTA (Evans, 1996). Although the sensitivity of MRI to nonhemorrhagic intracranial pathology after MTBI is well documented, the relationship of abnormal MRI to chronic residual impairment is not (Doezema et al., 1991; Fumeya et al., 1990; Levin et al., 1987, 1992; Mittl et al., 1994). In general, discrepancies between injury severity and severity of sequelae create confusion in labeling all levels of TBI. The correlation between initial injury severity and outcome is not a perfect one. A minority of cases with severe initial injury, as measured for instance by the Glasgow Coma Scale, recover with only mild sequelae. Conversely, a small percentage of cases of MTBI result in relatively severe and persistent cognitive and behavioral impairments. Confusion arises in lay, professional, and legal settings when TBI is described as *mild, moderate,* or *severe* based alternatively on initial injury severity or on severity of sequelae.

The initial diagnosis of TBI and its severity is important in determining acute treatment. Cases of moderate to severe TBI require more detailed emergency and acute evaluation, typically including neuroimaging and hospital observation. Many cases of MTBI do not require extensive emergency care. However, even in very mild cases, a diagnosis of MTBI initiates important preventive interventions that include counseling regarding avoidance of the risk of a second impact, PCS, and return to work and other activities.

If PCS are persistent for more than a month or two after MTBI, the diagnosis of persistent PCS and their etiology becomes a separate issue from the original diagnosis of MTBI. Persistent PCS may result from a number of factors including brain trauma, additional concurrent stressors, psychological and motivational processes, and nonbrain injuries, as well as preinjury adjustment, personality, and psychosocial influences. The ACRM BI-ISIG MTBI Committee proposed that the assessment of BI at all levels of initial injury severity recognize the multifactorial nature of brain injury sequelae.

A survey conducted by the ACRM BI-ISIG MTBI Committee (Harrington et al., 1993) indicated that a majority of rehabilitation professionals believe that there is a need for a grading system to differentiate the severity of the long-term sequelae of TBI from initial injury severity. Most rehabilitation professionals feel it would be desirable to be able to classify all types of brain injuries not only on the basis of initial injury severity but also in terms of consequent impairment and disability. In MTBI in particular, assessment of preinjury factors and concurrent medical and psychological conditions is paramount to the accurate diagnosis of PCS and appropriate treatment or management recommendations. Such a system was proposed by the ACRM BI-ISIG (Harrington, 1995; see Table 2.3).

RISK MANAGEMENT IN SPORTS

A number of authors have identified the risk of MTBI in contact sports (Alves, Rimel, & Nelson, 1987; Cantu, 1991; Fekete, 1968; Stricevic, Patel, Okazaki, & Swain, 1983; Wilberger, 1993). Kelly and Rosenburg (1997) reported an annual incidence of 100,000 concussions per year in all levels of football alone. The American Academy of Neurology (AAN; Quality Standards Committee, 1997) integrated and further developed previous recommendations (Cantu, 1992; Kelly et al., 1991) for the diagnosis and management of sports concussion.

Table 2.1 describes AAN recommendations for management of three grades of concussion. Grades 1 and 2 describe concussions without LOC in which PCS are present for varying lengths of time. After such mild brain trauma, the athlete may return to play if symptoms clear within 15 min. If symptoms persist longer than 15 min, the athlete should avoid play, practice, or other activities in which there is risk of additional head injury for 1 week. After a Grade 3 concussion, immediate transport to an emergency room is recommended for neurologic evaluation, with hospital admission, neuroimaging studies, and transfer to a trauma center as appropriate. Neurologic status of the athlete should be monitored at least on a daily basis until symptoms stabilize or resolve. Return to play is recommended only after 1 week without symptoms at rest and with exertion in cases with very brief (seconds) LOC and only after 2 asymptomatic weeks in cases of more prolonged LOC (minutes). At all grades, a second MTBI requires more careful medical monitoring of the athlete and greater caution in return to play. The presence of neuroimaging abnormalities prompts termination of play for the season and consideration of termination of future participation in sports in which there is significant risk of additional concussion. Recognition, dissemination, and implementation of the AAN recommendations will do much to reduce morbidity and mortality risk associated with sports concussion.

NEED FOR GUIDELINES FOR EMERGENCY ROOM AND ACUTE CARE

Well-accepted guidelines for emergency room practices for patients presenting with MTBI are currently not available. Controversies remain regarding optimal care of such patients (Vollmer & Dacey, 1991). Brockelhurst,

TABLE 2.3
Six Area Brain Injury Assessment System (6A-BIAS)

Area I: Etiology/pathology
  A. Traumatic
       1. With associated hypotension
       2. With associated hypoxemia
  B. Nontraumatic diagnosis
  C. Severity, specified by one or more of the following:
       1. Alteration or loss of consciousness
       2. Posttraumatic amnesia
       3. Glasgow Coma Scale
       4. Presence of injury/illness-related intracranial abnormalities on neuroradiologic
          studies
  D. Chronicity, i.e., time since injury/onset

Area II: Preinjury status
  A. Preinjury medical diagnoses, including prior brain injury(ies), psychiatric disorders,
       substance abuse disorders, or developmental disorders (e.g., ADHD)
  B. Functional status, e.g., mobility, ADLs
  C. Living independence, i.e., level of supervision or support
  D. Years of education
  E. Employment status
       1. Professional/technical vs. skilled vs. semi- or unskilled
       2. Duration of episodes of unemployment
  F. History of criminal convictions
  G. History of physical or sexual abuse/trauma
  H. Personality/coping style
  I. Family roles
  J. Social support system
       1. Extent
       2. Satisfaction
       3. Social roles
  K. Date of birth
  L. Gender

Area III: Injury/illness-related medical conditions
  A. Systems
       1. Neurologic, including autonomic
       2. Musculoskeletal
       3. Immunologic
       4. Endocrinologic
       5. Cardiovascular
       6. Other, e.g., vestibular
  B. Medication effects, therapeutic vs. undesired side effects
  C. Other conditions
       1. Sleep disorders
       2. Pain disorders
       3. Sexual dysfunction
       4. Psychiatric, including psychogenic conditions, malingering

(Continued)

TABLE 2.3
(Continued)

Area IV: Impairments (any loss or abnormality of psychological, physiological, or anatomical structure or function; WHO, 1980) secondary to I, II, and III
A. Sensory perceptual
B. Motor
C. Emotional
D. Behavioral
E. Cognitive, including language
F. Other somatic, as defined by *Guides to the Evaluation of Permanent Impairment* (American Medical Association, 1993)

Area V: Disability (any restriction or lack, resulting from an impairment, of ability to perform an activity in the manner or within the range considered normal for a human being; WHO, 1980) as assessed by:
A. Patient
B. Family/significant others
C. Professionals

Area VI: Handicap (a disadvantage for a given individual, resulting from an impairment or a disability, that limits or prevents the fulfillment of a role that is normal, depending on age, sex, and social and cultural factors, for that individual; WHO, 1980)
A. Indicators
　　1. Living independence
　　2. Vocational activity
　　3. Avocational activity
　　4. Psychosocial adjustment
　　5. Quality of life
B. Influences
　　1. Physical environmental
　　2. Social attitudinal
　　3. Financial
　　4. Legal
　　5. Social support
　　6. Stress

Gooding, and James (1987) recommended hospital admission if a skull fracture or reduced consciousness is present. Along these same lines, Dacey et al. (1986) noted that neurosurgical complications are rare if the GCS score is 15 and skull x-ray is normal. Servadei and colleagues (Servadei et al., 1988a, 1988b, 1989, 1993; Servadei, Staffa, Morichetti, Burzi, & Piazza, 1988) recommended CT scanning if skull x-rays are abnormal or GCS declines, and Mohanty, Thompson, and Rakower (1991) advised against routine CT scanning in MTBI. Other researchers (Shackford et al., 1992; Stein, O'Malley, & Ross, 1991; Stein & Ross, 1990, 1992) concluded that routine CT scanning will decrease unnecessary hospital admissions in patients with a history of LOC. Feuerman, Wackym, Gade, and Becker (1988) and Rosenorn, Duus, Nielsen, Kruse, and Boesen (1991) recommended that if

GCS is less than 15, or decreased mental status or focal neurological signs are present, CT scan should be ordered and the patient admitted. These authors find no additional benefit from skull films. In a retrospective study of 1,448 patients seen in the emergency room after MTBI, Borczuk (1995) reported that limiting CT scans to patients with focal neurologic deficits or GCS less than 15 would have missed 56 positive scans and 1 patient who required emergent neurosurgical intervention. Borczuk (1995) reported only 10 false negatives with no neurosurgical cases (91.6% sensitivity; 46.2% specificity) for a protocol in which CT scans are ordered for all MTBI patients with any of four features: (a) focal neurologic deficits, (b) basilar skull fracture, (c) cranial soft-tissue injury, or (d) age greater than 60. Even liberally applied, CT scanning in the emergency room may miss slowly evolving hematomas (Benoit et al., 1982).

Psychological prophylactic care (information, support, reassurance) on initial evaluation of MTBI has been recommended by a number of authors (Englander, Hall, Stimpson, & Chaffin, 1992; Mahon & Elger, 1989; Minderhoud, Boelens, Huizenga, & Saan, 1980; Saunders, Cota, & Barton, 1986). Alves, Macciocchi, and Barth (1993) and Barrett, Ward, Boughey, Jones, and Mychalkiw (1994) provided data suggesting that such intervention reduces the risk of persistent PCS. However, such care is not standard or accepted practice in most emergency rooms or urgent care settings.

EARLY IDENTIFICATION OF RISK
FOR PERSISTENT PCS

Studies that provide estimates of the number of cases with residual symptoms typically indicate that 20% to 25% of individuals who sustain a MTBI will have residual symptoms or disability (Edna & Cappelen, 1987; Fenton, McClelland, Montgomery, MacFlynn, & Rutherford, 1993; Jones, Viola, LaBan, Schynoll, & Krome, 1992; Wrightson & Gronwall, 1981). However, in a recent study of 587 patients with uncomplicated MTBI, Alves et al. (1993) estimated that as many as 40% have two or more PCS 1 year after injury. In a smaller study, Barrett and colleagues (1994) reported that 50% of 24 patients admitted after MTBI and 60% of 58 patients dismissed from the emergency room reported PCS at 3-month follow-up. In reviewing the Belfast studies, Jacobson (1995) reported that 48% of MTBI patients complained of either persistent or worsening PCS over the first 6 months after MTBI.

Reliable predictors of which individuals will have chronic residual symptoms following MTBI have not been identified through replicated research. Barth and associates (1983) and Bornstein, Miller, and van Schoor (1989) found that chronic residuals are unrelated to LOC, PTA, skull fracture, or seizures. Persistent symptoms have been reported to increase with the presence of an intracranial lesion (Williams et al., 1990) and with older age or prior head injury (Binder, 1986). Bohnen, Twijnstra, and Jolles (1992) reported that a prior brain injury or emotional problems are related to postinjury emotional but not cognitive residuals. In a subsequent study, Bohnen, Twijnstra, and Jolles (1993) identified an increased risk of PCS among MTBI patients with subclinical disturbances of water metabolism.

Several groups of researchers (Alves et al., 1993; Cicerone & Kalmar, 1995; Gerber & Schraa, 1995) reported no relationship between preinjury psychiatric history and PCS. Cicerone and Kalmar (1995) did find that the extent and type of PCS present at 3 months postinjury predicted long-term disability at 1 year postinjury. Fenton and colleagues (1993) found that older females and patients with preinjury social stress were more likely to experience chronic symptoms. Gerber and Schraa (1995) also reported that more emotional symptoms were elicited from female subjects and that preinjury stress was related to reported disability 6 months after MTBI. These authors further delineated how the method of assessment of PCS affects the extent of reported symptomatology: More complaints were elicited with a list of possible symptoms than were volunteered in response to an open-ended question. Only partially consistent with prior studies, Karzmark, Hall, and Englander (1995) reported an association between emotional distress after MTBI and PCS, but found no relationship between PCS and past history of brain injury or psychiatric disorder. Nonbrain injuries in addition to MTBI appear to contribute to poor neuropsychological and psychosocial outcomes (Dacey et al., 1991; Grosswasser, Cohen, & Blankstein, 1990).

Initial reports have indicated a degree of value for psychometric and psychophysical tests in predicting chronic residuals, such as a modified Stroop Interference Test (Bohnen, Jolles, & Twijnstra, 1992) and psychophysically assessed intolerance to light and sound (Bohnen, Twijnstra, Wijnen, & Jolles, 1991). Cicerone (1996) reported that decline in performance on an attention task with the introduction of distraction conditions discriminated MTBI patients from controls and, among MTBI patients, correlated with complaints of impaired concentration, sensitivity to sound, and reduced frustration tolerance.

The sensitivity of MRI to mild intracranial pathology has been well documented, but abnormal MRI has not been a reliable predictor of chronic residual impairment (Doezema et al., 1991; Fumeya et al., 1990; Levin et al., 1987, 1992). The utility of specialized electroencephalographic (EEG) procedures (i.e., P-300, spectral analysis) and SPECT scanning in cases of MTBI is also under active investigation (Ford & Khalil, 1996a, 1996b; Fumeya et al., 1990; Jacobs, Put, Ingels, & Bossuyt, 1994; Nedd et al., 1993; Soutiel, Hafner, Chistyakov, Barzilai, & Feinsod, 1995; Varney et al., 1995). For instance, Soutiel and associates (1995) reported a correlation between the occurrence of a longer NO component to middle latency auditory evoked potentials and the presence of memory or behavioral disturbances after MTBI. Using single-photon emission computed tomography (SPECT), Jacobs and colleagues (1994) identified all 6 patients with PCS of 25 following mild head trauma with only 3 false positive errors; combined with a follow-up SPECT scan, all 6 PCS patients were again identified with only 1 false positive error. Jacobson (1995) cautioned that depression associated with PCS may result in SPECT abnormalities. Any study of chronic MTBI residuals must consider base rates of PCS that have been found to be present in a substantial minority of the non-brain-injured population (Gouvier, Uddo-Crane, & Brown, 1988; Gouvier et al., 1992).

Recent research suggests that apolipoprotein ε (apo ε) may be an important genetic marker of vulnerability to brain trauma. β-Amyloid deposits signify one of the processes resulting in morbidity and mortality after TBI (Roberts et al., 1995). Apo ε genotype appears to moderate the formation of β-amyloid deposits. For instance, Nicoll, Roberts, and Graham (1995) demonstrated that, in their sample of persons with TBI, 100% of participants who were homozygous for the ε4 allele had deposits, compared to 25–27% who had one ε4 allele; 12% with two ε3 alleles, and 0% for ε2/3 and ε2/2 participants. Diffuse axonal injury as indicated by β-amyloid deposition can occur even in mild TBI. Blumbergs and colleagues (1994) found β-amyloid deposits in persons who died of other causes after mild TBI. Jordan and associates (1997) found greater evidence of brain damage in boxers with the apo ε4 allele.

ETIOLOGY OF PCS: PSYCHOSOCIAL, MOTIVATIONAL, AND ORGANIC FACTORS

Very accurate methods to distinguish among patients with mild head injury who have persistent PCS secondary to motivational or psychogenic factors, rather than on a neurogenic basis, are not presently available. Psychological disorders that may present with symptoms that are similar to post-MTBI residuals include depressive disorders, conversion disorder, somatoform disorder, pain disorder, posttraumatic stress disorder, other anxiety and adjustment disorders, factitious disorder, and substance abuse or dependency.

Reviewing the current clinical and research literature, Rattok, Boake, and Bontke (1996) concluded that, although rare, posttraumatic stress disorder (PTSD) can co-occur with MTBI. Some clinicians suggest that MTBI excludes the possibility of PTSD because disruption of memory associated with MTBI prevents the development of stress-related symptoms secondary to memory of the traumatic event. Supporting the conclusion that PTSD does not occur concomitantly with MTBI, none of 28 MTBI patients evaluated by Sbordone and Liter (1995) met criteria for PTSD. Ohry, Rattok, and Solomon (1996), however, found a third of their sample of 24 patients with TBI met criteria for a diagnosis of PTSD. Some traumatic events in which MTBI occurs, such as prolonged assault or torture, rape, and natural catastrophes, may extend beyond the brief time period in which memory is not functional. MTBI survivors may also have clear memory of events associated with injury subsequent to MTBI, such as coincidental death or severe injury of a loved one or medical evacuation and emergency room treatment of other injuries. Consequently, it seems reasonable to conclude that PTSD can accompany MTBI in some cases.

Affective disorders more commonly accompany MTBI and contribute to postconcussive symptomatology (Fann, Katon, Uomoto, & Esselman, 1995). MTBI and PCS can exacerbate a preexisting psychological or personality disorder. Our experience has been that patients whose elevated blood alcohol levels (BAL > 0.10 g/L) at the time of injury place them at high suspicion for alcohol problems tend to deny PCS and are difficult to follow up. Of the first 117 consecutive patients admitted with MTBI that Anne Moessner and I have studied through the Mayo Trauma Center, 50% of those with BAL > 0.10 were lost to follow-up compared to 29% with positive BAL < 0.10 and 20% with negative or absent BAL. However, only 16% of those followed with BAL > 0.10 reported PCS at 1-month follow-up, compared to 29% with positive BAL < 0.10 and 33% with negative or absent BAL. Substance-dependent patients may not distinguish PCS from the effects of substance abuse, and may avoid contact with the medical establishment in order to avoid confrontation of their dependency.

The percentage of cases in which malingering occurs has traditionally been estimated to be small, and a number of studies have found no association between litigation and PCS (Bornstein, Miller, & van Schoor, 1989; Gerber & Schraa, 1995; Gfeffer, Chibnall, & Duckro, 1994; Karzmark et al., 1995; Leininger, Gramling, Farrell, Kreutzer, & Peck, 1990). On the other hand, in their meta-analysis of studies of PCS, Binder and Rohling (1996) estimated that compensation concerns account for 23% of symptomatology after MTBI. Both motivational and psychogenic PCS are potentiated by lay persons' knowledge and expectations of the sequelae of MTBI (Aubrey, Dobbs, & Rule, 1989; Mittenberg, DiGiulio, Perrin, & Bass, 1992). As mentioned previously, the differential diagnosis of malingering, psychological disorder, or organic brain injury as causal in PCS remains an inexact science. A literature review by Franzen, Iverson, and McCracken (1990) failed to identify any highly accurate method for identifying malingering.

The potential costs of both false negatives and false positives in diagnosing malingering are significant. Inaccurate diagnosis of neurogenic impairment as malingering may result in:

1. Unavailability of appropriate treatment to the patient.
2. Unavailability of other needed financial resources and support services.
3. Further reduction of the individual's self-worth—already threatened by impairment—by labeling as immoral or criminal.

Inaccurate diagnosis of malingering as neurogenic impairment may result in:

1. The individual receiving undeserved financial compensation.
2. Unneeded or inappropriate treatment.
3. Avoidance of legal prosecution.

Although no perfectly accurate diagnostic procedure to determine the cause of PCS is currently available, some psychological testing procedures show promise. Rawling (1992) and Rawling and Brooks (1990) reported greater than 90% correct discrimination between simulators and persons with severe TBI using an index based on qualitative analysis of Wechsler Adult Intelligence Scale–Revised and Wechsler Memory Scale–Revised (WMS–R) responses. Mittenberg, Azrin, Millsaps, and Heilbronner (1993) reported 91% correct classification of simulators from individuals with organic brain damage with a discriminant function based on WMS–R subtests. Bernard, Houston, and Natoli (1993) reported 86%–88% correct classification of simulators from persons with closed head injury using discriminant functions based on the WMS–R, Auditory Verbal Learning Test, and Complex Figure Test. Millis (1992, 1994; Millis & Putnam, 1994) showed good results in a series of studies using discriminant function analysis of the Recognition Memory Test. In one study, Millis (1994) reported 93% correct discrimination of MTBI patients who returned to work from those with compensation claims. Current clinical practice recommends a combination of qualitative and quantitative analysis of psychometric test data and clinical impression in identifying a psychogenic or volitional basis for MTBI residuals.

NEED FOR COST-EFFECTIVE TREATMENT
FOR PERSISTENT PCS

A number of potentially effective treatments of PCS have been described (Conboy, Barth, & Boll, 1986; Evans, Evans, & Sharp, 1994; Gronwall, 1986; Katz & DeLuca, 1992; Kay, 1990, 1992, 1993; Kay, Newman, Cavallo, Ezrachi, & Resnick, 1992; McBeath & Nanda, 1994; Mittenberg & Burton,

1994; Mittenberg, Zielinski, & Fichera, 1993; Novack, Roth, & Boll, 1988). However, no well-controlled treatment study has been reported, nor has treatment cost-effectiveness been systematically evaluated. Kay and his colleagues (Kay, 1990, 1992, 1993; Kay et al., 1992) outlined treatments that appear to be effective on a clinical basis. Kay's group recommended the following interventions for individuals who demonstrate PCS shortly after MTBI:

1. Evaluation and education.
2. Behavioral symptom management.
3. Gradual reintegration into activities.
4. Potential referral for more intensive treatment.

Kay and associates recommended the following process for individuals with chronic PCS:

1. Problem identification and validation.
2. Systematic support, that is, rebuilding sense of self and family ties.
3. Neurobehavioral rehabilitation.
4. Redefinition of self and goals.

Compatible with Kay's recommendations, Jacobson (1995) recommended a cognitive-behavioral model for treatment planning. Application of such a model involves the case-specific analysis of organic, psychosocial, cognitive, and behavioral factors underlying PCS and their interactions. Nonorganic etiologic elements relevant to treatment include the patient's beliefs, attributions, coping style, operant factors, and cognitive capacities. Illustrating the potential role of beliefs and appraisals in PCS, Mittenberg and associates (1992) reported that normal controls—asked to describe effects of an imaginary head injury—reported symptoms that were virtually identical to PCS reported by a sample of persons with closed head injuries.

Cicerone and colleagues (1996) actualized a treatment program for persistent PCS that reflects previous clinical recommendations, and conducted a retrospective analysis of outcomes for 20 patients who entered the program 3 to 20 months postinjury. Treatment included cognitive rehabilitation, emphasizing attention and communication skill training; cognitive-behavioral psychotherapy, including desensitization of hypersensitivities and anxieties, and reappraisal of symptoms and self-efficacy; neurosensory retraining for visual-vestibular dysfunction; pharmacologic interventions for sleep disturbance and headache; functional skill training in compensation and self-management methods to improve performance of personal responsibilities; and vocational interventions. Although half of the patients benefited from this multimodal treatment program, the other half did not.

Cicerone's program defines the state of the art in the treatment of persistent PCS and is similar to our own treatment approach at Mayo. In my experience, early implementation of such an intervention before PCS become complicated by family and social dynamics or secondary gain increases the likelihood of a good outcome. Cicerone and colleagues, however, found no relationship between time since injury and treatment outcome. It may be that more detailed analysis of the operant qualities of PCS and other case-specific factors will enhance treatment effectiveness. Future research may profitably explore how personality, social, and injury-related factors interact with specific treatment interventions to produce optimal outcomes.

SUMMARY

MTBI is a relatively commonly occurring threat to health and adaptation. Although human beings have been sustaining and surviving MTBI throughout history, the last decade has seen a dramatic increase in clinical and research investigations of MTBI. One wonders whether this escalating interest in MTBI and its sequelae reflects the expanding demands of modern life on cognitive and emotional capacities that may be jeopardized by MTBI. Much of the care of the patient following MTBI remains controversial. Nonetheless, much has been learned in the last decade. Professional groups, such as ACRM and AAN, are actively involved in translating research and clinical findings into practice recommendations.

The initial diagnosis of MTBI is important to initiate appropriate medical care and counseling regarding PCS and reduction of the risk of additional TBI. The ACRM definition of MTBI facilitates this diagnosis. Initial counseling—to include information about TBI and PCS, support, and reassurance—appears to reduce the frequency and persistence of PCS. Specific recommendations for the management of concussion in sports have recently been developed by the AAN. These recommendations furnish reasonable guidelines for the management of non-sports-related concussions as well. When PCS persist or interfere with return to work or other activities, a more thorough evaluation is indicated, as outlined by the Six Area Brain Injury Assessment System (6A-BIAS; Table 2.3).

Persistent PCS or a postconcussional disorder occurs frequently enough after MTBI (20%–40% of cases) that routine follow-up of patients within the first 2 months of injury is warranted. In ours and in other trauma centers, such follow-up is often conducted by a nurse over the telephone with further medical or neuropsychological evaluations scheduled according to results of the telephone follow-up. To date, research findings do not provide for sufficiently accurate prediction of persistent PCS to allow specific patients to be targeted for follow-up. Neither do psychometric testing, specialized EEG procedures, and SPECT scanning currently appear accurate enough in the early identification of patients who will develop persistent PCS to recommend their routine use in this application. Patients with intracranial lesions on neuroimaging require neurological follow-up with attention to PCS. Patients with nonbrain injuries, a history of prior brain injury, concurrent stress or psychological disorder, and patients—particularly women—over 40 years of age appear to be at increased risk for persistent PCS. Counseling, education, support, and reassurance during emergency care and through follow-up in cases of MTBI appears beneficial and may reduce the frequency and persistence of PCS and associated disability.

In lay, professional, and legal settings, the classification of TBI based on initial injury severity continues to be confused with classification based on the severity of injury sequelae. In this same vein, some clinicians confound the diagnosis of MTBI with the diagnosis of persistent PCS. Persistent PCS do not necessarily evolve from MTBI. To the contrary, the majority of individuals appear to recover completely after MTBI. When present, persistent PCS may result from brain trauma, concurrent psychological features or medical problems, preinjury factors, on a motivational basis, or because of some interaction of these multiple influences. Very accurate methods for the determination of the etiology of persistent PCS do not exist. Nonetheless, misdiagnosis in PCS can have serious financial and social consequences and can result in inadequate or inappropriate medical and rehabilitative treatment. Psychometric testing often assists clinical judgment in confronting this difficult diagnostic challenge.

Limited research and clinical experience in the treatment of persistent PCS suggest that a multimodal program along the lines described by Cicerone and associates (1996) benefits some patients. There is much to be learned about prediction and diagnosis of persistent PCS. A better understanding of the evolution and maintenance of PCS after MTBI should assist in the development of more specific and individualized treatment methods.

REFERENCES

Alves, W., Macciocchi, S. N., & Barth, J. T. (1993). Postconcussive symptoms after uncomplicated mild head injury. *Journal of Head Trauma Rehabilitation, 8*(3), 48–59.

Alves, W. M., Rimel, R. W., & Nelson, W. E. (1987). University of Virginia prospective study of football-induced minor head injury: Status report. *Clinical Sports Medicine, 6*(1), 211–218.

American Medical Association. (1993). *Guides to the evaluation of permanent impairment* (4th ed.). Chicago: Author.

American Psychiatric Association. (1994). *Diagnostic and statistical manual of mental disorders* (4th ed.). Washington, DC: Author.

Annegers, J. F., Grabow, J. D., Kurland, L. T., & Laws, Jr., E. R. (1980). The incidence, causes, and secular trends of head trauma in Olmsted County, Minnesota, 1935–1974. *Neurology, 30*, 912–919.

Aubrey, J. B., Dobbs, A. R., & Rule, B. G. (1989). Laypersons' knowledge about the sequelae of minor head injury and whiplash. *Journal of Neurology, Neurosurgery, and Psychiatry, 52*(7), 842–846.

Barrett, K., Ward, A. B., Boughey, A., Jones, M., & Mychalkiw, W. (1994). Sequelae of minor head injury: The natural history of post-concussive symptoms and their relationship to loss of consciousness and follow-up. *Journal of Accident and Emergency Medicine, 11*, 79–84.

Barth, J. T., Macciocchi, S. N., Giordani, B., Rimel, R., Jane, J. A., & Boll, T. J. (1983). Neuropsychological sequelae of minor head injury. *Neurosurgery, 13*(5), 529–533.

Benoit, B. G., Russell, N. A., Richard, M. T., Hugenholtz, H., Ventureyra, E. C., & Choo, S. H. (1982). Epidural hematoma: Report of seven cases with delayed evolution of symptoms. *Canadian Journal of Neurological Science, 9*(3), 321–324.

Bernard, L. C., Houston, W., & Natoli, L. (1993). Malingering on neuropsychological memory tests: potential objective indicators. *Journal of Clinical Psychology, 49*, 45–53.

Binder, L. M. (1986). Persisting symptoms after mild head injury: a review of the postconcussive syndrome. *Journal of Clinical and Experimental Neuropsychology, 8*(4), 323–346.

Binder, L. M., & Rohling, M. L. (1996). Money matters: A meta-analytic review of the effects of financial incentives on recovery after closed head injury. *American Journal of Psychiatry, 153*, 7–10.

Blumbergs, P. C., Scott, G., Manavis, J., Wainwright, H., Simpson, D. A., & McLean, A. J. (1994). Staining of amyloid precursor protein to study axonal damage in mild head injury. *Lancet, 344*, 1055–1056.

Bohnen, N., Jolles, J., & Twijnstra, A. (1992). Modification of the Stroop Color Word Test improves differentiation between patients with mild head injury and matched controls. *Clinical Neuropsychologist, 6*, 178–184.

Bohnen, N., Twijnstra, A., & Jolles, J. (1992). Post-traumatic and emotional symptoms in different subgroups of patients with mild head injury. *Brain Injury, 6*(6), 481–487.

Bohnen, N., Twijnstra, A., & Jolles, J. (1993). Water metabolism and postconcussional symptoms 5 weeks after mild head injury. *European Neurology, 33*, 77–79.

Bohnen, N., Twijnstra, A., Wijnen, G., & Jolles, J. (1991). Tolerance for light and sound of patients with persistent post-concussional symptoms 6 months after mild head injury. *Journal of Neurology, 238*(8), 443–446.

Borczuk, P. (1995). Predictors of intracranial injury in patients with mild head trauma. *Annals of Emergency Medicine, 25*, 731–736.

Bornstein, R. A., Miller, H. B., & van Schoor, J. T. (1989). Neuropsychological deficit and emotional disturbance in head-injured patients. *Journal of Neurosurgery, 70*(4), 509–513.

Brocklehurst, G., Gooding, M., & James, G. (1987). Comprehensive care of patients with head injuries. *British Medical Journal (Clinical Research Edition), 294*(6568), 345–347.

Cantu, R. C. (1991). Minor head injuries in sports. *Adolescent Medicine: State of the Art Reviews, 2*, 141–148.

Cantu, R. C. (1992). Cerebral concussion in sport. Management and prevention. *Sports Medicine, 14*(1), 64–74.

Cicerone, K. D. (1996). Attention deficits and dual task demands after mild traumatic brain injury. *Brain Injury, 10*, 79–89.

Cicerone, K. D., & Kalmar, K. (1995). Persistent postconcussion syndrome: The structure of subjective complaints after mild traumatic brain injury. *Journal of Head Trauma Rehabilitation, 10*(3), 1–17.

Cicerone, K. D., Smith, L. C., Ellmo, W., Mangel, H. R., Nelson, P., Chase, R. F., & Kalmar, K. (1996). Neuropsychological rehabilitation of mild traumatic brain injury. *Brain Injury, 10*(4), 277–286.

Conboy, T. J., Barth, J., & Boll, T. J. (1986). Treatment and rehabilitation of mild and moderate head trauma. *Rehabilitation Psychology, 31*, 203–215.

Dacey, R. G., Jr., Alves, W. M., Rimel, R. W., Winn, H. R., & Jane, J. A. (1986). Neurosurgical complications after apparently minor head injury. Assessment of risk in a series of 610 patients. *Journal of Neurosurgery, 65*(2), 203–210.

Dacey, R., Dikmen, S., Temkin, N., McLean, A., Armsden, G., & Winn, H. R. (1991). Relative effects of brain and non-brain injuries on neuropsychological and psychosocial outcome. *Journal of Trauma, 31*, 217–222.

Doezema, D., King, J. N., Tandberg, D., Espinosa, M. C., & Orrison, W. W. (1991). Magnetic resonance imaging in minor head injury. *Annals of Emergency Medicine, 20*(12), 1281–1285.

Edna, T. H., & Cappelen, J. (1987). Return to work and social adjustment after traumatic head injury. *Acta Neurochirurgica (Wien), 85*(12), 40–43.

Englander, J., Hall, K., Stimpson, T., & Chaffin, S. (1992). Mild traumatic brain injury in an insured population: subjective complaints and return to employment. *Brain Injury, 6*(2), 161–166.

Esselman, P. C., & Uomoto, J. M. (1995). Classification of the spectrum of mild traumatic brain injury. *Brain Injury, 4*, 417–424.

Evans, R. W. (1996). The postconcussion syndrome and the sequelae of mild head injury. In R. W. Evans (Ed.), *Neurology and trauma* (pp. 91–116). Philadelphia: W. B. Saunders.

Evans, R. W., Evans, R. L., & Sharp, M. J. (1994). The physician survey on the post-concussion and whiplash syndromes. *Headache, 34*, 268–274.

Fann, J. R., Katon, W. J., Uomoto, J. M., & Esselman, P. C. (1995). Psychiatric disorders and functional disability in outpatients with traumatic brain injuries. *American Journal of Psychiatry, 152*(10), 1493–1499.

Fekete, J. F. (1968). Severe brain injury and death following minor hockey accidents: the effectiveness of the "safety helmets" of amateur hockey players. *Canadian Medical Association Journal, 99*(25), 1234–1239.

Fenton, G., McClelland, R., Montgomery, A., MacFlynn, G., & Rutherford, W. (1993). The postconcussional syndrome: Social antecedents and psychological sequelae. *British Journal of Psychiatry, 162*, 493–497.

Feuerman, T., Wackym, P. A., Gade, G. F., & Becker, D. P. (1988). Value of skull radiography, head computed tomographic scanning, and admission for observation in cases of minor head injury. *Neurosurgery, 22*(3), 449–453.

Ford, M. R., & Khalil, M. (1996a). Evoked potential findings in mild traumatic brain injury 1: Middle latency component augmentation and cognitive component attenuation. *Journal of Head Trauma Rehabilitation, 11*(3), 1–15.

Ford, M. R., & Khalil, M. (1996b). Evoked potential findings in mild traumatic brain injury 2: Scoring system and individual discrimination. *Journal of Head Trauma Rehabilitation, 11*(3), 16–21.

Franzen, M., Iverson, G., & McCracken, L. (1990). The detection of malingering on neuropsychological assessment. *Neuropsychology Review, 1*, 247–279.

Fumeya, H., Ito, K., Yamagiwa, O., Funatsu, N., Okada, T., Asahi, S., Ogura, H., Kubo, M., & Oba, T. (1990). Analysis of MRI and SPECT in patients with acute head injury. *Acta Neurochirurgica Suppl. (Wien), 51*, 283–285.

Gerber, D. J., & Schraa, J. C. (1995). Mild traumatic brain injury: searching for the syndrome. *Journal of Head Trauma Rehabilitation, 10*(4), 28–40.

Gfeffer, J. D., Chibnall, J. T., & Duckro, P. N. (1994). Postconcussion symptoms and cognitive functioning in post-traumatic headache patients. *Headache*, *34*, 503–507.

Gouvier, W. D., Uddo-Crane, M., & Brown, L. M. (1988). Base rates of post-concussional symptoms. *Archives of Clinical Neuropsychology*, *3*, 273–278.

Gouvier, W. D., Cubic, B., & Jones, G. (1992). Postconcussion symptoms and daily stress in normal and head-injured college populations. *Archives of Clinical Neuropsychology*, *7*, 193–211.

Gronwall, D. (1986). Rehabilitation programs for patients with mild head injury: Components, problems, and evaluation. *Journal of Head Trauma Rehabilitation*, *1*, 53–62.

Groswasser, Z., Cohen, M., & Blankstein, E. (1990). Polytrauma associated with traumatic brain injury: incidence, nature and impact on rehabilitation outcome. *Brain Injury*, *4*, 161–166.

Harrington, D. E. (1995). A universal nomenclature for brain injury (6A-BIAS). *Moving Ahead*, *9*(3), 1,3.

Harrington, D. E., Malec, J., Cicerone, K., & Katz, H. T. (1993). Current perceptions of rehabilitation professionals towards mild traumatic brain injury. *Archives of Physical Medicine and Rehabilitation*, *74*(6), 579–586.

Hayes, R. L., Povlishock, J. T., & Singha, B. (1992). Pathophysiology of mild head injury. In L. J. Horn & N. D. Zasler (Eds.), *Rehabilitation of postconcussive disorders* (pp. 9–20). Philadelphia: Hanley & Belfast.

Jacobs, A., Put, E., Ingels, M., & Bossuyt, A. (1994). Prospective evaluation of technetium-99m-HMPAO SPECT in mild and moderate traumatic brain injury. *Journal of Nuclear Medicine*, *35*, 942–947.

Jacobson, R. R. (1995). The postconcussional syndrome: physiogenesis, psychogenesis, and malingering. An integrative model. *Journal of Psychosomatic Research*, *39*, 675–693.

Jones, J. H., Viola, S. L., LaBan, M. M., Schynoll, W. G., & Krome, R. L. (1992). The incidence of post minor traumatic brain injury syndrome: A retrospective survey of treating physicians. *Archives of Physical Medicine and Rehabilitation*, *73*(2), 145–146.

Jordan, B. D., Relkin, N. R., Ravdin, L. D., Jacobs, A. R., Bennett, A., & Gandy, S. (1997). Apolipoprotein E epsilon 4 associated with chronic traumatic brain injury in boxing. *Journal of the American Medical Association*, *278*, 136–140.

Karzmark, P., Hall, K., & Englander, J. (1995). Late-onset post-concussion symptoms after mild brain injury: The role of premorbid, injury-related, environmental, and personality factors. *Brain Injury*, *9*, 21–26.

Katz, R. T., & DeLuca, J. (1992). Sequelae of minor traumatic brain injury. *American Family Physician*, *46*(5), 1491–1498.

Kay, T. (1990). Rehabilitation after minor head injury. *Rehabilitation Management, June/July*, 88–95.

Kay, T. (1992). Neuropsychological diagnosis: Disentangling the multiple determinants of functional disability after mild traumatic brain injury. *Physical Medicine Rehabilitation: State of the Art Reviews*, *6*, 109–127.

Kay, T. (1993). Neuropsychological treatment of mild traumatic brain injury. *Journal of Head Trauma Rehabilitation*, *8*, 74–85.

Kay, T., Harrington, D. E., Adams, R., Anderson, T., Berrol, S., Cicerone, K., Dahlberg, C., Gerber, D., Goka, R., Harley, P., Hilt, J., Horn, L., Lehmkuhl, D., & Malec, J. (1993). Definition of mild traumatic brain injury. *Journal of Head Trauma Rehabilitation*, *8*(3), 86–87.

Kay, T., Newman, B., Cavallo, M., Ezrachi, O., & Resnick, M. (1992). Toward a neuropsychological model of functional disability after mild traumatic brain injury. *Neuropsychology*, *6*, 371–384.

Kelly, J. P., Nichols, J. S., Filley, C. M., Lillehei, K. O., Rubinstein, D., & Kleinschmidt-DeMasters, B. K. (1991). Concussion in sports: guidelines for the prevention of catastrophic outcome. *Journal of the American Medical Association*, *266*, 2867–2869.

Kelly, J. P., & Rosenberg, J. H. (1997). Diagnosis and management of concussion in sports. *Neurology, 48,* 575–580.

Kraus, J. F., Black, M. A., Hessol, N., Ley, P., Rokaw, W., Sullivan, C., Bowers, S., Knowlton, S., & Marshall, L. (1984). The incidence of acute brain injury and serious impairment in a defined population. *American Journal of Epidemiology, 119,* 186–201.

Leininger, B. E., Gramling, S. E., Farrell, A. D., Kreutzer, J. S., & Peck, E. A. (1990). Neuropsychological deficit in symptomatic minor head injury patients after concussion and mild concussion. *Journal of Neurology, Neurosurgery, and Psychiatry, 53,* 293–296.

Levin, H. S., Amparo, E., Eisenberg, H. M., Williams, D. H., High, W. M., Jr., McArdle, C. B., & Weiner, R. L. (1987). Magnetic resonance imaging and computerized tomography in relation to the neurobehavioral sequelae of mild and moderate head injuries. *Journal of Neurosurgery, 66*(5), 706–713.

Levin, H. S., Williams, D. H., Eisenberg, H. M., High, W. M., Jr., & Guinto, F. C., Jr. (1992). Serial MRI and neurobehavioural findings after mild to moderate closed head injury. *Journal of Neurology, Neurosurgery, and Psychiatry, 55*(4), 255–262.

Mahon, D., & Elger, C. (1989). Analysis of post-traumatic syndrome following a mild head injury. *Journal of Neuroscience Nursing, 21*(6), 382–384.

Malec, J. F. (1996). DSM–IV postconcussional disorder: Recommendations (letter). *Journal of Neuropsychiatry and Clinical Science, 8*(1), 113–114.

McBeath, J. G., & Nanda, A. (1994). Use of dihydroergotamine in patients with postconcussion symptoms. *Headache, 34,* 148–151.

Millis, S. R. (1992). The Recognition Memory Test in the detection of malingered and exaggerated memory deficits. *Clinical Neuropsychologist, 6,* 405–413.

Millis, S. R. (1994). Assessment of motivation and memory with the Recognition Memory Test after financially compensable mild head injury. *Journal of Clinical Psychology, 50,* 601–605.

Millis, S. R., & Putnam, S. H. (1994). The Recognition Memory Test in the assessment of memory impairment after financially compensable mild head injury: a replication. *Perceptual and Motor Skills, 79,* 384–386.

Minderhoud, J. M., Boelens, M. E., Huizenga, J., & Saan, R. J. (1980). Treatment of minor head injuries. *Clinical Neurology and Neurosurgery, 82*(2), 127–140.

Mittenberg, W., Azrin, R., Millsaps, C., & Heilbronner, R. (1993). Identification of malingered head injury on the Wechsler Memory Scale–Revised. *Psychological Assessment, 5,* 34–40.

Mittenberg, W., & Burton, D. B. (1994). A survey of treatments for post-concussion syndrome. *Brain Injury, 8,* 429–437.

Mittenberg, W., DiGiulio, D. V., Perrin, S., & Bass, A. E. (1992). Symptoms following mild head injury: expectation as aetiology. *Journal of Neurology, Neurosurgery, and Psychiatry, 55*(3), 200–204.

Mittenberg, W., Zielinski, R., & Fichera, S. (1993). Recovery from mild head injury: A treatment manual for patients. *Psychotherapy in Private Practice, 12,* 37–52.

Mittl, R. L., Grossman, R. I., Hiehle, J. F., Hurst, R. W., Kauder, D. R., Gennarelli, T. A., & Alburger, G. W. (1994). Prevalence of MR evidence of diffuse axonal injury in patients with mild head injury and normal head CT findings. *American Journal of Neuroradiology, 15,* 1583–1589.

Mohanty, S. K., Thompson, W., & Rakower, S. (1991). Are CT scans for head injury patients always necessary? *Journal of Trauma, 31*(6), 801–805.

National Head Injury Foundation. (1993). Interagency Head Injury Task Force Reports. Washington, DC: National Institute of Neurologic Disorders and Stroke, National Institutes of Health.

Nedd, K., Sfakianakis, G., Ganz, W., Uricchio, B., Vernberg, D., Villanueva, P., Jabir, A. M., Bartlett, J., & Keena, J. (1993). 99*m*Tc-HMPAO SPECT of the brain in mild to moderate traumatic brain injury patients: Compared with CT—a prospective study. *Brain Injury,* 7, 469–479.

Nicoll, J. A. R., Roberts, G. W., & Graham, D. I. (1995). Apolipoprotein E e4 allele is associated with deposition of amyloid b-protein following head injury. *Nature and Medicine, 1,* 135–173.

Novack, T. A., Roth, D. L., & Boll, T. J. (1988). Treatment alternatives following mild head injury. *Rehabilitation Counseling Bulletin, 31,* 313–324.

Ohry, A., Rattok, J., & Solomon, Z. (1996). Post-traumatic stress disorder in brain injury patients. *Brain Injury, 10*(9), 687–695.

Quality Standards Committee, American Academy of Neurology. (1997). Practice parameter: The management of concussion in sports (summary statement). *Neurology, 48,* 581–585.

Rattok, J., Boake, C., & Bontke, C. F. (1996). Do patients with mild brain injuries have post-traumatic stress disorder, too? *Journal of Head Trauma Rehabilitation, 11*(1), 95–102.

Rawling, P. J. (1992). The Simulation Index: A reliability study. *Brain Injury, 6,* 381–383.

Rawling, P. J., & Brooks, D. N. (1990). The Simulation Index: A method for detecting factitious errors on the WAIS–R and WMS. *Neuropsychology, 4,* 223–238.

Roberts, G. W., Gentleman, S. M., Lynch, A., Murray, L., Landon, M., & Graham, D. I. (1995). Beta amyloid protein deposition in the brain after severe head injury: Implications for the pathogenesis of Alzheimer's disease. *Journal of Neurology, Neurosurgery, and Psychiatry, 57,* 419–425.

Rosenorn, J., Duus, B., Nielsen, K., Kruse, K., & Boesen, T. (1991). Is a skull X-ray necessary after milder head trauma? *British Journal of Neurosurgery, 5*(2), 135–139.

Saunders, C. E., Cota, R., & Barton, C. A. (1986). Reliability of home observation for victims of mild closed-head injury. *Annals of Emergency Medicine, 15*(2), 160–163.

Sbordone, R. J., & Liter, J. C. (1995). Mild traumatic brain injury does not produce post-traumatic stress disorder. *Brain Injury, 9,* 405–412.

Segalowitz, S. J., & Lawson, S. (1995). Subtle symptoms associated with self-reported mild head injury. *Journal of Learning Disabilities, 28,* 309–319.

Servadei, F., Ciucci, G., Morichetti, A., Pagano, F., Burzi, M., Staffa, G., Piazza, G., & Taggi, F. (1988a). Skull fracture as a factor of increased risk in minor head injuries. Indication for a broader use of cerebral computed tomography scanning. *Surgical Neurology, 30*(5), 364–369.

Servadei, F., Ciucci, G., Pagano, F., Rebucci, G. G., Ariano, M., Piazza, G., & Gaist, G. (1988b). Skull fracture as a risk factor of intracranial complications in minor head injuries: A prospective CT study in a series of 98 adult patients. *Journal of Neurology, Neurosurgery, and Psychiatry, 51*(4), 526–528.

Servadei, F., Staffa, G., Morichetti, A., Burzi, M., & Piazza, G. (1988). Asymptomatic acute bilateral epidural hematoma: Results of broader indications for computed tomographic scanning of patients with minor head injuries. *Neurosurgery, 23*(1), 41–43.

Servadei, F., Faccani, G., Roccella, P., Seracchioli, A., Godano, U., Ghadirpour, R., Naddeo, M., Piazza, G., Carrieri, P., Taggi, F., & Pagni, C. A. (1989). Asymptomatic extradural haematomas. Results of a multicenter study of 158 cases in minor head injury. *Acta Neurochirurgica (Wien), 96*(1–2), 39–45.

Servadei, F., Vergoni, G., Nasi, M. T., Staffa, G., Donati, R., & Arista, A. (1993). Management of low-risk head injuries in an entire area: Results of an 18-month survey. *Surgical Neurology, 39*(4), 269–275.

Shackford, S. R., Wald, S. L., Ross, S. E., Cogbill, T. H., Hoyt, D. B., Morris, J. A., Mucha, P. A., Pachter, H. L., Sugerman, H. J., O'Malley, K., Strutt, P. J., Winchell, R. J., Rutherford, E., Rhodes, M., Koslow, M., & DeMaria, E. J. (1992). The clinical utility of computed tomographic scanning and neurologic examination in the management of patients with minor head injuries. *Journal of Trauma, 33*(3), 385–394.

Sosin, D. M., Sniezek, J. E., & Thurman, D. J. (1996). Incidence of mild and moderate brain injury in the United States, 1991. *Brain Injury, 10,* 47–54.

Soutiel, J. F., Hafner, H., Chistyakov, A. V., Barzilai, A., & Feinsod, M. (1995). Trigeminal and auditory evoked responses in minor head injuries and post-concussion syndrome. *Brain Injury, 9,* 805–813.

Stein, S. C., O'Malley, K. F., & Ross, S. E. (1991). Is routine computed tomography scanning too expensive for mild head injury? *Annals of Emergency Medicine, 20*(12), 1286–1289.

Stein, S. C., & Ross, S. E. (1990). The value of computed tomographic scans in patients with low-risk head injuries. *Neurosurgery, 26*(4), 638–640.

Stein, S. C., & Ross, S. E. (1992). Mild head injury: A plea for routine early CT scanning. *Journal of Trauma, 33*(1), 11–13.

Stricevic, M. V., Patel, M. R., Okazaki, T., & Swain, B. K. (1983). Karate: Historical perspective and injuries sustained in national and international tournament competitions. *American Journal of Sports Medicine, 11*(5), 320–324.

Varney, N. R., Bushnell, D. L., Nathan, M., Kahn, D., Robert, R., Rezai, K., Walker, W., & Kirchner, P. (1995). NeuroSPECT correlates of disabling mild head injury: Preliminary findings. *Journal of Head Trauma Rehabilitation, 10,* 18–28.

Vollmer, D. G., & Dacey, R. G., Jr. (1991). The management of mild and moderate head injuries. *Neurosurgical Clinics of North America, 2*(2), 437–455.

Wilberger, J. E. (1993). Minor head injuries in American football. Prevention of long term sequelae. *Sports Medicine, 15*(5), 338–343.

Williams, D. H., Levin, H. S., & Eisenberg, H. M. (1990). Mild head injury classification. *Neurosurgery, 27*(3), 422–428.

World Health Organization. (1980). *International classification of impairments, disabilities, and handicaps.* Geneva: Author.

Wrightson, P., & Gronwall, D. (1981). Time off work and symptoms after minor head injury. *Injury, 12*(6), 445–454.

Forces and Accelerations in Car Accidents and Resultant Brain Injuries

Robert N. Varney
Palo Alto, California

Richard J. Roberts
Veterans' Administration Medical Center, Iowa City, Iowa

Classical physics principles can be employed to establish what actual physical forces are acting on the brains of vehicle occupants in many motor accidents. Such an application of classical mechanics has recently been described at length (Varney & Varney, 1995). In that report some 15 car accidents were selected for analysis because neuropsychological information on the injuries to the occupants and extensive details of the mechanics of the car accidents were simultaneously available. The estimated forces exerted on the brains of accident victims in this series of 15 case studies ranged from 30 to 1,500 times the weights of the elements involved (i.e., accelerations from 30 to 1,500 g). The physical analysis involved in these determinations is the subject of this chapter. Details concerning the personal injuries involved are given briefly, only enough to enable the reader to note the correlation between the brain injury and the acceleration. Biomechanical aspects of brain injury (i.e., how the forces of motor vehicle accidents effect brain tissue and brain structures) are the subject of chapter 4.

FORCES

The term *force* as used in this work is simply characterized as *push* or *pull*. The commonest force in everyday life is the force of gravity, or weight, that pulls every object downward. Almost four centuries ago, Galileo

(1564–1642) discovered that all bodies in free fall descend with the same constant acceleration. The acceleration amounts to approximately 32.2 feet per second per second, and is represented by the letter g. Regardless of an object's weight, the acceleration of every falling body is g.

Motor vehicle operation, in which drivers are continually speeding up or slowing down, makes the terms *acceleration* and *deceleration* familiar ones, although the true physical terms call for specification of how quickly the vehicle is speeded up or slowed down. The formal definition is: Acceleration is the rate of change of speed.

The famous *Principia* of Sir Isaac Newton (1642–1727), published in 1688, pointed out important correlations between forces and accelerations. Without force, accelerated motion does not occur. Force causes acceleration. Acceleration of any given body is proportional to the force causing the acceleration. If the body is identified by its weight w, Galileo's observation was that the force of gravity, acting on w, produces acceleration g. Any other force f acting on a weight w, gives it acceleration a. Hence, the constant proportionality of force and acceleration for a given weight gives the formula:

$$w/g = f/a \quad \text{or} \quad f = (w/g)a \tag{1}$$

This equation is a variant form of Newton's Second Law. (In practice, Equation 1 is used to more precisely define force.) Equation 1 then enables us to determine what force on any given weight w caused the acceleration a.

Acceleration rather than force is the quantity primarily measurable by physicists and hence becomes the subject of the present study of car accidents. Equation 1 enables us to determine what force on any given weight w has caused the acceleration a.

ACCELERATIONS

In mathematical form the definition of acceleration reads:

$$a = (v - v_0)/t \tag{2}$$

where a is the acceleration, v_0 is the speed at the start of the acceleration (i.e., at $t = 0$), v is the speed at the finish of the acceleration (i.e., at time t), and t is the time required for the acceleration to occur. The words *rate of change* in the definition of *speed*, as used by physicists, always mean that the change is to be divided by the time.

To illustrate the application of Equation 2 to the present problem, imagine that two identical cars are traveling at equal speeds in opposite directions and that they collide head on. Consider the motion of one of the drivers, who is securely belted into his seat. He is traveling before the collision at speed v_0 and is brought to rest in the collision (hence to $v = 0$) in a very short interval of time (t). It may be a matter of a few hundredths of a second (0.01 sec). Referring to the formula, it can be seen at once that if his initial speed was high and the time to come to a stop was very short, the resulting acceleration is a very large number.

A Practical Definition of Acceleration

From a practical point of view, Equation 2 is difficult to the point of impossibility to apply to everyday auto accidents. An observer not only needs to be present but also needs to be equipped with fast electronic timers and even high-speed movie cameras to watch and record the value of t in the collision. The actual direct observations of collisions rarely occurs at all; that the observer should also happen to be equipped with the necessary instruments is indeed unimaginable. Performing suitable tests in a laboratory or on a proving ground is unfeasible because deliberate and intentional injury of the vehicle operators is unthinkable. The difficulty can be circumvented by a simple mathematical process that is typically included in most freshman-level physics courses, which is to eliminate the time t and express the acceleration in terms of the stopping distance distance s that the car occupants traverse during the interval of the collision process. The resulting equation is:

$$a = (v^2 - v_0^2)/2s \tag{3}$$

There are at once two practical advantages to using Equation 3 instead of Equation 2: The displacement s in most ordinary collisions is in no sense a small quantity, such as t is, but is frequently of the order of magnitude of a foot and is thus measurable with simple rulers or tape measures. Furthermore, s can be measured by examination of the wreckage of the vehicles long after the accident has occurred and does not require an on-the-spot, instrumentally equipped observer.

Finally, it may be noted that in many collision studies, the moving objects come to rest at the end of the process, whence the final speed, v, is zero. In such cases, Equation 3 reduces to:

$$a = -v_0^2/2s \tag{4}$$

In this case, in which the vehicle comes to rest after the impact, all that is needed to determine the acceleration is the speed before the collision (v_0) and the distance s that the vehicle occupants moved during the collision process. The following section explains how this distance s can be determined.

Determination of S

Let us return to the previously presented example of two identical cars moving with equal speeds in opposite directions into head-on collision. Assume that the driver being studied is securely belted into his seat. At the instant before collision he is traveling at speed v_o, and he is at a distance b_o from his own front bumper. At the instant of collision, the two colliding front bumpers come to rest, but the belted-in driver, complete with his seat and belting, continues to move toward his front bumper because of the crumpling of the car under the impact. When the driver finally comes to rest ($v = 0$), he is closer to his front bumper than he was originally; call the new distance b. During the collision the driver has moved a distance $b_o - b$ in the forward direction, and this is exactly the value of s that we are seeking. We accordingly write:

$$s = b_o - b \qquad (5)$$

The value of b_o can be found from design data of the vehicle, and the value of b can be determined by measurements on the wreckage long after the actual accident. If the precollision speed is known, all the data are in hand for calculating the acceleration of the driver and of his brain.

The crushing distance s appears in the denominator of Equation 4 just as the crushing time t appears in the denominator of Equation 2. As a consequence, the more rigid the vehicle happens to be, the smaller s will be and the larger the acceleration and the force will be. From this point of view, an armored vehicle is actually highly undesirable if protection against brain injury is the objective, precisely because it is so rigid and resistant to crumpling on impact. An example of an armored vehicle accident is included in Varney and Varney (1995), and the reported injury to the vehicle occupant was indeed severe. Certain motor vehicle manufacturers are actually advertising that they are producing cars with "soft" front ends, expressly for the purpose of protecting passengers by maximizing the s value for any particular accident. The larger the "crumple zone" (i.e., the value of s), the lower the acceleration of the brain. Similarly, a very sturdy vehicle would have a small s value in a collision, resulting perhaps in smaller repair costs for the car but greater risk for central nervous system (CNS) damage for the occupants.

A Trial Example

Here is a typical hypothetical numerical example. Suppose that the speed before impact was 45 miles per hour. For calculating purposes it is necessary to express this speed as 66 feet per second. Suppose the front bumper is found to have been crushed in by a distance of 1 foot. Then using Equation 4:

$$a = -(66)^2/2 \times 1 \times 32.2 = 68 \ g \tag{6}$$

We have intentionally divided Equation 4 by $g = 32.2$ so that Equation 6 expresses the acceleration as a multiple of g. We have also omitted the minus sign on the result because it only concerns the direction of the acceleration and of the causing force and not their strengths. This then makes the force on any element of the driver's brain that weighs w pounds equal to 68 multiplied by w. Readers should consider the enormity of this force. For example, if a certain section of the driver's brain weighs 1 lb, such as an anterior frontal lobe, this lobe experiences a force of 68 lbs during the hypothesized collision.

As previously mentioned, how the force of acceleration (deceleration) acts on the brain is the subject of biomechanical studies; the results depend on the exact orientation of the driver's head relative to the direction of motion at the instant of the collision and on the location of skull surfaces relative to the brain element within the skull. There is, in addition, a possibility that the victim may be subjected to a twisting motion during the collision, and this can cause a centrifugal force on the victim's brain and complex internal forces that are beyond the scope of this chapter to analyze. However, these additional considerations do not detract from the basic point of this section, which is that when substantial accelerations of the brain occur, in accord with the laws of physics, they represent forces that will most certainly produce brain injury.

APPLICATIONS

In Varney and Varney (1995), the consequences of actual motor vehicle crashes were examined. For each, the accelerations that vehicle occupants experienced in various car accidents were computed, and the subsequent neuropsychological and medical observations on the occupants were detailed. The cases included head-on collisions, broadside collisions, rear-end collisions, sandwich-type collisions, single-vehicle accidents, armored car/tank collisions, low-speed accidents, and one case of an actual head impact accident to show that the calculations of the present chapter are equally applicable to other than closed head types of injury. Except for this single case, all the injuries reported disclosed no head impacts whatsoever. The findings of Varney and Varney (1995) are summarized in Table 3.1.

TABLE 3.1
Consequences of Actual Motor Vehicle Crashes (Varney & Varney, 1995)

Accelerations Reported	Brain Injuries Found
Head-on impact with stationary object, 120 g	Brief loss of consciousness. Amnesia for 24 hr, behavioral malfunction, inability to hold preaccident managerial positions, CT scan showing hemorrhage of right temporal lobe.
Rear-end collision, 50 g	Slight initial symptoms. Behavioral symptoms later. Seizures with left temporal focus. Disabled after 4 years.
Rear-end collision, 150 g	No immediate signs; after 3 months, behavioral symptoms, severe headaches, petit mal seizures, mania, forced retirement.
Single-car roll-over; two accelerations, 51 and 200 g	Driver killed, passenger thrown 180 ft. Severe behavioral problems. Some signs of recovery after 41 months.
Side impact; two accelerations, 68 and 270 g	No loss of consciousness. Behavior problem that increased over 18 months. Unable to continue work. Signs of cervical strain.
Single vehicle, 48 g	Amnesia for 3 days. Granted disability retirement for neuropsychological reasons.
Sandwich accident; two accelerations, 7.5 and 75 g	Cervical and whiplash injuries. Anterior frontal lobe syndrome.
Single-vehicle accident, 30 g	Seizures, behavioral symptoms. Frontal lobe injury.
Rear-end collision, 92 g	Neck pains, right side numbness. Unable to resume teaching work for a month. Four years later still showing behavioral symptoms. Indication of left-hemisphere damage.
Sandwich accident; two accelerations, 162 and 30 g	Victim walked away from accident. Later, whiplash symptoms. Orbital frontal cortex damage. Four years later severe behavioral symptoms. Complete loss of multilingual abilities.
Rear-end collision, 75 g	Unconscious for 45 min. Amnesia 3 to 5 days. Symptoms of marked passivity. Partial seizures. Attempt at suicide. Unemployable after graduating from college.
Collision of armored military vehicles, 1,550 g	At least 30 min amnesia. Cervical strain. Psychiatric ward for fights. Loss of earlier competence. Discharged from Army. Evidence of complete frontal lobe damage.
Low-speed collision, 34 g	Victim a commissioned Army officer. Received disability discharge for neurobehavioral symptoms. Unable to hold positions for which previously qualified. Partial seizures. Frontal lobe damage.
Head impact, 83 g	Gash on side of head. Grand mal seizure within ½ hr continuing 2 years. Posttraumatic dementia.

Examination of these findings reveals that no simple mathematical correlation between accelerations and subsequent brain injuries can as yet be computed. Nonetheless, accelerations as low as 30 g produce neuropsychological evidence of significant brain injury; on the other hand, accelerations as high as 1,500 g, although causing severe and permanent brain damage, are not necessarily fatal.

FURTHER CONSIDERATIONS

Equation 4, which contains collision speed v_0 and crushing distance s for the computation of the acceleration a, does not disclose that there is a further relationship between v_0 and s. That some such relationship exists is apparent from the following observation: In any given collision, the greater the speed at which the impact occurs, the greater the deformation will be. Conversely, the lower the collision speed for a given vehicle, the less the deformation will be. We rewrite Equation 4 here,

$$a = v_0^2 / 2s$$

and point out that a increases less than might be thought when v_0 increases, because s increases at the same time. Just how this connection between speed and crushing distance works is dependent on still other factors, such as the structure and the strength of the colliding bodies, and it may not be expressible analytically.

For the present considerations, the relationship between v_0 and s becomes particularly interesting in the case of quite low-speed collisions in which s may become so small that quite dangerous accelerations result, even though the speed is low. That is, a very rapid deceleration at low speed may be caused by a small s value and can be as dangerous as a protracted deceleration in a high-speed accident. Put simply, a low s value poses as great a danger as a high v value. This feature of collision accidents is illustrated in the analysis of cases 13 and 14 in Varney and Varney (1995).

AN ADDITIONAL CONSIDERATION

In the preceeding analysis the simplifying assumption has been made that the acceleration or deceleration occurring during a collision process was constant. Associated with this assumption was a further one, that the passenger in a colliding vehicle was fastened into his or her seat by a seatbelt and was totally immovable as a result. Neither of these assumptions is likely to be completely tenable. As to the latter, the passenger's neck will almost certainly bend during the impact, so that, in a head-on collision for example, his or her head will end up closer to the bumper than if the head had been fixed relative to the seat. Because the value of the distance called s was to be measured by comparing the distance from the head to the bumper before collision, called b_o, with the distance again from the head to the crushed-in bumper, called b, the value of $s = b_o - b$ will be larger than if the passenger's head had been fixed. As previously mentioned, a larger value of s makes for a smaller value of a. This result is consistent with the general idea that any sort of cushioning effect during a collision serves to protect the brain by diminishing the acceleration. Just how this flexibility of the passenger's neck modifies the acceleration depends on the direction in which the passenger was seated relative to the collision direction, with the neck being more flexible if bending forward, less if bending sideways, and possibly effectively negligible for backward bending, particularly if the vehicle has a good head rest.

There are additional concerns, however. The preceding discussion is based on the presumption of constant acceleration during the impact. In the extreme circumstance that the subject's head flies forward, in a head-on collision, with no restraint at all until the limit of bending of the neck is reached, there will be no acceleration at all initially; however, after the limit of bending is reached, the acceleration may be the same as or even greater than the value reached with the simplified assumption of neck rigidity. Actually, the value of b_o, the distance from the head to the bumper before collision, should probably be measured from the head in its advanced position after the neck bending, and the value of $s = b_o - b$ ends up the same as for the rigid-neck calculation.

If, for unspecified reasons, the acceleration simply is not constant throughout the impact process, then the average acceleration will be equal to the value obtained from the assumption of constant acceleration, so that no error arises from employing the constant acceleration obtained by use of Equation 3. On the other hand, the force on the victim's brain is the result of the peak acceleration and may thus be greater than that obtained from the average value. These conflicting possibilities leave us with the conclusion that the values as calculated in this chapter are likely to be reasonably near to the true values.

CONCLUSIONS

Ten of the victims of accidents listed in Table 3.1 showed clear and undeniable signs of permanent brain damage. The accelerations involved ranged from 34 g to 270 g with a single extreme case estimated to have been 1,550 g. As to the last, it is surprising that the victim survived the accident. Because the value of the critical quantity s was extremely small in that case, a relatively small error in assigning a value to it might make the acceleration less, perhaps by as much as a factor of four. In that case the acceleration would still have been nearly 400 g, certain to have caused severe but not necessarily fatal injury.

It must be concluded that accelerations in excess of 34 g can cause apparently irreversible brain injury. Whether it is possible to withstand such accelerations without brain damage remains to be determined, but as of this writing it seems highly unlikely.

REFERENCE

Varney, N. R., & Varney, R. N. (1995). Brain injury without head injury: Some physics of automobile collisions with particular reference to brain injuries occurring without physical trauma. *Applied Neuropsychology, 2,* 47–62.

Biomechanics of "Low-Velocity Impact" Head Injury

Y. King Liu
University of Northern California, Petaluma, California

The phrase *low-velocity impact* is a misnomer—an impact to any object produces an acceleration and an accompanying deformation of the body. For example, in a collision, a vehicle experiences a deceleration in a frontal impact or an acceleration in a rear-end impact. The kinematic (the study of motion without knowing the causes of motion) formula for the averaged acceleration is $\bar{A} = \Delta V / \Delta T$, where ΔV is the change in velocity and ΔT is the contact time duration. For a given value of $\bar{A}$, there are an infinity of values of ΔV and ΔT that will satisfy the equation. For example, if $\bar{A}$ is 1.5 g or 48.3 fps/sec, then for a 100-msec impact duration, the $\Delta V = 4.83$ fps or 3.3 mph. On the other hand, if the impact duration was 1 sec, then ΔV becomes 48.3 fps or 33 mph. Although it is easy to characterize 3.3 mph as a low change of velocity, it might be a little more difficult to do so for 33 mph. Viewed from another perspective, there is considerably more "ride-down" when going from 33 mph to a stop in 1 sec than from 3.3 mph to an extremely abrupt stop in 0.1 sec. Yet the averaged acceleration is exactly the same. If the contact impact duration is assumed constant, then the change in velocity, ΔV, is an equivalent measure of the impact severity, that is, the acceleration imparted to the vehicle as a result of the collision. This change of velocity is the input to the occupant(s) of the vehicle.

OCCUPANT KINEMATICS

The occupant responds to the input (vehicle acceleration) by moving in translation and rotation in conformity with the constraints imposed on the body. For so-called low-velocity impacts, the method of reconstructing the accident was well summarized by Szabo et al. (1994) and Bailey, Wong, and Lawrence (1995). Once the change of velocity is determined, the crucial question becomes whether this input to the vehicle can cause injury to its occupants. For example, in a rear-end impact, the seat back will push into the dorsal aspect of the occupant's torso, thus inducing a hyperextension and possibly followed by a hyperflexion of the head and neck relative to the seat. A recent study was done by McConnell et al. (1993). Similarly, in a frontal impact, the occupant will continue to translate forward while the vehicle is being decelerated. Unless appropriately restrained, the body may experience a second or even a third contact impact within the vehicle. Figure 4.1 illustrates a mathematical simulation, using the general-purpose dynamics program MADYMO, of a 50th percentile lap-belted male driver subjected to a relatively long (0.32 sec) frontal triangular 3 g deceleration pulse. Note that contact impact with the steering wheel is most likely.

Motor vehicle collisions are the major source of head injury. When the head receives a blow, the impact force produces (a) a local structural deformation wave, which gets propagated into the constituents of the head and (b) an angular and linear acceleration of the head and neck. If the impact is not sufficiently severe as to cause a local cratering, that is, no depressed skull fracture and tear of the dura mater, then any dysfunction or injury to the intracranial contents must be due to the deformation wave propagation into the brain and/or the translational and rotational acceleration of the head. When the motion of the head and neck is induced by the kinematics of the rest of the body, such as a hyperextension–hyperflexion or "whiplash" motion of the head and neck, then the mechanism of dysfunction or injury can only be due to the induced translational and rotational accelerations.

For so-called low-velocity impacts, once the vehicular change of velocity is determined, the crucial question becomes whether this input to the vehicle will injure its occupants; that is, what sort of transient acceleration time history (i.e., pulse) will cause acute and chronic dysfunction and/or injury to the intracranial contents? This was the question faced by a group of researchers at Wayne State University as early as the 1940s. These

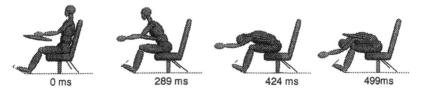

| 0 ms | 289 ms | 424 ms | 499ms |

FIG. 4.1. Occupant kinematics of a 50th percentile lap-belted male driver undergoing a frontal triangular 3 g deceleration pulse of 320 msec duration. Note the potential head contact with steering wheel between 289 and 424 msec.

researchers idealized the head as a one-degree-of-freedom linear, lumped-parameter system having inertia, stiffness, and damping subjected to an acceleration pulse. The solution of such an ordinary differential equation was given by Liu (1970). Given a typical impact situation, one can usually discern the following elements: mass, elasticity, dissipation, and the nature of the pulse. More specifically, in the head impact problem, the first mathematical model consisted of the skull stiffness (the spring) and the head mass with some dissipation always present (the damper). An acceleration pulse $a(t)$ applied to the head, assuming linear elements, would result in a motion governed by the well-known linear ordinary differential equation:

$$\ddot{x} + 2\zeta\omega\dot{x} + \omega^2 x = a(t) \tag{1}$$

where ω is the natural frequency, ζ is the damping ratio, and $x(t)$ is the absolute displacement of the skull. The solution of Equation 1 for an arbitrary $a(t)$ is in the form of a plot of the dynamic load factor, D, versus the ratio of the pulse duration t_1 to the natural period τ, with ζ as parameter. The dynamic load factor, D, also known as the amplification factor of "overshoot," is the ratio of the maximum dynamic spring force, F, to the product of the mass and the maximum skull acceleration. For purposes of illustration, let us consider an undamped case excited by a rectangular acceleration pulse; its governing differential equation is:

$$\ddot{x} + \omega^2 x = A_m[H(t) - H(t - t_1)] \tag{2}$$

where A_m is maximum value of the applied acceleration pulse and $H(t)$ is the Heaviside unit step function. The solution to Equation 2 can be found in many books, such as Thomson (1960) or Kornhauser (1962). For convenience of discussion the result is reproduced here:

$$D = \frac{kx_m}{mA_m} = \frac{\omega^2 x_m}{A_m} = \begin{cases} 2 & t_1/\tau \geq \tfrac{1}{2} & \text{(3a)} \\ 2\sin(\pi t_1/\tau) & t_1/\tau < \tfrac{1}{2} & \text{(3b)} \end{cases}$$

where k is the spring constant, m is the mass, and $\tau = \omega/2\pi$ is the natural period of the system. Notice that the force and acceleration of the spring are both proportional to maximum relative amplitude, x_m. Graphically, Equation 3 appears as Fig. 4.2. Its most striking feature is that the dynamic load factor, D, is 2 beyond the critical duration $t_1/\tau = \tfrac{1}{2}$. Below this critical pulse duration, consider a Taylor series expansion of Equation 3b,

$$D \approx 2[(\pi t_1/\tau) - 1/6(\pi t_1/\tau)^3 + \cdots] \tag{3b'}$$

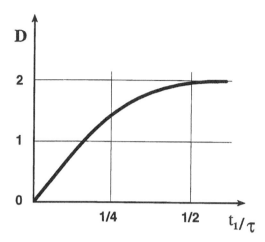

FIG. 4.2. Dimensionless dynamic load factor D as a function of the pulse width to natural period ratio.

For very small values of t_1/τ, that is, $t_1/\tau \ll \frac{1}{2}$, this can be approximated by:

$$D \approx 2\pi t_1/\tau \tag{3b''}$$

In the biodynamics literature, the term *dynamic response index* (DRI) is preferred (see Payne, 1965, and Stech & Payne, 1969). DRI was defined by Von Gierke (1962, 1964) as the ratio of the peak force in the spring to the body weight (mg). The relationship between DRI and D is expressed as

$$DRI = D(A_m/g)$$

In terms of the peak force, F, Equations 3a and 3b'' become

$$F = 2mA_m \qquad t_1/\tau \geq \tfrac{1}{2} \tag{4a}$$
$$F = 2\pi mA_m t_1/\tau \qquad t_1/\tau \ll \tfrac{1}{2} \tag{4b}$$

The implication of Equation 4b is that the peak force is approximately proportional to velocity change, that is, $\Delta V = A_m t_1$, if the pulse duration is much less than one-half the natural period of the dynamic system. Equation 4a states that the peak force is proportional to the peak acceleration of the input acceleration pulse when the pulse duration is greater than one-half the natural period of the system. When the pulse duration is less than but comparable to one-half the natural period, the peak force is found from Equation 3b to be nonlinearly related to pulse duration as follows:

$$F = 2mA_m \sin(\pi t_1/\tau) \quad t_1/\tau < \tfrac{1}{2} \tag{4c}$$

The results for the rectangular pulse can be generalized to an arbitrary pulse. The critical duration, t_c, if it exists, marks the boundary between two dynamic regions: (a) For $t < t_c$, the input pulse shape has no influence upon the system, but only the pulse area, which is equal to the imposed velocity change. (b) For $t > t_c$, the pulse shape is the important factor.

If one were to assume that the spring always breaks at a given peak force level, the so-called equal tissue strain assumption, it is then possible to relate the damage or injury, through the system response, to the parameters of the input pulse. For the rectangular pulse response given in Equations 4a, 4b, and 4c, let the damaging peak force be designated F_d; then we get

$$A_m = F_d/2m, \qquad\qquad t_1/\tau > \tfrac{1}{2} \tag{5a}$$
$$A_m = F_d\tau/2m, \qquad\qquad t_1/\tau \ll \tfrac{1}{2} \tag{5b}$$
$$A_m = F_d/2m \sin(\pi t_1/\tau) \quad t_1/\tau < \tfrac{1}{2} \tag{5c}$$

Plotting this result on a log-log scale, using the maximum acceleration, A_m, and the duration of the pulse, t_1, as variables, we get the theoretical tolerance curve as shown in Fig. 4.3. In Fig. 4.3, the "knee" represents the critical duration, t_c. To its left is the velocity change region and to the right the absolute acceleration peak regime. If damping were to be in-

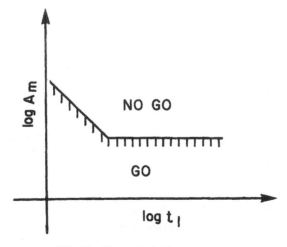

FIG. 4.3. Theoretical tolerance curve.

cluded as shown in Equation 1, the absolute value of the peak force overshoot would decrease and thereafter decrease exponentially with time, approaching the applied acceleration pulse magnitude, A_m, asymptotically. A smaller overshoot implies that a greater input acceleration can be applied before reaching the critical force threshold.

A massive program of experimental validations was performed on cadaveric and animal (in vivo) heads, as well as clinical data, to arrive at the Wayne State tolerance curve as shown in Fig. 4.4. The acceleration time history of a specimen's head was measured at a diametrically opposite point to the location of impact. The averaged acceleration, A, was plotted against the contact time, T. The data points, such as cerebral concussion or the absence of the same in canines and primates, appropriately scaled to human head size, were plotted onto the diagram. Similarly, data points found from cadaveric experiments and clinical observations were also plotted on to this diagram. These experimental data points indicated a falling tolerance to head injury as acceleration pulses of increasing duration were applied to the head. These data points were curve-fitted to a hyperbola. Theoretically, the hyperbola has two asymptotes: the horizontal asymptote expressed the concept that at some level of averaged acceleration, A, no injury would occur no matter how long

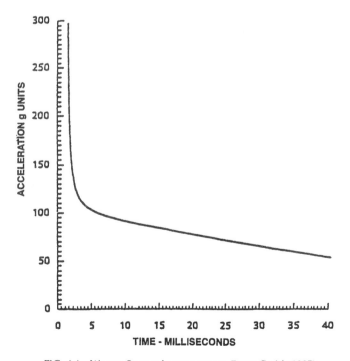

FIG. 4.4. Wayne State tolerance curve. From Gadd (1985).

the contact time, T. Similarly, there exists a vertical asymptote where at a sufficiently low contact time duration, T, an "infinite" averaged acceleration, A, can be theoretically tolerated. The left lower region bounded by the hyperbola and its two asymptotes are considered the safe region; that is, data points within this region are below the level of physiological injury, for example, no cerebral concussion. Outside this safe region is the unsafe region.

The reports of Eiband (1959), Lissner et al. (1960), Coermann (1961), Kornhauser (1962), and many other investigators were used by Gadd (1962, 1966) to arrive at a Severity Index. The log-log plot of plateau acceleration versus duration reiterated the concept that tolerable acceleration pulses diminished as the duration of the pulse increased, as shown in Fig. 4.5.

A straight line at $-1/2.5$ slope could be drawn midway between the "injured" and "uninjured" lines out to about 1 sec duration, as shown in Fig. 4.6. This insight led Gadd (1966) to formulate a single number criterion for head injury, known as the Severity Index (SI). The criterion used an exponential weighting factor for appraising acceleration impulses as measured on the object being struck. Such an acceleration impulse-integration procedure can more rationally account for the time duration and pulse intensity as given by the tolerance data, such as the NASA and JARI data as well as the Wayne State Curve shown in Figs. 4.4, 4.5, and 4.6. Mathematically, the Gadd Severity Index (SI) is given as:

$$SI = \int_0^T [a(t)]^{2.5} \, dt \tag{6}$$

where SI denotes the Severity Index as formulated by Gadd (1966), $a(t)$ is the acceleration pulse, T is the contact duration in milliseconds, and t is the time. The critical Gadd Severity Index (SI) is 1,000; that is, if the SI is less than 1,000, then the head impact is considered probabilistically safe, and vice versa.

A variant to the Gadd Severity Index for impacts where the impact pulse width is not definitive, the Head Injury Criterion (HIC), was proposed by Versace (1971):

$$HIC = \max(t_2 - t_1) \left\{ \frac{1}{t_2 - t_1} \int_{t_1}^{t_2} a(t) \, dt \right\}^{2.5} \leq 1,000 \tag{7}$$

where t_1 and t_2 are the initial and final time during the acceleration pulse $a(t)$ for which the HIC attains a maximum value.

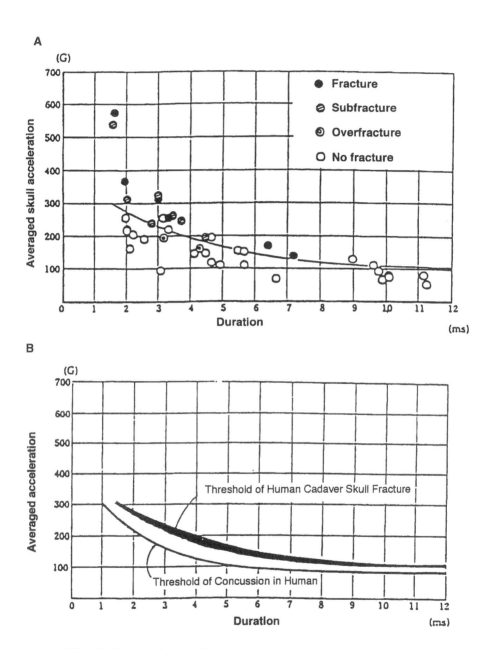

FIG. 4.5. (a) Experimental data for human cadaveric skull fracture in frontal impact. From JARI test data. (b) JARI test data for sagittal head impact.

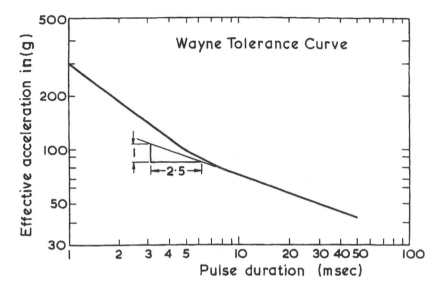

FIG. 4.6. Straight-line approximation to the Wayne State tolerance curve for head impact used by Gadd (1985).

One can view the threshold number of 1,000 as the peak of a probability distribution curve. For head injury, the nature of the normal probability distribution, that is, whether it is a sharply peaked or relatively flat curve, is not clearly delineated and reflects the inherent variability of most biological tolerance data.

Of course, there exists a parallel set of equations similar to Equations 1 to 6 for angular rotations. Rotational acceleration tolerance curves have been proposed by Gennarelli et al. (1982) based on rhesus monkey experimental data wherein they constrained the head to accelerate translationally and rotationally. For concussion, these curves reassemble the translational Wayne State tolerance criteria except that the coordinates were rotational acceleration and pulse duration. As yet, these proposals have not been approved or adopted. Part of the problem is the validity of scaling monkey tolerance data to human beings based on fluid-filled spheres when the neuroanatomy suggests otherwise.

Patrick, Kroell, and Mertz (1965) and Orne and Liu (1970) showed that because the head is attached to the neck, every induced motion, whether the result of inertial loading or direct contact impact, will have both translations and (angular) rotations. What combinations of translation and rotation will cause injury and/or dysfunction is not very clearly understood. A recent unauthenticated compilation, from the Proceedings of the IRCOBI (International Research Committee on Biokinetics of Impacts) and the Stapp Car Crash Conferences, of such combinations was given by

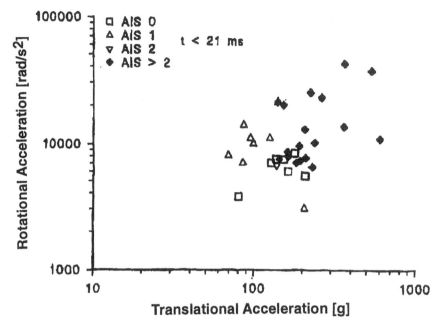

FIG. 4.7. Tolerance data for combined translational and rotational accelerations. From Schuller et al. (1993).

Schuller, Konig, and Beier (1993). It is reproduced here without prejudice as Fig. 4.7 for illustrative purposes only. The main conclusion of the article was, "a significant reduction of (the) limit for the translational headform deceleration, e.g., up to 120 g, would exclude critical rotational head acceleration in real impact situations" (p. 287). These results, if true, would suggest that the current protective helmet drop test standards [e.g., Department of Transportation (DOT) Federal Motor Vehicle Safety Standard (FMVSS) 218, Snell Memorial Foundation, etc.] should be significantly lowered to reduce head impact injury.

HOMEOMORPHIC FINITE-ELEMENT MODEL OF THE HUMAN HEAD AND NECK

Head injury may be sustained during impact and/or deceleration of the head and neck. The head is roughly a hard skull containing a fairly uniformly dense "Jello-like" brain floating in a bath of cerebrospinal fluid (CSF). The brain consists of two hemispheres of the cerebrum and the cerebellum. These entities are compartmentalized by tough membranes: the falx cerebri dividing the hemispheres, and the tentorium between the cerebrum and the cerebellum. The skull is 10–13 mm (⅜ to ½ in) thick and is approximately 165 mm (6.5 in) long in the antero-posterior direction and 140 mm (5.5 in) wide. The brain weighs about 1,500 g (3.3 lb). At the site of a blow to the scalp/skull, large compressive pressure gradients are produced by the linear acceleration of the skull and the inertia of the CSF-suspended brain material. The "pile-up" of the fluid and nervous tissue at the site of the blow causes a coup injury. As the deformation wave travels around the skull and along the fluid, the skull and the brain/fluid material will tend to separate at the opposite end of the diameter, causing a "rarefaction" or tensile stress and leading to cavitation and/or tearing injury. This rarefaction stress injury is called a *contrecoup*. Because the head sits atop the articulated neck, angular acceleration is inevitable. The relative angular motion between the skull and the fluid-like brain may introduce significant shear strains between the various layers, with straining and/or tearing of the interconnected structures, such as bridging veins, axons, and intracranial blood vessels.

Hosey and Liu (1982) constructed the most comprehensive finite-element model of the human head and neck, taking into account the gross neuroanatomy as well as the inertial and material properties of the head and neck. In a simulation of an occipital blunt impact, a half-sine contact force of 6,000 N (1,349 lb) spread over 10 occipital nodes for 4.0 msec yielded a contrecoup pressure of −23.0 kPa. The pressure distribution at maximum contrecoup pressure is illustrated in Fig. 4.8.

These results indicate that (a) the point of zero pressure is roughly located over the anterior portion of the foramen magnum, where the brain blends into the spinal cord, and (b) the maximum absolute negative pressure at the contrecoup site is higher in magnitude than at the coup site. When the contrecoup pressure reaches 1 negative (tensile) atmosphere (−101 kPa), cavitation ensues. Dissolved gases come out of solution in liquids at cavitation pressure, and voids and bubbles form and collapse, releasing enormous energy to produce the contrecoup injury or dysfunction. Using elementary engineering stress wave theory, Johnson and Mamalis (1978) estimated that an impact speed of 80 cm/sec (31.5 ft/sec or 21.5 mph) will be needed for cavitation, that is, contrecoup injury, to occur. Based on a finite-element model of the human brain, Elson and Ward (1994) suggested that to produce "mild" brain injury, the compressive stresses must be less than 233.6 kPa.

CRASHWORTHINESS

Johnson and Mamalis (1978) defined crashworthiness as (a) the capability of a (framed) vehicular structure to maintain a protective space around the occupants during a crash and (b) the ability to insure that any human occupant can tolerate the deceleration or retardation rate. The design of

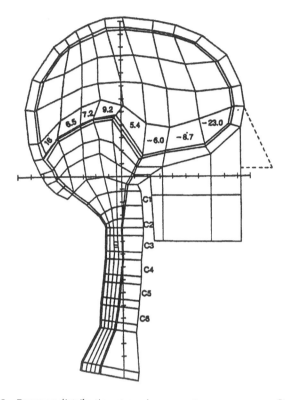

FIG. 4.8. Pressure distribution at maximum contrecoup pressure. Occipital impact of 6,000 N over nine nodes with half-sine pulse of 4 msec duration. From Liu (1986).

crashworthy vehicular framed structures must be coupled with knowledge and understanding of the loads that human occupants can withstand. For frontal and rear-end collisions, the bumpers are the structures that most often get deformed and/or damaged. Bailey et al. (1995) and Siegmund, Bailey, and King (1994) characterized automotive bumper components and specific bumpers in so-called low-velocity impacts.

REFERENCES

Bailey, M. N., Wong, B. C., & Lawrence, J. M. (1995). Data and methods for estimating the severity of minor impacts. In *Accident reconstruction, technology & animation V* (pp. 139–175). SAE Monograph SP-1083. Warrendale, PA: Society of Automotive Engineers (SAE paper 950352).
Coermann, R. R. (1961, November). Comparison of the dynamic characteristics of dummies, animals and man. *Proceedings of the National Academy of Sciences Symposium on Impact Acceleration Stress*, Brooks AFB, San Antonio, TX.

Eiband, A. (1959). Human tolerance to rapidly applied accelerations: A summary of the literature. NASA memorandum 5-19-59E.

Elson, L., & Ward, C. (1994). Mechanisms and pathophysiology of mild head injury. *Seminars in Neurology, 14*(1), 8–18.

Gadd, C. W. (1962). Criteria for injury potential. *Proceedings, Impact Acceleration Stress Symposium.* National Academy of Sciences, National Research Council, Publication no. 977.

Gadd, C. W. (1966). Use of a weighted-impulse criterion for estimating injury hazard. *Proceedings, Tenth Stapp Car Crash Conference* (pp. 164–174). Warrendale, PA: Society of Automotive Engineers.

Gadd, C. W. (1985). Development of head injury criteria. *Head Injury Prevention, Past and Present Research.* Detroit, MI: Wayne State University.

Gennarelli, T. A., Segawa, H., Wald, U., Czernicki, Z., Marsh, K., & Thompson, C. (1982). Physiological response to angular acceleration of the head. In R. G. Grossman & P. L. Gildenberg (Eds.), *Head injury: Basic and clinical aspects* (pp. 129–140). New York: Raven.

Hosey, R., & Liu, Y. K. (1982). A homeomorphic finite element model of the human head and neck. In Gallagher, Simon, Johnson, and Gross (Eds.), *Finite element methods in biomechanics* (pp. 379–401). New York: Wiley.

Johnson, W., & Mamalis, A. G. (1978). *Crashworthiness of vehicles.* London: Mechanical Engineering Publications.

Kornhauser, M. (1962). *Structural effects of impact.* Baltimore, MD: Spartan, Cleaver-Hume.

Lissner, H. R., et al. (1960). *Experimental cerebral concussion.* ASME Annual Meeting paper no. 60-WA-273.

Liu, Y. K. (1970). Distributed-parameter dynamic models of the spine. *Proceedings on Bioengineering Approaches to Problems of the Spine* (pp. 53–83). Bethesda, MD: Department of Health, Education, and Welfare.

Liu, Y. K. (1986, January). Finite element modeling of the head and spine. *Mechanical Engineering,* 60–64.

McConnell, W. E., et al. (1993). *Analysis of human test subject kinematic responses to low velocity rear end impacts* (SAE Paper 930889). Warrendale, PA: Society of Automotive Engineers.

Orne, D., & Liu, Y. K. (1970). A mathematical model of spinal response to impact. *Journal of Biomechanics, 4*(4). Also as ASME preprint No. 70-BHF-1, pp. 49–71.

Patrick, L. M., Kroell, C. K., & Mertz, H. J. (1965). Forces on the human body in simulated crashes. *Proceedings, Ninth Stapp Car Crash Conference.* Minneapolis: University of Minnesota.

Payne, P. R. (1965). *Personnel restraint and support system dynamics* (Rep. No. TR-65-12F). Wright-Patterson AFB, OH: Aerospace Medical Research Lab.

Schuller, E., Konig, W., & Beier, G. (1993, September). Criteria for head impact protection by motorcycle helmets. *Proceedings, 1993 IRCOBI Conference* (pp. 283–294). Eindhoven, The Netherlands.

Siegmund, G. P., Bailey, M. N., & King, D. J. (1994). *Characteristics of specific automobile bumpers in low-velocity impact* (SAE Paper 940916). Warrendale, PA: Society of Automotive Engineers.

Stech, E. L., & Payne, P. R. (1969). *Dynamic models of the human body* (Rep. No. AMRL-TR-66-157). Wright-Patterson AFB, OH: Aerospace Medical Research Lab.

Szabo, T., Welcher, J., Anderson, R., Rice, M., Ward, J., Paulo, L., & Carpenter, N. (1994). *Human occupant kinematic responses to low-speed rear-end impacts* (SAE Paper 940532). Warrendale, PA: Society of Automotive Engineers.

Thomson, W. T. (1960). *Laplace transformation.* Englewood Cliffs, NJ: Prentice Hall.

Versace, J. (1971, November). A review of the Severity Index. *Proceedings of the 15th Stapp Car Crash Conference* (SAE paper 710881, pp. 771–804). Warrendale, PA: Society of Automotive Engineers.

Von Gierke, H. E. (1962). Biomechanics of impact injury. *Proceedings, Impact Acceleration Stress Symposium (with Comprehensive Chronological Bibliography)*. Washington, DC: National Academy of Sciences, National Research Council (Publication No. 977).

Von Gierke, H. E. (1964). Biodynamic response of the human body. *Applied Mechanics Reviews, 17*, 961–968.

Neuroimaging in Mild TBI

Erin D. Bigler
Brigham Young University, Provo, Utah

Alexander (1995) provided an excellent overview of mild traumatic brain injury (TBI) wherein he discussed pathophysiology, natural history, and clinical management of this disorder. In his review of mild TBI, Alexander stated that "by common clinical agreement, neuroimaging studies are negative, but this defining characteristic may be more complex than just positive or negative findings on CT" (p. 1253). Accordingly, traditional neuroimaging in mild TBI usually does not demonstrate major abnormalities or structural defects; however, some abnormalities may be present, and new neuroimaging techniques or refinements of existing techniques have the potential to reveal subtle abnormalities associated with mild TBI. Because of potential complications associated with any TBI, the majority of mild TBI cases do receive standard neuroimaging at some point in the course of their clinical work-up. This chapter briefly reviews the status of neuroimaging in mild TBI. However, before neuroimaging of mild TBI is presented, the typical acute and chronic imaging findings in more severe injury are presented for comparison. This chapter only discusses neuroimaging findings from computerized tomography (CT), magnetic resonance (MR) imaging, and cerebral perfusion studies. These are currently the neuroimaging methods in use for clinical investigations for the effects of cerebral trauma. For details concerning imaging methods and clinical interpretation the reader is referred to Bigler (1996a, 1996b), Gean (1994), and Osborn (1994).

SEVERE TBI

Acute Neuroimaging Findings

The typical abnormalities associated with TBI during acute neuroimaging are in the form of hemorrhages (typically subdural, epidural, petechial, and/or contusion), presence of edema, and midline shift or herniation (Bigler, 1996c; Bigler & Clement, 1998; Gean, 1994; Osborn, 1994). Figures 5.1–5.3 provide several examples of these types of acute abnormalities observed with brain imaging. Acute neuroimaging addresses several important initial criteria with regards to injury severity. First, initial management decisions are made by the presence of neuroimaging findings (i.e, is there a neurosurgically treatable lesion, if edema is present should it be medically managed, etc.). Second, the presence of abnormalities assists in identifying the severity of injury (Katz & Alexander, 1994) and the presence of any traumatically induced lesion is certainly an objective indicator for the presence of brain injury. Typically, the severity of injury (as well as outcome) is in part related to the type of abnormalities observed in acute imaging studies (Ryser, Bigler, & Blatter, 1998). Based on human postmortem as well as animal work, the presence of such identifiable lesions typically is a benchmark for even greater ultrastructural defects (Bigler, 1997). Third, acute neuroimaging studies provide the baseline from which to monitor changes over time (Bigler, 1996c). As readily observed in Figs. 5.1 and 5.2, when the day-of-injury scan is compared to the follow-up scans, ventricular dilation and evidence of atrophy are apparent.

Neuroimaging in the Chronic Phase Following Severe TBI

Figure 5.4 presents the typical MR neuroimaging pattern of pathological changes observed during the chronic phase (greater than 6 months) following severe TBI. These changes are typically manifested in terms of increased sulcal width (i.e., cortical atrophy), ventricular dilation, and presence of signal abnormalities in white matter, particularly near the gray/white matter interface. These latter lesions are felt to represent sequela associated with shear injuries to the white matter. Also, typically the intensity of the signal differentiating white from gray may not be as clearly demarcated in some regions, particularly the frontal and temporal regions. These findings have been interpreted as indicators of diffuse axonal injury (DAI) and at times may be quite subtle in their detection.

In terms of DAI and white matter damage as a consequence of severe TBI, midsagittal MR views of the corpus callosum (CC) are particularly instructive (Gale, Johnson, Bigler, & Blatter, 1995). For example, Fig. 5.5 demonstrates generalized atrophy of the CC in a patient with severe injury.

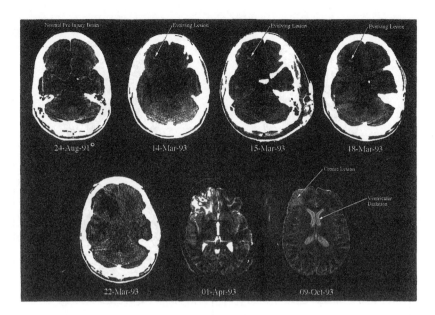

FIG. 5.1. Sequential CT imaging studies in the same patient who sustained a traumatic brain injury. Of particular interest in this imaging sequence is that this patient had been experiencing headaches and underwent CT imaging approximately a year and a half prior to sustaining a severe traumatic brain injury, secondary to a fall. The normal scan is shown in the upper left-hand corner. All scans are in the axial plane. On the day of injury (14 March 1993), the patient sustained frontal and temporal contusion as a consequence of a contracoup injury, wherein he struck the back of his head in a fall from a second-story balcony. On 14 March it is a little difficult to distinguish the hemorrhagic lesion as some are ill-defined on this day. However, by the next day (15 March), it is obvious that there are scattered areas of hemorrhage throughout the right frontal and temporal regions of the brain (all images are presented in the axial plane with right on the viewer's left). By 18 March, not only can the areas of hemorrhagic contusion and intraparenchymal hemorrhaging be identified, but there is surround edema and degradation of neural tissue, which, in turn, is seen predominantly on 22 March. By this time the actual blood by-products are substantially absorbed and removed from the region. By 1 April, magnetic resonance imaging demonstrates massive frontal encephalomalacic changes (white areas in the right frontal lobe). This magnetic resonance scan is what is referred to as a T2-weighted image, where the cerebral spinal fluid is depicted in white and the brain parenchyma is represented in various shades of gray. Also noted in this image is hemosiderin, which is a blood by-product that shows up on MR imaging as a doric region. Another MR image is presented from 9 October 1993, which demonstrates the chronic lesion with permanent necrotic changes in the right frontal lobe and uniform ventricular dilation. This sequence of scans is important to recognize because if the interpretation is taken at a single data point, one may not fully grasp the significance of the injury. For example, if imaging studies were done only on the day of injury, the full magnitude of this brain injury would not be recognized.

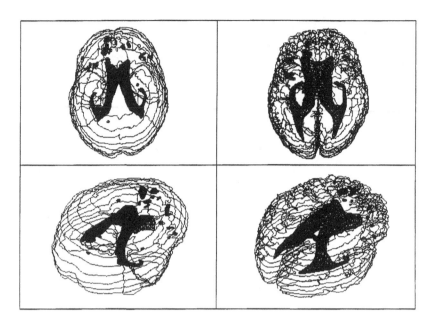

FIG. 5.2. The images presented in the left-hand column represent the primary focus of intraparenchymal and petechial type hemorrhages associated with acute severe TBI. Top upper left: This is a three-dimensional reconstruction of the brain with a wire-frame outline taken from the CT scan, which is depicted below (next page). Only the body of the lateral ventricle is presented in this image. Middle figure, left: This is an oblique posterior view of the same brain, showing multiple areas of hemorrhagic lesion, predominantly in the frontal temporal area. Bottom left (next page): This is CT imaging on the day of injury. The "white" areas scattered throughout the frontal region are focal hemorrhagic lesions. These have been colorized (in black) and presented in three-dimensional view in the two upper panels on the left. Upper right: A wire-frame outline of the outer rim of the brain, based on chronic MRI findings, is presented. As a consequence of tissue necrosis, there are regions of cavitation that develop in the frontal area, as well as signal abnormality on the magnetic resonance imaging studies (light spots noted in the frontal region). These lesions have been colorized and can be seen predominantly in the frontal temporal regions of the brain. It is also evident that there is significant ventricular dilation. Because the CT scan on the left establishes the baseline, these significant increases in ventricular size are indicative of hydrocephalus ex vacuo, wherein the ventricular system expands and responds to loss of surrounding brain tissue. Middle view, right: This is a right posterior oblique view to be compared with the CT oblique view to the left. Again, note the ventricular dilation and the location of the lesions. Bottom right: Axial MR imaging depicting ventricular dilation and areas of residual lesion in the frontal region (dark regions and signal hyperintensities—white areas).

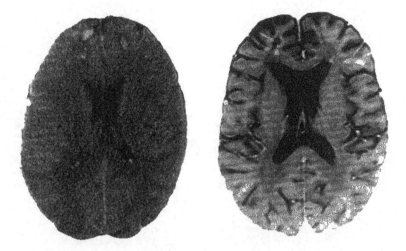

FIG. 5.2. *(Continued)*

Note that the atrophy is predominantly in the genu and anterior aspect of the CC body. These atrophic changes are representative of primarily frontotemporal wasting and DAI (Johnson, Bigler, Burr, & Blatter, 1994). In this same figure, the axial view demonstrates temporal horn dilation, which is a reflection primarily of temporal lobe atrophy with some contribution of trauma-induced hippocampal atrophy (Bigler et al., 1997).

Pathological changes induced by moderate to severe injury can be investigated by subjecting MR imaging studies to quantification (see Bigler, 1996c; Blatter et al., 1995, 1997). These studies have objectively demonstrated what has been discussed earlier, actually quantifying the degree of brain atrophy. With moderate to severe trauma, there is substantial volume loss of total brain parenchyma that starts within the first few weeks postinjury and is largely complete by 6 months postinjury, but some persistent atrophic changes may continue for over 3 years. These type of atrophic changes are objectively presented in Fig. 5.6.

With this background for comparison, the chapter next focuses on neuroimaging characteristics associated with mild TBI.

ACUTE NEUROIMAGING IN MILD TBI

Rarely are significant lesions found that require neurosurgical intervention. The norm for acute evaluation of the TBI patient is to scan with computerized tomography during the initial assessment, particularly if loss of consciousness (LOC) was present or when routine skull films or clinical assessment suggest skull fracture. Because the presence of signifi-

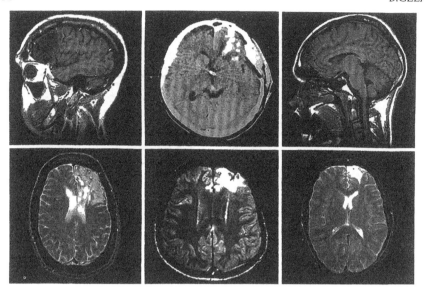

FIG. 5.3. Three cases of traumatic brain injury, all demonstrating different aspects of pathologic change in three different patients. Left column: This patient sustained a pronounced frontal injury as a result of depressed skull fracture to the left frontal lobe. This is clearly depicted on the axial T2-weighted image (bottom left). Note how the anterior aspect of the body of the lateral ventricle expands to where the lesion is present. The sagittal view in the upper left clearly demonstrates the massive change that accompanies this frontal trauma. Note the complete absence of definable brain tissue in the frontal region. Also note the encapsulation of the frontal lobe by the frontal and ethmoid/orbital frontal bone. It is this very encapsulation that may be at the basis for the greater likelihood of frontal injury following trauma. Middle figure, top: Axial CT done during acute injury phase. This CT demonstrates blood in the left frontal region of the brain. Note the obliteration of the anterior horn on the left. Notice also (dark area) the surround edema around this acute injury. The acute injury effects give way to chronic lesion in the frontal lobe as demonstrated below (center figure, bottom). This is a mixed weighted magnetic resonance scan that shows marked encephalomalacic changes in the frontal pole region of the brain. Top right: Sagittal view demonstrating encephalomalacic changes scattered across the left frontal pole. Note also some thinning of the genu of the corpus callosum. Bottom right: Axial T2-weighted image demonstrating the residual effects of the frontal lesion; note how it extends down into the white matter of the frontal lobe.

cant intracranial lesions is associated with greater severity of injury, by definition it is less likely that structural lesions will be observed in the patient with admitting GCS scores of 13 to 15. In fact, where no LOC is reported with no mental status changes noted on emergency room evaluation (i.e., GCS = 15), with no persistent anterograde amnesia, the patient may not even be scanned. Studies have demonstrated a very low yield

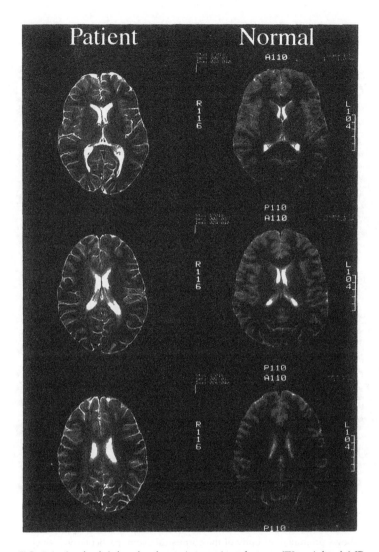

FIG. 5.4. In the left-hand column is a series of scans (T2-weighted MR scans) taken from a patient who was involved in an auto–pedestrian accident and sustained a severe traumatic brain injury. Note the increased CSF (white areas) across the frontal region and the more prominent sulcal indentation evidenced by increased cortical CSF. Note also the general increase in ventricular size when compared to the normal subject to the right. Also, in each image in the upper right frontal region (in the central white matter), note the white-matter hyperintensity lesion that likely represents a definitive shear injury. Also, note that the signal that is evident (particularly in the upper left and middle left illustrations) suggest that the signal emanating from the right frontal lobe does not match the signal from the left frontal lobe. A normal age-matched comparison is given at each level in the scan presented on the right.

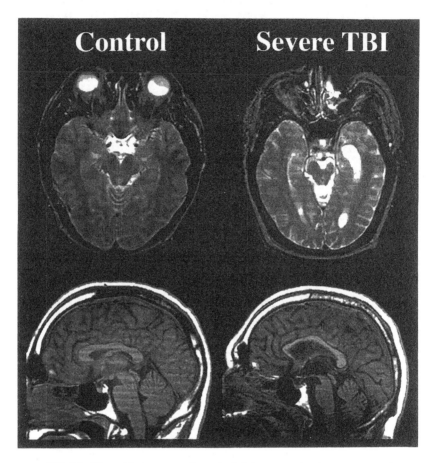

FIG. 5.5. The subject presented on the left is a control subject, compared
to a patient (right) with severe traumatic brain injury. The severe TBI subject
shows prominent atrophy of the corpus callosum, particularly at the genu
and anterior body region. It is felt that this is due to the predominant effects
of head injury to the frontal and temporal regions of the brain. In the axial
views presented for the patient with severe TBI, note the significant dilation
of the temporal horn region. This type of dilation is indicative of
surrounding temporal-lobe pathology and may also reflect wasting of the
hippocampus.

of demonstrable lesions in patients with such a clinical history (Alexander,
1995). When neuroimaging abnormalities are detected in the mild TBI
patient, the types of lesions typically are frontal- and temporal-lobe contusions, particularly at the anterior tip of the frontal lobe, orbital regions
of the frontal lobe, and the anterior as well as medial region of the
temporal lobe, and/or white matter shearing type lesions, usually at the
gray/white matter junction (see Fig. 5.7). Again, by definition, if lesions

SUBJECT 1-Parenchymal Changes

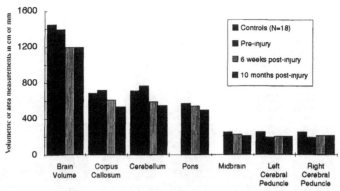

%=% Change from Pre-injury MR

SUBJECT 1-Ventricular Changes

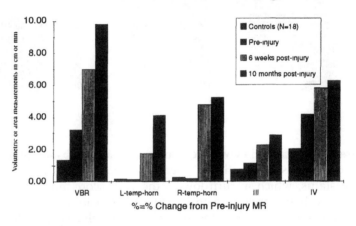

%=% Change from Pre-injury MR

FIG. 5.6. These MR images are from a subject who was scanned before injury and then followed at 6 weeks and 10 months postinjury. It is evident that there is increased CSF space, thinning of the corpus callosum, and particular prominence of the ventriculars, most notably at the level of the temporal horn. There is also evident hippocampal wasting. This patient's imaging studies were subjected to quantitative image analysis and the various regions were examined (total brain volume, corpus callosum volume, cerebellum, pons, midbrain, region of the cerebral peduncle, VBR, temporal horn, third ventricle, and fourth ventricle). It is evident that there are significant and dramatic changes that occur as a consequence of injury. There is an overall loss of brain volume of the magnitude of almost 200 cm^3. There is reduction in the corpus callosum, reduction in the cerebellum and pons, but minimal changes at the level of the midbrain and cerebral peduncle. The ventricle-to-brain ratio (VBR) goes up dramatically. The higher this ratio score is, the greater the likelihood is for significant atrophic and brain wasting changes. Also note the dramatic increase in the size of the temporal horns and that they continued to change, even after 6 weeks postinjury. Also note the increase in third and fourth ventricular size.

71

Pre   6 Weeks   10 Months

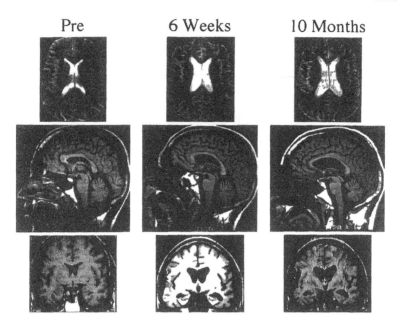

FIG. 5.6. *(Continued)*

are present typically they will be minimal, because substantial frontotemporal contusions or multifocal shearing lesions will significantly alter
mental status, which in turn lowers the GCS score, placing the patient
outside the boundaries of a mild TBI and in a in a more severe head
injury category. Some small foci of white matter change may be observed
as well (see Fig. 5.4; each axial view demonstrates the characteristic appearance of "shear"-type injury at the gray/white matter junction in the
right frontal lobe) or contusions in the inferofrontal region (see Fig. 5.8).
Also, small deposits of hemosiderin (a degraded blood by-product) may
be observed.

NEUROIMAGING IN CHRONIC PHASE OF MILD TBI

Bigler and Snyder (1995) were able to compare either CT or MR scans
obtained prior to mild TBI to scans obtained during the chronic phase
(more than 4 months postinjury) following mild TBI. This was an ideal
clinical study because each patient served as his or her own control.
Comparing neuroimaging studies prior to mild TBI with those obtained
postinjury demonstrated no quantitative changes. Thus, no gross structural atrophy or change in brain anatomy could be demonstrated as a

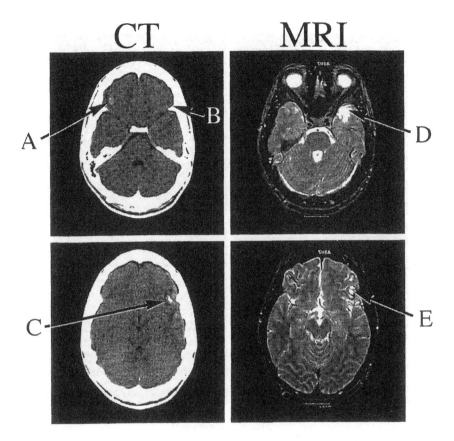

FIG. 5.7. The column on the left identified as "CT" represents the CT imaging studies on admission to the hospital following a significant traumatic brain injury. Note the presence of bifrontal hemorrhagic contusions (a, b, c). The areas of injury in the left frontal temporal have the most notable edematous changes as well. On follow-up with magnetic resonance (presented in the right hand column under MRI) there is a demonstration of the presence of predominant encephalomalacic changes in the inferior frontal and anterior temporal regions of the brain (d and e). The frontal injury depicted in (e) also shows hemosiderin deposit (the black ring around the encephalomalacic change). Because hemosiderin is a blood by-product only found after degradation of the blood deposit, this is a clear sign of significant injury. (f) The abnormality depicted is a distinct change in white matter signal and integrity in the position commonly seen following traumatic injury. Lastly, it should be evident that the patient's scans show a significant increase in ventricular size associated with some generalized wasting and loss of brain substance.

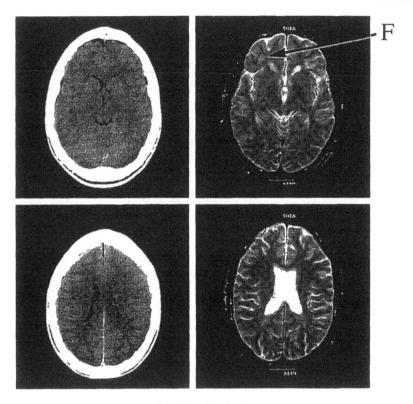

FIG. 5.7. *(Continued)*

consequence of mild TBI in the subjects investigated. These observations are consistent with the position that mild TBI typically does not result in detectable gross structural changes and that the locus of pathology is likely at the microstructural and/or neurochemical level (Maxwell, Povlishock, & Graham, 1997).

If abnormalities associated with mild TBI are associated more with microstrucutal and/or neurochemical changes, then neuroimaging methods that assess physiological integrity of the brain may show greater sensitivity. Accordingly, various metabolic, blood flow, or measures of neurophysiological function have demonstrated greater sensitivity in detecting cerebral dysfunction than the structural imaging offered by CT and/or MR. For example, both single-photon emission computed tomography (SPECT) and positron emission tomography (PET) have been used in evaluating the long-term effects of mild TBI (Kant, Smith-Seemiller, Isaac, & Duffy, 1997; Ruff et al., 1994; Varney et al., 1995). Although these studies have to be interpreted with caution (see "Assessment of Brain SPECT," 1996; *Journal of Nuclear Medicine*, 1996), the presence of SPECT or PET

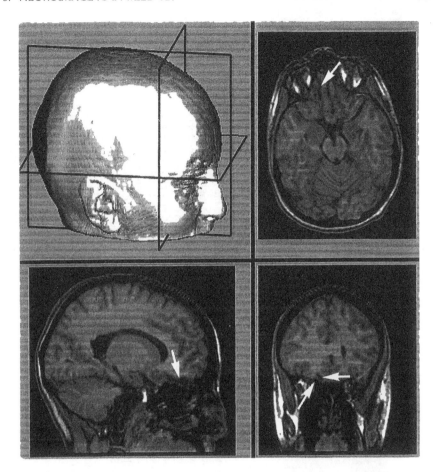

FIG. 5.8. Top left: Three-dimensional MR reconstruction of the brain showing the different planes where the image has actually been taken in this patient. Top right: Axial view showing a lesion (white arrow) at the level of the gyrus rectus. This injury is depicted in the coronal plane (bottom right) as well as sagittal plane (bottom left). Although this is a subtle neuroimaging abnormality, it is distinctly present; the signal from the MRI is abnormal at this level, and indicative of old inferior frontal hemorrhagic type contusion.

abnormalities that correlate with the clinical pattern typically observed (i.e., frontal and/or temporal abnormalities) likely is associated with the residual effects of mild TBI (Bigler, 1997). Other techniques such as functional magnetic resonance imaging (fMRI), diffusion-weighted MR imaging, magnetoencephalography, and sophisticated electrophysiological imaging (Bigler, 1997; Gevins, 1996) may all be useful in imaging the mild TBI patient. For example, the case presented in Fig. 5.9 is a classic case of frontal

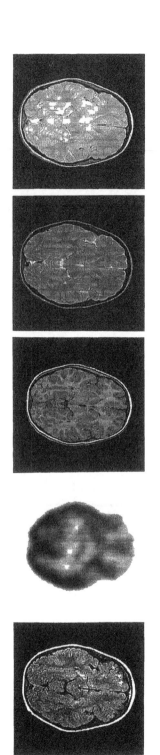

FIG. 5.9. This patient sustained what was considered to be a "mild" TBI. The three scans presented on the left were the clinical magnetic resonance scans (mixed weighted, T2 second from left, and T1-weighted, third from the left). These scans were interpreted as "normal" when read clinically. The patient clearly had behavioral and cognitive changes consistent with traumatic brain injury, and particularly frontal-lobe pathology, and SPECT imaging shows hypoperfusion in the anterior and inferior aspects of the frontal lobe. With SPECT imaging, there should be uniform perfusion around the outer rim of the brain where gray matter resides. When this is not observed or not observed bilaterally, it is an indication of a defect. With the SPECT imaging findings and the patient's clinical history clearly indicating frontal pathology, a diffusion-weighted MR scan was performed (as illustrated in the right panel). This demonstrates an abnormal signal in the right frontal region of the brain. If careful inspection is now done with the images presented in the first two panels on the left, it is evident that there are subtle signal irregularities noted in the right frontal region and that the signal characteristics are not uniform across the two frontal regions. Thus, sometimes even in imaging studies that have been interpreted as "normal," very careful review can detect and identify abnormalities.

76

injury associated with what would otherwise be characterized as "mild TBI." The clinical MR scans performed several months postinjury were negative; however, the SPECT studies clearly demonstrated inferior and anterior frontal hypoperfusion. Additionally, a diffusion-weighted scan clearly demonstrates additional signal abnormalities in the frontal region, lateralized to one hemisphere. If one refers back to the standard clinical images that were interpreted as "normal," there is a subtle difference in the signal intensity in the more affected frontal lobe (see Fig. 5.9). Thus, even with traditional imaging methods, careful examination of the scans may reveal subtle abnormalities that are clearly identified and consistent with the clinical history.

One clinical caveat needs to be mentioned and a cautionary note registered. The exact clinical significance of these newer techniques requires clinical correlation as well as additional research and clinical experience to establish valid relations with the effects of TBI. Unlike the pathognomonic significance of a CT- or MR-demonstrated cortical contusion, which can be directly attributed to the trauma, imaging abnormalities associated with various physiological indices do not necessarily have the same pathognomic implications.

NEUROIMAGING RESEARCH FINDINGS:
IMPLICATIONS FOR THE EFFECTS OF MILD TBI

Numerous animal studies have demonstrated the sensitivity of the hippocampal formation to the effects of trauma (see Tang, Noda, Hasegawa, & Nabeshima, 1997). Because the hippocampus is a critical structure for memory function and that the most frequent cognitive sequela associated with mild TBI is disruption in normal short-term memory function, it is not surprising that research would point to hippocampal involvement. Along these lines, we have shown hippocampal atrophy in TBI to be associated with severity of injury and degree of memory impairment (Bigler et al., 1997). It is also interesting to note that research has demonstrated a relationship between history of head injury (loss of consciousness of a minimum of 5 min) to be associated with subsequent development of Alzheimer's disease (AD) (Schofield et al., 1997). Because one of the major structures involved in AD is the hippocampus, the confluence of this clinical and research information points to hippocampal involvement in mild TBI. Potentially, with more sensitive functional and structural imaging methods (combined fMRI with special imaging parameters), hippocampal pathology will be elucidated. Also, Alzheimer's disease is felt to involve frontotemporal systems to a large extent, and because TBI typically involves a significant frontotemporal component this is probably a factor as well. Lastly, TBI involves some nonspecific injury elements, and Alzheimer's disease is considered to be a global dementia. All of these factors may be components of why head injury, even mild TBI, may play a role in the evolution of Alzheimer's disease.

With TBI, more severe head injury disproportionately affects white rather than gray matter, as can be demonstrated by contemporary MR imaging methods and quantitative analysis (see Fig. 5.9). Because white matter represents the interconnecting pathways in the brain, damage or disruption of white matter pathways is often thought to be the basis of slowed reaction time and speed of processing in TBI (Bigler, 1990). Recent neuropathological studies have demonstrated that perturbations in the integrity of the axon may occur even as a consequence of mild TBI, wherein the axon may not degenerate yet be rendered dysfunctional (see Maxwell et al., 1997). Although significant white matter changes can be detected with MR imaging technology, these types of microstructure changes may not be visualized with current technology. Hence, one can sustain a significant TBI yet have no demonstrable lesions or abnormalities demonstrated on contemporary structural or functional neuroimaging. Undoubtedly, new advances will probably permit objective identification of even these microstructure perturbations (see Fig. 5.9).

CONCLUSIONS

By definition, mild TBI is likely to be associated with few demonstrable abnormalities as visualized by contemporary clinical neuroimaging. When present, the most likely abnormalities are contusions in the frontal–temporal region of the brain and/or shear-type lesions noted in white matter. Although these are not frequent findings, MR imaging in mild TBI patients should be routinely reviewed for detecting any abnormality, often quite subtle, that might be present. Likewise, any imaging performed in the acute phase can be compared to imaging studies performed in the sub-acute and chronic stages for any changes. Imaging studies that capitalize on blood flow or metabolism may be the most sensitive indices of cerebral dysfunction in TBI. Accordingly, various functional neuroimaging techniques hold the greatest promise for the detection of cerebral abnormalities in mild TBI, but standards for this type of neuroimaging will likely take several years to develop.

REFERENCES

Alexander, M. P. (1995). Mild traumatic brain injury: Pathophysiology, natural history, and clinical management. *Neurology, 45,* 1253–1260.
Assessment of brain SPECT. (1996). *Neurology, 46,* 278–285.

Bigler, E. D. (1990). *Traumatic brain injury: Mechanisms of damage, assessment, intervention and outcome.* Austin, TX: Pro-Ed.

Bigler, E. D. (1996a). *Handbook of human brain function: Neuroimaging I. Basic science* (Vol. 1). New York: Plenum Press.

Bigler, E. D. (1996b). *Handbook of human brain function: Neuroimaging II. Clinical applications* (Vol. 2). New York: Plenum Press.

Bigler, E. D. (1996c). Neuroimaging and traumatic brain injury. In E. D. Bigler (Ed.), *Neuroimaging II: Clinical applications* (pp. 261–278). New York: Plenum Press.

Bigler, E. D. (1997). Brain imaging and behavioral outcome in traumatic brain injury. In E. D. Bigler, E. Clark, & J. E. Farmer (Eds.), *Childhood traumatic brain injury: Diagnosis, assessment, and intervention* (pp. 7–29). Austin, TX: Pro-Ed.

Bigler, E. D., Blatter, D. D., Anderson, C. V., Johnson, S. C., Gale, S. D., Hopkins, R. O., & Burnett, B. (1997). Hippocampal volume in normal aging and traumatic brain injury. *American Journal of Neuroradiology, 18,* 11–23.

Bigler, E. D., & Clement, P. (1998). *Diagnostic clinical neuropsychology.* Austin, TX: University of Texas Press.

Bigler, E. D., & Snyder, J. L. (1995). Neuropsychological outcome and quantitative neuroimaging in mild head injury. *Archives of Clinical Neuropsychology, 10,* 159–174.

Blatter, D. D., Bigler, E. D., Gale, S. D., Johnson, S. C., Anderson, C. V., Burnett, B. M., Parker, N., Kurth, S., & Horn, S. (1995). Quantitative volumetric analysis of brain MR: Normative database spanning five decades of life. *American Journal of Neuroradiology, 16,* 241–251.

Blatter, D. D., Bigler, E. D., Gale, S. D., Johnson, S. C., Anderson, C. V., Burnett, B. M., Ryser, D., Macnamara, S. E., & Bailey, B. J. (1997). MR-based brain and cerebrospinal fluid measurement after traumatic brain injury: Correlation with neuropsychological outcome. *American Journal of Neuroradiology, 18,* 1–10.

Gale, S. D., Johnson, S. C., Bigler, E. D., & Blatter, D. D. (1995). Trauma-induced degenerative changes in brain injury: A morphometric analysis of three patients with preinjury and postinjury MR scans. *Journal of Neurotrauma, 12,* 151–158.

Gean, A. D. (1994). *Imaging of head trauma.* New York: Raven Press.

Gevins, A. (1996). Imaging the neurocognitive networks of the human brain. In E. D. Bigler (Ed.), *Handbook of human brain function: Neuroimaging I. Basic science* (Vol. 1, pp. 133–159). New York: Plenum Press.

Johnson, S. C., Bigler, E. D., Burr, R. B., & Blatter, D. D. (1994). White matter atrophy, ventricular dilation, and intellectual functioning following traumatic brain injury. *Neuropsychology, 8,* 307–315.

Journal of Nuclear Medicine (1996). 37, 1256–1258.

Kant, L., Smith-Seemiller, L., Isaac, G., & Duffy, J. (1997). Tc-HMPAO SPECT in persistent post-concussion syndrome after mild head injury: Comparison with MRI/CT. *Brain Injury, 11,* 115–124.

Katz, D. I., & Alexander, M. P. (1994). Traumatic brain injury: Predicting course of recovery and outcome for patients admitted to rehabilitation. *Archives of Neurology, 51,* 661–670.

Maxwell, W. L., Povlishock, J. T., & Graham, D. L. (1997). A mechanistic analysis of nondisruptive axonal injury: A review. *Journal of Neurotrauma, 14,* 419–440.

Osborn, A. G. (1994). *Diagnostic neuroradiology.* St. Louis, MO: Mosby.

Ruff, R. M., Crouch, J. A., Tröster, A. I., Marshall, L. F., Buchsbaum, M. S., Lottenberg, S., & Somers, L. M. (1994). Selected cases of poor outcome following a minor brain trauma: Comparing neuropsychological and positron emission tomography assessment. *Brain Injury, 8,* 297–308.

Ryser, D. K., Bigler, E. D., & Blatter, D. (1998). Clinical and neuroimaging predictors of post TBI outcome. In J. Ponsford, P. Snow, & V. Anderson (Eds.), *International perspectives in traumatic brain injury* (pp. 79–83). Bowen Hills: Australian Academic Press.

Schofield, P. W., Tang, M., Marder, K., Bell, K., Dooneief, G., Chun, M., Sano, M., Stern, Y., & Mayeux, R. (1997). Alzheimer's disease after remote head injury: An incidence study. *Journal of Neurology, Neurosurgery and Psychiatry, 62*, 119–124.

Tang, Y., Noda, Y., Hasegawa, T., & Nabeshima, T. (1997). A concussive-like brain injury model in mice (II): Selective neuronal loss in the cortex and hippocampus. *Journal of Neurotrauma, 14*, 863–873.

Varney, N. R., Bushnell, D. L., Nathan, M., Kah, D., Roberts, R., Rezai, K., Walker, W., & Kirchner, P. (1995). NeuroSPECT correlates of disabling mild head injury: Preliminary findings. *Journal of Head Trauma Rehabilitation, 10*, 18–28.

6

Mild Head Injury:
The New Frontier in Sports Medicine

Jeffrey T. Barth
University of Virginia School of Medicine

Robert N. Varney
Palo Alto, California

Robert A. Ruchinskas
Temple University

Joseph P. Francis
Naval Medical Center, Portsmouth, Virginia

Multiple mild concussions in high-profile, professional football players in the mid 1990s and the resultant media feeding frenzy have ushered in a new era in the study of mild head injury in athletics. In particular, Troy Aikman, Steve Young, *Sports Illustrated*, ESPN, and *CNN Sports*, among others, have begun a cascade of events including a new appreciation for and concern over the immediate and long-term effects of the invisible sports injury. This new focus is predicated on the newsworthy nature of this injury involving sports celebrities, its potential for disability and career termination, and the obvious liability and financial implications. These concerns are shared by athletes, their families, school officials, team physicians, coaches, athletic trainers, franchise owners, athletic directors, player agents, insurance companies, and the public. Sensitivity to the effects of mild head injury on the playing field has created a need for information and expertise in factors critical to the identification of mechanism, prevalence, and severity of injury. These factors, along with treatment, recovery curves, long-term outcome, and prevention, all parallel the concern over sports spinal-cord trauma and orthopedic injuries in earlier years. The natural inclination has been to turn to the clinical/medical and scientific literature in an attempt to find similarities and answers to questions regarding sideline medical assessment of severity, and criteria for return to play or termination of athletic career after multiple mild head injuries.

Decades earlier, modern medicine concerned itself with the sequelae of moderate and severe traumatic brain injury in the clinical population with little attention paid to mild head trauma. This lack of focus on mild injury was predicated on the belief that such trauma was not of clinical significance, nor could it directly result in long-term disability. This popular position was not espoused by the entire scientific community, as noted by Symonds (1962), who stated that "it is questionable whether the effects of concussion, however slight, are ever completely reversible" (p. 4), and Oppenheimer (1968), who discovered postmortem microscopic brain lesions in presumed mild head injured patients, with no clinical/neurologic impairment. Nevertheless, medical interest focused on moderate and severe brain injury in clinical populations (i.e., NINCDS Traumatic Coma Data Bank, etc.) and sports, with a natural gravitation toward the study of boxing, because it is one of the few sports where the goal is to "inflict brain damage, cause a concussion or render the opponent unconscious" (Jordan, 1987, p. 453). In a review of intracranial injuries in boxing by Ryan (1987) and specific studies and analyses by Casson et al. (1984), Corsellis, Bruton, and Freeman-Browne (1973), Johnson (1969), Jordan (1987), Jedlinski, Gatarski, and Szymusik (1970), Lampert and Hardman (1984), Martland (1928), Mendez (1995), Roberts (1969), Ross, Casson, Siegel, and Cole (1987), Serel and Jaros (1962), and Unterharnscheidt (1972), it is clear that professional boxers can experience severe cerebral trauma (hemorrhage, edema, axonal tearing). More chronic and insidious degenerative neurologic conditions (chronic boxers' encephalopathy and cerebral atrophy) from multiple concussive and subconcussive blows to the head can result in various forms of neurocognitive decline (dementia pugilistica, and punch drunk syndrome). Determining who will develop such disorders is difficult and likely relates to issues of individual vulnerability as well as severity and frequency of concessions. Unfortunately, this literature has only limited application to the issue of mild head injury in sports.

Seminal clinical investigations of mild head injury began in the late 1970s and proceeded through the 1980s and 1990s with the work of Gronwall and Wrightson (1974, 1980), Wrightson and Gronwall (1980), Rimel, Giordani, Barth, Boll, and Jane (1981), Barth et al. (1983), Dikmen, McLean, and Temkin (1986), Levin, Lippold, Goldman, Handel, High, Eisenberg, and Zelitt (1987), Levin, Mattis, Ruff, Eisenberg, Marshall, and Tabbador (1987), Ruff et al. (1989), Leininger, Gramling, Forrel, Kreutzer, and Peck (1990), Ruff et al. (1994), and Alves, Macciocchi and Barth (1993). The New Zealand studies by Gronwall and her colleagues, as well as those initiated at the University of Virginia (Rimel et al., 1981; Barth et al., 1983) and at the Medical College of Virginia (Leininger, Gramling, Ferrel, Kreutzer, & Peck, 1990), revealed neurocognitive deficits in selected mild head injured patients with some postconcussion syndrome symptoms. Research by Dikmen et al. (1986), Levin, Lippold, et al. (1987), and Levin, Mattis, et al. (1987) indicated neuropsychological impairments at 1 month post mild head injury in a significant number of patients, with almost complete recovery 2 months later. Ruff et al. (1989) reported memory deficits in mild head injury patients at various posttrauma intervals, and Levin, Amparo, Eisenberg, Williams, High, McArdle, and Weiner (1987) found parenchymal lesions on magnetic resonance imaging (MRI) in mild and moderate head injuries. Alves et al. (1993), in a study of 587 patients, noted few postconcussion syndrome symptoms in an uncomplicated mild head injured population at 1 year postinjury. A neuropsychological positron emission tomography (PET) study of 9 mild head injured patients and 43 controls (Ruff et al., 1994) noted neurocognitive deficits and glucose uptake abnormalities in all mild head trauma patients, compared to normal findings in the control group.

The question of identifiable neurologic lesion associated with such mild injuries was initially addressed by Gennarelli, Adams, and Graham (1981) in their classic study of mild head injury in primates. Injuries characterized by brief loss of consciousness from linear acceleration–deceleration resulted in brainstem axonal tearing. These findings provided evidence for possible underlying histological impairment in individuals who suffer mild traumatic head injury (Jane, Steward, & Gennarelli, 1985). Further elaboration of this model and review of the animal and human research in this area is provided by Povlishock and Christman (1995).

Although the early human studies all differ in a number of critical experimental design features, such as patient demographics and inclusion criteria, neuropsychological assessment procedures, test intervals, statistical applications, and use of control groups, in sum, they suggest that most mild head injured patients typically make good recoveries, yet some can suffer at least temporary neurocognitive deficits. Further, it appears that extent and speed of recovery are related to individual vulnerability: factors that are unique to the individual, such as age, education, severity of injury, premorbid health and cognitive ability, pain, previous psychiatric condition or neurologic problems, substance abuse, existence of postconcussion syndrome symptoms, socioeconomic supports, pending litigation, and information provided by the health care system (Barth, Diamond, & Errico, 1996).

In an attempt to better understand the effects of mild deceleration head injury in humans, and to control for several of the factors which often effect outcome, Barth et al. (1989) found the American football field to be an ideal, relatively controlled laboratory setting. Their 4-year study of

2,350 college football players (and controls) from 10 northeastern universities is, to date, the most extensive prospective study of neurocognitive outcome following very mild head injury in young, healthy, motivated athletes. Brief neuropsychological assessment at preseason and postseason, for all players, and repeat testing at 24 hr, 5 days, and 10 days post mild head injury (usually without loss of consciousness, but rather with subtle alteration in mental status), and similar evaluations of red-shirted and roommate controls, revealed mild cognitive decline at 24 hr postinjury, with general recovery of function by most at 5 days postinjury and no statistical difference between head-injured players and controls 5 days later. These findings provided further support for the notion that very mild deceleration head injury (amnestic dings, Yarnell & Lynch, 1993) in young, healthy, well-motivated, bright college athletes results in temporary neurocognitive deficits and a rapid recovery curve (5 to 10 days).

This study created the foundation for sports mild head injury research, which has recently gained new momentum. This new surge in interest in mild head injury in sports is attributable to:

1. A new sensitivity to mild concussion in the professional sports community and the media, resulting in a search for answers regarding questions of mechanism and severity of injury, course of recovery, guidelines for return to play (or termination of play), and the effects of multiple mild injuries.
2. A recognition of an opportunity by medical researchers to study mild head injury in a partially controlled laboratory setting.
3. A fascination with sports and a wish to identify with celebrities, which afflicts so many of us (let's face it, it's fun to assess and hang out with football and hockey players, etc.).

DEFINING THE INJURY

Defining mild head injury in the clinical population is problematic, and the complications increase when considering the sports context. The research criteria for the traditional study of mild head injury include a Glasgow Coma Scale score of 13 to 15, less than 20 min loss of consciousness (or no loss of consciousness), less than 48 hr hospitalization (no physical complications), and no neuroimaging evidence of impairment (Levin, Eisenberg, & Benton, 1989; Rimel et al., 1981). In the clinical environment, it is not unusual to find individuals who meet the first three of these criteria but show some mild neuroimaging abnormality (i.e, skull fracture or small hematoma, etc.). These patients, along with those who demonstrate high levels of individual vulnerability to mild head trauma, are often slow to recover, may exhibit postconcussion syndrome, and are categorized as "complicated" mild head injuries (Alves et al., 1993). According to Alves et al. (1993), it is unlikely that someone with an uncomplicated mild head injury will experience more than two or three postconcussion syndrome symptoms (such as headache, dizziness, memory and attentional deficits, lowered frustration tolerance, irritability, depression, sleep disturbance, fatigue, diplopia, tinnitus, and slowed and inefficient mental processing).

In 1993, the American Congress of Rehabilitation Medicine reported its definition of mild traumatic brain injury, which has striking similarities to the previously cited research criteria for mild head injury, yet more specifically describes the cognitive and neurologic implications. That definition includes a Glasgow Coma Scale of 13 to 15 (after 30 min), less than 30 min loss of consciousness, and 24 hr or less of posttraumatic amnesia. This definition also includes at least one of the following: loss of consciousness, retrograde or posttraumatic amnesia, altered mental state at the time of the trauma, and transient or permanent focal neurologic deficits (American Congress of Rehabilitation Medicine, 1993). This definition of mild traumatic brain injury allows for no loss of consciousness (merely an alteration in mental function), the possibility of temporary to permanent identifiable neurologic impairment, and further possible long-term disability. This definition of mild traumatic brain injury is consistent with that of mild head injury, yet it utilizes the term *brain injury*, which implies greater specificity than the term *head injury*, which may or may not reference brain dysfunction. Of course, the research criteria for mild head injury also imply at least temporary neurologic dysfunction (Glasgow Coma Scale $\geq$ 13). The definitions of mild head injury and mild traumatic brain injury are now quite similar and make less obvious the distinction between *head injury*, which does not necessarily imply significant insult to the brain, and *brain injury*, which does make such assumptions and can imply permanent impairment and some level of disability.

In the sports literature, it is much more common to come across the terms *concussion* and *mild concussion*. Traditional concussion was defined by Gennarelli (1987) as temporary and reversible neurologic impairment and loss of consciousness for less than 6 hr, as a result of trauma to the head. He went on to describe mild concussion as a temporary disturbance or alteration in neurologic function without full loss of consciousness. As in mild traumatic brain injury, there is a direct reference to at least temporary alteration in mental state without necessarily having complete loss of consciousness. In the sports context, the terms *mild head injury* and *mild concussion* are often used interchangeably, with *mild traumatic brain injury* more often being linked to the clinical literature. In this chapter we use the more generic terms *mild head injury* and *mild concussion*.

More mild head injuries and mild concussions occur in the general population than moderate and severe head injuries combined (Rimel et al., 1981). Kraus and Conroy (1984) reported over 300,000 mild head injury hospitalizations per year, with many more occurring that do not require medical observation or intervention. From a clinical perspective, it appears that most mild head injured individuals either experience no significant neurocognitive deficits following their trauma, or experience impairments that are short-lived (days, weeks, or 2–3 months). It is, however, also recognized that there is a "miserable minority" (Ruff, Camenzuli, & Mueller, 1996) that may experience longer periods of disability, which are related to individual recovery curves or individual vulnerability. With the exception of boxing and equestrian sports, moderate and severe head trauma are of low incidence in relationship to other bodily injury in sports. Mild head injury and mild concussion, on the other hand, are likely quite common in the sports arena, yet go unrecognized due to their less visible features and the athletes' tendency to cover up due to their credos of "play with pain" and "you can't make the club in the tub."

MECHANISMS AND SEVERITY OF INJURY

Mild concussion in sports typically involves acceleration and rapid deceleration from direct or indirect impact, creating linear or rotational forces on the brain. As noted earlier, many in the scientific community have long believed that insufficient forces are exerted on the brain in typical mild head injury to cause persistent problems—a view that, until recently, has been accepted in the sports community. There are, however, fundamental Newtonian physics formulas and theoretical models that can be utilized to determine the probable acceleration–deceleration energy that can come to bear on brain tissue under specified conditions. Varney and Varney (1995) proposed such a model for predicting severity of head injury in motor vehicle accidents, where accelerations (decelerations) from 37 g to 270 g (with no direct head impact) were found to result in significant neurocognitive deficits. A similar sort of analysis may be applied to sports concussions, in which at least temporary brain injury appears to occur even when no direct head contact is noted. The analysis depends on arriving at an acceleration or deceleration experienced by the player and deducing from it what brain forces would likely have occurred. This approach to brain forces via computation of accelerations appears to be a highly practical route to follow when calculating potential for significant injury.

Accelerations (or decelerations, which are simply accelerations with a negative sign and are proportional to the forces causing them in the same way as for positive signs) can be determined from a simple relationship found in almost any elementary physics textbook, namely:

$$a = (v^2 - v_0^2)/2s$$

or

$$a = (v^2 - v_0^2)/2sg$$

The latter form is to be used if the acceleration is to be expressed as a multiple of the acceleration of gravity, g, which is 32.2 ft/sec^2. In this formula, a is the acceleration, v_0 is the speed at the start of the acceleration, v is the speed at the end of the acceleration, and s is the distance traveled during the period of the acceleration. The formula is even simplified in most cases of interest here in that if the player is brought to rest at the end of the acceleration, the value of v is zero, making the formula read:

$$a = -v_0^2/2sg$$

Thus, for example, if a football player running at 10 ft/sec speed collides with another player and is brought to a stop in a distance of 2 in (or 0.167 ft) the acceleration becomes:

$$a = -10^2/2 \times 0.167 \times 32.2 = 9.3 \ g$$

If it is indeed the player's head that is stopped in this short distance, the forces acting on any elements of his brain are 9.3 times the weight of that element. Just what this force will do to the brain depends on many factors, such as the direction of the force, and whether the element of the brain is moved by the force relative to its neighbors, thereby creating shear strain or axonal injury (Holburn, 1943).

The problem to be faced in sports injuries to the brain is to evaluate (a) what the values of v_0, the speed at impact, and s, the stopping distance, are, and (b) how this accumulated force is transmitted to the head and brain of the player. In many cases, this reduces to the problem of evaluating the stopping distance (s), which is, in the case of football, affected by the helmet, which "cushions" impacts to the head (which amounts to increasing the value of s). Similarly, the role of "pillow" gloves in boxing is also to increase the distance s over which the victim's head moves during the actual impact.

Four types of sports (football) acceleration–deceleration models are classified next, recognizing that no single injury may fall exactly into one of these classifications. For the purpose of simplification, only impacts occurring between two individuals are considered:

Model 1. Both players initially at rest. This basically becomes a pushing match, and significant shock to the brain does not typically occur. To be sure, one of the players may be hurled to the ground hard enough to incur injury, but this is taken up in another case.

Model 2. Player A is in motion and Player B is at rest. In this case a question at once arises as to which player may incur injury. In the Barth et al. (1989) college football study, in many cases, there were more significant injuries sustained by those performing tackles and blocks than by those being tackled or blocked:

(a) Player B fully expects the collision with Player A and plants himself firmly. Let us assume that in addition, B is considerably heavier than A. In this subcase, Player B may suffer no acceleration at all whereas Player A is brought to a dead stop in the impact. If A hits B with his head or shoulder, A's head (and brain) may be brought to a quick stop and the value of s will be small. A's deceleration may thus be quite large with significant brain acceleration. If B should tackle A below A's waistline, A will probably be brought to a stop over a considerably longer distance (s larger) and no significant injury arises (yet such a tackle may actually increase the acceleration of the head like a whiplash, and increase the possibility of severe injury).

(b) Player B is caught completely unaware, has not braced himself at all, and is knocked hard into the direction of A's speed, v_o. If A holds onto B, and if the two players have approximately the same weights, both will end up with a final speed of about half of v_o. If on the other hand, A simply knocks B forward and stops himself, B may acquire virtually all of the speed v_o. Because A is well prepared for the collision, he may protect himself so that no sensitive area of his body takes the blow. Player B, on the other hand, is likely to experience a whiplash if the impact is below his neckline. In crude terms, his head will simply lag behind the speed acquired by the rest of his body until his neck is bent to its extreme angle. His head will then "snap" into the new speed in a very short distance between the end of its backward lag and the full speed in the new direction. In other words, s may be quite small and the consequent acceleration quite large. Thus under these circumstances, A may suffer no trauma and B may be critically injured.

Model 3. Players A and B are both in motion when they collide. For simplicity it will be assumed that they have the same speeds but in different directions.

(a) Head-on impact. Both players will experience the same decelerations (unless one is much heavier than the other). If they hit head to head or shoulder to shoulder, both players are likely to have considerable brain accelerations. If instead, for example, A low-tackles B so that A passes under B, both players will doubtless stop over long distances s, decreasing the likelihood of significant injury.

(b) The two players hit each other at an angle. Because the players' heads are not likely to collide in this case, there is less danger of injury to either, although shoulder-to-shoulder impact may give accelerations to their heads. Again, the question of the advance awareness of each player is important; most notably, if one is not expecting the collision at all, one is likely to encounter a whiplash at the oblique angle at which the other hit, and because of the lesser flexibility of the neck in a sidewise direction, the value of s may be small and the acceleration and potential neurologic injury worse.

Model 4. A single player hits the ground. If he simply falls down, there may be no problem. If he is running at top speed and has his feet tackled or simply stumbles, he may hit the ground with most of his forward running speed. There are then two factors: first, what part of his body first touches the ground, and second, how hard is the ground (clearly there are implications with regard to artificial versus natural turf). The standard question arises, namely, in how short a distance (s) is his head brought to a stop.

As an extreme example of the forces that could be at work, let us consider a fast runner moving at a speed of nearly 30 ft/sec. As a possible extreme value of the stopping distance s, we take about 1 in, or rounded off, 0.1 ft. Using the formula $a = v_o^2/2sg$, we arrive at:

$$a = 30^2/2 \times 0.1 \times 32.2 = 140 \; g$$

It is highly probable that this deceleration in the case of a motor vehicle accident would produce permanent neurologic impairment under certain conditions. This value is doubtless the worst possible case for a football injury and is relatively unlikely to occur, yet a more likely case would be a speed of 15 ft/sec and a stopping distance of 0.2 ft, yielding a deceleration (g) of 17.5 g. Such a force is still considerable, but one not as likely to cause permanent neurologic dysfunction in a single event.

The previous considerations are further complicated by the issue of multiple mild concussions and second impact syndrome. Saunders and Harbaugh (1984) explained some catastrophic neurologic injuries that occur following successive mild head injuries as being related to increased intercranial pressure and vascular congestion, which can be triggered by loss of cerebral autoregulatory capacity (Second Impact Syndrome). Theoretically the first injury impairs the system, and without sufficient time to recover between traumas, the second injury further compromises the system and creates a more serious malfunction. Although such cases are rare, and experimental data are generally lacking to verify this theory, common sense would dictate that suffering multiple mild head injuries in close temporal proximity may result in synergistic effects and poor outcome.

ASSESSMENT OF MILD HEAD INJURY AND RETURN TO PLAY

Several sports medicine researchers and team physicians have developed methods for assessing the severity of mild head injury and criteria for return to play, based on the little scientific literature available, neurological principles, and clinical/practical experience. Polin, Alves, and Jane (1996) provided a comparison of four concussion severity assessment systems or guidelines (Cantu, 1986, 1991; Torg, Beer, & Vesgo, 1980; Colorado Medical Society, 1991, and Kelly et al., 1991; Virginia Neurological Institute, in Polin et al., 1996), most of which categorize mild head injuries from Grade 1 to Grade 3 (least to most severe). The Colorado Medical Society guidelines were eventually summarized by Kelly and Rosenberg (1997) and further explicated in a Neurology Practice Parameter article (see Practice Parameter, 1997). In general, these systems consider a Grade 1 mild head injury to include brief (or no) loss of consciousness, little or no posttraumatic amnesia (or other amnesia), or confusion. Grade 2 injuries typically involve less than 5 min loss of consciousness (or no loss of consciousness), some posttraumatic (up to 24 hr) or retrograde amnesia, and some confusion. Finally, Grade 3 is characterized by brief loss of consciousness (less than 5 min), greater than 24 hr posttraumatic amnesia, a Glasgow Coma Scale score of 13 or 14, and confusion.

The Cantu, Neurology Practice Parameter, and Virginia Neurological Institute severity grading systems also provide practical guidelines for return to play after one, two, or three successive injuries in a season and with reference to the grade of the mild head injury (Polin et al., 1996). For example, the Cantu guidelines (1986, 1991) suggest that an athlete may return to play when asymptomatic (no neurologic or postconcussion syndrome symptoms) and if this is his or her first Grade 1 mild head injury that season. After a second Grade 1 injury, the player may return to games and practices in 2 weeks if asymptomatic for 1 week. Cantu went on to suggest that the athlete's season be terminated with a third mild head injury, regardless of grade. In contrast, he suggested that an individual may return to play if asymptomatic for 1 week after the first

Grade 2 mild head injury, and in 1 month if asymptomatic for 1 week after a single Grade 3 injury. The latter criteria are applied to return to play after a second Grade 2 mild head injury, and Cantu advised termination of the athlete's season after the second Grade 3 injury. These guidelines are an outgrowth of Quigley's Rule (Schneider, 1973), which was supported by the work of Gronwall and Wrightson (1975), which cited evidence of cumulative effects of successive blows. The rule recommends that athletes should discontinue participation in sports after receiving three cerebral concussions, and Maroon, Steele, and Berlin (1980) added that neuroradiological abnormalities are also sufficient to terminate sports participation.

An assessment of neurologic integrity and postconcussion symptoms is often necessary at the time of potential injury. McCrea, Kelly, Kluge, Ackley, and Randolph (1997) developed the Standardized Assessment of Concussion (SAC), which is a sideline mental status assessment that can be utilized for this purpose by the athletic trainer or team physician in conjunction with the brief physical neurological examination. The SAC can assist in determining the likelihood of an athlete having experienced a mild head injury, the necessity for terminating play at that time, and the need for further monitoring of neurocognitive functions and postconcussion symptomatology.

Neurocognitive outcome assessment of mild head injury in sports poses unique challenges for the neuropsychologist. First, the athletic establishment (players, coaches, athletic trainers, physicians, etc.) must be convinced of the need for preseason and serial postinjury evaluations to determine severity of impairment and rate and extent of recovery, using the player as his or her own control, and having comparison groups of other athletes assessed at identical intervals. Second, the assessment measures must be sensitive and broad-based enough to elucidate the neurocognitive effects of very mild head injury. And third, the assessment must be of short duration, because players and coaches typically have little tolerance for disruption of athletic routines. Because it is difficult to address each of these issues in sports mild head injury outcome research, most investigations of boxing, football, soccer, rugby, ice hockey, and equestrian sports have been retrospective and epidemiological in nature and typically rely on athlete self-report, observations, and medical record reviews, with little formal prospective neuropsychological evaluation and no use of control groups (Bixby-Hammett, 1992; Foster, Leiguarda, & Tilley, 1976; Gerberich, Priest, Boen, Staub, & Maxwell, 1983; Gibbs, 1993; Haglund & Bergstrand, 1990; Haglund, Edman, Murelius, Oreland, & Sachs, 1990; Haglund & Persson, 1990; Hamilton & Tranmer, 1993; O'Brien, 1992; Pelletier, Montelpare, & Stark, 1993; Tegner & Lorentzen, 1996; Tysvaer, Storli, & Bachen, 1989; Zemper, 1989).

These challenges to neuropsychological assessment were first met in the previously described 4-year, many-subject investigation of college football players (Barth et al., 1989), which now stands as a model for sports mild head injury research. The test battery was short (17 min), incorporated four neurocognitive tests (WAIS Vocabulary, Trail Making A & B, Paced Auditory Serial Addition Task, and Symbol Digit; Lezak, 1995), and was considered valuable by the coaches, athletic trainers, and team physicians for its potential to assist all concerned in developing better rules for determining return to play. It should be noted that tolerance for this project would have been tested by all parties if the test battery had been much longer, and such a large undertaking would have been impossible without significant funding from a granting agency.

Similar neuropsychological assessments have been employed by Abreau, Templer, Schuyler, and Hutchison (1990) and Witol (1996) in smaller studies of high school, college, and professional soccer players. In these investigations of 62 and 60 soccer players, respectively, neuropsychological test performance was negatively associated with age, number of games played, and heading frequency, particularly when compared to a small control group in the later study. Other brief neurocognitive assessment models have been applied to soccer (Tysvaer, 1992; Tysvaer & Einar, 1991) and amateur boxing (Brooks et al., 1987; Haglund & Eriksson, 1993; Heilbronner, Henry, & Carson-Brewer, 1991; McLatchie et al., 1987; Thomassen, Juul-Jensen, Olivarius, Braemer, & Christensen, 1979). The most extensive neuropsychological investigation of mild head injury in amateur boxing to date comes from a study funded by the U.S. Olympic Foundation and the National Institute of Neurological Disorders and Stroke, carried out by the Johns Hopkins University Department of Epidemiology, School of Hygiene and Public Health (Stewart et al., 1994). In this 4-year study of 484 amateur boxers (baseline and 2-year reassessments), a comprehensive battery of 12 neuropsychological tests was utilized, in addition to gathering intake interview information and samples of brainstem auditory evoked potentials, electroencephalographic readings, an ataxia/vestibules test battery, and urine drug screens. Their results indicated a relationship (trend) between memory, visuoconstructional ability, and perceptual-motor functions and number of bouts pre baseline testing. In a much smaller study utilizing MR and neurocognitive assessments, Levin, Lippold, et al. (1987) found few neurobehavioral deficits and no MR abnormalities in a group of 13 amateur boxers when compared to 13 matched controls. Both of these investigations suggest that amateur boxers are at considerably less risk for neurocognitive disruption than their professional counterparts.

Recent trends in the assessment of sports-related mild head injury have generally focused on refinements of the brief neuropsychological testing model with college and professional football, soccer, and ice hockey, with some efforts also directed at high school athletics. As examples, studies at Pennsylvania State University directed by Dr. Rubin Echemendia and his colleagues employ 10 neuropsychological test procedures over a 45-min session, administered preseason to all football, soccer, ice hockey, and basketball players who wish to participate. Further evaluations take place at 48 hr, 1 week, and 1 month postconcussion, as well as at the end of the athlete's playing career at Penn State. At the professional level, Drs. Mark Lovell, Julian Bailes, and Joseph Maroon are spearheading efforts in the National Football League to recognize the value of neuropsychological assessment of mild concussion, with their work being piloted with the Pittsburgh Steelers. The Hopkins Memory Test, Stroop Word Color Test, Digit Span, Symbol Digit, Controlled Oral Word Association Test, and Trail Making Test (Lezak, 1995) comprise the Pittsburgh Steelers' brief 20-min neurocognitive battery. The similarities in these assessments reflect a learning from previous and current research efforts, as well as a cooperative spirit and desire to create a common language and meaningful dialogue within the sports medicine and neuropsychology/neurology communities.

FUTURE DIRECTIONS

With substantial progress over the last decade in the study of sports-related mild head injury, we continue to search for answers to what remain very basic questions—questions that will continue to guide our research into the 21st century. These questions include: How do we measure the relative severity and effects of mild concussion? What is the typical recovery curve for sports mild head injury and how is this different from clinical populations? When is it safe for a player to return to play and practice? What are the acute and chronic effects of multiple mild concussions and what are the critical recovery periods between concussions to avoid synergistic deficits or second impact syndrome? When (after how many concussions in what period of time) should an athlete terminate play for a season or for a career? What individuals and sports should we study? What experimental design and assessment procedures should we use in the study of sports mild head injury? How do we fund this research, and for whom do we ultimately work when providing these neuropsychological assessments?

In our attempts to address these issues, we have found that an interdisciplinary approach to mild head injury investigation, which involves medical/neurological and neuropsychological assessment, provides the most broad-based and comprehensive severity and outcome evaluation. Most of the research to date suggests that there is a very rapid recovery curve (hours to days) for Grade 1 (very mild) concussion in the majority of single injury cases, but there are few data regarding multiple head injuries in a single season or over longer periods of time. Return-to-play guidelines presently utilized in many sports, although logical, and based on conservative clinical judgment, reference little scientific foundation, and should be subjected to the scrutiny of sound, controlled research.

It is fortunate that neuropsychologists, neurologists, neurosurgeons, and trainers who are interested in sports mild head injury have various interests and levels of access to athletes and sports organizations. For this reason, present research spans high schools, colleges, and professional teams from football and soccer to boxing and equestrian sports. Mild head injury in sports is undoubtedly multidimensional and differs across factors such as age, level of participation, and type of potential injury mechanisms; thus, research efforts in each of these areas would appear advantageous.

The question of experimental design and neuropsychological test protocols is more complex than it seems at first glance. It appears obvious that if we all adhered to one experimental design procedure (e.g., preseason, postseason, and 24 hr, 5 days, and 10 days posttrauma assessments) and one brief but broad-based neuropsychological test battery, data could be pooled, statistical analyses would be robust, and answers would be forthcoming and definitive with regard to the questions of interest. On the other hand, using one experimental design and one set of assessment procedures increases the risk of measuring the wrong variables at the wrong time, just as only focusing on college football players might provide us with a skewed view of sports mild head injury. For this reason, it may be best to focus our collective efforts on several experimental designs and assessment procedures, and pool data within each of these approaches.

The neuropsychological assessment procedures utilized in our future research efforts, although they may be varied, should be well-standardized, valid, reliable measures with solid normative bases. They should also be sensitive to the functions that are likely to be affected by mild neurologic insult (new, rapid problem solving, attention, concentration, memory, abstract reasoning, reaction time/discrimination, etc.), and we should attempt to study the ecological validity of these measures within the sports context. Practice effects must be considered along with adequate controls, and the assessment must be brief and cost-effective. In consideration of these later issues, self-administered, computerized assessment procedures, perhaps specifically designed for this sports application, and direct involvement of the athletic trainers with the neuropsychologist will likely be the evaluation method of choice.

Addressing these issues in a rigorous, scientific fashion will require a philosophical and practical commitment by the athletes, their families, coaches, team physicians, trainers, administrators/owners, players advisors, insurance companies, and perhaps even the fans (public). Without cooperation from all involved, and some funding resources, which may come from those with the most vested interest and/or risks, our progress in answering these practical questions will likely be haphazard and slow. Fortunately, with the rising awareness of the risks of multiple mild concussions created by the media, there has been a concomitant increase in interest in these issues in the high school, college, and professional communities, as well as the insurance industry. Now, more than at any time in the past quarter century, we are well positioned to develop a comprehensive sports initiative to systematically collect data using two or three overlapping experimental designs and neuropsychological assessment batteries for a National Sports Mild Head Injury Data Bank.

REFERENCES

Abreau, F., Templer, D. I., Schuyler, B. A., & Hutchison, H. T. (1990). Neuropsychological assessment of soccer players. *Neuropsychology, 4,* 175–181.

Alves, W. M., Macciocchi, S. N., & Barth, J. T. (1993). Post concussion symptoms after uncomplicated mild head injury. *Journal of Head Trauma Rehabilitation, 8,* 48–59.

American Congress of Rehabilitation Medicine. (1993). Definition of mild traumatic brain injury. *Journal of Head Trauma Rehabilitation, 8,* 86–87.

Barth, J. T., Alves, W. M., Ryan, T. V., Macciocchi, S. N., Rimel, R. E., Jane, J. A., & Nelson, W. E. (1989). Mild head injury in sports: Neuropsychological sequelae and recovery of function. In H. S. Levin, H. M. Eisenber, & A. L. Benton (Eds.), *Mild head injury* (pp. 257–275). New York: Oxford.

Barth, J. T., Diamond, R., & Errico, A. (1996). Mild head injury and post concussion syndrome: Does anyone really suffer? *Clinical Electroencephalography, 27,* 183–186.

Barth, J. T., Macciocchi, S. N., Boll, T. J., Giordani, B., Jane, J. A., & Rimel, R. W. (1983). Neuropsychological sequelae of minor head injury. *Neurosurgery, 13,* 529–533.

Bixby-Hammett, D. M. (1992). Pediatric equestrian injuries. *Pediatrics, 89,* 1173–1176.

Brooks, N., Galbraith, S., Hutchinson, J. S. F., McLatchie, G., Melville, I., Teasdale, E., & Wilson, L. (1987). Clinical neurological examination, neuropsychology, electroencephalography and computed tomographic head scanning in active amateur boxers. *Journal of Neurology, Neurosurgery, and Psychiatry, 50,* 96–99.

Cantu, R. C. (1986). Guidelines for return to contact sports after a cerebral concussion. *Physician and Sportsmedicine, 14,* 75–83.

Cantu, R. C. (1991). Criteria for return to competition after a closed head injury. In J. S. Torg (Ed.), *Athletic injuries to the head, neck, and face* (pp. 323–330). St. Louis, MO: Mosby Year Book.

Casson, I. R., Siegel, O., Sham, R., Campbell, E. Q., Tarlau, M., & DiDomenico, A. (1984). Brain damage in modern boxers. *JAMA, 251,* 2663–2667.

Colorado Medical Society. (1991). *Report of the Sports Medicine Committee: Guidelines for the management of concussion in sports (revised).* Denver: Colorado Medical Society.

Corsellis, J. A. N., Bruton, C. J., & Freeman-Browne, D. (1973). The after-math of boxing. *Psychologie Medicale, 3,* 270–303.

Dikmen, S., McLean, A., & Temkin, N. (1986). Neuropsychological and psychological consequences of minor head injury. *Neurosurgery, 48*, 1227–1232.

Foster, J. B., Leiguarda, R., & Tilley, P. (1976). Brain damage in national hunt jockeys. *Lancet, i*, 981–983.

Gennarelli, T. A. (1987). Cerebral concussion and diffuse brain injuries. In P. R. Cooper (Ed.), *Head injury* (2nd ed., pp. 108–124). Baltimore, MD: Williams & Wilkins.

Gennarelli, T. A., Adams, J. H., & Graham, D. I. (1981). Acceleration induced head injury in the monkey: I. The model, its mechanical and physiological correlates. *Acta Neuropathologica (Berlin) (Suppl.), 1*, 23–25.

Gerberich, S. G., Priest, J. D., Boen, J. R., Staub, C. P., & Maxwell, R. E. (1983). Concussion incidences and severity in secondary school varsity football players. *American Journal of Public Health, 73*, 1370–1375.

Gibbs, N. (1993). Injuries in professional rugby league: A three year prospective study of the South Sydney Professional Rugby Football Club. *American Journal of Sports Medicine, 21*, 696–700.

Gronwall, D., & Wrightson, P. (1974). Delayed recovery of intellectual function after minor head injury. *Lancet, 2*, 604–609.

Gronwall, D., & Wrightson, P. (1975). Cumulative effect of concussion. *Lancet, 2*, 995–997.

Gronwall, D., & Wrightson, P. (1980). Duration of post-traumatic amnesia after mild head injury. *Journal of Clinical Neuropsychology, 2*, 51–60.

Haglund, Y., & Bergstrand, G. (1990). Does Swedish amateur boxing lead to chronic brain damage? 2. A retrospective study with CT and MRI. *Acta Neurologica Scandinavica, 82*, 297–302.

Haglund, Y., Edman, G., Murelius, O., Oreland, L., & Sachs, C. (1990). Does Swedish amateur boxing lead to chronic brain damage? 1. A retrospective medical, neurological, and personality trait study. *Acta Neurologica Scandinavica, 82*, 245–252.

Haglund, Y., & Eriksson, E. (1993). Does amateur boxing lead to chronic brain damage? A review of some recent investigations. *American Journal of Sports Medicine, 21*, 97–109.

Haglund, Y., & Persson, H. E. (1990). Does Swedish amateur boxing lead to chronic brain damage? 3. A retrospective clinical neuropsychological study. *Acta Neurologica Scandinavica, 82*, 353–360.

Hamilton, M. G., & Tranmer, B. I. (1993). Nervous system injuries in horseback-riding accidents. *Journal of Trauma, 34*, 227–232.

Harbaugh, R. E., & Saunders, R. L. (1984). The second impact in catastrophic contact-sports head trauma. *JAMA, 252*, 538–539.

Heilbronner, R. L., Henry, G. K., & Carson-Brewer, M. (1991). Neuropsychologic test performance in amateur boxers. *American Journal of Sports Medicine, 19*, 376–380.

Holburn, A. H. S. (1943). Mechanics of head injuries. *Lancet, 2*, 438–444.

Jane, J. A., Steward, O., & Gennarelli, T. (1985). Axonal degeneration induced by experimental noninvasive minor head injury. *Journal of Neurosurgery, 62*, 96–100.

Jedlinski, J., Gatarski, J., & Szymusik, A. (1970). Encephalopathica pugilistica (punch drunkenness). *Acta Medica Polana, 12*, 443–451.

Johnson, J. (1969). Organic psychosyndromes due to boxing. *British Journal of Psychiatry, 115*, 45–53.

Jordan, B. D. (1987). Neurologic aspects of boxing. *Archives of Neurology, 44*, 453–459.

Kelly, J. P., Nichols, J. S., Filley, C. M., Lillehei, K. O., Rubinstein, D., & Kleinschmidt-DeMasters, B. K. (1991). Concussion in sports: Guidelines for the prevention of catastrophic outcome. *JAMA, 226*, 2867–2869.

Kelly, J. P., & Rosenberg, J. H. (1997). The diagnosis and management of concussion in sports. *Neurology, 48*, 575–580.

Kraus, J. F., & Conroy, C. (1984). Mortality and morbidity from injuries in sports and recreations. *Annual Review of Public Health, 5*, 163–192.

Lampert, P. W., & Hardman, J. M. (1984). Morphological changes in brains of boxers. *JAMA*, *251*, 2676–2679.

Leininger, B. E., Gramling, S. E., Ferrel, A. D., Kreutzer, J. S., & Peck, E. A. (1990). Neuropsychological deficits in symptomatic minor head injury patients after concussion and mild concussion. *Journal of Neurology, Neurosurgery, and Psychiatry, 53*, 293–296.

Levin, H. S., Amparo, E. G., Eisenberg, H. M., Williams, D. H., High, W. M., McArdle, C. B., & Weiner, R. L. (1987). Magnetic resonance imaging and computerized tomography in relation to the neurobehavioral sequelae of mild and moderate head injuries. *Journal of Neurosurgery, 66*, 706–713.

Levin, H. S., Eisenberg, H. M., & Benton, A. L. (1989). *Mild head injury*. New York: Oxford University Press.

Levin, H. S., Lippold, S. C., Goldman, A., Handel, S., High, W. M., Jr., Eisenberg, H. M., & Zelitt, D. (1987). Neurobehavioral functioning and magnetic resonance imaging findings in young boxers. *Journal of Neurosurgery, 67*, 657–667.

Levin, H. S., Mattis, S., Ruff, R. M., Eisenberg, H. M., Marshall, L. F., & Tabaddor, K. (1987). Neurobehavioral outcome following minor head injury: A 3-center study. *Journal of Neurosurgery, 66*, 234–243.

Lezak, M. (1995). *Neuropsychological assessment* (3rd ed.). New York: Oxford Press.

Maroon, J. C., Steele, P. B., & Berlin, R. (1980). Football head and neck injuries—An update. *Clinical Neurosurgery, 27*, 414–429.

Martland, H. S. (1928). Punch-drunk. *JAMA, 19*, 1103–1107.

McCrea, M., Kelly, J. P., Kluge, J., Ackley, B., & Randolph, C. (1997). Standardized assessment of concussion in football players. *Neurology, 48*, 586–588.

McLatchie, G., Brooks, N., Galbraith, S., Hutchinson, J. S. F., Wilson, L., Melville, I., & Teasdale, E. (1987). Clinical neurological examination, neuropsychology, electroencephalography and computed tomographic head scanning in active amateur boxers. *Journal of Neurology, Neurosurgery, and Psychiatry, 50*, 96–99.

Mendez, M. F. (1995). The neuropsychiatric aspects of boxing. *International Journal of Psychiatry in Medicine, 25*, 249–262.

O'Brien, C. (1992). Retrospective survey of rugby injuries in the Leinster province of Ireland 1987–1989. *British Journal of Sports Medicine, 26*, 243–244.

Oppenheimer, R. D. (1968). Microscopic lesions in the brain following head injury. *Journal of Neurology, Neurosurgery, and Psychiatry, 31*, 299–306.

Pelletier, R. L., Montelpare, W. J., & Stark, R. M. (1993). Intercollegiate ice hockey injuries: A case for uniform definitions and reports. *American Journal of Sports Medicine, 21*, 78–81.

Polin, R. S., Alves, W. M., & Jane, J. A. (1996). Sports and head injuries. In R. W. Evans (Ed.), *Neurology and trauma* (pp. 166–185). Philadelphia: W. B. Saunders.

Povlishock, J. T., & Christman, C. W. (1995). The pathobiology of traumatically induced axonal injury in animals and humans: A review of current thoughts. *Journal of Neurotrauma, 12*, 555–564.

Practice Parameter: The management of concussion in sports [summary statement]. Report of the quality standard subcommittee. (1997). *Neurology, 48*, 581–585.

Rimel, R. W., Giordani, M. A., Barth, J. T., Boll, T. J., & Jane, J. A. (1981). Disability caused by minor head injury. *Neurosurgery, 9*, 221–228.

Roberts, A. H. (1969). *Brain damage in boxers. A study of the prevalence of traumatic encephalopathy among ex-professional boxers*. London: Pitman Medical and Scientific.

Ross, R. J., Casson, I. R., Siegel, O., & Cole, M. (1987). Boxing injuries: Neurologic, radiologic, and neuropsychologic evaluation. In J. S. Torg (Ed.), *Clinics in sports medicine: Head and neck injuries* (pp. 41–52). Philadelphia: W. B. Saunders.

Ruff, R. M., Crouch, J. A., Tröster, A. I., Marshall, L. F., Buchsbaum, M. S., Lottenberg, S., & Somers, L. M. (1994). Selected cases of poor outcome following a minor brain trauma:

Comparing neuropsychological and positron emission tomography assessment. *Brain Injury, 8,* 297–308.

Ruff, R. M., Camenzuli, L. F., & Mueller, J. (1996). Miserable minority: Emotional risk factors that influence the outcome of mild traumatic brain injury. *Brain Injury, 10,* 551–556.

Ruff, R. M., Levin, H. S., Mattis, S., High, W. M., Marshall, L. F., Eisenberg, H. M., & Tabaddor, K. (1989). Recovery of memory after mild head injury: a three center study. In H. S. Levin, H. M. Eisenberg, & A. L. Benton (Eds.), *Mild head injury* (pp. 176–188). New York: Oxford Press.

Ryan, A. J. (1987). Intracranial injuries resulting from boxing: A review (1918–1985). In J. S. Torg (Ed.), *Clinics in sports medicine: Head and neck injuries* (pp. 31–40). Philadelphia: W. B. Saunders.

Saunders, R. L., & Harbaugh, R. W. (1984). The second impact in catastrophic contact-sports head trauma. *JAMA, 252,* 538–539.

Schneider, R. C. (1973). *Head and neck injuries in football: Mechanisms, treatment, and prevention.* Baltimore, MD: Williams & Wilkins.

Serel, M., & Jaros, O. (1962). The mechanisms of cerebral concussion in boxing and their consequences. *World Neurology, 3,* 351–358.

Stewart, W. F., Gordon, B., Selnes, O., Bandeen-Roche, K., Zeger, S., Tusa, R. J., Celentano, D. D., Shechter, A., Liberman, J., Hall, C., Simon, D., Lesser, R., & Randall, R. D. (1994). Prospective study of central nervous system function in amateur boxers in the United States. *American Journal of Epidemiology, 139,* 573–588.

Symonds, C. (1962). Concussion and its sequelae. *Lancet, 1,* 1–5.

Tegner, Y., & Lorentzon, R. (1991). Ice hockey injuries: Incidence, nature, and causes. *British Journal of Sports Medicine, 25,* 87–89.

Thomassen, A., Juul-Jensen, P., Olivarius, B. D. F., Braemer, J., & Christensen, A. L. (1979). Neurological, electroencephalographic and neuropsychological examination of 53 former amateur boxers. *Acta Neurologica Scandinavica, 60,* 352–362.

Torg, J. S., Beer, L. A., & Vesgo, J. (1980). Head trauma in football players with infectious mononucleosis. *Physician and Sportsmedicine, 8,* 107–110.

Tysvaer, A. T. (1992). Head and neck injuries in soccer: Impact of minor trauma. *Sports Medicine, 14,* 200–213.

Tysvaer, A. T., & Einar, A. L. (1991). Soccer injuries to the brain: a neuropsychologic study of former soccer players. *American Journal of Sports Medicine, 19,* 56–60.

Tysvaer, A. T., Storli, O. V., & Bachen, N. I. (1989). Soccer injuries to the brain. A neurologic and electroencephalographic study of former players. *Acta Neurologica Scandinavica, 80,* 151–156.

Unterharnscheidt, F. J. (1972). Head injury after boxing. *Scandinavian Journal of Rehabilitation Medicine, 4,* 77–84.

Varney, N. R., & Varney, R. N. (1995). Brain injury without head injury. Some physics of automobile collisions with particular reference to brain injuries occurring without physical head trauma. *Applied Neuropsychology, 2,* 47–62.

Witol, A. (1995, August). *Neuropsychological deficits associated with differing exposure to heading and experience in soccer.* Paper presented at the American Psychological Association Annual Convention, Washington, DC.

Wrightson, P., & Gronwall, D. (1980). Duration of post-traumatic amnesia after mild head injury. *Journal of Clinical Neuropsychology, 1,* 51–60.

Yarnell, P. R., & Lynch, S. (1973). The "ding": Amnestic states in football trauma. *Neurology, 23,* 196–197.

Zemper, E. D. (1989). Injury rates in a national sample of college football teams: A two year prospective study. *Physician and Sportsmedicine, 17,* 100–113.

7

Discipline-Specific Approach Versus Individual Care

Ronald M. Ruff
University of California, San Francisco

The following nine chapters of this volume address how diverse disciplines evaluate mild traumatic brain injury (MTBI). The range includes the physical perspective (electophysiological correlates, epilepsy, orbitofrontal syndrome), cognitive aspects (executive dysfunctioning, tests of malingering), and the emotional domain (mood disorders). Given this discipline-specific approach to evaluating MTBI, the aim of the present chapter is to explore how such discipline-specific approaches are anchored to a host of implicit assumptions about how we gain clinical knowledge.

The study of knowledge or knowing (epistemology) has historically been rooted in the longstanding controversy between the philosophies of rationalism and empiricism (Gardner, 1985; Mahoney, 1991). Indeed, the field of science is directly aligned with empiricism, adhering to the thesis that all knowing essentially emanates from the gradual process of induction through observation. Thus, the scientific study of MTBI is based on the process of discovering and internalizing the facts as they emerge from experiments and careful observations. Knowledge is declared valid by the verifiable observations. Let us examine the built-in limitations of the assumptions that underlie the empirical approach. The reason for this examination is based on the notion that diagnosticians and therapists should gain an understanding for the multiple underlying implicit assumptions that make up their knowledge base.

DISCIPLINE-SPECIFIC APPROACH

Discipline-Specific Schemas

Clinicians examining MTBI patients are basically trained as scientists, and thus as empiricists their knowledge is based on specific observations. However, the key point is to recognize that these observations are typically embedded in discipline-specific schemas. In the evaluation of MTBI, it is not a stretch to claim that individuals trained in specific disciplines will use the schemas that they mastered within their disciplines. These schemas in general serve specific functions: they (a) facilitate recognition, recall, and comprehension; (b) influence speed of information processing and problem solving; (c) gather information into meaningful and more easily retrieved units; (d) enable the individual to fill in missing information; and (e) provide greater confidence in prediction and decision making (Winfrey & Goldfried, 1986). Thus, when a patient is observed by a clinician, specific schemas are in place, and information that is schema congruent is processed more quickly and is viewed as more relevant. Indeed, it is the skill of a specialized diagnostician to attend with a high degree of acuity to discipline-specific symptom complexes, while ignoring those outside of the boundaries of the discipline, in order to achieve discipline-specific diagnoses.

A neurosurgeon who is highly trained to assist TBI patients with survival will view a patient with MTBI in terms of a neurosurgical schema, which includes decisions on whether or not surgery is required and whether neuroimaging indicates further follow-up. The diagnostic classification schema of the Glasgow Coma Scale (GCS; Teasdale & Jennett, 1974), which evaluates TBI based on a severity scale, has served the international neurosurgical community well, and is applied on a daily basis. However, if your focus on differentiating the symptom complex of MTBI is psychiatry, then the GCS provides an insufficient categorization schema. Thus, psychiatrists have developed their own classification schema for MTBI that describes a postconcussional disorder in the *DSM–IV*. This diagnostic framework incorporates the schemas of psychiatrists, who are typically not part of the initial evaluation in the emergency room. Instead, patients are as a rule referred on an outpatient basis, and therefore the *DSM–IV* classification is only to be applied to MTBI patients whose symptoms have persisted for at least 3 months. Thus, the GCS and the *DSM–IV* schemas are like night and day for a neuropsychologist who sees patients at the acute and postacute phases. Neither of the schemas are of much use for a longitudinal classification of MTBI over these critical time points.

In addition to the different focus across time, the thinking in specific disciplines can also lead to a "bias" of establishing one's own discipline in the center. For example, for a neurosurgeon (see Fig. 7.1), the physical symptoms make up the core symptomatology, and all other symptoms are relegated to the periphery. However, a clinical psychologist or psychiatrist will replace the physical symptoms in Fig. 7.1 with the emotional symptoms, because feelings are viewed by these disciplines as essential for health. As a cognitive psychologist and neuropsychologist, I have my bias of placing cognition in the center. After all, this is based on a rich philosophical tradition dating back to René Descartes' statement, "I think, therefore I am." A further argument that could place cognition in the center is that it is cognition that separates humans from lower species because, for example, bears' or lions' bodies are at least as sophisticated as human bodies. The key difference is the brain, and there is no doubt that the brain's key output is cognition. I don't want to elaborate on these biases any further, other than to demonstrate by example that all clinicians have a tendency to place their discipline in the center of their universe. This viewpoint does in turn determine both discipline-specific research and clinical experience. No doubt these biased schemas play a role in how MTBI patients are diagnosed by the different disciplines.

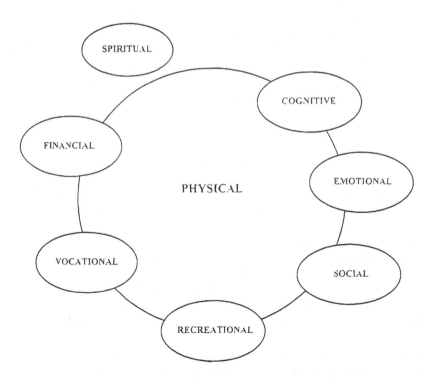

FIG. 7.1. Diagnostic approach to MTBI: medical model.

Lack of Integration

Disciplines have evolved in a more or less arbitrary fashion. No doubt, there are reasonable historical reasons for training health care professionals in the disciplines of psychiatry, psychology, neurology, and neurosurgery. However, no conceptual model exists by which these disciplines can integrate their knowledge base. As a rule, a specific language or jargon within the discipline evolves, which further distinguishes (or separates) the disciplines. Indeed, it is ironic that we expect brain-injured patients to integrate the information from the various disciplines when we as professionals are unable to integrate ourselves in a unified fashion for the patient's sake. Thus, MTBI is viewed differently by neurosurgeons, psychiatrists, and neuropsychologists, in large part due to different schemas, which are influenced by discipline specific research and observations. It is naive to assume that the observations from different disciplines will fall together like pieces into a puzzle without an a priori conceptual model. Philosophers of science have pointed out the pitfalls of this atomistic assumption for centuries. Among the analogies used, the question is posed, what would happen if you placed strings of wool on a floor? Would you expect to come back the next day and find a rug? Similarly, two-dimensional strings of data within a discipline will not weave themselves into a three-dimensional reality of a patient's life without a conceptual integration. Given this insight from philosophy of science, the limits of side-by-side data collections that fill our journals each year become evident.

Clinician-Specific Biases

In addition to the already mentioned biases derived from schemas of our discipline, clinicians evaluate MTBI patients from their unique viewpoints. Some clinicians view themselves as rescuers, wanting to assist and help the victims of MTBI, versus other clinicians who view themselves as skeptics or detectives who are critically searching for the "real truth." I have also found that certain clinicians, particularly surgeons, are used to making decisions, and sooner or later they want to reach the bottom line, versus others who see themselves as explorers and who enjoy raising more and more questions as they turn each corner in the diagnostic exploration. Litigation can also cast clinicians in the role of the plaintiff. Then, of course, there are those "humble" clinicians who assert that they "go down the middle," insinuating that they do not have a bias. This "objective" viewpoint can be dangerous—because their biases are likely to go unrecognized. However, these individuals cannot escape being in a role, even if they are, for example, consistently attempting to place their opinion in the middle of the road. In short, it is safe to say that we all have our biases, and it is time that all scientists/clinicians explore both their discipline-specific and their uniquely personal biases.

INDIVIDUAL CARE

So far, I have emphasized that each scientist/clinician must become aware of his or her framework for the evaluation. The time has also come for us to go beyond listing the various deficits within our disciplines. In addition, we must search for conceptual models by which we can integrate the symptom complex. In the remaining portions of this chapter, a conceptual model is proposed for integrating the multiple layers of MTBI symptoms.

Constructivist Approach

The constructivist approach will serve as the philosophy of science for the proposed integration. Although empirical research remains an important dimension for understanding MTBI, the notion that the scientific method is the only correct source of true knowledge (i.e., scientific positivism) is rejected. As mentioned earlier, the atomistic assumption (i.e., scientific facts will fall automatically into place) is also rejected. Thus, the following issue remains: What underlying assumption can we make that will enhance our clinical knowledge base of MTBI?

The constructivist's approach assumes that realities are basically a dynamic human invention. As opposed to empiricism, which views reality as a single stable and knowledgeable category, constructivism views knowing as inherently flawed. Thus, the constructivist's perspective recognizes that all knowledge is potentially fallible, and thus revisions and modifications are best viewed in terms of its present viability. The constructivists' meta-theory reflects a number of overlapping theoretical frameworks, which include the formative influence by Piaget (1954, 1970), the contemporary theory of self-organization (Mahoney, 1991), and the study of evolving knowledge by Popper (1972) and Campbell (1974). In summary, this approach provides the freedom to postulate a viable construct that can be used as a system to explain the phenomena observed and reported by our MTBI patients.

Patient-Specific Approach

I propose that the underlying framework for evaluating a patient with MTBI should focus on the patient's symptoms and symptom interactions. Thus, our discipline-specific diagnostic schemas should be subordinated so that we are not trapped in reductionism. It is essential that cross-disciplinary interactions are explored as they relate to the viability of our patients' symptom presentations. Using a constructivist's framework, the physical domain as well as the emotional and cognitive domains are viewed as different ways of knowing, and each of the different ways of knowing are inherently just as valuable to an individual as any other. Moreover, the clinician no longer accepts the underlying assumptions that perpetuate fragmentation, because the effectiveness of a clinician is proportionate to the ability to sort through the complexity of the symptoms presented by each patient. In short, the proposed viewpoint for achieving this integration is as follows: Let us focus on the patient and the patient's symptoms and symptom interactions, and let us subordinate the discipline-specific diagnostic schemas. To achieve this individually based care, the following model is proposed (Fig. 7.2).

In this model, the emotional, cognitive, and physical domains overlap and are of equivalent significance for the intrapersonal dynamic. This intrapersonal dynamic, however, is interactive within a social and recrea-

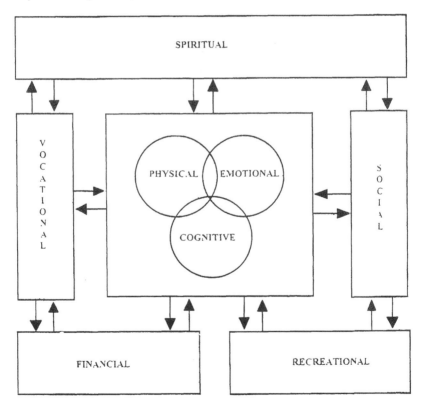

FIG. 7.2. Individual care model.

tional network, which is also dependent on vocational and financial components. A meaning in life, or a spiritual direction, rounds out the picture. If, for example, an accident results in loss of employment, this can in turn affect the finances, which can affect the recreational outlet or social life, which can in turn negatively influence the emotional well-being of the individual. In another example, when an individual's concussion results primarily in emotional lability and depression, this leads to a lack of initiation for social interactions, which in turn reduces the patient's confidence and desire to return to work. These types of dysfunctional loops, as described by Kay, Newman, Cavallo, Ezrachi, and Resnick (1992), can lead to poor functional outcome tied to a variety of interactions.

The model proposed above is not claimed to be the Truth, but rather a schema or construct that allows clinicians to evaluate the interactions among different factors that can influence the outcome following a mild TBI. This approach does not negate or replace the discipline-specific measures; however, it perpetuates the attitude that information outside of one's own discipline is not relegated to "noise." Thus, an integration is constructed between parallel static measures, and these interactions are best served if the interactions are based on the patient's symptoms and perceived problems caused by the trauma. Let us now explore how our schemas for classifying a concussion could be integrated.

Searching for a Transdisciplinary Definition

As alluded to earlier, neurosurgeons typically use the schema of the GCS to define MTBI. This tool is particularly useful in the early stages (Jennett & Teasdale, 1981). The GCS scale allows for a classification between severe, moderate, and mild head injuries along a scale ranging from 3 to 15. Mild TBI is classified by scores 13 to 15, and the three target behaviors that are rated are eye opening, motor response, and verbal response. If the GCS is administered on the patient's admission to the emergency room and the score is 15, this does not exclude the possibility that the patient was nonresponsive at the scene of the accident. Thus, this scale by itself does not capture the presence or absence of an MTBI. It does not reflect the retroactive status of a patient at the scene, but rather describes the status at the time of administration.

To my knowledge, neurologists have not come up with a uniformly recognized definition. However, the psychiatrists in the *DSM–IV* have proposed a definition for postconcussional disorder, although they have neglected to introduce a definition that would classify severe, moderate, and mild brain trauma. Instead, the *DSM–IV* definition implicitly establishes a rather conservative definition for MTBI. Although the *DSM–IV* does state that the definition needs to be further refined by research, the criteria that have been suggested include (a) a period of unconsciousness lasting more than 5 min, (b) a period of posttraumatic amnesia that lasts more than 12 hr subsequent to the closed head injury, and (c) a new onset of seizures or marked worsening of preexisting seizure disorder that occurs within the first 6 months. A further criterion is that on neuropsychological testing, difficulties in attention and memory must be demonstrated. The definition also includes that three or more symptoms persist for at least 3 months, and these include becoming fatigued easily, disordered sleep, headache, vertigo or dizziness, irritability or aggression on little or no provocation, anxiety, depression, or affective lability, changes in personality (e.g., social or sexual inappropriateness), apathy, or lack of spontaneity.

A third definition that has been established by the American Congress of Rehabilitation Medicine (ACRM, 1993) delineates the following four inclusion criteria, of which at least one must be manifested: (a) any period of loss of consciousness; (b) any loss of memory for events immediately before or after the accident; (c) any alteration of mental state at the time of accident (e.g., feeling dazed, disoriented, or confused); and (d) focal neurological deficit(s) that may or may not be transient. The following three exclusion criteria are delineated: (a) loss of consciousness exceeding approximately 30 min; (b) after 30 min the GCS falling below 13; and (c) posttraumatic amnesia (PTA) persisting longer than 24 hr. The marked differences between the latter two definitions are highlighted in Table 7.1.

Our patients are simply ill served by the application of these discrepant definitions. The time has come to establish MTBI as a uniform construct. Because one of the hallmark features of TBI in general is that the severity can range significantly, it is important that we become fine tuned to the differences in severity. For example, within the population of severe TBI patients, defined by a GCS score ranging between 3 and 8, the Traumatic Coma Data Bank demonstrated that patients with GCS scores in the lower ranges (3 and 4) have a much poorer outcome than patients with a GCS between 7 and 8 (Marshall et al., 1991). However, within the mild TBI

TABLE 7.1
Comparison of Definitions of MTBI

	ACRM	DSM–IV
LOC	Any period of alteration in mental state	>5 min LOC
PTA	Any loss of memory for events before and after the event	>12 hr
Neurological deficits	Focal (no time parameters)	Three or more that persist for at least 3 months

TABLE 7.2
Classifications for MTBI

	Type I	Type II	Type III
LOC	Altered state or transient loss	Definite loss with time unknown or <5 min	Loss 5–30 min
PTA	1–60 sec	60 sec–12 hr	>12 hr
Neurological symptoms	One or more	One or more	One or more

population defined by a GCS score of 13 to 15, no similar differences have emerged between the patients with a score of 13, 14, or 15 (Kraus & Nourjah, 1989). Indeed, it is my impression that the GCS scores of 13, 14, and 15 are not sufficiently sensitive to establish a transdisciplinary classification system for MTBI. Thus, I propose a subclassification, which is shown in Table 7.2, that incorporates the ACRM definition as well as the implicit *DSM–IV* definition as a continuum rather than two parallel definitions of MTBI.

Type I falls in line with the lowest entry criteria as established by ACRM, and Type III basically is aligned with the *DSM–IV* classification. Type II bridges the two discrepant definitions. These three proposed subtypes are presently being evaluated in an ongoing research protocol to establish whether the symptom presentation varies among the three types of severity within MTBI. Based on our experience, we have found that classification according to the number of neurological symptoms is rather unwieldy. We have therefore changed the number of neurological symptoms to one or more, even for Type III, which in this respect deviates from the *DSM–IV* definition. The hallmark features for the distinction among the three types are loss of consciousness (LOC) and posttraumatic amnesia (PTA). If any of the two criteria of LOC and PTA for Type I are met, then this classification is made. For Type III, criteria for both LOC and PTA have to be met, and all ratings that fall between the two are classified as Type II.

Let us now identify the underlying assumptions that are part of this classification schema. It is essential that when classifying TBI, we separate the severity of the brain trauma from the severity of the posttraumatic symptoms that follow. Thus, the symptom complex 3 months following the concussion should not define the severity of the MTBI. In Table 7.2, we are attempting to define the initial organic deficit (i.e., concussion), and in a later section we discuss a model for defining the postconcussional symptoms. The information that we typically use for the proposed classification is comprised of (a) a review of the medical records, (b) a clinical interview, and (c) the administration of the Galveston Orientation and

Amnesia Test, which retrospectively estimates both LOC and PTA (Levin, Benton, & Grossman, 1982).

Evaluating Outcome

Since my involvement in the three-center study (Levin et al., 1987), it has become evident that not all individuals with a single uncomplicated mild TBI have a poor outcome. Indeed, it has been estimated that approximately 80%–90% of all MTBI patients enjoy a favorable recovery (Kay et al., 1992; Wong, Regennitter, & Barrios, 1994). Thus, in the future a method needs to be developed by which the clinicians can predict the 10%–20% of the MTBI population who will have a poor outcome (i.e., the Miserable Minority).

In establishing a division between those who have a favorable outcome and the Miserable Minority, it is essential that we construct a schema and measurement for "poor outcome." To achieve such a division, there is a tendency for physicians to select physical outcome variables in much the same way that neuropsychologists select neurocognitive outcome variables, and so on. Again, it is my suggestion that we avoid such discipline-specific conceptualizations of outcome. Instead, outcome needs to be viewed as a construct that incorporates multiple aspects, and we must become aware of how the selection of variables is dependent upon the concept (see Fig. 7.3).

To date, no generally accepted outcome measure for MTBI has emerged. However, if such an outcome measure could identify the Miserable Minority, the task still lies before us to determine the extent to which the problems reported subsequent to the injury are (a) neurogenic, (b) psychogenic, (c) due to comorbid medical complications (i.e., neck injury, vestibular problems, etc.), (d) financial gain, or (e) premorbid factors. Thus, much future work is called for. In the interim, the term *postconcussional disorder* is applied, although pitfalls can be expected with this classification.

Postconcussional Disorders

After an MTBI has been diagnosed, the term *postconcussional disorder* refers to acquired physical, emotional, and cognitive symptoms that occur as the direct consequence of the cerebral concussion (Alves, Colohan, O'Leary, Rimel, & Jane, 1986). Indeed, to render this diagnosis it makes sense that at least 3 months has passed since the trauma. Even after 3 months, some

(Premorbid) (Severity of TBI) (Comorbid) (Treatment) (Selection of Variables)

_____

Concept

FIG. 7.3. Components of outcome.

improvement due to spontaneous recovery is possible. However, if the postconcussional disorders persist after 12 months, then it may become useful for us to use the term *prolonged postconcussional disorder* because, as mentioned earlier, only a small portion of the MTBI patients present with a postconcussional disorder 1 year postinjury. Even though it is only a small portion, one needs to remember that of all the TBI patients, mild brain traumas are by far the most common. Epidemiological evidence suggests that each year in the United States alone over 1,300,000 individuals sustain an MTBI (Kay et al., 1992). Thus, if even a small portion (10%–20%) present with persistent problems, between 130,000 and 260,000 individuals fall into the category of Miserable Minority each year in the United States.

Let us identify the key symptoms that most frequently follow MTBI. Note that the subsequent list is not exhaustive. The most common physical symptoms associated with a postconcussional disorder include headache, fatigue, disordered sleep, vertigo, and dizziness. Less common residua include nausea, numbness, visual problems (e.g., diplopia), hearing problems (e.g., tinnitus, hyperacusis), seizure disorder, and alcohol intolerance. Typical emotional residua include irritability (aggression on little or no provocation), anxiety, depression, and affective lability; somewhat less frequently, symptoms include personality changes (social inappropriateness), and apathy or lack of spontaneity. The most pronounced cognitive impairments include difficulties with attention (concentration, shifting focus of attention, performing simultaneous cognitive tasks) and memory (learning or recalling information); less frequently observed declines can also occur in the executive functions (problem solving, avoiding perseverations) and a general slowing in information processing. There are two particularly difficult issues that face the clinician when diagnosing postconcussional disorder: (a) differentiating among the potential contributors that can compound the symptom presentation, and (b) determining the interactions among the symptoms.

Determining the Contributing Causes

In Table 7.3, the potential causes for postconcussional syndrome are grouped into three categories separated by a timeline. We have found this separation to be clinically useful in gathering the pertinent information. Estimating preexisting or premorbid risk factors is essential in order to relate the present functioning levels to the estimated preexisting functioning levels. Only this relative comparison allows one to answer the key question: Is there a decline in functioning between the estimated premorbid levels and the present levels? Among the physical risk factors, one needs to ascertain the family medical history, rule out genetically transmitted deficits or conditions, and evaluate the developmental milestones. One also

TABLE 7.3
Contributing Causes for Postconcussional Syndrome

Preinjury	TBI	Postinjury
Risk factors	Brain-based change	Recovery
Physical	Non-brain-based injuries	Decompensation
Emotional	Facial or head injuries	Persistent symptoms
Cognitive	Whiplash injury	
Social	Bodily pain	
Vocational		
Financial		
Spiritual		

needs to rule out preexisting neurological illnesses, including prior MTBIs or major illnesses, and treatments that may have had an impact on cerebral functions. From an emotional perspective, it is important to determine preexisting psychiatric illnesses, and one should also evaluate whether the patient had a particularly vulnerable personality style in order to determine how the clinician would have expected this individual to react to the TBI. From a cognitive perspective, one should assess the preexisting strengths and weaknesses and evaluate premorbid history of serious alcohol or substance abuse, or any other medical illnesses that could have compromised cognitive functioning. Degree of educational influence and opportunity should be established. From a psychosocial perspective, it is essential to appraise the family structure, their ability to cope with crisis situations, the role assigned to specific family members, and how the family members resolve the psychosocial conflicts. Vocational and financial issues need to be explored, and the importance that the patient assigned to work or vocational status must be ascertained (were the patient's work habits erratic or inconsistent, was the patient a workaholic, etc.). With respect to the financial situation, it is essential to assess whether the patient was living with an unreasonable debt or close to the edge without financial buffers. For a more comprehensive review of estimating premorbid functioning, see Ruff, Mueller, & Jurica (1996).

In addition to evaluating the severity of the cerebral concussion with a variety of tools such as neuroimaging, neuropsychological testing, clinical interview, and so on, it is essential to evaluate comorbid factors such as whiplash injuries, vestibular injuries, and other orthopedic injuries that can result in chronic pain. These comorbid factors can have a significant impact on emotional, psychosocial, vocational, and financial functioning. The challenge is to determine the degree to which these nonorganic injuries contribute to the symptomatology.

With respect to the postinjury residuals that persist, it is important to delineate the extent to which the patient has suffered from specific deficits versus disabilities that affect day-to-day functioning. A certain amount of improvement is expected to occur within the first 3 months. However, if symptoms persist or decompensate after 3 to 6 months, contributing etiologies other than the concussion need to be explored.

Determining the Interactions Among Symptoms

In most TBI patients, there are a number of difficulties or disorders that can cluster in an overlapping fashion; however, as a rule there are unique features to each patient's presentation. Moreover, it is essential that the clinician be open to new combinations of interactions. The message of this chapter is that a model needs to be constructed to sort through these interactions. According to the model (Fig. 7.2), a convergence can be clinically explored with the focus on multiple levels of interactions between the MTBI patient and his or her environment. The goal of this model is to bridge the gap between isolated observations. Thus, discipline-specific schemas can still be applied; however, I believe it is the role of the treating clinician to also look at the overall picture, the gestalt, to establish a conceptual cohesion even if it is hypothetical or an interpretation. This integration has to be viewed across time periods, as well, by estimating the types of interactions that existed before the accident and what changed interactions are taking place subsequent to the MTBI.

For example, we have encountered a patient who, after a mild TBI in a skiing accident, suffered from a catastrophic reaction. In our exploration of her premorbid issues, we uncovered that in her childhood she had been physically and verbally abused by an alcoholic mother, who also minimized her complaints to such an extent that she was rarely treated even for serious illnesses such as pneumonia. Thus, in order to be heard by the clinician even years later with respect to her symptoms of MTBI, she presented with seizure-type episodes. With electroencephalographic (EEG) telemetry in place during these episodes, it was verified that these episodes were not epileptiform in nature. It appeared instead that these episodes were elicited by a feeling of helplessness. This example illustrates the richness with which certain premorbid issues can interact with an MTBI. This case and other examples that explore the interactions that can occur in the Miserable Minority have been described elsewhere (Ruff, Camenzuli, & Mueller, 1996).

Integration of Therapies

In reviewing the literature on MTBI, it is my impression that far more energy is spent on the diagnostic differentiation with relatively little emphasis placed on interventions. Obviously, a good diagnostic workup is critical for planning a therapeutic regimen. However, some of the interactions that evolve over time between the symptom complexes can best be understood if the clinician has the opportunity to see the patient over a prolonged period of time. Obviously we need to be aware of the cost–benefit ratio, and it is essential that early and appropriate interventions are provided for those patients that fall in the category of Miserable Minority. It is for this Miserable Minority that I recommend an analysis of interactions among pre- and comorbid factors in order to determine whether permanent brain damage can be diagnosed with a reasonable degree of certainty. As a clinician, I have found it helpful to list the problems and then explore the various interactions. Thereafter, the patient together with the therapist sets priorities for which interactions and problems can best be addressed with what type of treatment. Finally, our treatments need to be selectively targeted with an eye on avoiding iatrogenic problems.

REFERENCES

Alves, W. M., Colohan, A. R. L., O'Leary, T. J., Rimel, R. W., & Jane, J. A. (1986). Understanding posttraumatic symptoms after minor head injury. *Journal of Head Trauma Rehabilitation, 1*, 1–12.

American Congress of Rehabilitation Medicine. (1993). Definition of mild traumatic brain injury. *Journal of Head Trauma Rehabilitation, 8*(3), 86–87.

Campbell, D. T. (1974). Evolutionary epistemology. In P. A. Schilpp (Ed.), *The philosophy of Karl Popper* (Vol. 14 [I and II], pp. 416–463). LaSalle, IL: Open Court.

Gardner, H. (1985). *The mind's new science: A history of the cognitive revolution.* New York: Basic Books.

Jennett, B., & Teasdale, G. (1981). *Management of head injuries.* Philadelphia: F. A. Davis.

Kay, T., Newman, B., Cavallo, M., Ezrachi, O., & Resnick, M. (1992). Toward a neuropsychological model of functional disability after mild traumatic brain injury. *Neuropsychology, 6*, 371–384.

Kraus, J. F., & Nourjah, P. (1989). The epidemiology of mild head injury. In H. S. Levin, H. M. Eisenberg, & A. Benton (Eds.), *Mild head injury* (pp. 8–22). New York: Oxford University Press.

Levin, H., Benton, A. L., & Grossman, R. G. (1982). *Neurobehavioral consequences of closed head injury.* New York: Oxford University Press.

Levin, H., Mattis, S., Ruff, R. M., Eisenberg, H. M., Marshall, L. F., Tabaddor, K., High, W. M., & Frankowski, R. F. (1987). Neurobehavioral outcome following minor head injury: A three-center study. *Journal of Neurosurgery, 66*, 234–243.

Mahoney, M. J. (1991). *Human change processes.* New York: Basic Books.

Marshall, L. F., Gautille, T., Klauber, M. R., Eisenberg, H. M., Jane, J. A., & Luerssen, T. G. (1991). The outcome of severe closed head injury. *Journal of Neurosurgery, 75*, S28–S36.

Piaget, J. (1954). *The construction of reality in the child.* New York: Basic Books.

Piaget, J. (1970). *Psychology and epistemology: Toward a theory of knowledge.* New York: Viking.

Popper, K. R. (1972). *Objective knowledge: An evolutionary approach.* London: Oxford University Press.

Ruff, R. M., Camenzuli, L. F., & Mueller, J. (1996). Miserable Minority: Emotional risk factors that influence the outcome of a mild traumatic brain injury. *Brain Injury, 10*, 551–565.

Ruff, R. M., Mueller, J., & Jurica, P. (1996). Estimation of premorbid functioning after traumatic brain injury. *NeuroRehabilitation, 7,* 39–53.

Teasdale, G., & Jennett, B. (1974). Assessment of coma and impaired consciousness: A practical scale. *Lancet, 2,* 81–84.

Winfrey, L. P. L., & Goldfried, M. R. (1986). Information processing and the human change process. In R. E. Ingram (Ed.), *Information processing approaches to clinical psychology* (pp. 241–258). New York: Academic Press.

Wong, J. L., Regennitter, R. P., & Barrios, F. (1994). Base rate and simulated symptoms of mild head injury among normals. *Archives of Clinical Neuropsychology, 9,* 441–426.

8

Posttraumatic Anosmia
and Orbital Frontal Injury

Nils R. Varney
Veterans' Administration Medical Center, Iowa City, Iowa

Damage to orbital frontal cortex is common following traumatic brain injury (TBI) and is, therefore, of particular concern in the evaluation of TBI patients. The mechanism of injury typically involves abrasions, lacerations, and contusions to tissue on the inferior aspect of the frontal lobes as a result of contact with the cribriform plate (cf. Gurdjan & Gurdjan, 1976; Jennette & Teasdale, 1981). This rough bony structure, which supports the frontal lobes, has irreverently been referred to as "the dashboard of the brain." Injury to orbital frontal cortex may have impact on executive functioning, psychosocial competency, ability to maintain employment, and reliable conduct of adult activities in daily living (Damasio, 1979; Lezak, 1978; Martzke, Swan, & Varney, 1991; Stuss & Benson, 1984; Stuss & Gow, 1992; Varney & Menefee, 1993). Thus, the patient with orbital frontal damage, despite having a "mild" head injury (at least from an emergency room perspective), may nevertheless have a catastrophic outcome with very disagreeable life-altering consequences.

One problem presented by the "typical" patient with orbital frontal damage is that despite marked personality changes, mental inertia, loss of initiative, loss of psychosocial competencies, and related problems, such patients may nevertheless perform well on standard psychological tests (cf. Brown, 1984; Damasio, 1979). A second problem is that posttraumatic orbital frontal damage can be difficult to demonstrate with structural neuroimaging technologies, computerized tomography (CT) and magnetic resonance imaging (MRI) in particular (cf. Newberg & Alavi,

1996). Thus, the patient with orbital frontal damage may simultaneously show normal IQ, memory, and language, as well as normal CT, MRI, and electroencephalograph (EEG), while nevertheless having life-altering, disabling psychosocial symptoms that impair his or her ability to meet the demands of adult life.

The attention being paid to posttraumatic anosmia in this chapter reflects more than interest in a simple sensory function. Rather, posttraumatic anosmia can be an indication of damage to orbital frontal cortex and as such is also of value in drawing inferences or raising questions about a head injured patient's neuropsychological well-being and long-term vocational status (cf. Varney & Bushnell, 1998). As shown in this chapter, posttraumatic anosmia is a reasonably reliable means for identifying patients (a) who have orbital frontal damage, (b) who are at high risk for a characteristic constellation of symptoms (i.e., "an orbital frontal syndrome"), and (c) who have vocational limitations or disabilities not readily apparent in the immediate postacute recovery phase.

MECHANISMS AND ASSESSMENT OF ANOSMIA

Because the olfactory nerves (the first cranial nerves) are located on the inferior aspect of the frontal lobes, damage to the olfactory nerves is an occasional correlate of closed head injury, even minor head injury without loss of consciousness (LOC) or posttraumatic amnesia (PTA), as is noted, among other places, in the AMA *Guides for the Determination of Disability* (American Medical Association, 1993) and *DSM-IV* (APA, 1994). In particular, the coup–contrecoup movement of the brain over the cribriform plate makes these fragile structures vulnerable to damage, particularly when the blow is to the posterior aspect of the skull (cf. Sumner, 1976; Zusho, 1982).

With injury to the olfactory nerves by abrasion, contusion, or laceration, the affected patient may develop total anosmia, partial anosmia, or parosmia. In total anosmia, the patient is unable to identify common odors of any type and also suffers a severe diminution in sense of taste (ageusia). All patients with true posttraumatic anosmia have ageusia. Indeed, many will be far more aware of their diminished sense of taste than their loss of sense of smell (cf. Sumner, 1976; Varney, 1988).

Partial anosmia can often take the form of the patient losing sense of smell in one nostril (in association with diminished sense of taste). Keep in mind with such cases that the olfactory nerves do not decussate, so that damage to the left olfactory nerve will cause a left-sided anosmia, and a left-sided anosmia would indicate damage to the left olfactory nerve. Obviously, another type of partial anosmia would involve bilateral diminution of sense of smell, once again with loss of sense of taste. With parosmia, sense of smell is distorted such that normal odors and flavors take on highly disagreeable qualities (e.g., coffee tasting like urine). Please note that any injury to the olfactory nerve will cause losses in both sense of taste and smell. Other types of injury to or obstruction of olfactory apparatus (e.g., a head cold, a broken nose) could leave the patient with a nearly normal sense of taste and would not count as a true posttraumatic anosmia. Also note that it is important not to use stimuli such as formaldehyde, ether, ammonia, odors suspended in alcohol (e.g., artificial vanilla), or other fifth nerve irritants. These can be felt in the nasal passages and thus may give the impression of being smelled.

It is important to note that anosmia can occur for many reasons and that it is particularly important to insure that the patient under examination has not experienced very high fevers (over 40°C), exposure to toxic chemicals, hypoxia, and related events.

THE NEUROPATHOLOGICAL SIGNIFICANCE OF ANOSMIA

Autopsy studies dating back to the 19th century have indicated that posttraumatic anosmia is very often associated with damage to orbital frontal cortex, even in cases with apparently mild head trauma (Sumner, 1976). However, four studies concerned with neuropsychological outcome measures in anosmic TBI patients have involved very few subjects with abnormal CT or MRI findings (at least among those with mildly to moderately severe head injuries) (Martzke et al., 1991; Varney, 1989; Varney & Bushnell, 1998; Varney & Menefee, 1993). That CT and MRI are so frequently unremarkable in patients with posttraumatic anosmia is not unexpected because (a) autopsy study had indicated that the injury to orbital frontal cortex typically involved contusions, lacerations, and abrasions—injuries not readily apparent with CT or MRI—and (b) the bony irregularities in the orbital frontal area and resultant artifact make the imaging of all but very substantial lesions very difficult (cf. Newberg & Alavi, 1996).

It has recently been established that neuroSPECT scanning with Te-99m-HMPAO can reveal central nervous system (CNS) injuries/functional abnormalities that are not readily apparent on CT or MRI (Goldenberg, Oder, Spatt, & Podereka, 1992; Gray et al., 1992; Newton et al., 1992; Varney et al., 1995; Varney & Bushnell, in press). It has also been shown that patients who have suffered apparently minor head injuries with disabling neuropsychological deficits may also show neuroSPECT abnormalities in anterior mesial temporal (Varney et al., 1995) and anterior orbital frontal regions (Varney & Bushnell, 1998). The damage demonstrated in such patients typically involved hypometabolism (vs. no CNS activity at all) in the affected regions. Closely similar findings have been obtained from quantitative PET studies (cf. Anosmia and Functional Neuroimaging section of this chapter for details). Thus, the neuropsychological deficits shown by these patients were the result of reduced CNS activity (vs. a three-dimensional "dead zone") in areas at high risk for injury in TBI.

ANOSMIA AND TESTS OF EXECUTIVE FUNCTIONING

There have been many studies on "frontal lobe damage" and neuropsychological testing (cf. Brown, 1984; Damasio, 1979; Lezak, 1983). However, most of these studies have concentrated on the patient with lateral frontal injury. Although tests such as the Wisconsin Card Sorting Test (Heaton, 1981) or Porteus Mazes (Porteus, 1965) may be reliably associated with lateral frontal damage, they are not closely associated with orbital frontal damage (cf. Martzke et al., 1991).

The fact that orbital "frontal tests" show such low hit rates in patients with orbital frontal injury is not as mysterious as it might first appear. The frontal lobes represent about 38% of whole brain, of which there are many distinct subsections, which, when damaged, produce different characteristic symptoms. For example, it has been demonstrated that mesial frontal lobe injury results in a very specific and distinctive disorder highlighted by an amnestic syndrome with wild confabulation. Thus, for the patient with mesial frontal injury, memory testing is as directly relevant to frontal injury as card sorting, and confabulatory amnesia is as much a frontal lobe syndrome as pseudopsychopathy. Thus, what constitutes characteristic symptoms of orbital frontal injury are not and need not be like other frontal syndromes, either on tests or in clinical presentation.

Probably 90% or more of the literature on frontal lobe testing concerns lateral frontal injured patients. The major set of studies that have concerned orbital frontal damage involved transorbital leukotomy patients evaluated in the 1930–1950 period. In more than 20 distinct studies involving possibly as many as 500 patients, before versus after leukotomy testing indicated no loss of IQ, memory, or language skill (cf. Brown, 1984; Hecaen & Albert, 1978; Luria, 1966; Seron, 1978). At the same time, the surgery had profound effects in quieting psychosis and "tranquilizing" psychotic patients. It was taken for granted in the era of frontal lobotomy that the behavior of the patient (and his or her symptoms) would be substantially to manifestly changed although testing would not be changed.

The degree of orbital frontal disconnection/malfunction in these lobotomy cases is far greater than posttraumatic orbital frontal injury. Thus, it is not at all unexpected that TBI patients with known or suspected orbital frontal injury typically perform adequately in "routine" psychological testing. A new category of testing has developed, concerned with "executive functioning," which has shown promise in the evaluation of orbital frontal injured patients (cf. chap. 9 for a detailed discussion of executive function testing). For this chapter, two specific pieces of information are relevant in this regard. First, some tests are more sensitive than others (e.g., Design Fluency, Tinker Toy Test vs. Card Sort or Trails; Varney et al., 1996). Second, the most sensitive "executive functioning" tests currently available are failed by no more than 50% of patients with manifest orbital frontal syndromes, as indicated by highly dysfunctional activities of daily living (ADLs). Thus, in mild TBI, at least half of patients with orbital frontal symptoms that are manifestly evident at work and in the home will pass any test, even the latest or most sophisticated "frontal lobe" task (cf. Martzke et al., 1991).

COLLATERAL INTERVIEW AND MILD TBI

As noted earlier, patients with TBIs, particularly mild TBIs, may perform normally on a wide variety of neuropsychological measures and can appear relatively normal within the structure of standard psychological interviews (cf. Lezak, 1978). At the same time, they are often substantially impaired in independent, self-determined "adult" behaviors and activities of daily living (cf. Varney & Menefee, 1993). Thus, there has been increasing recognition of the importance of obtaining information from collateral informants who are familiar with the patient (e.g., parents, spouses, siblings, coworkers). In addition to being able to elaborate on nature and severity of more traditional cognitive deficits (e.g., reliability of memory), collaterals have a unique vantage point from which to assess the social, behavioral, and interpersonal changes the individual might have experienced as a result of a head injury because they see the patient in his or her day-to-day living environment. In addition, the typical collateral informant is likely to have spend hundreds if not thousands of hours in the company of the head injury patient both before and after the injury. There is no way that psychological testing, imaging studies, chart review, or even patient interview can provide such a rich archive of information about behavior change.

Information obtained from collaterals may often differ markedly from information given by the patient. TBI patients may provide inaccurate histories, over- or underreport symptomatology, and lack insight concerning their behavior and its effect on singificant others in their environment. Because these individuals are likely to fall within normal ranges on traditional batteries of neuropsychological tests and may appear "normal" during a psychological interview, critical psychosocial symptoms (which often render the individual defective in daily functioning) may be overlooked by the most astute observer without collateral interviews.

The Iowa Collateral Head Injury Interview (ICHII) is a structured interview that assesses psychosocial symptoms commonly reported after TBI and that are closely associated with orbital frontal injury (Varney, 1989). Collaterals are asked to assess whether specific psychosocial behaviors were present or have become worse following TBI. It is intended to offer an at least somewhat quantified, standardized, and systematic procedure for detecting what may be serious neuropsychological sequelae of TBI that are otherwise difficult to unearth. A complete copy of the protocol is contained in the Appendix.

A question that could be raised at this point concerns the frequency at which ICHII symptoms are found in the "normal" population. First, it should be pointed out that many of the symptoms inquired about are indeed present in some normals (e.g., absentmindedness). However, the structure of the interview is such that the collaterals are asked about change, not the simple presence or absence of a symptom. Second, we have been able to standardize the test on a population of 40 particularly challenging "normals": the parents of children receiving care from a child guidance clinic. Here, the children were the patients and had behavior problems (e.g., attention deficit hyperactivity disorder [ADHD], eating disorders) requiring the participation of their parents for therapy. Presumably there were unusual stressors in the home, making the parents more likely to have "psychological symptoms" and relationship stressors than traditional standardization samples. At the same time, the parents were not themselves neurologically or psychiatrically ill (those with histories of psychiatric care or TBI were excluded). Each parent was interviewed with regard to the other on the ICHII. The mean score on the test was slightly above 1 point and the worst score was 6, with the maximum possible score being 42 (Fig. 8.1). Thus, even in this somewhat troubled population, endorsement of change as tested in the ICHII was relatively rare.

These findings underscore the importance of interviewing collaterals as part of the neuropsychological workup of patients with mild TBI. In many cases, the findings obtained may offer a unique perspective on specific neurobehavioral disabilities that might escape our attention in formal testing and interview with the patient himself. The ICHII is offered as an example of how to attack this problem. It has the advantage of being quantified, standardized, and field tested. However, in an area where knowledge is rapidly expanding (indeed, the test itself has been

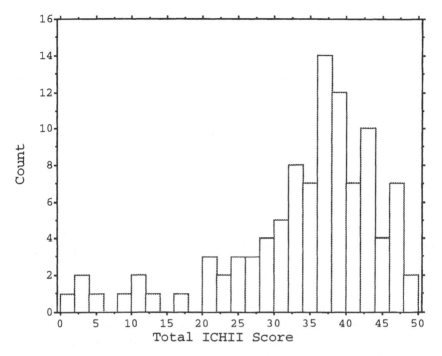

FIG. 8.1. Distribution of ICHII scores from 100 patients with posttraumatic anosmia.

substantially modified twice since the initial field testing was performed in 1989), it may be best to view it as an instrument with practical applications today but that will likely be rendered obsolete and/or incomplete with further study.

ANOSMIA AND PSYCHOSOCIAL OUTCOME

In a recent study of the ICHII, the interview was given to 98 collaterals of TBI patients with posttraumatic anosmia who had suffered an LOC of sufficient duration to be noted in emergency room reports, but no longer than 20 min (Varney & Menefee, 1993). The TBI patients consisted of 57 males and 41 females. The mean age of this group was 34.9 years (range 30 to 60 as per study design), the mean education was 12.5 years (range 8 to 16), and the mean Full Scale IQ was 105 (range 83 to 138). None had history of psychiatric illness, substance abuse, or developmental disability. All were old enough to have clearly established that they were reliable in the workplace. Thus (oddly), the demographics of this set of mild TBI patients makes them substantially different from the modal TBI patient, who is, by some reports, a young, intoxicated, poorly educated, dyslexic male with antisocial personality traits (i.e., a *DSM–IV* Axis II diagnosis).

Figure 8.1 shows the distribution of the total score on the ICHII for 100 mild head injury patients with partial or total anosmia. As can be seen, the results are skewed badly to the right, with a majority of collaterals endorsing more than half of the items available (i.e., scores >25). Only four obtained scores clearly within the normal range (0–6). The symptoms clearly cluster around total score 38. The distribution and clustering of scores strongly suggests that the symptoms shown by anosmic patients constitute a syndrome (i.e., a constellation of characteristic symptoms).

These findings underscore the simultaneously elusive yet devastating nature of the deficits shown by patients with orbital frontal syndromes. On the one hand, these patients were, for the most part, normal appearing both on tests and in structured interviews. On the other hand, the deficits they showed most frequently, such as poor judgment, absentmindedness, indecisiveness, and so on, rendered these patients unemployable and/or disabled. As has been pointed out by Lezak (1978, 1983) such patients are also socially and interpersonally "difficult." Indeed, it was not uncommon for family members to use the expression "invasion of the body snatchers" in reference to their head injured relative. That is, they looked the same, but had become totally different persons.

ANOSMIA AND VOCATIONAL OUTCOME

A preliminary indication of the importance of anosmia as a marker for orbital frontal damage and associated psychosocial deficits can be found in a study (Varney, 1988) that examined vocational outcome in apparently recovered patients with posttraumatic anosmia. All had been cleared for return to work at least 2 years prior to evaluation of their vocational status. All were physically healthy, and none showed significant neuropsychological deficits. Nevertheless, 92% of those with total anosmia suffered chronic employment problems (active employment less than 25% of the time since being cleared for work over a period of at least 2 years). Among partial anosmics, 64% showed chronic employment problems. Factors listed most frequently as forming the basis for these patients' unemployability were absentmindedness, poor planning and anticipation, indecisiveness or faulty decision making, erratic quality of work output, unreliability in work attendance, an inability to learn from errors, and an inability to get along socially with coworkers and particularly supervisors. The conclusion was that "post traumatic anosmia, used as a sign of orbital frontal damage, has quite negative implications for vocational prognosis

... despite (the patients) having no clear neurologic, intellectual or memory deficits" (p. 253).

A second study of patients with total anosmia (Varney & Menefee, 1993) offered similar findings with regard to the prognostic significance of post traumatic anosmia for vocational outcome. However, this population was particularly interesting in that all (a) had minor head injuries with less than 30 min LOC or less than 48 hr PTA, (b) were an average of 31 years of age at time of injury, thus establishing their premorbid work histories as good, (c) had an average of 10 years of following their head trauma prior to examination, and (d) had, as a group, above average intelligence and average memory. In this population, 80% suffered chronic unemployment and the remainder either worked for relatives or were in work therapy or related subsidized programs.

In a third group (reported here), numbering 100 partial and total anosmics in which assessment of vocational outcome took place at least 5 years following injury, 81 were unemployed and had worked less than 25% of the time during the previous year. It is interesting to note the pattern of unemployment these patients showed. Only 8 had never returned to work following their accident. This means that the rest ($n = 73$) had tried and failed to return to former employment. Most of these attempted to obtain employment between 1 and 69 times following their first dismissal. The typical pattern was one in which the patients got and lost jobs (i.e., not chronic inactivity). Most eventually were awarded disability status, but often with a key piece of evidence being the number of jobs they had been fired from since their head injury. This "hired and fired" history following head injury is typical for most anosmics until, after a number of years, their own history of employment failure becomes a substantial obstacle to being hired again.

FUNCTIONAL IMAGING AND ANOSMIA

Autopsy and neuropsychological studies strongly suggested that posttraumatic anosmia is a sign of orbital frontal damage (Sumner, 1976; Zusho, 1982). This has been corroborated in a recent functional neuroimaging study that found orbital frontal hypometabolism to be closely associated with posttraumatic anosmia (Varney & Bushnell, 1998). It is noteworthy when comparing these findings with CT or MRI research that the functional neuroimaging studies found very little evidence of three-dimensional structural lesions. Thus, rather than showing that there was a hole in orbital frontal cortex, the results indicated that the target area was functioning, but far below minimal normal levels.

Subjects were 18 individuals with a history of mild head injury at least 5 years prior to being involved in the study. None had premorbid problems with substance abuse, mental disorder, or arrest for any reason. All subjects had been gainfully employed for at least 5 years prior to their head trauma. This latter criterion was adopted to establish that each subject most probably had a productive and well-adjusted premorbid history. Control subjects consisted of five age-matched hospital employees.

Anosmic subjects were identified from a sample of about 200 patients at the Iowa City VA Medical Center who had mild head injuries that resulted in posttraumatic anosmia. All potential subjects were clinically referred patients. That is, their initial injuries and report of symptoms were sufficiently credible that they were referred for neuropsychological evaluation by hospital medical staff in a setting where, under most circumstances, the evaluation had no relevance to litigation (as VA staff are only rarely permitted to testify in court). Obviously, litigation would not affect a neuroSPECT. However, the absence of litigation potential is mentioned here because it underscores the clinical concern of the referral source. That is, these were not trivial "bump on the head" cases even though their head injuries were classified as mild. For each subject, 20 mCi of 99m-Tc hexamethylpropyleneamine oxime (HMPAO) was administered intravenously while the individual was resting in a supine position in a room with low-level ambient light and minimal background noise. Single-photon emission computed tomography (SPECT) images were obtained using a triple detector system (PRISM 3000, Picker Int.) with ultrahigh-resolution collimators. Total Imaging time was 25 min for each SPECT study. SPECT images were reconstructed using a Weiner filter and displayed in transverse, coronal, and sagittal planes.

A quantitative analysis was performed in which HMPAO count density ratios were calculated for six regions of interest (ROIs) using a sagittal cut:

1. Orbital frontal cortex.
2. Inferior frontal pole.
3. Superior frontal pole.
4. Posterior superior frontal lobe.
5. The parasagital area.
6. The occipital pole.

ROIs were also established for both the right and left hemispheres using sagittal SPECT slices that bisected the frontal lobes at approximately the level of the olfactory nerve at the anterior end and the level of the occipital poles at the posterior end (cf. Fig. 8.2 for a representative sagittal cut with each ROI, outlined in white). Ratios of each region to whole brain hemisphere slice activity were generated for both the right and left hemispheres in all subjects.

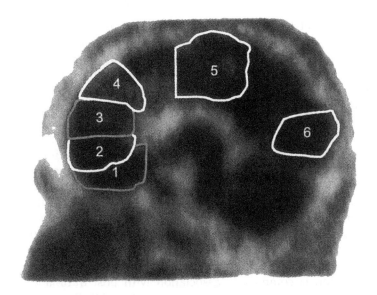

FIG. 8.2. Sample neuroSPECT image with regions of interest identified. ROI legend: 1 = orbital frontal cortex, 2 = inferior frontal pole, 3 = superior frontal pole, 4 = posterior superior frontal lobe, 5 = parasagital region, 6 = occipital pole.

Initial evaluation of SPECT images was done via visual inspection of each scan in coronal, axial, and sagittal planes. Control scans were mixed with brain injured scans, and all were read "blind." All control scans were correctly classified as normal, as were 6 of the head injured patients' scans. All of the remaining 12 scans had abnormalities to visual inspection in one or both anterior mesial temporal lobe regions. Among these, 4 also had visually apparent abnormalities in the orbital frontal region. Additional, individual specific abnormalities were noted on 5 of the scans.

A quantitative SPECT analysis was performed in which target area (i.e., ROI 1, orbital frontal cortex) to whole brain count density ratios were calculated for each ROI in the right and left hemispheres. Statistical analysis via t-test indicate that count ratios were significantly lower in orbital frontal cortex for anosmics versus controls ($t = 2.81$; $p < .01$). No other between-group comparison involving the remaining five ROIs was significant. Virtually identical findings were obtained repeating the analysis using the Mann–Whitney U-test. Once again, comparison of orbital frontal findings was significant ($Z = -2.83$; $p < .01$), whereas all other comparisons fell well short of significance. For the purpose of analysis of individual data, the count ratios for the anosmic head injury subjects were classified as being abnormal if they fell at least two standard deviations below the level of the lowest control subject on the right or left. This criterion was set to be sure that findings designated as abnormal and indicating hypometabolism were clearly different from findings subsumed within the control group. Twelve of the 18 anosmic patients (67%) showed abnormally low counts in one or both orbital frontal ROIs.

There were 12 individual count ratios below 0.80 from among the 216 count ratios computed for anosmic patients on the right and left for all ROIs. This represents the lowest 5% of count ratios computed for head injured subjects regardless of the ROI location. Eleven (92%) of these particularly low count ratios were in orbital frontal cortex. It is also worth noting that the lowest count ratio was 0.51. That is, none was close to zero. Thus, the lowest count ratios were clustered in orbital frontal cortex, but no subject showed obliteration of orbital frontal cortex. Rather, orbital frontal metabolism in these posttraumatic anosmics was "unhealthy" rather than "dead." It is, therefore, understandable that all of these same subjects had normal MRI scans.

The results of the study are clear in indicating that orbital frontal hypoperfusion is common in association with post traumatic anosmia. For posttraumatic anosmics as a group, Tc-99*m* HMPAO neuroSPECT produced significantly lower orbital frontal counts than was found among controls. This was the only one of six areas (i.e., ROIs) in which anosmic patients differ significantly from controls. In addition, a clear majority of individual patients with posttraumatic anosmia had significantly abnormal orbital frontal findings. Abnormal individual count ratios were relatively uncommon in the other five ROIs. In addition, among the 12 most abnormal scores obtained from any patient in any ROI, 11 were in orbital frontal cortex. By implication, the presence of anosmia in a head injured patient could indicate substantial risk for orbital frontal injuries.

IMAGING AND OUTCOME

Employing neuroSPECT and collateral interview data from subjects as well as controls, a significant correlation (rho $= -.64$; $p < .001$) was obtained between orbital frontal count and the score obtained on the ICHII. Correlations for the remaining five ROIs with collateral ratings did not reach significance. It is also noteworthy in this regard that correlation coefficients involving the ICHII and 27 neuropsychological test scores were all below $r = -.25$. The neuropsychological tests involved ranged from IQ, memory, and language to "frontal" tests such as Design Fluency and the Tinker Toy Test. Thus, while there may be distinct elements to the syndrome noted in these head injury patients, they are not simply a reflection of "general mental impairment" and actually appear quite independently in relation to traditional mental abilities or disabilities.

CONCLUSION

Patients with TBI, particularly when this involves a relatively minor head injury and/or orbital frontal damage, may appear normal, claim to be normal, and perform well on tests. Nevertheless, they suffer a potentially devastating syndrome involving a constellation of disabilities, which are, in large part, consistent from patient to patient. These symptoms include mental inertia, indecisiveness, an inability to plan or anticipate, and a marked inclination to make errors of omission. Unfortunately, many of the component symptoms of this syndrome are difficult to demonstrate relying only on formal testing. Even the most state-of-the-art testing fails 50% of the time or more to identify the manifestly disabled. Thus, it is essential that collateral informants be interviewed and vocational histories obtained from sources other than the patient.

It could be argued that the presence of anosmia seems to be a "slender reed" on which to base predictive diagnostic conclusions. Similarly, the use of collateral interviews may seem to some like "soft-science." Nevertheless, multiple studies involving more than 200 subjects have indicated that vocational outcome and psychosocial symptomology are quite consistent for mild TBI patients with anosmia. In addition, functional neuroimaging shows that these patients have "real" injuries to the orbital frontal cortex. Finally, a significant correlation was found between number and severity of symptoms reported by collaterals and orbital frontal count ratios in neuroSPECT. In combination, these findings offer a solid foundation for viewing anosmia (with ageusia) as a posttraumatic symptom of substantial clinical importance.

It should also be pointed out that clinical knowledge about human orbital frontal symptomology, both phenomenological and empirical, is still in a relatively early stage. It can be hoped that substantial advances will be made over the next few years to better elucidate and understand the nature of this complex and catastrophic disability. At the same time, the reader should be cautioned that TBI can involve a wide variety of central nervous system pathologies, and that the eventual etiology of the complex of psychosocial and executive deficits shown by the head injured may reflect multiple etiologies.

ACKNOWLEDGMENT

Preparation of this manuscript was funded in part by the Department of Veterans' Affairs.

APPENDIX: IOWA COLLATERAL HEAD INJURY INTERVIEW

NOTE TO INTERVIEWER: The interview is concerned with a set of psychosocial symptoms often seen in association with frontal lobe damage, particularly that following closed head injury. The general title or name of each symptom is listed in boldface. Also included are initial questions for each item. Interviewers are to start with these general questions, but may be required to elaborate in order to facilitate the informant's understanding. Collateral informants should always be advised that many of the symptoms discussed occur in "normals" and that our concern is if there has been a significant change for the worse. Collaterals are encouraged to avoid false positives by being told to respond yes only if they are sure that the behavior is worse than prior to the injury. Finally, because the majority of head injured patients are male, the masculine nouns and pronouns were chosen to be used in the interview questions to simplify the questionnaire. Obviously, when one is interviewing a female, the feminine nouns and pronouns should be substituted.

SCORING: Give 2 points if change is reported to be substantial. Give one point if change has clearly occurred but is only a modest problem. Give no points if there is no change or the reported change poses no problems to the informant and/or the patient's life. For 100 control subjects: Mean = one point. Fifth %ile = 6 points. Scores of 10 or more can be regarded as clearly abnormal. Scores above 30 should be viewed with suspicion since four test items are foils.

1. **ABSENTMINDEDNESS:** Is your husband absentminded or could he be called a scatterbrain? That is, rather than simply having a bad memory, does he remember things at the wrong time or in a haphazard manner which makes his memory inefficient? For example, you might send him out to buy bread, and he will return with a full tank of gas and other errands completed, but spontaneously remembers bread only after returning home.
(These patients are clinically notable for being able to narrate long lists of things they have forgotten, very much unlike Amnestic Syndrome or the memory disturbance of SDAT.)

2. **INDECISIVENESS:** Does your husband have difficulty making even the most simple of decisions? For example, can it take him an unreasonable length of time to get dressed in the morning? Does he let you make decisions for him now, that he might not have before the injury? In this regard, do you sometimes feel responsible for most of the daily household decision making as well as the larger decisions (e.g., what to watch on TV, what to have for dinner)?

3. **NON-SPONTANEITY:** Does your husband seem to initiate fewer behaviors on his own? Does he have a hard time directing his own activities, even trivial ones, with directions? If left to himself, would he just lie around,

doing little, if anything, for hours at a time? For example, lights emit a certain amount of light. People emit a certain amount of behavior. Does your husband just emit less behavior? If he was a 100 watt light bulb before, what is he now?

4. **PERPLEXITY:** Can your husband become very confused by small changes of plan or topics of conversation because he has a "one track mind?" That is, he cannot change with changes in the environment.

5. **APPARENT LOW MOTIVATION:** While we realize that your husband may express and even feel highly motivated to return to work or "be normal again," does he appear lazy, unambitious or unambitious to others?

6. **DISORGANIZATION:** Does your husband have difficulty getting organized to complete even the simplest of tasks because he is inefficient, doesn't carry out plans that are made, etc.? Even if it is something he used to be able to do quite easily? Is he unable to complete a task that he was previously able to complete, such as tune the car, even if someone tells him to do so?

7. **INFLEXIBILITY:** Does your husband insist that things are done the same way every time, over and over again? And if there is any deviation from how things are traditionally done, is he inappropriately upset?

8. **POOR PLANNING & ANTICIPATION:** To your knowledge, does your husband ever form any reasonable plans? Or, to put it another way, does he often act in a manner that suggests that he made a plan of action?

9. **FAILURE TO LEARN FROM EXPERIENCE:** Does your husband seem to make the same mistakes over and over again? In other words, does he fail to learn from experience?

10. **POOR JUDGMENT:** We all make many little decisions every day, such as the order in which daily chores are to be performed, what to purchase at the store, or how our time should be allocated. Does it seem as though your husband routinely makes poor decisions in these activities of daily living? For example, even though he may have good intentions, does he choose an inappropriate, undesirable, or inefficient means of completing some task when a better option was clearly available?

11. **NON-REINFORCING:** Does your husband seem to have a rather neutral attitude toward you? While not meaning to be rude, does he fail to do all of those "little things" which make a person feel appreciated or loved? Please note that our emphasis is on absent positive behavior. Rudeness or temper would not count in this category.

12. **RISK SEEKING BEHAVIOR:** Does your husband seem to enjoy taking unnecessary risks "just for the fun of it" (this may be particular evident in his driving)?

13. **DISINHIBITION:** Does your husband do things in public that embarrass you? Are these things that might be described as "things he just couldn't seem to resist doing?"

14. **IMPULSIVITY:** Does your husband sometimes act impulsively? In other words, does he sometimes act first, and think later; or not consider the consequences of his actions until after he has acted? This may be particularly evident in his driving, spending, or casual conversation.

15. **STIMULUS-BOUND BEHAVIOR:** Have you noticed that while your husband may be generally non-responsive, certain objects or events, some relatively trivial, may compel him to act (e.g., repetitively changing channels with the remote control)? Do you ever notice that your husband will use an object (e.g., a pen, a spoon, a hammer) just because the object happened to be there, not because he needed to use the item?

16. **IMPOLITIC SPEECH:** Does your husband stick his foot in his mouth more often than he used to? Does he tend to talk first and think later?

17. **IMMATURITY/CHILDLIKE DEPENDENCE:** Do you feel as if there is one more child in your home since your husband's injury? Do you sometimes feel as if you are the only parent or responsible adult at home? How old would a child be if that child acted the way your spouse has been acting since the injury?

18. **NEUTRAL AFFECT:** Does your husband usually have no affect or emotion at all? Is he inanimate, sort of like a piece of furniture is inanimate?

19. **POOR INSIGHT:** Does your husband have a poor understanding of himself, his emotions and limitations? In particular, does he seem unable to comprehend in any way the psychological or mental changes he has suffered from his head injury?

20. **POOR EMPATHY:** Since the injury, is your husband worse at understanding how you are feeling? Does he have a harder time taking your perspective on things? Does he seem to not even consider that you might have feelings or opinions on certain subjects?

21. **SELF-CENTEREDNESS:** Has your husband become very self-centered, without becoming highly selfish? That is, while appreciating his own point of view or needs, does he fail to appreciate that others may have similar feelings?

This interview has been reprinted from Varney (1991) and Varney and Menefee (1993).

REFERENCES

American Medical Association. (1993). *Guides to the evaluation of permanent disability*. Chicago: American Medical Association.

American Psychiatric Association. (1994). *Diagnostic and statistical manual of mental disorders* (4th ed.). Washington, DC: American Psychiatric Association.

Brown, J. (1984). Frontal lobe syndromes. In G. Vinken, G. Bruyn, & H. Klwanas (Eds.), *Handbook of clinical neuropsychology* (Vol. 45, pp. 23–42). Amsterdam: Elsevier.

Damasio, A. (1979). The frontal lobes. In K. Heilman & E. Valenstein (Eds.), *Clinical neuropsychology* (pp. 360–404). New York: Oxford University Press.

Goldenberg, G., Oder, W., Spatt, J., & Podereka, I. (1992). Cerebral correlates of disturbed executive function and memory in survivors of severe closed head injury: A SPECT study. *Journal of Neurology, Neurosurgery, & Psychiatry, 55*, 362–368.

Gray, B., Ichise, M., Chung, D., Kirsh, J. C., & Franks, W. (1992). Technetium-99m-HMPAO SPECT in the evaluation of patients with a remote history of traumatic brain injury: A comparison with computed tomography. *Journal of Nuclear Medicine, 33*, 55.

Gurdjan, E., & Gurdjan, E. (1976). Cerebral contusions: Reevaluation of the mechanisms of their development. *Journal of Trauma, 16*, 35–51.

Heaton, R. (1981). *A manual for the Wisconsin Card Sorting Test*. Odessa, FL: F. A. Davis.

Hecaen, H., & Albert, M. (1978). *Human neuropsychology*. New York: Wiley.

Jennett, B., & Teasdale, G. (1981). *Management of head injuries*. Philadelphia: F. A. Davis.

Lezak, M. (1978). Living with the characterologically altered brain injured patient. *Journal of Clinical Psychiatry, 57*, 592–598.

Lezak, M. (1983). *Neuropsychological assessment* (2nd ed.). New York: Oxford University Press.

Luria, A. (1966). *Higher cortical functions in man*. New York: Basic Books.

Martzke, J., Swan, C., & Varney, N. (1991). Post traumatic anosmia and orbital frontal damage: Neuropsychological and neuropsychiatric correlates. *Neuropsychology, 5*, 213–225.

Newberg, A., & Alavi, A. (1996). Neuroimaging in patients with traumatic brain injury. *Journal of Head Trauma Rehabilitation, 11*, 65–79.

Newton, M. R., Greenwood, R. J., Britton, K. E., Charlesworth, M., Nimmon, C. C., Carroll, M. J., & Dolke, G. (1992). A study comparing SPECT with CT and MRI after closed head injury. *Journal of Neurology, Neurosurgery, and Psychiatry, 55*, 92–94.

Oder, W., Goldberg, G., Spratt, J., & Podereka, I. (1992). Behavioral and psychosocial sequelae of severe closed head injury and regional cerebral blood flow: A SPECT study. *Journal of Neurology, Neurosurgery, and Psychiatry, 55*, 475–480.

Porteus, S. (1965). *Porteus Maze Test*. Palo Alto, CA: Pacific Books.

Seron, X. (1978). Analyse neuropsychologique des lesions préfrontales chez l'homme. *L'Année Psychologique, 78*, 183–202.

Stuss, D., & Benson, D. (1984). Neuropsychological studies of the frontal lobes. *Psychological Bulletin, 95*, 3–28.

Stuss, D., & Gow, C. (1992). "Frontal dysfunction" after traumatic brain injury. *Neuropsychiatry, Neuropsychology, and Behavioral Neurology, 5*, 272–282.

Sumner, D. (1976). Disturbances in sense of smell and taste after head injuries. In P. Vinken & G. Bruyn (Eds.), *Handbook of clinical neurology* (pp. 1–24). New York: Elseiver.

Varney, N. (1988). The prognostic significance of anosmia in patients with closed head trauma. *Journal of Clinical and Experimental Neuropsychology, 10*, 250–254.

Varney, N. (1989). Iowa Collateral Head Injury Interview. *Neuropsychology, 5*, 223–225.

Varney, N. R., & Bushnell, D. (1998). NeuroSPECT findings in patients with post-traumatic anosmia: a quantative analysis. *Journal of Head Trauma Rehabilitation, 13*, 63–92.

Varney, N. R., Bushnell, D., Nathan, M., Kahn, D., Roberts, R., Rezai, K., Walker, W., & Kirchner, P. (1995). NeuroSPECT correlates of disabling "mild" head injury: Preliminary findings. *Journal of Head Trauma Rehabilitation, 10*, 18–28.

Varney, N. R., & Menefee, L. (1993). Psychosocial and executive deficits following closed head injury. *Journal of Head Trauma Rehabilitation, 8*, 32–44.

Varney, N. R., Struchen, M., Hanson, T., Franzen, K., Connell, S., & Roberts, R. (1996). Design fluency among normals and patients with closed head injury. *Archives of Clinical Neuropsychology, 11*, 345–535.

Zusho, H. (1982). Post traumatic anosmia. *Archives of Otolaringology, 108*, 90–92.

9

Executive Function: Some Current Theories and Their Applications

Tessa Hart
MossRehab Hospital and Moss Rehabilitation Research Institute, Philadelphia

Myrna F. Schwartz
Moss Rehabilitation Research Institute and Temple University School of Medicine, Philadelphia

Nathaniel Mayer
MossRehab Hospital and Temple University School of Medicine, Philadelphia

Executive functions are the neurocognitive operations that enable purposeful behavior as it unfolds in time. By this we mean behavior above the level of reflex or instinct, organized by purposes (goals) at multiple levels of complexity and abstractness. This definition embodies three central themes that we wish to highlight. The first is the idea of *goals, or end-states, guiding or directing behavior.* This theme is of course a familiar one in conceptualizations of executive function. The importance of cortical regulatory mechanisms that use in some way representations of goals to plan, initiate, maintain, and adjust behavior was emphasized by Bianchi (cited in Benton, 1991) and Luria (1966), among others. These investigators based their ideas largely on both subtle and dramatic breakdowns in the structure of goal-directed activity observed in monkeys and humans, respectively, with brain lesions primarily affecting prefrontal cortex. Such observations were influential because the loss of goal-directedness, or purpose, to behavior appeared to occur in the absence of more basic or primary deficits in sensory or motor function. Thus there must be separate—probably frontal—cortical systems specialized for this type of behavioral control.

This theme is carried on in the work of current theorists such as Duncan (1986), who emphasized the controlling role of purpose in guiding the selection of behaviors from a large "store" of potential actions. Duncan and colleagues also studied the conditions under which behavior fails to be controlled by goals in both uninjured and brain injured subjects ("goal neglect"; Duncan, Emslie, Williams, Johnson, & Freer, 1996). Most clinically based conceptualizations of executive function also incorporate the concept of "planning," which includes generation of alternative actions, maintenance of attention during the action sequence, and online adjustment of behavior to achieve the goal (e.g., Lezak, 1993).

Second, theories and conceptualizations of executive function must account for the *temporal organization of behavior*. As one moves up the phylogenetic scale, and most of all for human beings, the action series that achieve goal states become increasingly protracted. If executive functions subserve purposeful behavior, they must supply the mechanisms by which goal-directed behavior sequences are selected, enacted, and sustained over time. Fuster (1991, 1995) contributed extensive work on the temporal organization of behavior and its reliance on prefrontal systems involved in retrospective (memory) and prospective (preparatory set) mechanisms. According to Fuster (1989), the longer the span of time over which a plan of action must be deployed, the more its completion will depend upon this specialized prefrontal circuitry. From a clinical standpoint, consistency or predictability of human behavior over spans of time is one of the hallmarks of the construct of "personality," changes in which are frequently linked to frontal lobe pathology (Stuss, Gow, & Hetherington, 1992).

The third theme implied by our definition is that of the necessary *flexibility* of behavior that is complex and purposeful. Protracted sequences of behavior that achieve goals must be adaptable in order to deal with variances in the environments and contexts in which they are embedded. For example, if any one step in the action sequence is subverted by a circumstance in the environment, executive mechanisms enable the action to switch to new procedures that capitalize on the circumstances that are present, or effect a change in the circumstances, or seek a new environment more conducive to the plan. By definition, executive functions do not enter into behaviors that are "hard-wired" or expressed in the same way regardless of circumstances.

This last property of executive functions helps to account for their elusive nature in clinical assessment. Even if the demands on the executive system are manageable within the constraints of one situation, such as a testing session, there could still be revealed breakdown in purposeful behavior in other, "real-world" situations that present unexpected and changing circumstances. It has become familiar that some brain-injured patients do well on neuropsychological tests, even those that require planning and other presumably executive operations, yet experience failure when they attempt to achieve real-life social and vocational goals (Eslinger & Damasio, 1985). To maximize validity, some authors have urged situational assessments for patients suspected of frontal injury or dysfunction in executive systems (e.g., Hart & Jacobs, 1993). However, without a theory of what executive functions are and how they are expressed in behavior, such assessments are difficult to interpret. Ultimately, executive functions must be explained in terms of specific cognitive mechanisms instantiated in neural networks. But what are the cognitive mechanisms, and where are the neural networks?

In this chapter we examine three recent theories that have attempted to explain some of the specific cognitive mechanisms that may underlie executive function. Each of the three has generated intriguing lines of research, and each has offered some clarification of the anatomical substrate of these complex operations. Moreover, each has stimulated the development of at least one evaluation method that is easily adaptable to the clinical setting, and that holds promise both for understanding and assessing the specific cognitive mechanisms involved in executive function.

SUPERVISORY ATTENTION

An influential theory put forward by Norman and Shallice (1985) attributes the control of purposeful nonroutine action to a mechanism, associated with conscious volition, termed *supervisory attention* (SA). According to the theory, SA operates by biasing the activation levels of the learned programs—schemas—that collectively control routine actions. The conditions under which SA comes into play are stated very precisely; it is involved in tasks that:

1. Involve planning or decision making.
2. Necessitate monitoring for error.
3. Contain novel action sequences.
4. Are judged to be dangerous or technically difficult.
5. Require overcoming a strong habitual response, or resisting temptation.

The Norman and Shallice theory was based on several lines of evidence. These included studies of the attentional lapses that induce "slips" of everyday action, as well as observations of the breakdowns in purposeful behavior that occur following brain injury. Regarding the latter, Norman and Shallice argued that the characteristic disorders of action control following injury to prefrontal cortex resulted from breakdown of SA, which depends on frontal mechanisms. Specifically, they noted intact performance on simple or overlearned routines, but disorganized, distracted, and/or perseverative behavior when the task demanded novel actions, or error monitoring and correction. This pattern of behavioral breakdown particularly affecting nonroutine action was later characterized as the *dysexecutive syndrome* (Baddeley, 1986).

The supervisory attention theory provides a reason for the already mentioned failure of neuropsychological tests to detect real-life deficits in purposive behavior. Such tests rarely instantiate the conditions that call forth SA (however, see Duncan, Burgess, & Emslie, 1995, for a discussion of the relationship between measures of fluid intelligence and executive function). A practical and valuable by-product of the theory has been the development of new methods of assessment specifically designed to incorporate some or all of the conditions in which SA is required for appropriate action.

The Six Element Test is one of several behavioral assessments developed by Shallice and his colleague Paul Burgess to challenge SA (Shallice & Burgess, 1991). A variant of the Six Elements was used in a recent study by Levine et al. (1998). This test requires the subject to work independently on three activities: picture naming, arithmetic, and figure copying. Within each activity, some items are worth 15 points, and others are worth 1 point. Items are arranged in blocks of two, and subjects are not allowed to complete both blocks of one task in immediate succession. Subjects are told to earn as many points as possible in 5 min, which is too short a time to complete all the activities. The strategy subjects devise and implement to maximize their score is the feature of interest. SA is involved in a successful strategy because the task requires planning (number 1 on Norman and Shallice's list of conditions) and overcoming the strong habitual tendency to complete both blocks of a high-scoring activity in succession (condition 5).

The original Six Element Test (Shallice & Burgess, 1991) was given to three patients who, many years after traumatic brain injury (TBI), showed real-life behavioral deficits suggestive of SA dysfunction but scored well on standard neuropsychological measures. As predicted, on the Six Element Test the patients earned fewer points than controls and produced more rule violations and more inefficiencies. Levine et al. confirmed these findings in a larger group of chronic TBI patients, using a quantitative measure distinguishing strategic from nonstrategic behavior. TBI patients were more likely than controls to behave nonstrategically; so, too, were patients with focal frontal lobe lesions. However, the nonstrategic pattern was also found with focal nonfrontal lesions, and Levine et al. concluded that right-hemisphere involvement was a better predictor of this pattern of behavior than frontal injury. Furthermore, although Six Element Test performance did correlate with several traditional measures of executive function, it was also related to other measures taken to reflect generalized speed or capacity of attentional resources (e.g., the control conditions of the Stroop task).

In our laboratory at MossRehab, we have used a variant of the Six Element Test to study errors of everyday action in patients with TBI (Schwartz et al., 1998). By *errors of action* we mean things like applying shaving cream to one's toothbrush, or attempting to pour from an closed container. We first determined that TBI patients at different points on the severity spectrum differ in their vulnerability to errors of action. We then sought to determine whether patients with relatively few such errors under routine task conditions would still show an increased tendency to err when the supervisory attentional demands were increased. We imposed these demands by the compounding of tasks and the imposition of rules, as in the Six Element Test procedure.

Our version of the Six Element Test is called the 2 × 3. Subjects are instructed to perform three familiar, naturalistic tasks: Make a slice of toast with butter and jam; wrap a gift as a present; and pack a child's lunchbox with a sandwich, a snack, and juice. Each task must be performed twice, but not in succession; for example, the wrapping of the second gift cannot be performed concurrently with, or immediately following, the wrapping of the first. One or more steps from a different task must intervene. As in the Six Element Test, this constraint was imposed to necessitate planning. In addition, we limited the supply of materials such as gift wrap, juice for the thermos, and so on, which also required the subject to plan more carefully. Finally, as a challenge to working memory, we added the requirement to press a buzzer following completion of each of the six tasks.

We studied the performance of patients with recent, severe traumatic brain injury who nonetheless had performed well on various other versions of these naturalistic tasks without the added demands on planning and working memory (see Schwartz et al., 1998). As anticipated, and consistent with the findings of the Six Element Test studies, these relatively high-functioning TBI subjects committed more "executive" errors on the 2 × 3 task compared to uninjured controls. That is, they more frequently violated the rule governing the order of task completion, and they also had significantly more buzzer-press omissions. The more surprising finding was that the TBI subjects also made more errors of action *on the basic tasks themselves* when these tasks were performed under the challenging conditions of the 2 × 3. For example, they omitted more key steps (e.g., failing to insert the gift into the box before wrapping), and committed more sequence errors (e.g., closing the lunchbox before all items had been packed) and object substitutions (e.g., packing a single slice of toast, rather than the sandwich, into the lunchbox).

This finding is interesting in several respects. It demonstrates that the tendency to commit errors of action on familiar, naturalistic tasks is a general feature of TBI and is not limited to the most severely impaired patients. Whether or not this tendency is realized depends on the situational and cognitive context in which the task is embedded. Thus, our less impaired TBI patients committed errors of action in excess of normal controls on the 2 × 3, but not when these same naturalistic tasks were performed singly or in pairs. On the other hand, the more severely compromised patients committed errors at higher than normal rates even under the less complex condition.

Is the causal basis for errors of action the same for patients at different levels of severity? We believe that it is. Can the cause be attributed to defective supervisory attention? Not without undermining the dichotomy between familiar and novel activities that is central to the supervisory attention theory (as well as many other theories of executive function). According to the theory, disruption of the SA would not be expected to compromise the performance of a familiar task like making a slice of toast. For defective SA to account for the failure in routine tasks under "executive" demands, we would have to argue that the imposition of additional cognitive demands made the task novel, in effect, by forcing the subject to perform it under new conditions (i.e., with multiple task constraints in mind).

However, there is another explanation for errors of action in TBI that is better supported by our data in this and other experiments (Buxbaum, Schwartz, & Montgomery, 1998; Schwartz et al., 1998; Schwartz et al., 1999). The alternative proposal is that action errors arise from some nonspecific consequence of cerebral damage—such as reduced capacity of attentional resources or slower rate of information processing—which does not localize to the frontal lobes but is correlated with the extent of damage. In our studies of naturalistic action breakdown, we have found impressive similarities across etiologies of injury (i.e., TBI, left-hemisphere stroke, right-hemisphere stroke) and a strong association between overall error rate and clinical severity. Whether or not the damage extends into the frontal lobes has not been found to affect the strength of this association. However, right-hemisphere damage does confer an extra disadvantage, which is consistent with an account based on diminished attentional resources (e.g., Coslett, Bowers, & Heilman, 1987).

In the Levine et al. study described earlier, performance on the Six Element Test correlated with measures of generalized speed and attentional capacity, as well as with measures of executive function. It may be that behavioral measures that challenge SA also challenge general attentional and other processing resources. Thus, behavioral measures alone may be incapable of distinguishing the performance of executive systems from the resources they control. Nonetheless, Six Element-type tests may have specific utility in the assessment of patients with otherwise "clean" test profiles and manifest deficits of purposeful behavior in real life.

WORKING MEMORY

The supervisory attention theory is related conceptually to another highly influential model, which is based on the concept of *working memory*. The original working memory model, proposed by Baddeley and Hitch (1974), was developed in reaction to the "staged" memory models that had been dominant for several decades. As an alternative to a short-term memory system that acted as a staging area for long-term memory, Baddeley and Hitch proposed a three-component system specialized for simultaneously storing and operating on information for relatively short periods of time. Two of the components were modality-specific buffer systems for temporary storage of information in articulatory–phonological and visuospatial formats, respectively. The third component was a central executive (CE), responsible for regulating the flow of information within the limited-capacity buffer systems as well as retrieving information as needed from long-term stores. Thus, the representations in working memory are not only of stimuli in the recent environment, but also of past information—that is, from semantic or episodic memory—that are "highlighted" in the workspace to bear on current decisions and actions. As stated by Baddeley (1992), working memory

> provides a system for representing the past in a way that allows the organism to reflect on it, and actively choose a further action, rather than simply responding to the highest probability . . . it (also) offers the capacity to set up and utilize models to predict the future. (p. 282)

Although the working memory model has motivated a great deal of research, the superordinate or controlling aspect of the system—the CE—initially received much less attention than the two modality-specific buffer systems. Baddeley himself (1986) proposed equating the CE with Norman and Shallice's SA, described in the previous section. As the SA system was presumed to be mediated by prefrontal cortex, this placed the CE in the frontal lobes. However, Baddeley doubted that the CE would prove to be a unitary mechanism akin to a homunculus or "agent." Rather, he speculated that it consists of subsystems responsible for specific controlling mechanisms, differing on the basis of modality and/or type of cognitive operation (Baddeley, 1992). Shallice and his colleagues took the SA construct in a similar direction, identifying such subprocesses as monitoring, energizing, inhibiting, and if–then logic (Stuss, Shallice, Alexander, & Picton, 1995).

The possible subsystems of working memory, their anatomical locations, and how they relate to the executive control of action have been the focus of much study in recent years. One line of research was stimulated by studies in nonhuman primates by Goldman-Rakic (1987) and Fuster (Fuster & Alexander, 1971). These investigators showed that fields of neurons in the dorsolateral frontal cortex (area 46) responded during specific components of delayed-response tasks. In a delayed-response task, a stimulus is presented and then removed. Following a delay, a response is required that is contingent on some aspect of the initial stimulus (e.g., its identity, spatial location, etc.). Working memory is presumably what allows information about the stimulus to be held in mind, after it has been removed, for long enough to guide the response. The work of Goldman-Rakic (for review see Goldman-Rakic, 1995) and her colleagues suggested that there were specific prefrontal cells functioning as the temporary storage units of the visuospatial component of working memory. Later work revealed that different stimulus attributes relevant to the response (e.g., object identity vs. location) activated cells in separate, adjacent areas in the monkey prefrontal cortex (Wilson, Scalaidhe, & Goldman-Rakic, 1993). In humans, information on object identity and spatial location may activate working memory networks in the left and right hemispheres, respectively (Smith et al., 1995). With improved resolution of imaging techniques, the regions of the human cortex specialized for working memory operations on different kinds of information are being "mapped." For example, in humans the region specialized for spatial working memory may be superior and posterior to area 46, which seems more critical in nonhuman primates (Courtney, Petit, Maisog, Ungerleider, & Haxby, 1998).

The question remains: Is there a functionally separate CE controlling and coordinating these working memory operations, and if so, where is it? Goldman-Rakic (1995) took the position that the CE does not exist as a separate entity, favoring the idea of "multiple working memory domains—that is, multiple special purpose systems organized in parallel rather than the concept of a central panmodal executive processor to account for the diversity and complexity of the human thought process" (p. 80). A similar view was expressed by Kimberg and Farah (1993), who argued that the cognitive deficits typically seen in patients with frontal lobe injury can be explained with one mechanism—the weakening of connections among working memory representations—without recourse to a separate or superordinate executive controller.

Although the human frontal lobes cannot be studied with single-cell methods as in the monkey, techniques such as positron emission tomography (PET) and functional magnetic resonance imaging (fMRI) show much promise for the exploration of the CE and other working memory components. As mentioned previously, the improved resolution of these imaging methods has allowed investigators to explore the areas involved in storage and rehearsal mechanisms of working memory, as in performance of delayed-response tasks. Imaging studies are also being used to determine what parts of the brain are most activated while subjects are engaged in tasks thought to involve the controlling functions of the CE. The *dual-task paradigm* is one approach that has been used for this purpose. In the dual-task paradigm, subjects practice a task that is within their capacity to perform at a low error rate, such as repeating digit strings at their maximum successful span. A second task in a different modality, such as visually tracking and crossing out a series of boxes on a page, is also practiced. Then the two tasks are performed at the same time. The decrement in accuracy on one or both tasks is taken as a measure of the challenge to the CE, which coordinates simultaneous processing by allocating attentional resources (Della Sala, Baddeley, Papagno, & Spinnler, 1995). This interpretation of dual-task performance assumes that the two tasks use separate input/output mechanisms; that is, that there is little or no overlap between the sensory and motor demands of performing them. If this assumption is met, then performance decrements must be due not to demands on task- or domain-specific resources, but to demand on a system that allocates general-purpose attentional resources to both tasks. Disproportionate decrements in dual- versus single-task accuracy have been shown in patients with Alzheimer's dementia (Baddeley, Bressi, Della Sala, Logie, & Spinnler, 1991) and severe diffuse traumatic brain injury (McDowell, Whyte, & D'Esposito, 1997). Imaging studies with uninjured control subjects have demonstrated bilateral dorsolateral frontal and cingulate cortex activation during dual-task performance (D'Esposito et al., 1995).

Studies using different tasks thought to engage the CE have also shown dorsolateral frontal activation. For example, Petrides, Alivisatos, Meyer, and Evans (1993) demonstrated similar activation on PET when the subject was required to generate random series of verbal or nonverbal stimuli, a task previously implicated in CE function (Baddeley, 1993). As tasks are developed that isolate cognitive components of executive function, they appear to depend on different portions of prefrontal cortex. For example, Owen, Evans, and Petrides (1996) found different patterns of PET activation in tasks requiring active stimulus comparison and response organization (e.g., reproducing a spatial sequence) versus active manipulation or monitoring of information (e.g., judging whether a stimulus has occurred in an ongoing series). These processes were associated with greater activity in mid-ventrolateral and mid-dorsolateral regions, respectively.

Is there a connection between these studies of working memory, and the clinical phenomena seen with frontal lobe injury or disease? Recent research suggests that a deficit in dual-task performance—putatively, a dysfunction of the CE—is correlated with at least some of the behavioral dysfunctions of the dysexecutive syndrome. Baddeley, Della Sala, Papagno, and Spinnler (1997) classified a series of patients with focal frontal lobe lesions as "dysexecutive" or "nondysexecutive" on the basis of documented behavioral changes such as inertia or disinhibition; inability to complete simple activities autonomously; and need for constant supervision. Patients were tested on the dual-task procedure described previously (digit span + visual tracking) and on two neuropsychological tests traditionally associated with frontal lobe function: controlled verbal fluency and the Wisconsin Card Sorting Test. Although both of the latter tests were sensitive to the frontal injuries in this sample, neither discriminated the behaviorally impaired from the unimpaired group. In contrast, the patients with behavioral dysfunction performed significantly worse on the dual-task paradigm than the group without significant behavioral disturbance. Baddeley et al. speculated that behavioral control may require cognitive components similar to those of the dual task, in that social behavior demands simultaneous attention to the cues and priorities of others in addition to one's own. This group recently began an attempt to develop norms for an easily administered paper-and-pencil version of the dual task (Baddeley, Della Sala, Gray, Papagno, & Spinnler, 1997).

According to another influential theory of executive function that emphasizes social behavior—the somatic marker hypothesis, described later—a special type of working memory may help to account for the ability to prioritize actions, decide which goals are important or preferred, and choose the means that are most likely to satisfy them. Any full understanding of executive function must include the idea that control of behavior means selecting some actions and rejecting others. These choices are made, presumably, to maximize personal success. Moreover, adaptive behavior always includes social behavior: We internalize the values of others through learning, and we consider the priorities of others, as well as our own, when we select our actions.

THE SOMATIC MARKER HYPOTHESIS

Antonio Damasio and his colleagues articulated a theory, known as the somatic marker hypothesis, to describe how actions are selected in favor of one another as we enact momentary decisions and judgments in our behavior. This hypothesis (Damasio, 1994, 1996) states that as human beings experience and learn about the consequences of their behaviors, representations of bodily states associated with pleasurable and aversive consequences become part of the stored experience of the consequences of particular actions. These state representations—called somatic markers—are called up automatically and below the level of conscious choice when, in the stream of action, different behaviors could be enacted that would lead to different outcomes. The process by which such representations are called up could be an example of a specific form of working memory (Damasio, 1994). According to the theory, a somatic marker associated with a potentially good outcome "flags" that potential behavior as better than another alternative, and increases the probability that that behavior will be chosen. Conversely, a state associated with a negative outcome would provide a marker saying to the actor, in effect, "don't do it." In the words of Damasio, somatic markers

> have been connected, by learning, to predicted future outcomes of certain scenarios. When a negative somatic marker is juxtaposed to a particular future outcome the combination functions as an alarm bell. When a positive somatic marker is juxtaposed instead, it becomes a beacon of incentive. (Damasio, 1994, p. 174)

The somatic marker hypothesis has been built on the study of patients with relatively focal injury to the ventromedial frontal cortex, who appear to lose the ability to make advantageous decisions because they fail to attach behaviors with their emotional "valences." A series of patients beginning with the now-famous EVR (Eslinger & Damasio, 1985) have been reported who fail miserably at real-life decision making, but score within normal limits on tests of intelligence, memory, and concept formation. These patients make ruinous business decisions, associate with people who blatantly take advantage of them, and fail to learn from their mistakes. Their postinjury social behavior stands in dramatic contrast to their preinjury status. Most strikingly, they can verbalize knowledge of the probable negative consequences of their behavior, stating accurately what they *should* do instead, even as they act against their own best interests.

In their search for the mechanism of this deficit in purposive behavior, Bechara, Damasio, Damasio, and Anderson (1994) developed a task with which they were able to quantify it in the laboratory. As the authors noted, this task simulates real-life problem solving in that it incorporates reward and punishment for responses whose outcomes (consequences) are uncertain at the outset, but become clearer with experience. Both "EVR-like" and uninjured subjects were given four decks of cards and $2,000 in "play money" with which to gamble. They were told to turn over the cards from any of the decks, one by one, in such a way as to maximize their winnings. After each card was turned, the subject received a monetary bonus or penalty according to a schedule arranged in advance by the experimenters. Two of the decks paid high returns, but also exacted high penalties at staggered intervals. If a subject only used these "bad" decks, he or she would progressively lose money and end the game with a negative balance. The other two decks paid modestly but exacted much lower penalties; a subject who stuck with the "good" decks would end up with a net gain.

The performances of the two groups was dramatically different. Uninjured subjects first sampled more from the immediate-payoff decks, but eventually learned to avoid these "bad" decks in favor of the "good" ones. Subjects with ventromedial frontal injury selected significantly fewer "good" and significantly more "bad" cards compared to controls. In a follow-up study (Bechara, Damasio, Tranel, & Damasio, 1997), subjects were monitored for autonomic arousal using the skin conductance response (SCR) during the gambling task. Normal control subjects, as usual, began by sampling heavily from the "bad" decks that provided immediate payoffs, but high penalties at random intervals. As the task progressed, however, they began to display SCR responses before sampling from the "bad" decks. These autonomic responses occurred even before the subjects were able to articulate the consequences of sampling from any deck—that is, they developed an anticipatory emotional response to the possible consequence, even before they "knew" about it consciously. In contrast, the patients with ventromedial frontal injury did not develop SCR responses to the "bad" decks, and (as in the previous study) did not change their behavior as the task went on—even when they were able, later in the task, to articulate the probabilities of success associated with each deck of cards. Thus, there was a dissociation between their knowledge of what they should do to maximize their success, and what they actually did—just as had been observed in their everyday lives.

It remains to be seen whether this task will prove to be useful for the assessment of patients with TBI. Rolls, Hornak, Wade, and McGrath (1994) used a similar contingency learning task with a mixed group of TBI subjects and patients with vascular injuries, some of whom were selected for documented ventral frontal injuries or dysexecutive symptoms (disinhibition, irritability, inflexibility, etc.). The ventral frontal group showed a deficit in learning new reward contingencies to visual stimuli, despite IQ and memory test scores within the normal range. In addition, ratings of behavioral dysfunction were related to the contingency learning task, such that subjects who were rated as more behaviorally impaired had more difficulty mastering the contingency. However, there was no relationship between behavioral ratings and more traditional neuropsychological test scores. Reminiscent of the findings of Bechara and colleagues, many subjects who were unable to perform well on the contingency task could nonetheless articulate what they should have done. Certainly from a clinical standpoint, the dissociation between judgment at a verbal level, and actual behavior requiring judgment, is a familiar one to those working with patients with TBI.

EXECUTIVE FUNCTION AND MILD TBI

The study of executive function seems to be moving toward greater specificity in identifying and locating the cognitive operations subserving the broad aims of purposeful behavior. The three theories we have discussed are examples of this trend. The construct of supervisory attention is undergoing fractionation (Stuss et al., 1995), and experiments on working memory are localizing the frontal circuits responsible for holding specific stimulus attributes in cognitive work space. The somatic marker hypothesis attempts to qualify and quantify an apparently isolated deficit in social behavior in persons with relatively circumscribed injuries.

Although the trend toward specificity has begun to enhance our understanding of the cognitive mechanisms that compose executive functions, we are still a long way from knowing how to apply such research findings to the clinical evaluation of patients with severe, diffuse injuries and multiple cognitive and behavioral symptoms. Still less do we know whether, and how, research on specific executive functions will inform the evaluation of patients with mild TBI. However, there is reason to believe that a subset of patients with mild TBI may have difficulties in executive function without significant impairment in other cognitive functions. For example, Varney and colleagues (Varney et al., 1995; Varney & Bushnell, 1998) have described patients with very brief loss or alteration of consciousness, who perform relatively well on standard tests of neuropsychological function yet report persistent posttraumatic changes in life circumstances (e.g., unemployment, divorce). The clinical evaluation of such patients may ultimately be enhanced by the research on specific cognitive mechanisms of executive function; already, the theories discussed in this chapter have led to new tests adaptable to the clinical setting. These procedures may prove sensitive to the real-life difficulties of patients with mild TBI, as they have with more severely injured patients. Performance on the original Six Element Test, for example, correlated with real-life difficulties that were not predicted by routine evaluation (Shallice & Burgess, 1991). Some of the behavioral deficits of the dysexecutive syndrome were predicted by poor performance on a paper-and-pencil version of the dual-task paradigm (Baddeley, Della Sala, Gray, Papagno, & Spinnler, 1997), as well as a contingency learning procedure similar to the gambling task generated by the somatic marker hypothesis (Rolls et al., 1994). These types of tasks illustrate the ways in which research on the basic cognitive mechanisms of executive function might enrich the clinical care of persons with both mild and severe TBI.

ACKNOWLEDGMENT

This work was supported in part by a grant from the National Institute for Neurological Diseases and Stroke (RO1 NS31824) to M. F. Schwartz.

REFERENCES

Baddeley, A. (1986). *Working memory.* Oxford: Oxford University Press.
Baddeley, A. (1992). Working memory: The interface between memory and cognition. *Journal of Cognitive Neuroscience, 4,* 281–288.
Baddeley, A. (1993). Working memory or working attention? In A. Baddeley & L. Weiskrantz (Eds.), *Attention: Selection, awareness and control* (pp. 152–170). Oxford: Oxford Science Publications.
Baddeley, A., Bressi, S., Della Sala, S., Logie, R., & Spinnler, H. (1991). The decline of working memory in Alzheimer's disease: A longitudinal study. *Brain, 114,* 2521–2542.
Baddeley, A., Della Sala, S., Gray, C., Papagno, C., & Spinnler, H. (1997). Testing central executive functioning with a pencil-and-paper test. In P. Rabbitt (Ed.), *Methodology of frontal and executive function* (pp. 61–80). East Sussex, UK: Psychology Press.
Baddeley, A., Della Sala, S., Papagno, C., & Spinnler, H. (1997). Dual-task performance in dysexecutive and nondysexecutive patients with a frontal lesion. *Neuropsychology, 11,* 187–194.
Baddeley, A., & Hitch, G. (1974). Working memory. In G. A. Bower (Ed.), *The psychology of learning and motivation* (pp. 47–89). New York: Academic Press.
Bechara, A., Damasio, A. R., Damasio, H., & Anderson, S. W. (1994). Insensitivity to future consequences following damage to human prefrontal cortex. *Cognition, 50,* 7–15.
Bechara, A., Damasio, H., Tranel, D., & Damasio, A. R. (1997). Deciding avantageously before knowing the advantageous strategy. *Science, 275,* 1293–1295.
Benton, A. L. (1991). The prefrontal region: Its early history. In H. Levin, H. Eisenberg, & A. L. Benton (Eds.), *Frontal lobe function and dysfunction* (pp. 3–32). New York: Oxford University Press.
Buxbaum, L. J., Schwartz, M. F., & Montgomery, M. W. (1998). Ideational apraxia and naturalistic action. *Cognitive Neuropsychology, 15,* 617–643.
Coslett, H. B., Bowers, D., & Heilman, K. (1987). Reduction in cerebral activation after right hemisphere stroke. *Neurology, 37,* 957–962.
Courtney, S. M., Petit, L., Maisog, J. M., Ungerleider, L. G., & Haxby, J. V. (1998). An area specialized for spatial working memory in human frontal cortex. *Science, 279,* 1347–1351.
Damasio, A. R. (1994). *Descartes' error: Emotion, reason and the human brain.* New York: Avon Books.
Damasio, A. R. (1996). The somatic marker hypothesis and the possible functions of the prefrontal cortex. *Philosophical Transactions of the Royal Society of London—Series B: Biological Sciences, 351,* 1413–1420.
Della Sala, S., Baddeley, A., Papagno, C., & Spinnler, H. (1995). Dual-task paradigm: A means to examine the central executive. In J. Grafman, K. J. Holyoak, & F. Boller (Eds.), *Structure and functions of the human prefrontal cortex* (pp. 161–171). New York: New York Academy of Sciences.

D'Esposito, M., Detre, J., Alsop, D., Shin, R., Atlas, S., & Grossman, M. (1995). The neural basis of the central executive system of working memory. *Nature, 378,* 279–281.

Duncan, J. (1986). Disorganisation of behaviour after frontal lobe damage. *Cognitive Neuropsychology, 3,* 271–290.

Duncan, J., Burgess, P., & Emslie, H. (1995). Fluid intelligence after frontal lobe lesions. *Neuropsychologia, 33,* 261–268.

Duncan, J., Emslie, H., Williams, P., Johnson, R., & Freer, C. (1996). Intelligence and the frontal lobe: The organization of goal-directed behavior. *Cognitive Psychology, 30,* 257–303.

Eslinger, P. J., & Damasio, A. R. (1985). Severe disturbance of higher cognition following bilateral frontal lobe ablation: Patient EVR. *Neurology, 35,* 1731–1741.

Fuster, J. M. (1989). *The prefrontal cortex* (2nd ed.). New York: Raven Press.

Fuster, J. M. (1991). Role of prefrontal cortex in delay tasks: Evidence from reversible lesion and unit recording in the monkey. In H. Levin, H. Eisenberg, & A. L. Benton (Eds.), *Frontal lobe function and dysfunction* (pp. 59–71). New York: Oxford University Press.

Fuster, J. M. (1995). Temporal processing. In J. Grafman, K. J. Holyoak, & F. Boller (Eds.), *Structure and functions of the human prefrontal cortex* (pp. 173–181). New York: New York Academy of Sciences.

Fuster, J. M., & Alexander, G. (1971). Neuron activity related to short-term memory. *Science, 173,* 652–654.

Goldman-Rakic, P. S. (1987). Circuitry of primate prefrontal cortex and regulation of behavior by representational memory. In F. Plum (Ed.), *Handbook of physiology: The nervous system* (pp. 373–417). Bethesda, MD: American Physiological Society.

Goldman-Rakic, P. S. (1995). Architecture of the prefrontal cortex and the central executive. In J. Grafman, K. J. Holyoak, & F. Boller (Eds.), *Structure and functions of the human prefrontal cortex* (pp. 71–83). New York: New York Academy of Sciences.

Hart, T., & Jacobs, H. E. (1993). Rehabilitation and management of behavioral disturbances following frontal lobe injury. *Journal of Head Trauma Rehabilitation, 8,* 1–12.

Kimberg, D., & Farah, M. (1993). A unified account of cognitive impairments following frontal lobe damage: The role of working memory in complex, organized behavior. *Journal of Experimental Psychology: General, 122,* 411–428.

Levine, B., Stuss, D., Milberg, W. P., Alexander, M., Schwartz, M., & Macdonald, R. (1998). The effects of focal and diffuse brain damage on strategy application: Evidence from focal lesions, traumatic brain injury and normal aging. *Journal of the International Neuropsychological Society, 4,* 247–264.

Lezak, M. D. (1993). Newer contributions to the neuropsychological assessment of executive functions. *Journal of Head Trauma Rehabilitation, 8,* 24–31.

Luria, A. R. (1966). *Higher cortical functions in man.* New York: Basic Books.

McDowell, S., Whyte, J., & D'Esposito, M. (1997). Working memory impairments in traumatic brain injury: Evidence from a dual-task paradigm. *Neuropsychologia, 35,* 1341–1353.

Norman, D. A., & Shallice, T. (1985). Attention to action: Willed and automatic control of behavior. In R. J. Davidson, G. E. Schwartz, & D. Shapiro (Eds.), *Consciousness and self-regulation: Advances in research* (Vol. IV, pp. 1–18). New York: Plenum Press.

Owen, A. M., Evans, A. C., & Petrides, M. (1996). Evidence for a two-stage model of spatial working memory processing within the lateral frontal cortex: A positron emission tomography study. *Cerebral Cortex, 6,* 31–38.

Petrides, M., Alivisatos, B., Meyer, E., & Evans, A. C. (1993). Functional activation of the human frontal cortex during the performance of verbal working memory tasks. *Proceedings of the National Academy of Sciences USA, 90,* 878–882.

Rolls, E. T., Hornak, J., Wade, D., & McGrath, J. (1994). Emotion-related learning in patients with social and emotional changes associated with frontal lobe damage. *Journal of Neurology, Neurosurgery and Psychiatry, 57,* 1518–1524.

Schwartz, M. F., Buxbaum, L. J., Montgomery, M. W., Fitzpatrick-DeSalme, E., Hart, T., Ferraro, M., Lee, S., & Coslett, H. B. (1999). Naturalistic action production following right hemisphere stroke. *Neuropsychologia, 37*, 51–66.

Schwartz, M. F., Montgomery, M. W., Buxbaum, L. J., Lee, S., Carew, T. G., Coslett, H. B., Ferraro, M., Fitzpatrick-DeSalme, E., Hart, T., & Mayer, N. (1998). Naturalistic action impairment in closed head injury. *Neuropsychology, 12*, 13–28.

Shallice, T., & Burgess, P. W. (1991). Deficits in strategy application following frontal lobe damage in man. *Brain, 114*, 727–741.

Smith, E., Jonides, J., Koeppe, R., Awh, E., Schumacher, E., & Minoshima, S. (1995). Spatial versus object working memory: PET investigations. *Journal of Cognitive Neuroscience, 7*, 337–356.

Stuss, D. T., Gow, C. A., & Hetherington, C. R. (1992). "No longer Gage": Frontal lobe dysfunction and emotional changes. *Journal of Consulting and Clinical Psychology, 60*, 349–359.

Stuss, D. T., Shallice, T., Alexander, M. P., & Picton, T. W. (1995). A multidisciplinary approach to anterior attentional functions. In J. Grafman, K. J. Holyoak, & F. Boller (Eds.), *Structure and functions of the human prefrontal cortex* (pp. 191–212). New York: New York Academy of Sciences.

Varney, N., & Bushnell, D. (1998). NeuroSPECT findings in patients with post-traumatic anosmia: A quantitative analysis. *Journal of Head Trauma Rehabilitation, 13*, 63–72.

Varney, N., Bushnell, D., Nathan, M., Kahn, D., Roberts, R., Rezai, K., Walker, W., & Kirchner, P. (1995). NeuroSPECT correlates of disabling mild head injury: Preliminary findings. *Journal of Head Trauma Rehabilitation, 10*, 18–28.

Wilson, F., Scalaidhe, S., & Goldman-Rakic, P. S. (1993). Dissociation of object and spatial processing domains in primate prefrontal cortex. *Science, 260*, 1955–1958.

Neuropsychiatric Evaluation of the Closed Head Injury of Transient Type (CHIT)

Vernon M. Neppe
Pacific Neuropsychiatric Institute, Seattle, Washington,
St. Louis University, St. Louis, Missouri,
and University of Washington, Seattle, Washington

Glenn T. Goodwin
Pacific Neuropsychiatric Institute, Seattle, Washington

NEUROPSYCHIATRY

The long historical relationship between neurology and psychiatry impacts the area of transient traumatic head injury. This neuropsychiatric link impacts both the actual brain injury facets and the psychological elements. Historically, physicians interested in the central nervous system focused either globally on behavior or more specifically on demonstrated pathology of the central nervous system, reflecting such terms as *posttraumatic* and *postconcussional* in the brain injury context and interpretations of etiology that were polarized. Most practitioners in the area have had very little exposure, if any, to neuropsychiatry.

Three specialties have approached the area, but from rather diverse origins and conceptual frameworks. Behavioral neurologists define brain behavior relationships often through the single case study with generalizations made about the anatomical basis of the manifested behavior and specific localization of similar types of behavior. Neuropsychiatrists emphasize the phenomenology of behavioral disorders and how these correlate with diseases in neurology and the neurologic aspects of behavioral disorders (Tucker & Neppe, 1988). In head injury, the psyche and the brain are recognized as interplaying with each other. Finally, neuropsychologists employ standardized and objective assessments of intellectual, cognitive, and psychological functioning, emphasizing a more actuarial and statistical methodology of evaluating behavior.

Although each group appears to look at different aspects of the same animal, each has identified important areas of knowledge that are missing in traditional psychiatric, psychological, and neurologic training. We focus here primarily on the comparison of behavioral neurology and neuropsychiatry and make the case for a time-based neuropsychiatric approach applied to the head injury population.

In the context of head injury, exacerbation of preexisting conditions commonly occurs. In this context, neuropsychiatrists recognize that marked behavior disturbance may correlate with paroxysmal discharges in the temporal lobe on the electroencephalogram (Tucker & Neppe, 1994). Although these patients would not be considered to have a seizure disorder by most behavioral neurologists, many neuropsychiatrists believe these patients represent a form of seizure disorder, which we for nonprejudicial reasons have called *paroxysmal neurobehavioral disorder* (Neppe & Blumer, 1998). We have characterized the individual events as "atypical spells" (Neppe & Tucker, 1992, 1994; Tucker & Neppe, 1991). Many of these patients respond to anticonvulsant treatment. Similarly, a patient on neuroleptic medication who develops an atypical movement disorder with neuroleptic medication different biochemically or clinically from extrapyramidal reactions may still be labeled "tardive dyskinesia" with a recommendation that the medication be stopped by the behavioral neurologist; the neuropsychiatrist may be prepared to recognize such atypicality and delineate movement disorders different from those of tardive dyskinesia.

There is a need to incorporate the neuropsychiatric approach to the often misunderstood population of patients with closed head injury (Tucker & Neppe, 1991). A gap exists in the evaluation and management of patients with closed head injury primarily because of the differences in approach between neurology and neuropsychiatry. The neuropsychiatric emphasis can be a practical and helpful adjunct to the primary health care providers (neurologists and neuropsychologists) who are primarily responsible for services provided to the closed head injury population. The purpose of this chapter is to discuss the neuropsychiatric approach and offer some clinical ideas to assist health care providers in providing a more comprehensive and thorough evaluation.

CONTROVERSIES OF MILD TRAUMATIC BRAIN INJURY

The experimental and scientific understanding of mild traumatic head injury (MTHI) has evolved over the past 20 years, with a plethora of research being generated and documented within the scientific literature. At the same time, clinical experience across multidisciplinary lines has increased as health care professionals have continued to interact with this population of patients. It has recently been estimated that approximately 2 million people annually in the United States experience closed head injury (Brown, Fann, & Grant, 1994). Closed head injury represents a significant cause of morbidity and mortality, especially within the younger populations. This has resulted in a considerable increase in health problems associated with the residual sequelae of closed head injury.

Epidemiological studies have documented that within the incidence of closed head injury in general, injuries that are classified as mild or minor typically account for the greater percentage of cases evaluated in emergency room and outpatient settings (Goodwin, 1989). This is also the case outside the United States, where estimates range as high as 80% (Cohadon, Richer, & Castel, 1991).

Although the current body of research literature and experience from clinical practice has provided a greater understanding of MTHI, there continues to be controversy with respect to definition and classification (Kibby & Long, 1996). Any approach for neuropsychiatric and/or neuropsychological evaluation of MTHI must take into account the confusion that exists in understanding this injury as it is differentiated from more severe injuries and from other neuropsychiatric disorders. Earlier attempts at defining the parameters of MTHI have been seen in the research literature (Colohan, Dacey, Alves, Rimel, & Jane, 1986; Davidoff, Kessler, Laibstain, & Mark, 1988). The Mild Traumatic Brain Injury Committee of the Head Injury Interdisciplinary Special Interest Group of the American Congress of Rehabilitation Medicine has proposed definitive guidelines, which have been utilized by the research community in more recent studies (Kay et al., 1993). More current proposals for classification of the spectrum of MTHI have also been suggested (Esselman & Uomoto, 1995).

Despite the clearer definitive guidelines, there continues to be clinical confusion in evaluating and understanding the pathophysiology, symptomatology, and differential diagnosis of MTHI. The terms *postconcussive syndrome* (PCS) and *posttraumatic syndrome* (PTS) have been used to describe the pattern of symptom presentation seen in this population of patients. However, this has not led to a clearer understanding of MTHI with respect to evaluation and assessment. In addition, there have been suggestions that mild head injuries should be differentiated from mild brain injuries. Furthermore, there is often the development of secondary psychiatric disorders that may have a physiological and/or psychosocioenvironmental basis, typically referred to among clinicians as psychological overlay, that complicate the clinical presentation of MTHI and make the evaluative process more complex.

Clearly, the greatest scientific and clinical controversy has been associated with the postconcussive nomenclature (Alves, Macciocchi, & Barth, 1993; Binder, 1986; Kibby & Long, 1996; Lowden, Briggs, & Cockin, 1989).

In general, PCS has been understood to represent the synergistic and interactive effects of physical, cognitive, and psychological symptoms seen on clinical presentation. The assumption is made that there may be physiologic, pharmacologic, psychologic, socioenvironmental, circumstantial, and medicolegal bases underlying the perpetuation of symptomatology. There is also typically a presentation of chronic pain syndrome that may have both physical and psychological factors contributing to the pattern of symptoms and complaints. Neuropsychiatric and neuropsychological evaluation of these patients presents the clinician with a complex task of deciding how to explain the nature of PCS and, more importantly, what to recommend with respect to treatment.

There is also disagreement among researchers and clinicians as to the duration of PCS and what factors predispose individuals to developing a persistent PCS. Within this context, the issue of premorbid factors such as personality characteristics, past psychiatric history, previous substance abuse, prior incidence of MTHI, and general health problems certainly appears to have an influence on the chronicity of symptoms (Goodwin, 1989).

Because of the confounding issues inherent in the diagnostic assessment of the MTHI patient, a comprehensive time-based neuropsychiatric evaluation is proposed to clinically deal with the complexities seen in this patient population. Such a time-based evaluation process may not always be necessary, but in cases where there are confusing diagnostic differentials, a time-based approach will be helpful in guiding the clinician through the evaluation process. The time-based approach is presented later in this chapter.

We further propose a neuropsychiatric nomenclature and classification based on the practical aspects of evaluation, which are more meaningful to the clinician in everyday practice. These clinical distinctions should not be considered distinct entities, but rather as clinical aspects of a dynamic post head trauma spectrum that can be useful in guiding the clinician in the evaluation process. We attempt to integrate current research findings and clinical experience into a methodology for neuropsychiatric evaluation that first of all is useful to the patient and second reflects clinical acumen and multiclinical diversity.

A NEUROPSYCHIATRIC CLASSIFICATION OF CHIT: A NEW TERMINOLOGY

We have chosen to modify the definition proposed by the Interdisciplinary Special Interest Group of the American Congress of Rehabilitative Medicine (Kay et al., 1993). Proposed instead is the use of the term *closed head injury of transient kind* (CHIT) to describe a traumatic-induced psycho-physiologic event that occurs to the head that produces initially little or no unconsciousness, limited retrograde and anterograde amnesia, and alteration of consciousness that does not last longer than a day. We feel the term *closed* head injury should be used because injuries involving skull fractures and open exposure of the brain have their own special characteristics such as infection, vascular phenomena, and focal disease. We prefer terms like *head* to *brain* because this way psychiatric sequelae are not necessarily implied to have a definite organic base. We understand that there is an observable and diagnosable cluster of physical, cognitive, and psychological symptoms that is associated with CHIT and is most usefully defined as posttraumatic CHIT syndrome (PTCHITS). Because *injury* usually implies "traumatic," we see redundancy in using terms like *traumatic* (brain or head) *injury*: Injury will suffice. Finally, and most important, we feel it is important to be nonprejudicial at the outset—hence the term *transient*. CHITs are often reported to be of *mild* severity, but the mildness is not invariably so and the trauma may lead to significant sequelae. Conversely, many so-called mild injuries are more severe because of the lack of available compensation by the brain. We believe terms like *mild* (or for that matter *minor*), *moderate*, *severe*, and *profound* should be confined to severity of outcome and not assumed on the basis of initial duration of unconsciousness. Consequently, we do not like the term *brief*, preferring *transient*. Although the two are similar, *brief* is more unidimensional in the context of implying some unconsciousness and not commenting on duration of clouding or altered consciousness. *Transient* implies an injury but unconsciousness may not be proven, and it takes this into account. On the one hand, such an injury can occur without distinguishable disruption of brain function and yet still be considered as a traumatic event. Some call this *posttraumatic syndrome*. Alternatively, such an injury can result in a disruption of brain function and thus be considered transient traumatic brain injury—some call this *postconcussional syndrome*. Additionally, Kurt Goldstein's dichotomy of "pathogenetic" changes based on the actual injury and "pathoplastic" compensations by other areas of the brain or by psychological adaptation introduces a situation of health as opposed to disease into the equation (Neppe & Tucker, 1988a). Consequently, we prefer *transient* in CHIT, which we contrast with *prolonged* and the term *CHIP—closed head injury of prolonged type*, in which there is clinically significant retrograde or anterograde amnesia, extended confusion or clouded consciousness over more than a day, or prolonged unconsciousness of more than a day. *Transient* implies an apparent blow to the head with no, momentary, or very short consciousness impairments, with the amnesia and confusion ranging from momentary to up to a day. In this regard, CHIPs can always be further subdefined descriptively: A CHIP with 2 days of coma as opposed to CHIPs with half an hour of unconsciousness but 2 weeks of confusion.

Seen within the CHIT syndrome are three subsyndromes, which can occur together: postconcussive, posttraumatic, and focal residual. It is assumed by definition that with the postconcussive subsyndrome, the brain has been concussed and there is a predominant physiologic basis for primary symptoms and secondary psychologic processes that contribute to the manifestation of symptom patterns. With the posttraumatic subsyndrome, there is a predominant feature of acute or chronic posttraumatic stress that represents the primary cluster of symptoms. With both the postconcussive and posttraumatic subsyndromes is typically an overlay of pain syndrome that may have physiologic and/or psychologic factors that affect the pain behavior. The focal residual syndrome involves focal dysfunction such as the development of episodic or paroxysmal atypical spells or seizure-type phenomena. These usually impact on the cerebral cortex or manifest as a pain syndrome.

POSTCONCUSSIVE SUBSYNDROME (PCCHITS) IN CHIT

The PCCHITS as described here refers to physical, cognitive, and psychological symptoms that typically occur concurrently following an alleged concussive episode. Since 1992, the clinical existence of postconcussive syndrome has obtained further verification and has become more widely accepted as a legitimate phenomenon (Gouvier, Cubic, Jones, Brantley, & Cutlip, 1992). Brown et al. (1994) more recently have suggested that there has been sufficient research generated to establish that postconcussive symptoms do occur and they have a predictable configuration. These are typically acute symptoms of nausea and/or vomiting, dizziness, blurred vision, ringing in the ears, problems with thinking clearly and quickly, and complaints of cervicocranial pain.

The concussive effect to the brain can occur with or without direct impact to the head, and there may be no documented loss of consciousness. There may be a transient change in consciousness with confusion and disorientation. This mild injury to the brain may not be observable on routine neurological examination, and typically CT and MRI scanning show no macroscopic findings. The injury underlying the PCCHITS is microscopic in nature and can occur diffusely throughout the brain. There is a high preponderance of involvement in the frontopolar, orbitofrontal, and anterior temporal regions of the brain. These areas are more susceptible to the effects of acceleration/deceleration, rotational, and coup/contrecoup injury, which is often the underlying pathophysiologic mechanism of the concussive episode. The PCCHITS develops primarily as a result of the disruption of normal brain functioning.

Physiologic Subgroup

Within the PC subsyndrome we distinguish those patients with focal neuropsychiatric signs from those with more generalized symptoms and complaints (Tucker & Neppe, 1994). Patients in this *physiologic subgroup* have more physical symptoms that predominate, although there may also be secondary cognitive and psychological features. These patients complain of posttraumatic headaches, myalgias, photophobia, dizziness, ringing in the ears, balance problems, numbness and tingling in the extremities, sleep disturbances, and often atypical disorientations or derealizations described as spells (Goodwin, 1989).

Cognitive Subgroup

We also see a *cognitive subgroup* of PCCHITS patients with primarily intellectual and cognitive changes upon initial presentation. These patients typically exhibit measurable deficits in attentional processes, sustained and focused concentration, memory, problem solving, cognitive flexibility, speed of information processing, and cognitive stamina. Although there may be concomitant psychological sequelae and physical symptoms along with pain problems, the chief complaints by patients are typically cognitive in nature.

Psychologic Subgroup

We also observe a *psychologic subgroup* of PC subsyndrome with predominantly psychological changes characterized by susceptibility to developing anxiety and depressive disorders, increased irritability, low frustration tolerance, emotional volatility, and a reduced ability to cope and deal with everyday life stressors. These patients present with a chief complaint of feeling different since the injury. They are typically aware of this perceived sense of change, and the changes are also observed by significant others.

POSTTRAUMATIC SUBSYNDROME IN CHIT (PTCHITS)

The posttraumatic subsyndrome represents a spectrum of posttraumatic symptoms commonly referred to within the context of *DSM–IV* as acute stress disorder and posttraumatic stress disorder. This constellation of symptoms is considered functional in nature and represents a psychological reactivity to the traumatic event. It is assumed that when an individual experiences trauma to the head during an event such as assault, moving vehicle accident, slip and fall, or other traumatic circumstances, there is the potential, inherent in these situations, for the development of predictable characteristic symptoms considered to be posttraumatic in nature.

The primary basis for the development of posttraumatic symptoms is a functional response by the individual to the traumatic event. There may be other physical findings associated with the event that may occur as a consequence of the trauma, but these are considered secondary with respect to etiology. It is obviously of clinical importance for the clinician to differentiate posttraumatic subsyndrome from postconcussive subsyndrome. Although many patients with postconcussive symptoms also may develop posttraumatic symptoms, clearly there are those patients, who experience trauma to the head, which is not concussive in nature, and present with minimal changes in intellectual and cognitive functioning, but seem to develop posttraumatic symptomatology.

The most appropriate methodology for differentiating this potential diagnostic overlap is to have the patient complete neuropsychological testing, in order to provide a more comprehensive diagnostic assessment of cognitive functioning. Patients with posttraumatic symptoms may have some cognitive difficulties, but not of the same frequency or intensity as patients who have experienced mild to moderate brain injury. Neuropsychological testing is fairly robust in being able to reveal primary cognitive impairment versus cognitive problems that may be associated with a posttraumatic disorder.

FOCAL RESIDUAL BRAIN SYNDROMES IN CHIT (FRCHITS)

There is a *frontal lobe syndrome* often seen within this psychologic subgroup of PCCHITS with more dramatic personality changes. This pattern of personality changes often becomes more observable as the acute effects of the PC injury resolve. These patients may lack the ability to be fully aware of how they have changed. They may seem indifferent and apathetic and may even describe themselves as being less bothered by the stresses and strains of life. These patients lack insight and become more passive. Amotivation is often a major problem. Alternatively, the frontal lobe manifestation may be an increase in aggressivity and explosive behavior. These patients exhibit diminished judgmental ability and are often described as impulsive. In both frontal lobe groups there may be measurable deficits in intellectual and cognitive functioning, for which the patient may only be minimally aware. Occasionally these patients exhibit frontal lobe release reflexes (e.g., pout, snout) on examination.

Seizure-like disorders and atypical spells fit within the framework of what Neppe and Blumer have called *paroxysmal neurobehavioral disorder* (Blumer & Neppe, in press). This is dealt with later.

Moreover, the central nervous system has a limited number of ways of responding to stressors and injuries. Consequently, similar behaviors are caused by a number of different etiologies.

FOCAL BRAIN INJURY AFTER TRANSIENT CLOSED HEAD INJURY

Neuropsychiatric evaluations should pay careful attention for the presence of focal episodic features that may be elicited by such instruments as regular wake–sleep electroencephalograms and ambulatory electroencephalograms but also clinically using such instruments as the INSET, BROCAS SCAN, and neurologic examination. Focal features that may appear after a CHIT include:

Visual object agnosia—left occipital.

Prosopagnosia—right temporal, old; right parietal, new.

Color agnosia—left occipital.

Simultognosia—left parieto-temporal-occipital.

Autotopagnosia—diffuse bilateral.

Visuospatial—right parietal.

Finger agnosia—left parietal.

Nominal aphasia—left parieto/temporal.

Gerstmann's syndrome of dysgraphia, dyscalculia, finger agnosia, right–left disturbance—left parietal.

Anosognosia—right parietal.

Hemisomatognosia—right parietal.

Unilateral inattention, unavailability, negligence—right parietal.

Right–left disturbance—left hemisphere.

MIXED SUBGROUP OF CHIT

Finally, there is a subgroup of PCCHITS with more classical postconcussive complaints representing the interactive and synergistic effects of physiologic, cognitive, and psychologic changes. This subgroup probably represents the greatest percentage of CHIT patients and the group most often encountered in general clinical practice. These patients may have focal residual features as well. We call them *MCHITS* or *mixed CHIT syndrome*.

This neuropsychiatric classification system provides a practical, clinical-based approach for beginning the evaluation process. An understanding of the differentiating features of CHITS can give the health care provider more specific direction when beginning evaluation. The predominant features of MCHITS presented during diagnostic interviewing can be classified and differentiated into more specific subcategories, which can be used to determine the specificity of the neuropsychiatric evaluation.

Most patients with primary psychiatric illness have some seeds of previous psychiatric symptoms in their histories. When the patient presents with a good premorbid social history, a good work history, and a warm and supportive family, and changes in behavior, particularly abrupt changes in personality, mood, or ability to function, occur after CHIT, the CHIT must be considered a prime etiologic candidate. Similarly, the patient who presents with rapid fluctuations in mental status or rapid variable motor behavior frequently suggests something other than the typical psychiatric disorders; it is unusual for schizophrenics to be hallucinating and delusional in the morning and clear in the afternoon (Neppe & Tucker, 1989).

THE TIME-BASED NEUROPSYCHIATRIC EVALUATION

Simply stated, the time-based evaluation presupposes that traditional evaluation procedures may not always be sufficient in properly understanding the etiology and manifestations of the CHITS. The traditional neuropsychiatric evaluation has routinely consisted of a diagnostic interview process, review of background information, mental status examination, and possibly some lab testing. This is often accomplished in a single session or over two sessions with the patient. If predominant cognitive sequelae exist, a referral to a neuropsychologist is often made.

The neuropsychologist or neuropsychiatrist in turn completes another one-time clinical interview, administers a battery of neuropsychological tests, reviews available medical and other pertinent records, and forms a clinical impression based on this limited time with the patient. At times, there may be additional collateral information obtained from significant others, usually obtained during a single session.

This traditional process of evaluation gives the clinician a sample of the patient's physical, cognitive, and psychological behavior that is essentially a snapshot view, much like the instant results obtained from the

Polaroid picture. The information obtained from this snapshot approach gives the clinician a small slice of how the patient is functioning at a given point in time. This represents a very limited sample of the patient's behavior.

Yet as health care providers, we continue to evaluate patients with CHITS in this way, and we make inferential leaps and generalizations affecting our conclusions and our recommendations. Although this approach may be sufficient in assessing many clinical syndromes, it can lead to many false positives and false negatives within the population of head trauma patients. The current database of research findings and multidisciplinary clinical experience would suggest that this snapshot approach does not give the evaluator enough information to clearly understand the dynamics presented in many patients with CHIT.

There are obviously many cases of CHIT where the findings derived from a single snapshot approach to evaluation will be sufficient to make appropriate recommendations. However, clinical experience has shown that there is often a need to defer final clinical impression until the clinician has had more time with the patient. This is encountered frequently among clinicians who work with the head injured patient on a daily basis.

When clinicians begin the evaluation process with a patient, we often make underlying assumptions with respect to the patient's abilities as a historian. We usually collect our data directly from the patient's report. We fail to realize that with patients experiencing head trauma symptoms, there is usually a diminished ability to be aware of oneself, and insight is often reduced. Furthermore, there are concurrent deficits in expressive speech that limit the patients in their attempts to completely express the full range of their ideas and recollections about their functioning. These patients almost always complain of difficulty expressing their thoughts and ideas and formulating a self-analysis of their behavior. When the very part of us as human beings that we refer to as "self" is experienced as changed because of underlying pathophysiological disruption, it is difficult to fully appreciate the meaning and effects of this change, let alone try to express this clearly and cogently during the brief time period of diagnostic interviewing. We must always remember that when we refer to head trauma we are also referring to trauma to the mind and its ability to experience and cope with the aftereffects of the trauma and in turn communicate these aftereffects to health care providers.

When these patients present their complex constellation of physical, cognitive, and psychological changes following head trauma, the clinician needs to give them the time to render a comprehensive self-report. Because of diminished awareness and insight, a patient may not be able to fully convey the qualitative aspects of his or her complaints. The patients also may not be able to remember everything they need to tell the provider.

Memory problems are typically one of the chief complaints in the CHIT syndrome. This makes it difficult for patients to organize and recall their experience of changes in their perception of self.

With a time-based approach, we interact with the patient over a number of sessions, allowing for the time to obtain a filmstrip version of the patient's experiences, symptoms, and complaints. This approach minimizes the tendency to over- or underdiagnose and increases the validity and reliability of the data collected from the diagnostic interviewing.

The clinician gathers data from a variety of the patient's life experiences over time and establishes greater validity to the spectrum of symptomatology. Patterns of symptoms and complaints become clearer as the patient interacts within the familial, social, and occupational environment over the course of days and weeks. The health care provider begins to obtain a time-based sample from the diverse topography of everyday life. This topographic elicitation of symptom manifestation within the context of the patient's personal ecology of life circumstances gives a three-dimensional perspective of symptomatology over time, across situations, and within different environments. We refer to this as time-based topographic validity. More simply stated, this validity is based on the presupposition that there is no substitute for time when it comes to case formulation of the dynamics involved in CHIT.

Over the course of time spent with the patient, we advocate utilizing a variety of assessment procedures to attempt to substantiate the patterns of physical, cognitive, and psychological problems being presented.

In essence, premorbid and predisposing features are often missed with single evaluations. Undetected problems are regarded as not existing instead of not diagnosed because evaluations are too short. In some instances, particular conditions are especially undiagnosed: In our experience, many have complex partial seizures (CPSzs) that remain undetected, and moreover, false reassurance by practitioners doing such single or cursory evaluations ultimately may harm the patient: The condition is not diagnosed and the patient regards his or her symptoms as psychological when there is a good physical base. Moreover, sometimes when symptoms have persisted over months, the patient is investigated neuroradiologically and when no positive findings are found, this is in error could be regarded as proof of the posttraumatic syndrome etiology and the absence of organicity. In actuality, invariably changes that may have been detected neuroradiologically early on in the first month no longer can be found, and this implies not psychological etiology but incorrect timing of the neuroradiologic evaluation.

Finally, we emphasize the real-world approach. Neuropsychological testing in a quiet office, with encouragement and one-on-one testing with one single task at a time, may be insensitive to the subtle changes that a bustling office of multitasked demands may bring. Many people require such multitasking in their regular occupation (e.g., physicians).

EVALUATION

The following is a regular model that we follow for a Comprehensive Complex Neuropsychiatric Evaluation in CHIT. It includes several time-based interviews allowing a longitudinal perspective with several cross-sectional views, including detailed history; physical and neurologic examination; mental status and cerebral cortical examination; testing including ASH, MMPI, SCL-90, INSET BROCAS SCAN, FMMSE, NRBRPS; and electroencephalography and labs, as required.

The patient is seen on several occasions (usually four to six) for comprehensive consultation. In general, the following order is followed:

On the first meeting, the major focus is the main complaint, focus of referral, a detailed pharmacologic history, and history of investigations and of associated features.

On the second meeting, more details about medical history are obtained, as well as physical and neurologic examination.

The third evaluation includes integration of test results and provisional diagnosis.

The fourth evaluation stresses recommendations and pharmacologic treatment options and also includes feedback.

Further consultations have a focus on symptom and etiology removal through psychopharmacologic integration and/or responsiveness, as well as any further details pertaining to tests or clinical information that have come to light later.

Mental status is assessed on each occasion.

At the conclusion, an extremely detailed report is produced reflecting historical data, medical evaluation, examination of higher brain functions, and investigation information. This allows for a detailed multiaxial neuropsychiatric diagnosis and a road map for present and future management, both pharmacologic and nonpharmacologic. To facilitate the report being properly read, although all areas may be important, some areas are emphasized in italics, and there are tables of investigations, pharmacology, and diagnosis; the recommendations headers allow quicker initial perspective on our findings.

The following order of the report is followed, which reflects information obtained, mostly following a solid medical and psychological history and examination model.

1. Major dates of evaluation are noted and codes relating to duration and complexity noted.

2. Demographic information is listed in as complete a fashion as possible as listed in Table 10.1.

3. Basic medical information *is elicited from several* sources of information: (a) Referring physician with date of discussion, report, referral reason and core issues. (b) Detailed notes from other medical colleagues and psychologists are requested and when available examined. (c) Family members are interviewed as to their perception of the problems and any observations they may have made. In possible seizure disorders, particularly, this is critical because even patients who are excellent historians may not be aware of certain events happening to them. (d) Information is then obtained directly from the patient.

4. *Main complaints* of patient and reason for the consultation are amplified. This is described in the patient's own words, as well as elicited listings and details of the main complaints of patient. This follows with history of main complaint, age of onset of each problem including the CHIT, history of current and past functionality, family history both psychiatric and neurologic, and the patient's self-perceived positive strengths.

5. A *special investigation history* follows. Specifically elicited are details on previous investigations such as EEGs, MRIs Head, CTs Head, SPECTs Head, PETs Head, spinal tap, neuroradiological procedures in the neck and back, electromyography and nerve conduction studies, electrocardiograms, polysomnography, Minnesota Multiphasic Personality Inventory (MMPI), and neuropsychological testing. When available, source material is examined. These tests often suggest that the CHIT was not the first major neuropsychiatric event the patient encountered.

6. *Blood and urine tests* are ordered during the course of the evaluation unless they have already been done. The following blood tests are the most usual procedures in CHIT, often done to eliminate or diagnose alternative or additional conditions: erythrocyte sedimentation rate, glucose, serology and HIV status, renal functions, electrolytes, complete blood count, vitamin B_{12}, folate, electrolytes (sodium, potassium, chloride, magnesium, bicarbonate, calcium, phosphate), hepatic functions, lipid profile (cholesterol, triglycerides, low-density lipoprotein [LDL], high-density lipoprotein [HDL]), and neuroendocrine status including thyroid functions (thyroid-stimulating hormone [TSH], thyroxin, and T_3) and sometimes adrenal status (cortisol) and pituitary and gonadal screens (prolactin, follicle-stimulating hormone [FSH], testosterone). It is usually sufficient to test the patient's urine biochemically at the office level for

TABLE 10.1
Demographic Information

Name					
Date of birth	Age	Sex	Social Security #		
Phone number	Home area:		Home language	Ethnicity	
Pharmacy name and phone:					
# Marriages:	Marital status:		Current relationship in years:		# children:
# children at home:					
Education and formal training:					
Occupation and current employment status					
Religion and religiosity:					
Referral physician and follow-up physician					
Allergies to medication	None mentioned.				
Insurance					
Spouse's occupation	Formal training and employment status		Employed		

protein, glucose, ketones, pH, blood, and bilirubin. If these are normal, and the patient has no genitourinary symptoms, one need not progress to sending urine specimens away for cell examination and microscopy, culture and sensitivity.

7. *Pharmacologic history* is the next critical area. Current medications are listed, and these frequently on first interview have not been prescribed by the evaluating physician, complicating interpretations because there is a need to rely on the patient or family as a historian. This constitutes a record of other medications for baseline and information purposes. The duration of each, onset of prescription, varied dosages, and combinations at varied times in the recent past are elicited. Degree of responsiveness and side effects are critically detailed and onset and offset of these effects are noted. Later interpretations as to whether events were drug related are made. Family history of response and nonresponse to specific medications and allergies and side effects are also listed. Differentiation of generic and trade preparations is made. The pharmacologic history ultimately leads to the most critical single determining factor for recommendations, so that this is done in great detail. A similar process is followed for spontaneously eliciting information pertaining to what the patient previously was taking. From this the patient's and also family members' opinions are elicited as to what medications the client did best with and did worst with historically.

Thereafter the patient is asked to complete a rather lengthy questionnaire listing all known commonly used psychotropics, pain medications, hormones, anticonvulsants, and muscle relaxants and even asking about experimental agents. Known common side effects are asked about, as well as any positive responses to medication. Dosage, duration of treatment, and therapeutic effects are also emphasized (Table 10.2). Again responsiveness and compliance are elicited with regard to each medication, as well as general impressions of best responsiveness and improving compliance.

8. *Nonprescription and recreational drug abuse history* is then elicited using the same principles as before. Duration, combinations, dosage, effects both good and bad, side effects, compliance, addictiveness, and dependency issues are all asked about. Relevant is the way the patient handled the specific recreational drug and whether this may have predisposed to the CHIT or its consequent severity.

9. *Nonprescription drugs* specifically asked about include all the varieties of marijuana, LSD, amphetamines, mescaline, cocaine, phencyclidine, heroin, and narcotics. Additionally, critical to the evaluation are the impacts of alcohol, caffeine, cigars, pipes, cigarettes, and other more socially acceptable, legal drugs of abuse.

All the preceding information (items 1–9) is generally elicited on first interview. Later consultations commonly amplify such information.

10. *Neuropsychiatric symptomatology* is then evaluated. Originally the measuring instrument used was the Neppe Temporal Lobe Questionnaire, derived from researching the symptoms of temporal lobe dysfunction from the literature, as most of the major historical organic brain symptoms as opposed to physical signs derive from or impinge on the temporal lobe. This was later revised to a new instrument, which we routinely use on all patients, namely, the Inventory of Neppe of Symptoms of Epilepsy and the Temporal Lobe (INSET). This is a paper-and-pencil test amplified by a detailed face-to-face interview. The INSET involves screening for possible temporal-lobe, epileptic, and organic symptoms and spells. Thereafter the symptoms are categorized into several headers: nonspecific symptoms, possible and controversial temporal-lobe symptoms, seizure related, and other focal features. The test is based on the subject and/or the subject's family responding to questions, which are thereafter elaborated in greater clinical detail. The INSET is contained in Appendix 1 and is a copyrighted instrument. The INSET has two sections: a broad demographic and screening section, and a second specific question section where responses are at two time levels—current, plus the most common frequency in the remote past. The patient ranks frequency from "never" through "more than daily" (i.e., 0–6). Questions in the INSET have been based on the earlier Neppe Temporal Lobe Questionnaire, which itself derived from an intensive literature review on the topic (Neppe, 1983a, 1983b, 1984a, 1984b).

TABLE 10.2
Medications Screen

Buspirone (Buspar)

Beta-blockers: nadolol (Corgard), propranolol (Inderal), atenolol (Tenormin), pindolol (Visken)

Alpha-adrenergic agents: clonidine (Catapres), guanfacine (Tenex)

Lithium carbonate (Eskalith, Lithobid, and others)

Hormones: thyroxin (Synthroid), triiodothyronine (liothyronine, Cytomel), thyroglobulin (Proloid), thyroid (Armour thyroid), bovine thyroid, prednisone, cortisone, androgens, estrogen (Premarin, Estrace, Ogen, Estratab), progesterone (Provera)

Anticonvulsants:
 Carbamazepine (Tegretol)
 Valproate (Depakote as divalproex sodium)
 Phenytoin (Dilantin)
 Lomotrigine (Lamictal)
 Gabapentin (Neurontin)
 Phenobarbital (Donnatal)

Antidepressants:
 Tricyclic antidepressants: nortriptyline (Pamelor), amitriptyline (Elavil), imipramine (Tofranil), desipramine (Norpramin), doxepin (Sinequan), clomipramine (Anafranil), trimipramine (Surmontil)
 Serotonin reuptake inhibitors: fluoxetine (Prozac), sertraline (Zoloft), paroxetine (Paxil), fluvoxamine (Luvox)
 Non-SSRI, non-TCA antidepressants: venlafaxine (Effexor), nefazodone (Serzone), trazodone (Desyrel), bupropion (Wellbutrin)
 Monoamine oxidase inhibitors: phenelzine (Nardil), tranylcypromine (Parnate), isocarboxazid (Marplan)

Other psychotropics
 Benzodiazepines: lorazepam (Ativan), alprazolam (Xanax), clonazepam (Klonopin), chlordiazepoxide (Librium), diazepam (Valium), triazolam (Halcion), Clorazepate (Tranxene)
 Neuroleptics: haloperidol (Haldol), chlorpromazine (Thorazine), perphenazine (Trilafon), trifluoperazine (Stelazine), thioridazine (Mellaril), thiothixene (Navane), pimozide (Orap), risperidone (Risperdal), fluphenazine (Prolixin) for use psychiatrically, or prochlorperazine (Compazine), metoclopramide (Reglan) for use for nausea or gastroesophageal reflux for prolonged periods of time

Zolpidem tartrate (Ambien)

Melatonin

Psychostimulants: methylphenidate (Ritalin), deanol (Deaner), pemoline (Cylert), dextroamphetamine (Dextrostat)

Antiparkinsonian/Anticholinergic agents: benztropine (Cogentin), trihexyphenidyl (Artane), biperiden (Akineton), orphenadrine (Norflex), levodopa/carbidopa (Sinemet), bromocriptine (Parlodel), amantadine (Symmetrel), hyoscyamine (Levsin), diphenhydramine (Benadryl), pergolide (Permax), selegeline (Eldepryl)

Antimigraine/headache/pain and other preparations:
 codeine, Ergotamine (Ergostat) (with caffeine Cafergot), cyproheptadine (Periactin), dihydroergotamine (DHE), sumatriptan (Imatrex), ibuprofen (Motrin), methysergide (Sansert), verapamil (Calan, Isoptin), diltiazem (Cardizem), other experimental psychotropic agents

---

The INSET listed in Appendix 1 is actually the Short INSET. This is a noncomputerized version not going into detail into any specific positive answers, although the scoresheet is completed rather clumsily on computer. Another more detailed instrument that should be computerized but currently is not is the Long INSET. This is derived from the items of the Short INSET but with detailed amplification. We have not found this noncomputerized form of practical utility, and there are enormous costs to convert it to a more useful computerized version. The INSET plus medical history are major determining factors as to whether to order follow-up specialized electroencephalograms such as an ambulatory EEG in the CHIT patient.

11. *Examples of uncommon paper-and-pencil neuropsychiatric instruments.* We have also developed several less commonly used paper-and-pencil neuropsychiatric instruments which are applied when appropriate. One is the *Neppe narcolepsy screen,* which has not been well researched. Narcolepsy is a rare condition itself (incidence possibly one in several thousand individuals). However, the questionnaire is far more versatile, probing sleep disturbance as well as anomalistic experiences, and these are common in the CHIT patient. Unfortunately, the questionnaire needs to be scored by paper and pencil at this stage and there are no norms, so that although highly relevant history information is obtained at a clinical level, a clinician needs to interpret the results.

The *Neppe Déjà Vu Questionnaires* are other screening history instruments seldom used in clinical practice. However, the major value of this well-validated instrument is to demonstrate how we cannot interpret symptoms not elicited in detail as the same. Using a phenomenological analysis, Neppe was able to demonstrate that the symptom of déjà vu, commonly regarded as symptomatic of temporal lobe epilepsy, indeed had a very special phenomenologic quality in patients with temporal-lobe epilepsy (Neppe, 1983a). This involves its association with postictal features such as sleepiness, headache, and clouded consciousness and its link in time with these features. This association provides an excellent clue to the existence of temporal lobe epilepsy, but déjà vu is a normal phenomenon occurring in 70% of the population, and unless such phenomenological detail is obtained, patients' symptomatology may be misinterpreted (Neppe, 1983a). Neppe similarly did such a study with olfactory hallucinations (Neppe, 1983b, 1984b). A specific type of temporal-lobe epilepsy olfactory hallucination could not be demonstrated, although there were suggestive features. A major message, therefore, may be the relevance of adequately assessing in detail the symptomatology of patients presenting with CHIT. If déjà vu occurs, temporal-lobe epileptic déjà vu must be specifically sought. Such detail may be as relevant as electroencephalographic monitoring (Neppe, 1983a).

12. *Historical Base.* The next consultation interview series focuses on increasing databases obtained by questionnaires and computers. This develops the longitudinal perspective of change over time, again essential in head injury patients to understand predisposing features. Any program involving detailed historical and medical responses should be adequate. At the Pacific Neuropsychiatric Institute we use information based on the patient's responses to the Automated Social History, the ASH, which has over 300 demographic, personal, social, and family history items, medical and psychiatric history questions, questions pertaining to recreation and drug misuse, and self-esteem items. It derived from assessments in the prison and justice system. Added to the ASH are more than 100 medical and pharmacologic questions that we developed at the Pacific Neuropsychiatric Institute. These produce an automated report, and significant time is then spent checking data and amplifying all positive information. The automated report has significant limitations, partly due to the way the answers in the ASH program are written, as well as insufficient detail. Particular attention should be paid to clarifying for example current and previous misuse of recreational drugs. Moreover, this cautious interpretation in regard to histories of alcohol and drug use sometimes produce automated interpretations based on group symptoms, which can be misconstrued where patterns of behavior unrelated to alcohol or drug use may be misinterpreted as linked. Results are then combined in general with additional tests and further detailed clarification done thereafter. The responses should be interpreted with care as the questions asked are broad and the possibility exists of incorrect information, particularly as patients may not be computer sophisticated or may make errors in answering paper-and-pencil forms. This is another reason for checking all positive data.

13. *Psychological and psychiatric diagnostic evaluations.* At this stage, the evaluation shifts to more formal standardized evaluations. Routinely at our institute, we evaluate patients using two computerized psychological instruments: the MMPI or its adolescent version, and the Symptom Check List 90 (SCL-90). There is strong support to use personality evaluations, and some would debate that the Millon Clinical Multiaxial Inventory (MCMI) should be used instead of or in addition to the MMPI. We believe it useful to screen current psychological symptoms—hence the use of the SCL-90. We do not find this an ideal instrument and recognize its significant limitations both in lack of detail and in selectivity of questions. Both these tests are not well standardized in the brain injured populations, but with the INSET and other organic screens (e.g., BROCAS SCAN, discussed later), we believe they are valuable. We have also considered adding the SCID to our instrumentation. We precede the test discussions with some background.

ASSESSMENT OF PERSONALITY

Within the head trauma population, perhaps the area that is the most difficult to understand for both patient and provider, and often the most complex, is the assessment of personality. Early research in this area (Thomsen, 1974) revealed that families of head trauma patients reported changes in personality to be more of a burden to them than residual physical problems. Goethe and Levin (1984) concluded that family complaints about head injured patients center around personality and behavior changes rather than physical disabilities, and family tensions typically increase with time, even up to 2 years following an injury.

Assessing potential changes in personality obviously cannot be accomplished properly within an hour or hour-and-a-half diagnostic interview with the patient. Understanding the subtle yet complex changes that can occur in personality dynamics following head trauma is primarily the basis for advocating a time-based evaluation process. Far too often, misdiagnosis is made with respect to the presence or absence of personality disorders. As clinicians, we simply need to humble ourselves and not be so quick to make clinical judgments based on limited time with the patient.

In the 1970s through the 1980s, the epidemiological, neurological, and neuropsychological evaluation of minor traumatic head injury produced a greater awareness of the changes that can occur in intellectual and cognitive functioning. In the 1990s there continued to be research generated on the definitions and neuropsychological aspects of minor head trauma (Alves et al., 1993; Cohadon et al., 1991; Esselman & Uomoto, 1995; Kibby & Long, 1996; Lowdon et al., 1989). There was, however, much less research and clinical literature written on the neuropsychiatric aspects of head trauma. McAllister (1992) discussed neuropsychiatric sequelae of head trauma in terms of pathophysiology, cognitive sequelae, behavior, effects of age, and treatment. Also, recent studies emphasizing personality issues following head trauma have increased our awareness of the need to understand this aspect of the head trauma spectrum (Middleboe, Birket-Smith, Anderson, & Friis, 1992; Miller, 1992). There is a great need within the health profession to appreciate the subtle yet significant changes in personality that can occur with head trauma, and to get beyond the purely clinical aspects of assessing these changes to recognize the trauma to the self. Clinicians who work day in and day out with head trauma patients will attest to the difficulties these patients experience when their equilibrium of self has been altered by trauma and brain injury.

In addressing this issue, it must be reiterated that to fully evaluate these changes in personality takes time. Initially, the patients are often preoccupied with problems with pain and are not yet aware of changes in themselves. As recovery progresses, there is more awareness of the cognitive and psychological problems. When patients begin to feel better physically, they attempt to get back in the swing of things, and this is usually the time period when they begin to notice that they do not feel the same. As cognitive sequelae resolve, they return to work and reintegrate into social and leisure activities. However, continued reduction in tolerance, irritability, emotional volatility, and mental and emotional fatigue are experienced on a daily basis.

These subtle residuals are typically difficult to assess in the clinical setting. Yet, time spent with these patients will often reveal the struggle they experience in trying to cope with everyday life. They are constantly reminded by the difficulties they encounter that they have changed and that they feel different. There is often a longing to be like they used to be and get their life back to what it used to be. But the truth of the matter is that many of these patients will never regain the old self and be able to capture the sense of being who they were.

Patients with more dysfunctional personality styles often develop secondary psychiatric problems, which can considerably complicate the clinical picture. This psychological overlay is often misjudged by inexperienced health providers as simply a manifestation of a personality disorder, when in fact it is a manifestation of impaired coping and the expression of futility at being unable to deal with life effectively. There is the constant experience of reduced cognitive stamina even though many frank cognitive symptoms have resolved. This usually takes the form of inability to keep up with the demands of life and inability to enjoy the process of living. There is often an anhedonic experience of going through the motions of living but without the ability to fully enjoy life events. These patients will often feel like they are on the outside looking in and not really participating. They feel detached and surrealistic about living.

Patients with a primary concussive injury and patients with predominant posttraumatic reaction can experience these changes in their sense of self. As a starting point for adequately assessing these issues, it is usually helpful to have a psychological consultation incorporating some standardized, objective measures such as the MMPI–2 and the MCMI–III (Millon Clinical Multiaxial Inventory). This is useful in differentiating predominantly posttraumatic symptomatology from postconcussive complaints. The MMPI–2 is helpful in assessing primary features of psychological functioning and can be supplemented with the MCMI–III to gain a more in-depth analysis of personality traits and style. This can guide the clinician in how to approach treatment. Patients with more extreme elevations on the MMPI–2 are typically experiencing greater distress and there may be a need for psychopharmacologic intervention. Examining personality style from the MCMI–III can give the clinician valuable information on how the expression of symptomatology will be seen by others and the relative strengths and weaknesses in personality structure.

Minnesota Multiphasic Personality Inventory

We use the adult clinical system interpretive report (based on several authors; we have been using Butcher's broad interpretations and modifying from there).

The MMPI–2 interpretation can serve as a useful source of hypotheses about patients. This report is based on objectively derived scale indexes and scale interpretations that have been developed in diverse groups of patients. The personality descriptions, inferences, and recommendations still need to be verified by other sources of clinical information because individual patients may not fully match the prototype. Moreover, the interpretations are based on statistically quantified results, and every individual is different enough to allow only relative norms. Some of the questions of the MMPI are difficult to answer yes or no to, which further complicates individual interpretation. Additionally, diagnostic hypotheses generated by the MMPI are only relevant in the appropriate clinical context.

Adolescent Minnesota Multiphasic Personality Inventory

This is the adolescent clinical system interpretive report (again, e.g., based on Butcher).

The Adolescent MMPI–2 interpretation can serve as a useful source of hypotheses about teenage patients in the age range 13 through 18 years. Outside this range, cautious interpretations should be made with the awareness that the test is technically invalid or of limited validity. This report is again based on objectively derived scale indexes and scale interpretations that have been developed in diverse groups of patients and that need to be verified by other sources of clinical information because individual patients may not fully match the prototype.

Symptom Checklist 90–R (Derogatis)

The SCL-90–R is a multidimensional self-report inventory developed by Leonard Derogatis. It was designed as a screening instrument for psychopathology in psychiatric, medical, and nonpatient populations. The scoring profile is expressed in percentile rankings across the 90 items, and following this is the Derogatis interpretation of scores. For patients below age 19 years, cautious interpretations should be made with the awareness that the test is technically invalid or of limited validity. Again, the interpretations are based on statistically quantified results, and every individual is different enough to allow only relative norms. Some of the questions of the SCL-90 are difficult to answer, which further complicates individual interpretation. In our experience, many patients are interpreted as having obsessive-compulsive symptoms on this test, probably far more than are warranted. Additionally, diagnostic hypotheses generated by the SCL-90 are only relevant in the appropriate clinical context.

MCMI–III—The Millon

The MCMI–III can be a rich source of information regarding how a given patient may be contributing to the postconcussive or posttraumatic syndrome by the way the patient may be reacting to injury and its effects. This clinical data often gives valuable insight into areas of personality vulnerability, which are usually attenuated after head trauma. When used in combination with the MMPI–2, a more comprehensive basis for understanding personality issues can be laid, with hypotheses being made for further evaluation.

It should be pointed out that traditional interpretative approaches for the MMPI–2 and MCMI–III are inadequate and often lead to erroneous conclusions when applied to the head trauma population. Too often, computerized printouts of MMPI–2 and MCMI–III results are misused by clinicians unfamiliar with the dynamics of head trauma, and these patients are assessed inaccurately. Interpretation of these psychological instruments should be made within the context of background information, details of the injury event, symptomatology, and collateral information. Psychological assessment should be considered a starting point and not the only source of evaluation.

The MMPI–2 and MCMI–III are also useful in understanding issues of symptom magnification and exaggeration or minimization of symptoms. These issues are usually inherent in medicolegal cases. Both the MMPI–2 and the MCMI–III can be helpful in detecting a mind set toward overreporting or underreporting symptomatology. Verifying these issues is difficult, and a conservative approach should be taken. Clinicians should look to the overall case presentation when making clinical judgment regarding the intentions of a given patient during an evaluation process.

Underreporting of symptoms can often be related to the denial that is seen in patients with head trauma. These patients are acutely aware of problems in cognitive and psychological functioning, but often minimize these problems, hoping they will just go away. During a cursory initial clinical interview, the clinician can be misled into concluding that the patients are not in any significant distress, when in actuality they are often presenting themselves in a favorable light because it is too difficult for them to admit to the type of symptoms they are experiencing. Patients are often embarrassed to admit to having problems in their cognitive functioning. There is also a tendency to minimize problems with irritability, emotional volatility, and reduced tolerance, as these problems may not be consistent with how they would like things to be. When there is consistency between psychological testing and clinical impression, this issue can be the catalyst to initiate a realistic acceptance of these problem areas so that recovery can be further facilitated.

On the other hand, overreporting of symptomatology is a much debated issue whenever there are potential sources of secondary gain, such as the case being in litigation. After ruling out other possible explanations of extreme elevations in clinical profiles from the MMPI–2 and less often the MCMI–III, the clinician can often detect this mind set toward exaggeration and be in a better position to explain the basis of persisting symptoms. This issue is almost always a part of the postconcussive spectrum and should be thoroughly evaluated. More often than not, patients may be magnifying symptoms rather than outright malingering. In addition, many patients magnify symptoms because of their need to convince the clinician that they really are having a legitimate problem. Intentional magnification of symptomatology is far less common than typically thought of among health care professionals and the legal community. Again, it should be pointed out that clarifying these issues takes time, and the most valid and reliable assessment of underreporting or overreporting, regardless of the results of psychological testing, is to see the patient over a number of sessions to document the consistency of their symptom presentation.

We now resume listing items of inventory.

14. *Relevant medical history data.* A detailed screening medical history involving specific medical systems such as neurologic, cardiovascular, respiratory, genitourinary, gastrointestinal, endocrine, and musculoskeletal systems (including pains) is then taken. Information in this regard is based on any basic medical textbook and is not further amplified here, although, of course, any positive features should be followed through. Allergy history is also elicited, as well as injuries including the CHIT that may be the current main complaint. For most patients this should be performed by a medical practitioner, although nurses and physicians' assistants often obtain this history. The requirement is obvious but worth emphasizing, as often psychiatrists particularly ignore taking a detailed medical history and miss critical information.

15. *Physical examination.*

16. *Neurologic examination, included in physical examination.* A single physical examination, generally on our second time-based examination, is then performed. Factors that may vary from time to time, such as labile

blood pressure, tachycardic pulse, areas of tenderness, and limitations in movement, may be repeated on several occasions. The neurological examination is particularly critical and part of the physical examination.

The following would reflect a prototype negative physical and neurological examination listed here to cover all the areas of such an evaluation:

General

Well-developed, well-nourished person.

Looks age, in no acute physical distress.

Blood pressure 125/85 (sitting, left arm).

Pulse (radial) 72/min, rhythmic, reasonable volume, pedal pulses palpable, no cranial or cervical bruits.

Weight 154 lbs, height is 5 ft 9 in.

Respiratory rate is 18/minute.

Scars: none.

Color is good—not pale, cyanotic, jaundiced or plethoric.

Extremities reveal no clubbing or edema.

Specific

Mouth, nose, and face appear within normal limits.

No masses in the neck.

No lymphadenopathy.

Skin is within normal limits—supple and not dry, no significant skin lesions.

Hair development appropriate.

Heart reveals regular sinus rhythm without murmurs, rubs, or gallops and grossly of normal size.

Lungs are clear.

Abdomen reveals no masses.

Neurological examination

Mental status: Alert. Clear consciousness. See next item for detail.

Cranial nerves: The cranial nerves appear intact.

Smelt 3/3.

Ophthalmoscopic exam reveals sharp disks bilaterally.

Vision is adequate grossly bilaterally.

Visual fields are full on both sides.

Pupils are equal and react consensually and to accommodation. No nystagmus.

Eye movements are full. Maintains closed eyes against pressure.

Facial sensation broadly intact.

No facial asymmetries.

Normal Weber and Rinne tests. Hearing is appropriate.

Gag reflex intact.

Palatal movements are appropriate and symmetrical.

Speech does not exhibit dysarthric elements.

Trapezius strength normal.

Tongue movements adequate.

Motor exam:

Gait is within normal limits. With ambulation, there is normal arm swing.

Tandem walk forward is within normal limits. Tandem walk backward is within normal limits.

There is normal facial expressivity.

No tremor at rest even with clenching and activation tests. No intention tremor.

Finger-nose-finger testing is normal. Tapping is normal.

No involuntary movements are noted facially, axially or trunkally.

Posture is within normal limits grossly neurologically.

Gets up from a chair without using hands without difficulty.

There is normal tone in the limbs. No clonus can be elicited.

Motor strength appears within normal limits peripherally and axially.

Reflexes:

There are no altered postural reflexes.

Deep tendon reflexes are symmetrical and within normal limits.

Down-going toes to plantar stimulation, and absent primitive reflexes—pout, snout, palmomental. There is no Romberg.

Sensory exam:

Normal light touch, proprioception and vibration in toes, limbs, and face.

Graphesthesia is within normal limits, simultognosis visual and tactile is within normal limits, two point discrimination is within normal limits.

17. *Mental status examination.* Just as neurologic evaluation is critical to finding subtle deficits, mental status evaluation is the key to a successful

psychiatric evaluation and can reflect pathology that may be symptomatic of the CHIT. This is performed sequentially on several occasions along the time-based examination. There are many different ways of performing the mental status examination in neuropsychiatry. No one technique is necessarily better than another. We approach mental status by making sure the major aspects are prioritized. The special structure involves mnemonics as a helpful means to recall items otherwise forgotten.

In mental status evaluations, the special skill is to be as flexible as possible. Some mental status headings are ambiguous, as you can, for example, describe certain signs under a person's appearance and very often, the same features could equally well relate to the patient's affect—the appearance of the patient may be sad, and that same sadness should be picked up with regard to the person's emotions.

The mental status examination in psychiatry is the equivalent of the physical examination in general medicine. Both logically follow the taking of a medical history. This elicits as much information as possible and prioritizes what needs to be evaluated; then you examine the patient. There is a fundamental difference, however: Much of the psychiatric examination is performed by taking a history—this is a special skill itself, as the two functions of history and examination are therefore performed simultaneously and sequentially.

Often the mental status examination is confused with history taking. For example, when the patient gives historical information, he or she may not admit to any hallucinations; this may or may not be true; and this is not part of the mental status examination. It is part of the mental status *evaluation*. It is clearly important to inquire about hallucinatory experiences, but asking about hallucinatory experience may get the response, "No, I never hear voices," when the patient is floridly hallucinating. The patient may or may not tell you about the voices he or she is hearing. Alternatively, the patient may describe voices he or she does not hear to ensure conscious or unconscious gains like admission to hospital (and a warm bed and caring environment) as well as fulfilling dependency needs. In the CHIT patient, where medicolegal facets are often relevant, particular attention should be paid to possible dissimulation or malingering.

We should distinguish between the *historical mental status evaluation*, which consists of the symptom cluster descriptions relevant to mental status, and the *mental status examination*, that component of evaluation often relating to the historical data but eliciting physical signs about mental status.

History taking involves probing. This is often facilitated by basic techniques or maneuvers that occur during the interview. Very often, history taking involves eliciting both symptoms and signs; to do so, the skilled examiner, as required by the demands of the situation, shifts his or her

TABLE 10.3
Mental Status Examination

A	Appearance: impact?	
C	Consciousness = psychiatry/medical ward?	
C	Cognition = diagnosis of psychopathology?	
L	Lesion localization: neuropsychiatric?	
A	Affect: Severity Index?	
I	Insight and judgment: psychosis?	
M	Motor-motivation: success? labeling?	
E	Ego-environment: psychotherapy?	
D	Danger-disability: hospital?	

interaction with the patient. This involves performing frequent probes, and keenly observing the response that results. These have both content and process components.

The single major mnemonic for mental status is ACCLAIMED (Table 10.3). In the CHIT we evaluate the nine major subheadings of AC-CLAIMED. These nine major subheadings imply the essence of every facet of the mental status examination. The order of this mnemonic was empirically derived from the most logical direction to do the mental status examination; it is not contrived with headings made to fit the mnemonic. ACCLAIMED constitutes a priority system for the larger of the headings of mental status examination.

The following is an example of a normal mental status examination in a high-functioning CHIT patient without posttraumatic features.

Appearance—well dressed and appropriately groomed; posture is within normal limits psychiatrically; gait shows no special psychiatric overtones; see neurologic exam.

Speech—Coherent and relevant. Normal rate, intensity, prosody and inflections.

Consciousness is clear. Orientated for time, place, person, space and passage of time.

Cognition: Intelligence appears in the normal range. Within that framework: Normal concentration.

Content of thinking is normal and appropriate for the interactional context: not overtly hallucinated.

Expressed no delusional ideation.

The patient's ability to abstract is reasonable.

Able to move well between topics.

Normal associations—quantity appropriate, logical links.

The patient describes no current rituals, obsessive or intrusive thoughts.

No overt malingering.

Registration, retention, recall, and recognition are all normal.

Lesion localization: In the BROCAS SCAN evaluation of higher cerebral cortical functioning.

Affect: anxiety level appropriate, normal autonomic reactivity based on blood pressure, pulse, sweating components, not overtly distressed, not exhibiting helplessness or uncertainty

The patient's affect is appropriate, not distressed, congruous and euthymic.

Normal level confrontativeness at times.

No major alienation of affect.

Affect quality is stable—nonlabile and nonblunted

Insight and judgment: Not psychotically impaired, reasonable judgment.

Ego syntonic for suffering and aware of difficulties.

No major ego-boundary distortions.

Motivation and motoric behavior:

No psychomotor retardation. Agitation level is within normal limits.

Impulse control: adequate.

Appears motivated for treatment.

Long-term goals are reasonable.

Environmental interaction: Normal level distress, appropriate withdrawal, responds to encouragement, able to experience warmth.

Makes reasonable eye contact.

Compliance with medication should be reasonable.

Adequate perspective at this time on problems.

Dangerousness:

Suicide risk—appears low at this time and probable average long-term risk for this condition.

Does not give evidence for homicidal, assaultative, and destructive intent currently.

18. *Cerebral cortical and neuropsychiatric evaluation.* No adequate screening evaluation of higher brain function appears in the literature. Screening evaluation of the head injured patient using available bedside screening instruments is limited at present. The most widely used test (Naugle & Kawczak, 1989), the Mini Mental Status Examination (FMMSE) (Folstein,

Folstein, & McHugh, 1975), is quickly administered and requires little training, but has little predictive power for diagnosis or classification of coarse neurobehavioral syndromes, and is not designed to detect mild cortical deficits (Naugle & Kawczak, 1989). Half of the MMSE's 30 questions emphasize orientation and calculation; focal pathology is not effectively screened. Only 30% of multi-infarct dementia patients (Babikian, Wolfe, Linn, Knoefel, & Albert, 1990) and 68% of Alzheimer's dementia patients scored below the recommended cutoff of 24/30 on the MMSE, raising questions about the test's sensitivity (Galasko et al., 1990). Even more seriously, 85% were false positive for the diagnosis of dementia, raising questions about its use in a geriatric community setting (Gagnon et al., 1990). The MMSE also correlates poorly with basic everyday living skills (Katz ADL Scale) (Ferrell, Ferrell, & Osterweil, 1990), education and intelligence level, right-hemisphere dysfunction, and mild cognitive dysfunction (Ferrell et al., 1990; Gagnon et al., 1990; Gurland, Cote, Cross, & Toner, 1987).

CHITS, CHIPS, dementia, focal cerebral cortical abnormalities, pseudo-dementia, and other coarse neurocognitive brain syndromes are frequently evaluated using neuropsychological batteries such as the Halstead–Reitan and the Luria–Nebraska. Neuropsychological evaluation is often helpful in gathering a comprehensive standardized sample of cognitive and intellectual functioning. When the practical demands of practice make it prohibitive to have a patient complete the often lengthy neuropsychological testing process, there is an alternative that is less formal but clinically quite useful, as follows.

NEUROPSYCHOLOGICAL EVALUATION

The BROCAS SCAN

The most promising such clinical instrument is our bedside screening test, the Screening Cerebral Assessment of Neppe (BROCAS SCAN), which we spent the late 1980s refining and the 1990s developing data on and using (Neppe, Chen, Davis, Sawchuk, & Geist, 1992) (scoresheets, Appendix 2). This is a test of higher cerebral cortical functions used as a bedside screening instrument.

The BROCAS SCAN permits a quantified behavioral neurologic examination by providing clinical personnel with a focal and global assessment of a patient's mental status. Focal assessments include gnosis, praxis, and sensory-motor-reflex skills, which are not adequately addressed by the MMSE and bedside tests, including the Neurobehavioral Cognitive Status Examination (NCSE) (Schwamm, Van Dyke, Kiernan, Merrin, &

Mueller, 1987). The BROCAS SCAN is a more valid and more sensitive indicator of pathology than the FMMSE, results that we have seen hundreds of times clinically over numerous neuropsychiatric diagnoses and also demonstrated in our research (Neppe et al., 1992).

The BROCAS SCAN is readily learned, administered, and scored and has high interrater reliability (Neppe et al., 1992), even when administered by psychology students. It is versatile—40% of neuropsychiatric patients who had the BROCAS SCAN were considered unable to tolerate longer neuropsychological batteries (Neppe et al., 1992). A SCAN on patients with CHITS should take 10 to 40 min. Screening questions eliminate unnecessary follow-up when the item is answered correctly.

The acronym BROCAS spells out the relevant scoring categories. "B" is for behavior rating: a revised form of the Brief Psychiatric Rating Scale (BPRS) of Overall and Gorham (1962; Overall & Beller, 1984)—the Neppe Modification of the BPRS, or NMBPRS (Appendix 3). Despite the frequent use of the BPRS, this is the least quantifiable category and the only one requiring specialized assessment. The remaining 10 categories comprise the ROCAS profile: "R" for recall and recognition, "O" for orientation and organization, "C" for concentration and calculation, "A" for apraxia and agnosia, and "S" for speech and sensory-motor-reflex. Each ROCAS category is scored from zero (no impairment) to 10 (gross impairment). The 40 items that compose the 10 ROCAS categories are tabulated on a two-dimensional score sheet (Appendix 2). The result is expressed as the BROCAS profile (Behavior + ROCAS), which reflects clinical and neuropsychiatric features.

The first half of the test is basic screening items, which compose the Core score; the second half is subtle items, which compose the Fine score. A Total SCAN score, ranging from 0 to 100, is the sum of the Core and Fine scores. Two versions of the BROCAS SCAN, labeled A and B, allow for retesting without contamination. Scoring involves the patient's performance. A perfect score is zero, and the normal-intelligence individual without major psychopathology generally scores <15. The maximum score for the very grossly impaired is 100.

Because the BROCAS SCAN test concentrates on physical signs, areas of the cerebral cortex such as the temporal lobe and limbic system involving predominantly symptom profiles are not evaluated in detail; this is done with the INSET evaluation.

Two validity scores are obtained. The first is the rater's validity scale (0 = highest level of validity; 4= very dubious). The second, the subjective validity scale, is the patient's ranking of difficulty in such areas as anxiety, concentration, and language understanding, and uses the same items as the rater's validity scale. This is currently used clinically and helps to give insight into the patient's perception of his or her illness.

TABLE 10.4
Examples of Scoring of BROCAS SCAN in
Normals (NI) and Closed Head Injured Patients (HI)

Patient	NI	HI	Comments on the HI patient
Core score	4	17	Commonly outside normal range but not invariably
Fine score	1	3	Focality may change fine score markedly
Total score	7	20	Usually falls in the mild cognitively impaired range
MBPRS score 18	2	6	Usually mild psychopathology
MBPRS score COP	0	2	Some concentration difficulty
MBPRS frustration score	0	2	Some frustration common
MBPRS score total	2	10	Sum of above
Rater's validity score	0	0	Usually valid
Subjective validity score	0	1	Concentration noted defective
MBPRS validity score	0	0	Invariably no rater dilemmas

Category	Scan items	N	CHIT	Comment
R	Spontaneous recall	1	3	(usually 0–2)
R	Cued recognition	0	1	(usually 0)
O	Orientation	0	0	(usually 0–1)
O	Organization	1	2	(usually 0–2)
C	Concentration	1	3	(usually 0–2)
C	Calculation	1	2	(usually 0–2)
A	Apraxia	2	4	(usually 0–4)
A	Agnosia	0	1	(usually 0–2)
S	Speech	1	1	(usually 0)
S	Sensory motor reflex	0	0	(usually 0)

Table 10.4 reflects two typical SCANs. The NI column reflects a normal profile, and the HI column may reflect a patient with a CHIT 3 months postinjury. Table 10.5 reflects the interpretations on these patients.

Mini-Mental Status Examination

The subject's mini-mental status examination score based on Folstein et al. (1975) (FMMSE: /30) and adding the World score (5) (/30–35) is usually done in our evaluations for comparison only. Because this test is suspect for sensitivity, specificity and reliability, it is listed here only because of its common use. *The scores alone should not be used to base any clinical decision.*

Neppe Modification of the Revised Brief Psychiatric Rating Scale (NMBPRS)

This test generally uses a 0 to 6 (occasionally 7) ordinal ranking scale of each of 18 basic items, plus 3 cognitive (COP) items and an additional frustration score. The original Overall and Gorham test has been subject

TABLE 10.5
Examples of Interpretation of Scoring of BROCAS SCAN in Normals
(NI) and Closed Head Injured Patients (HI)

Memory as reflected by recall and retention:
The patient did not perseverate.
Mild verbal but no obvious visual difficulties were present on spontaneous recall or
cued recognition.
Recall and recognition are inappropriate for age and intelligence.
Normal recall/recognition implies adequate eventual registration (measured, in part,
more acutely by concentration) and retention of information.
In this instance, impaired recall with reasonable recognition may imply difficulty with or-
ganizing retained information.
Orientation for time, space, and passage of time was within normal limits.
(Passage of time is selectively impaired in certain psychoses; spatial impairment may im-
ply organicity.)
Organization as reflected by abstraction of proverbs and ability to coherently put ele-
ments together appears within normal limits, taking cultural elements into account.
(The measure in this instance unfortunately has more cultural elements than any other
part of this test.)
Communication skills were unimpaired.
Concentration: The patient was able to concentrate but only poorly and outside normal
limits.
Calculation: Simple calculation skills as measured by subtraction appear appropriate for
the overall profile.
(Calculation difficulties may reflect specific impairments including preexisting learning
difficulties and focal impairments of either parietal or frontal lobe or generalized concentration disturbance.)
Praxic skills pertaining, inter alia, to copying, construction, and sequential movements
scored at the upper limits of normal.
(Many normal people have significant difficulties with tests of complex sequences. Separation of the motor impairment from the perceptual gnosic difficulties is at times very
difficult clinically.)
Gnosic elements testing both perceptual modality (auditory, visual, tactile) and organiza-
tion of information is within normal limits.
(The test involves relatively simple tasks so abnormality reflects significant pathology or
limited attention to detail.)
Speech pronunciation was normal.
Comprehension of complex English phrases was appropriate.
Naming of body parts, colors, and objects appears within normal limits.
Speech generation as reflected by spontaneous word generation using stipulated criteria
was normal.
(Tests broadly cover the spectrum of receptive and expressive speech.)
Sensory-motor-reflex elements: No evidence for impaired gait or posturing,
The patient has no obvious motor weakness in the upper limbs with nor arm sway and
no flexor-extensor weakness, and the lower limb strength appears adequate.
Motor tone appears adequate.
No tremor occurs on either side either at rest or on writing.
No obvious sensory loss exists.
No primitive reflexes were demonstrated by this test.
Because broad elements only are tested, this is no substitute for a detailed neurologic examination.

TABLE 10.6
Patient Performance on the NMBPRS Scoring,
Based on the HJ Example of Table 10.5

The patient scored 6 on the first 18 items, averaging 0.3, reflecting mild distress throughout. Particular loading occurred on anxiety items.

The single item frustration score is 2.

The score is 2 on the three COP items (concentration, orientation, perplexity) for higher
cerebral function.

The total score on the MBPRS is 10; this is a composite of the above 22 items.

The rater's validity score is 0 (0 is the highest level of validity) and subjectively 1 (concentration).

The Overall Clinical Impression Score is 1 (this item is the rater's overall impression of
psychopathology).

---

to numerous variations and used a great deal in evaluating change in
psychopathology scores over time, although interrater reliability may be
questioned. In this instance, the frustration score is an additional item not
found in the usual BPRS, and in addition to orientation, a score of on the
COP items—concentration, orientation, perplexity—is developed for
higher cerebral function. To ensure greater scoring consistency than in
the original BPRS, the essence of each item is summarized on a scoresheet
and the criteria in the PANSS of Kay and Fiszbein are used. Also, a
"validity score" based on whether particular items could be ranked accurately is used, as well as an Overall Clinical Impression Score.

The NMBPRS as recorded involves several assessments over each
interview and observation period during testing. The NMBPRS score may
be more exaggerated at times of evaluating distinct psychopathology and
in a nonstructured environment; hence, our tendency is to evaluate at a
time-based level and put in several scores. A subtest interpretative report
is then prepared. Table 10.6 reflects the NMBPRS results of the CHIT
patient in Table 10.5. (See Appendix 3.)

From the data of the ROCAS and B items (i.e., the BROCAS SCAN
and NMBPRS scores), a provisional attempt is made to analyze scores by
combining these profiles. Conclusions pertain to evidence of organic brain
dysfunction reflecting frontal-, parietal-, or temporal-lobe disease, current
marked dynamic or psychopathologic elements, any direct evidence for
possible psychotic preoccupation, although this is not specifically focussed
on, and evidence of a generalized organic brain syndrome. Finally, a
global perspective of range of normal limits or mildly, moderately and
severely impaired is made.

Here we resume our list of items of inventory.

19. *Movement disorder evaluation: The STRAW.* Movement disorders are
not generally of great significance in CHIT or CHIP but may be so,

depending on impacts on different parts of the brain. Moreover, many of these patients may be receiving major tranquilizer (i.e., neuroleptic, also called antipsychotic) medication, sometimes in small doses. Organicity may predispose to tardive dyskinesia, and thus it would then be mandatory to do such an evaluation for abnormal involuntary movements.

STRAW is an acronym for a new technique of evaluating involuntary movements, particularly tardive dyskinesia. Neppe developed the STRAW in the early 1990s because of the nonavailability of adequate measures that would reliably differentiate subtle differences in tardive dyskinesia and that could be easily scored within a 10% range by several different raters. The STRAW has two components: a timing component, and a severity component. The STRAW timing system involves equal scores of 50 for activation and rest. The key to the STRAW is the timed component. This component is scored out of 100 based on a time period using the criterion of presence. Tremor and epileptic seizure are not included as involuntary movements. Half the time is at rest—the "S" is for sitting at rest while relaxed, not under stress and standing; the score is a rest score. The 5 evaluations during activity are each out of 10, making up 50 for activity (the TRAW), loaded equally with the 50 for rest (the S of STRAW).

Three body sections are measured for severity: the head, the axial skeleton, and the limbs. Each body section is rated between 0 and 10 in severity. In practice, the most severe of these three rankings is the one that is most closely followed over a period of time for tardive dyskinesia. The STRAW timing system is multiplied by the STRAW severity, giving a total score out of 1,000. It is thereafter divided by 10 to score out of 100. This gives an index of both severity and duration of particular physical signs. Table 10.7 reflects a scoresheet of a typical CHIT patient, that is, with no movements.

20. *The PBRS.* The Problem Behaviors Rating Scale of Neppe and Loebel (PBRS) is only useful in the context of inpatients. Thus it may have more relevance acutely in a CHIP or in a situation of permanent sequelae. We have found it particularly useful to monitor change closely over time in that it is unambiguous and usable even by nurses' aides. It is still being researched, however.

The PBRS is a 33-item rating scale developed for nurses and related professionals in a nursing geriatric, neuropsychiatric, or other inpatient environment. This ranks patients' behavioral changes over a defined period of time (a day or a week). Each scale scores range from a normal of 0 to an extreme of 3, producing a total of 99, making a range from 0 to 99 (or 100 with 1 more for inpatients). These criteria are based on unambiguous clinical mental status features using the mental status mne-

TABLE 10.7
STRAW Examination for Involuntary Movements

AT REST
S—SITTING AND STANDING—out of 50; SCORED 0
ACTIVATION PROCEDURES; SCORED
T—TAPPING WITH RIGHT AND LEFT HAND—out of 10; SCORED 0
R—READING—out of 10; SCORED 0
A—ARMS OUTSTRETCHED—out of 10; SCORED 0
W—WRITING—out of 10; SCORED 0
W—WALKING—out of 10; SCORED 0
STRAW TIMING SCORE TOTAL IS 0
SEVERITY score is 0
COMBINED SEVERITY TIMING STRAW SCORE
= TIMING* SEVERITY/10 = 0

Note. This is a timed and severity neurologic evaluation for involuntary movements. When scores increase above zero, movements may be voluntary and related to anxiety.

monic ACCLAIMED covering areas broadly translated under appearance, consciousness and concentration, cognitive function, localization of cortical pathology, affect, insight and judgement, motivation and motoric elements, ego–environment interaction, and dangerousness and disability. A copy is listed in Appendix 4.

21. *Routine electroencephalogram (EEG).* (Both sleeping and waking versions are possible, with activating procedures such as hyperventilation and photic stimulation in the absence of medical conditions contraindicating these.) This is a reasonable procedure in CHIT given any possible temporolimbic features, episodic nature of symptoms, and history of atypical spells. Sleep records have been well demonstrated to more likely find focal pathology than waking EEGs. However, waking EEGs have a high pick-up rate, and sleeping EEGs cannot be interpreted without the waking EEG (Neppe, 1999).

It is interesting that prior to the development of the EEG (by the neuropsychiatrist Dr. Hans Berger in the 1930s), all seizure disorders were classified with mental disorders (Neppe & Tucker, 1988a, 1988b, 1992). EEG technology remains rather primitive, and reflections of brain waves from the perspective of analysis of psychopathology are somewhat limited. Nevertheless, the only definitive way of demonstrating that a symptom or physical sign—such as, for example, an olfactory hallucination—is definitely epileptic is the demonstration of correlates of seizure phenomena on EEG, such as spike-wave paroxysms, while the person is having that experience. This is unusual unless the seizure phenomena are relatively uncontrolled. Even in the event of the person having such an experience, the EEG correlate may not necessarily be of a spike kind but, depending on location, it could be normal or show a marked slowing, with a nonspecific theta rhythm generally of limited help unless focal, or a delta rhythm, which is frankly abnormal unless the patient is asleep (theta is 4 to 7 cycles per second; delta is less than 4). It is occasionally extremely difficult to localize such features on scalp EEG even when firing is occurring because symptoms may occur from the mesial temporal or deep structures within the brain, which do not easily manifest on surface EEGs (Tucker & Neppe, 1988).

Special electrode placements. Special techniques have been used to overcome this problem. One commonly used technique was nasopharyngeal electrodes, but the increased yield with nasopharyngeal electrodes is insubstantial. A second placement is sphenoidal electrodes, which unfortunately, require time, expertise, and discomfort, limiting availability. A recent new suggestion has been the placement of electrodes on the buccal skin surface in the area of the submandibular notch—possibly as effective in picking up foci as sphenoidal placements. Finally, cerebral cortical placements during neurosurgery procedures may show firing, for example, in patients with temporal-lobe epilepsy and psychosis, in the region of the hippocampus. The direct placement of intracranial electrodes shows how commonly spike firing may be occurring in this area with no correlate of any kind on surface EEGs (Neppe & Tucker, 1988a, 1988b, 1992).

Sleep EEG records. There are several methods that are used for evoking electroencephalographic abnormalities. Sleep records increase the potential delineation of focal abnormality such as a temporal-lobe focus by approximately fourfold. The administration of chloral hydrate, 1 to 3 grams, as premedication prior to the sleep record is useful as it induces little change of significance in the electroencephalogram and does not prevent the demonstration of focal abnormalities. Certain medications should be particularly avoided in this regard. The first is the benzodiazepine group, which may have, by virtue of their very strong antiepileptic effects, profound effects in normalizing the EEG. Such effects at a receptor level may last weeks, even with the apparently short-acting benzodiazepines, so that the yield of demonstrating epilepsy after the patient has had benzodiazepines administered apparently decreases substantially, although adequate data in this regard are not easily available (Neppe, 1984a). Photic stimulation and hyperventilation are also important evokers of abnormality in EEGs (Neppe, 1999).

22. *Home ambulatory electroencephalogram (EEG).* Developments in this regard have been rapid over the past few years. *EEG telemetry* involves prolonged monitoring over periods of time varying from 12 hr to 2 weeks while the patient is generally confined to a particular room. Cable telemetry is most commonly used. This involves, for example, a 25-ft cable connected to the EEG montage on the patient's head. Very often no seizure manifestations are picked up for prolonged periods of time

because seizures only occur paroxysmally. Moreover, those patients evaluated in a specialized center with EEG telemetry are invariably so atypical that the hypothesized seizure originates deep within the brain. The apparatus costs over $100,000, and the costs involved in monitoring patients are thousands of dollars per day at times for 2 weeks. Instead, home ambulatory electroencephalograms are easily available (Neppe & Tucker, 1988a, 1988b, 1992).

Ambulatory electroencephalogram (EEG) with the patient not modifying medication is a valuable test when the patient's symptomatology needs to be monitored day and night in the natural environment of home using computerized filtering of artifact. The advantage of this technique is to establish if any scalp electrode can detect events such as atypical spells alerted to by pushbuttons reflecting deep brain electrical activity. It has limited availability at this point, but its pick-up rate for atypical spells and seizures is high (Neppe, 1999).

Recent advances in EEG technology may ultimately change the whole perspective in its use in psychiatry. *Computerized EEG monitoring* allows breakdown of wave forms and allows correlation with evoked potentials including cognitive evoked potentials. It also facilitates demonstrations of changes in particular areas of the brain, which can be easily delineated at a visual level. This should prove to be a useful psychophysiological correlate of psychopathology. Indeed, this may be the beginning of an important new era. However, at this point in time it is still experimental.

23. *Other investigations.* Structural lesion investigations are sometimes necessary during the acute phase to ensure that secondary bleeding has not occurred. Usually, this is clear, based on neurologic deficits or deterioration of some kind. However, if neuroradiologic anatomic tests are not done in the first month, the likelihood that abnormalities will be picked up are considerably diminished. Thus depending on symptomatology, neuroradiologic investigations such as magnetic resonance imaging (MRI) of the head may be a useful consideration. The balance is one of cost versus computerized tomography (CT) scan, but the yield may be more with MRI. Additionally, CT is accessible and indicated when magnetic clips make MRI contraindicated and bony lesions or acute blood extraversations exist. This should be done with contrast material unless allergy contraindicates. However, it cannot demonstrate as well tiny lesions, lesions of the pituitary (where gadolinium contrasting on MRI should be performed), small vessel vascular disease, and white matter lesions such as demyelinating and degenerative disease.

Functional lesions that are not necessarily structural and detected on MRI or CT may be found on *single-photon emission computerized tomography (SPECT)*. This will demonstrate differences in regional cerebral blood flow and hot and cold areas of hyperflow and hypoflow. The differences in laterality and particular areas of the brain may have great clinical significance, but the interpretations are limited by lack of adequate diagnostic base.

Tests such as positron emission tomography (PET) are still experimental, very expensive, and not easily available in humans.

Similarly, measures such as computerized EEG, like BEAM or Spectrum, involve technology that has outstripped research, which means clinical meaning may be difficult to interpret.

24. *Symptom monitoring.* The patient and family should monitor episodes of symptoms of anger/aggression/irritability/anxiety/depression/memory/distress level. This will be based on a daily grade evaluation. Patient ranking and/or family ranking is listed in a table under the headings date, time, and approximate duration, with severity level at nil 0, mild 1, moderate 2, severe 3, and profound 4. Rank irritability, concentration, and memory.

For the *overall ranking for the day,* mark out of 10 every day. (This is individualized by the patient depending on impairments. One patient chose the following: "10 excellent, 0 very poor. with: 10 going to the store—walking; 8 still little trouble; 1 very impaired but can make coffee.")

A *sleep chart* may facilitate sleep monitoring so as to establish progress. The patient or family should list total amount of sleep for a 24-hr period, ending in morning on waking.

The patient should list time of day *when feeling worst,* eliciting diurnal variations in depression and fatigue.

25. *Collateral information.*

Collateral Information

We have stated previously that the patient with head injury symptoms is likely to have difficulty expressing thoughts and ideas. This may be due to expressive deficits, a reduction in self-awareness, or secondary to memory problems. Many patients with postconcussive symptoms experience a reduction in spontaneous word production and are unable to communicate the full extent of the changes in cognitive and psychological functioning. Patients with expressive problems often come up short in trying to explain the daily problems they are encountering. There may be dysnomia, poverty of thought content, and loss of their train of thought. This can result in inadequate clinical information being given to the health care provider, who in turn may under diagnose due to the appearance of minimal symptom presentation.

Concurrently, there may be an inability to fully appreciate the extent of cognitive problems or psychological changes. This can be due to denial and/or loss of ability to be aware of self and to engage in insightful introspection or self-analysis. This is often seen with the frontal dysexecutive syndrome. These patients do not fully appreciate the changes in cognitive and psychological functioning that significant others are keenly aware of.

On the other hand, many patients go through a phase of denial, where they minimize their postconcussive problems and may present themselves in the most favorable light. This is often the case where patients have been inappropriately reassured by medical personnel that they will be back to normal within a relatively short period of time, or that there is nothing to worry about, or that their symptoms will gradually diminish with time and there is very little that can be done to treat them. When they continue to experience difficulty in cognitive functioning, continue to have problems with pain, and are unable to cope effectively, they experience cognitive dissonance because of their belief that they should be improving. They may deny or try to hide or minimize their difficulties with the hope that it will just go away. There may be embarrassment with regard to their cognitive problems, irritability, and emotional volatility. These problems may often be obscured by the patients telling others that they just don't feel well.

Most patients with head trauma symptomatology experience memory problems. Impairments in memory processing may be due to concussive injury or as part of the spectrum of posttraumatic disorder or depression. These patients simply forget how they are doing from day to day. They may be experiencing a multiplicity of problems, but are unable to retrieve this information during the time spent with the health care provider. This may lead to the impression that a given patient is not experiencing any significant problems because he or she has not been able to adequately remember the instances of cognitive dysfunctioning or emotional overreactivity on a day-to-day basis.

It is for these reasons that it is crucial to interview significant others or acquaintances who have known the patient for some time before the injury and have been in regular contact with the patient following the injury. Where possible, these friends and family members should have had routine contact with the patient before the injury and be able to describe their premorbid behavior. These individuals will be able to document any changes that have taken place by way of their regular interactions with the patient. This collateral information is often more accurate than information given by the patient. The clinician should be careful to ask about physical, cognitive, and psychological functioning. The most important issue to establish is whether or not the significant other or acquaintance has observed changes in the patient's behavior following the traumatic event.

A review of the patient's physical functioning from someone who is around the patient on a daily basis can provide valuable information regarding the frequency, intensity, and duration of complaints. It is important to ask about changes in the patient's sense of smell and taste, because there is often a loss or partial loss of olfactory processes. This is often an overlooked symptom in the mild to moderate head injury population. Information should be gathered as to any complaints the patient may be making regarding more subtle changes in functioning such as sensitivity to bright light (sunlight or night driving), the sensation of obscurity to visual acuity, ringing in the ears, intolerance to noise or distractions during active concentration, problems with coordination and tactile dexterity, poor proprioception, and sensation. Review of the patient's pain behavior is essential in understanding the factors that may be influencing the experience of pain.

During a review of the patient's cognitive functioning, the clinician should ask about situational manifestations of cognitive problems. The clinician needs to know how the patient is functioning across different situations and within a variety of environments. It is important to know if the patient's cognitive changes are obvious to others and whether or not the patient is relying on others to compensate for his or her cognitive difficulties.

Primary care group members should be asked about the patient's flow of thinking, including speed of information processing, attention, and concentration. The clinician should try to ascertain whether the patient is able to maintain and sustain attention and concentration and if there is distractibility. Memory processing should be thoroughly evaluated to establish a pattern of memory problems that is specific to that patient. It is not enough to just document the presence or absence of memory problems. It is also important to review the patient's problem-solving abilities, organizational skills, reasoning, and the ability to perform sequential activities and make schedules and plan ahead. Mental arithmetic reasoning should be asked about, regarding the patient's ability to keep up with finances, make change, and estimate necessary everyday calculations. The clinician should ask about the patient's ability to express himself or herself, word-finding difficulties, losing the train of thought, and the style of speech. The patient's comprehension and receptive language abilities should also be reviewed, including reading comprehension, the ability to follow TV programs, and how well the patient understands and responds to others.

Perhaps the most important reason for obtaining collateral information is to document and describe the changes in psychological functioning. Head trauma patients typically are better historians with respect to their physical functioning, but have more difficulty describing changes in themselves. Individuals who know the patient well are often able to notice changes in mood and affect more readily than the patient. It is important to know how the patient is responding to stress. The clinician should determine whether the patient is more irritable, is less patient with others, has low frustration tolerance, and whether there have been episodes of emotional volatility. Questions should also be asked about frontal-lobe behavior, especially increased passivity or aggressivity. Routine questions should also be included to assess other areas of psychological functioning in consideration of secondary psychological problems such as anxiety or depression.

DIAGNOSTIC EVALUATION

Based on the preceding findings, provisional ideas begin to develop. In the course of the time-based evaluation these may change. We have found that a multiaxial schema is critical taking into account an amplification of *DSM–IV* psychiatrically and an equivalent schema neurologically. These are reflected in Fig. 10.1 under two major sections: neurologic and neuropsychiatric. This example is of a prototype patient with CHIT. The complexity of all these elements in this way can be perceived.

CONCLUSIONS

Evaluations of closed head injuries of transient kind are therefore areas for fertile research, as what was previously regarded as irrelevant is now realized to be significant. Many patients with CHITS have not been regarded as ill when, in actuality, they were so impaired that their day-to-day functioning was interfered with. Only by detailed, time-based, cross-sectional evaluations can one develop enough longitudinal perspective to be able to manage the patient appropriately and to appreciate better their strengths and their limitations. Certain pointers on management are dealt with later (Neppe, chap. 19, this volume).

ACKNOWLEDGMENT

We gratefully acknowledge the permission of the Pacific Neuropsychiatric Institute (www.pni.org) to publish the full version of this chapter plus the copies of the appendices.

DIAGNOSIS

Evaluation Based on the above findings, the following provisional ideas seem appropriate.

PREDOMINANT DIAGNOSIS	Closed head injury of transient kind (CHIT)
	Mixed elements:
	Post traumatic syndrome , Post concussional syndrome
	Possible contrecoup injury with frontal lobe features (residual focal)
	Secondary sexual dysfunction
	Secondary Pain syndrome predominantly hips.
	Tinnitus chronically
	Abnormal EEG with right lateral temporal structural abnormality
	Headache and dizziness both improving
	Obesity

NEUROLOGIC LABEL :

1n	**Neurologic overview**	CHIT with PTS, PCS, Focal syndrome
1s	**Seizure Classification**	possible minor temporal lobe features: structural on EEG and clinically correlates with tinnitus? and headache?
1m	**Movement disorder**	no evidence at this time
1e	**Neuro-endocrine disorder**	no evidence at this time
1s	**Dyssomnia**	intermittent initial insomnia (mild, secondary to psychological elements)
1h	**Higher cortical elements**	high functioning individual previously; now Significant organizational - integration impairment with frontal lobe elements
1p	**Perceptual distortions**	tinnitus - chronic persistent since accident.
1h	**Pain syndrome**	headaches when tired
1g	**General neurologic**	CHIT
1pn	**RELEVANT MEDICAL CONDITIONS**	no evidence at this time
1fn	**Family history**	No neurologic family history

FIG. 10.1. Prototype example of CHIT patient diagnosis, followed by neuropsychiatric framework of diagnosis.

2 l	Learning style	No evidence of pre-existing learning disability
2 n	Premorbid Intelligence:	Normal range.
3 p	Physical condition	As per examination, main complaints, social history
3 n	Links of Neurologic events to presentation	Probably significant. Dynamically different coping styles exist. Organically different compensations for deficits occur.
3 c	Cerebral Localization	Temporolimbic phenomena not triggered or mobilized by hallucinogen or stimulant use
4	Special investigations	as listed above
4 e	Electroencephalographic	sleep and wake EEG 1993 slightly abnormal with bitemporal spiking ambulatory EEG right lateral temporal
4 n	Neuroradiologic	tests as above MRI 1995 apparently normal
5 n	Other test features:	apparently normal blood tests
	Course :	
	Deteriorating or not	Non-deteriorating
	Chronicity degree	Not chronic
6 n	Neuropharmacologic Response	Carbamazepine has helped the explosive anger but not assisted with the amotivation and dysexecutive phenomena
	Compliance	By history, expected to be reasonable
7 n	Neurologic onset age	since head injury on 4/7/97

NEUROPSYCHIATRIC FRAMEWORK:		
1 p	Psychopathology: DSM IV	Post-traumatic episodes
	Descriptive Psychopathology:	atypical depression and anxiety confusional episodes
1 fp	Family history	family history negative except for one aunt

2 a	Addictive disorder	no evidence of alcoholism or drug dependency or abuse
2p	Personality Elements:	No relevant characterologic deficits *Anankastic personality features accentuated post-injury possibly as coping mechanism*
3p	Relevant Physical disorders:	conditions above are major components to current psychopathologic manifestations
	Symptomatic relevance:	major components to current psychopathologic manifestations
	Relatedness to illness:	significant
4p	Psychosocial components:	&&&&&&&&&&&&&&
	Family support	reasonable
	Patient Strengths	self-perceived : "trying to get better"
	Predisposing factors :	Constitutional diathesis. Environmental experience Aggravating cerebral trauma
	Precipitating stressors:	No significant new stressors. Chronic difficulties linked with impaired function
	Perpetuating factors:	Predisposing elements
	Problem areas	listed above
5p	Functionality:	&&&&&&&&&&&&&&
	Maximum expected in future:	limited
	Highest functionality before insult:	reasonable: normal day's work
	Functionality currently:	limited by deficits and unable to work though does daily chores
6p	Psychopharmacologic:	
	Psychopharmacologic Responsiveness:	as listed above: buspirone has helped irritability and concentration
	Psychopharmacologic Compliance:	historically reasonable
7p	Age of onset of major psychopathology:	since head injury on 4/7/97

FIG. 10.1. *(Continued)*

193

The INVENTORY OF NEPPE OF SYMPTOMS OF EPILEPSY OF THE TEMPORAL LOBE

The questions below refer to times when you have not been using alcohol or pleasure drugs.

There are two columns marked C and P. You will be writing a number into both of them which will allow us to know how often the symptom or event has happened to you. The left column under P refers to the greatest frequency in the past (ie: frequency at which it occurred at its worst); the column under C refers to your current experience (how often it has happened recently - today, this week, month, or year-if rare).

| 0=never, 1=less than once per year, 2=yearly or more, 3=monthly or more, 4=weekly or more, 5=daily, 6=more than daily. |

Indicate how often the event occurs by writing the frequency number into columns P and C. So if the symptom has never happened, you will write in 0 under C and P. If another symptom has been happening currently every day, you would fill in 5 under C. Let's imagine an example to make things clearer - Mr. Smith answered question #24 like this: P C

| 4 | 0 | 24)How often does time seem to be (x)speeded up or ( )slowed down or (x)not existing for periods (x)of minutes, ( )up to several hours? |

He did so because: He remembers that in the past when the symptom was at its worst, time seemed to speed up for minutes every week (=4).However, it does not happen currently (=0). He writes the most frequent number under each column. (i.e. #4 for past, under P and zero (0) for current, under C) . Even though it does not currently happen, he still fills in the 0 because otherwise his physicians may think he just ignored the question . He wants to let his physicians know that time was speeded up. that it lasted for minutes, and that there was also a sense of timelessness, so he checked each of those brackets. Also, in the past time was speeded up weekly(=4) while time was not existing yearly(=2). He wrote "4" under P because it was the most frequent number for this symptom in the past (i.e. weekly(=4) more frequent than yearly(=2).
PLEASE RE-READ THESE INSTRUCTIONS TO RE-INFORCE HOW TO ANSWER BELOW?

P	C	(remember C is currently happening to you, P is any time in the past but not the current. time)
		1)How often do you have episodes of ( )fits, ( ) seizures or ( )"peculiar spells"?
		2)How often have you had a blackout or lost consciousness for a short time like seconds or minutes ? Do not include times when you were knocked unconscious or fainted?
		3)How often have you or are you told that : you at times lose contact with ( )staring spells or ( )episodes where you have a blank look on your face ( )for seconds or ( )minutes?
		4)How often do you find that you suddenly feel confused or perplexed (you don't know where you are, or why you are there, or what time or date it is) and then have the feeling pass in a few minutes?

5)How often have you for a very short time like seconds or minutes been **completely unaware** that you did or been told that you did any of the following: ( )odd behaviors like ( )buttoning / unbuttoning; ( ) chewing / mouth movements or ( ) other unusual movements or ( )doing very strange things or ( ) saying strange things or ( ) finding yourself in places you don't remember going to ?	
6)How often do your ( )moods, ( )feelings or ( )thoughts fluctuate within minutes for no reason (like ( ) very happy then very sad) ? .	
7)How often do you...( )have clear cut gaps in your memory during which you cannot remember anything for 5 minutes or more; ( )miss major sections of TV shows you have been watching; ( )find yourself driving without remembering how you got there or where you are going; ( )do strange things automatically?	
8)How often have you...( )lost control of yourself due to anger; ( )easily become very irritable over 'nothing'; ( )become extremely angry; ( )got into an extremely bad temper; ( )been told by others about an anger episode of yours that you do not remember; ( )been told that you become violent or aggressive and you have no recollection of this?	
9)How often do you have a ( )strange sensation or ( )pain in your stomach, belly or upper abdomen <u>not</u> related to eating?	
10)How often have you come across a smell when there is **nothing to cause it**? (If so, what kind (check applicable)? ( )medicine; ( )steak; ( )perfume; ( )flowers; ( )burning; ( )rotting; ( )synthetic; ( )vomit; ( )incense; ( )musty; ( )grass; ( )bitter; ( )sweet; ( )cake; ( )mustard; ( )other _____)	
11)How often have you seen any of the following? Check all applicable. ( )dots; ( )lights; ( )patterns; ( )shapes; ( )wrong size; ( )movements; ( )distorted; ( )things moving; ( )stars; ( )bugs; ( )threads; ( )insects;; ( )other _____ (Were these in front of your eyes or in your side vision or both? ( )front vision; ( )side vision; ( )both)	
12)How often do you encounter tastes in your mouth which you cannot explain? (If so, what quality? ( )metallic; ( )bitter; ( )salt; ( )sweet; ( )sour; ( )other	
13) How often do you hear any of the following, when there is no-one or nothing to cause it? Check all applicable. ( )buzz; ( )ring; ( )hiss; ( )tap; ( )songs; ( )whistling; ( )music; ( )single word; ( )arguing; ( )names; ( )voices; ( )jumble; ( )message; ( )instructing; ( )radioTV; ( )phone;; ( )other	
14)How often do you have odd sensations in part of your body like ( )floating, ( )turning or ( )moving when you were doing none of those?	
15)How often do you have episodes of sudden, unexplained dizziness?	
16)How often do you feel strange sensations or crawling in your skin without reason? ( )insects; ( )other _____	
17).How often have you been in a **familiar** place and had the impression that you have <u>never</u> been in that place before? (the opposite of déjà vu called jamais vu – not recognized at all, totally unfamiliar)	

195

APPENDIX 1 (Continued)

18)How often do you find familiar persons or places: ( )strange, ( )foreign, or ( )different,?		
19)How often have you had déja` vu: You have ( ) gone somewhere, ( ) met someone, ( ) heard words, ( ) thought something, or ( ) said something, for the first time and felt it was familiar - as if you had been through it before?		
20)How often have you found that, for no apparent reason, you are actually reliving things in the past (as if the past flows like a movie screen before you)?		
21)How often do you have an overwhelming feeling that things are ( )weird, or ( )wrong, or ( )distorted?		
22)How often do you feel you ( )are not yourself, or ( )are just watching yourself, or ( )are not part of yourself?		
23)How often have you felt possessed by some kind of being or alien or something not yourself?		
24)How often do you feel someone is ( )watching, ( )observing or ( )plotting specifically against you?		
25)How often does time seem to be ( )speeded up or ( )slowed down or ( )not existing for periods ( )of minutes, ( )up to several hours?		
26)How often do you have sudden, unexplained or uncontrollable attacks of intense fear for no apparent reason?		
27) How often have you ( )had episodes of intense religious feeling, for example ( )you felt at one with the world or ( )felt that in some special way God had touched or had spoken to you or ( )felt as though you were close to a powerful spiritual life force?		
28)How often have you had repeated and unreasonable thoughts that you cannot stop from thinking even though you try - they keep coming into your mind?		
29)How often have you had episodes of compulsive sexual behavior that was out of character for you?		
30)How often have you had episodes of ( )compulsive eating (binge eating with or without vomiting) of such intensity that you felt out of control and could not stop or of ( )deliberate (not religious) starving of yourself?		
31)How often do you write the events in your life in detail down in a diary?		
32)How often do you hear what is being said, yet you cannot understand or make sense of it?		
33)How often do you discover that: ( ) your pronunciation or word order in your home language is wrong or ( )you are misplacing figures (digits) or ( )you have difficulty finding the right word or ( )while talking you have not made any sense?		
34)How often do you find that you are ( )slurring your speech or ( )cannot talk, when not due to alcohol or other drugs?		

		35) How often do you have *difficulty concentrating?* (Has it become worse every year? ( )yes; ( )no)
		36) How often do you feel ( )depressed or ( )anxious or ( )tense ?
		37) How often do you have severe headaches? (If so : Do you get ( )nauseous or/and ( )see stars /funny /blurred with them? ( )most times /( )rarely)
		38) How often do you get a ( )pain or ( ) sensation *in your head* which you would *not* classify as a *"headache"*?
		39) How often do you have *double vision?*
		40) How often do you ( )get *very tired even when you had enough sleep* or ( )sleep so soundly during the day that no one can arouse you?
		41) How often do you snore ( )so loudly or ( )for so long that others notice?
		42) How often do you ( )wake three or more times in the night or ( )lie awake three or more hours trying to sleep?
		43) How often do you *dream?*
		44) How often do you have *exactly the same repetitive dream and/or frightening nightmares?*
		45) How often have you had *"psychic", intuitive or paranormal experiences which prove correct?*
		46) How often have you ( )seen events that happened at a great distance as they were happening or ( )felt as though you were in touch with someone when they were far away from you?
		47) How often have you felt you have left your body?
		48) How often have you been close to death *and* been aware of a strange experience? (If so, was it like you had died and come back (so-called near-death experiences)
49) Do you find there are any specific things which trigger any one of the symptoms/ experiences discussed (e.g. ( )lights flashing or a sudden or special ( )sound, ( )smell)? ( )yes; ( )no. If yes, which ones (give the item numbers from above questions)? Numbers:
50) Which symptoms began only after a head injury or other problem like encephalitis, meningitis or a car accident? Please list (give the item numbers from above questions). Numbers:

198

BROCAS SCAN SCORESHEET -CORE

SCREENING CEREBRAL ASSESSMENT OF NEPPE

NAME : _____

DATE _____ Hospital ID#: _____ Age: _____ Code#: _____

START TIME : _____ VERSION A or B _____ Intv: _____ Scorer _____ Validity rating /SRS Sc

IF SCORE ON CORE BROCAS SCAN IS > 50 , OR > .5HOUR : end the SCAN . RIGID DIFF SC/#ITEMS/ADD-ON

TEST ITEM Task **CORE** **BROCAS** FMMSE30- /35- // 30+/TIME

Perf. _____ [✓] (Max score within column = 10) TOTAL RBPRS/ BPRS $CORE

(Max score per line=5) COP /FRUSTR / VAL RBPRS

SCORE TIME TAKEN

Core Sc

Fine

TOTAL

TEST ITEM	BEHAV	RECL	RECG	ORI	ORG	CONC	CALC	APRX	AGNOS	SPCH	SENS/MOT/RFLX	ITEM TOTAL
1 GAIT (Before) (Or if worse , After)								:1:			:1:	1
2 HANDS											:1: :1:	2
3 VERB MEM CONT REG name,place,car,color					:1:							3
4 VERB/VIS CONT REG objects in room					:1:							4
5 COPYING (Copy)							:1:		:1:		:1:	5
6 COPYING REGIST (Differences)		:1:					:1:					6
7 CLOCK CONSTRUCTION								:1:		:1:		7
8 TIME ORIENTATION PLACE ORIENTATION			:1: :1:									8
9 MOTOR TONE (ELBOW) ▨ R L											:1: :1:	9

	RECL	RECG	ORI	ORG	CONC	CALC	APRX	AGNOS	SPCH	SENS/MOT/RFLX	TOTAL

10 POWER (WRIST) R

11 PRIMITIVE REFLEXES — Glab / Pout / Other

12 MOTOR SWAY (1min) R / L

13 DIGITS FORWARD (start with 6)

14 DIGITS BACKWARD (start with 5)

15 ARITHMETIC (−13,−14) (errors use) (−7) (still errors to) (−3)

16 SEQUENTIAL (Difficult3) MOVEMENTS (Complex 3) (Simple 2)

17 GNOSIS/PRAXIS finger, face, other side

18 SPEECH FLUENCY

19 VERB RETENT. #3above (Recogn.)

20 VERB/VIS RETENT. #4above (Recogn.)

21 COPYING (Later)

22 COPYING (recog) ⊕(2,4) ◁⊜(3,2)

PART A (Core) TOTAL

End time (Core) : _____

NAME _____ BROCAS SCAN SCORESHEET – FINE (PAGE 2) DATE _____

SCREENING CEREBRAL ASSESSMENT OF NEPPE (BROCAS SCAN) CODE #: _____

TEST ITEM   INTERVIEWER: _____
                                                                     SCORER: _____

(Max score per line=5)   Perf. Task   BROCAS
(Circle flexible scores) [✓] BEHAV   (Max score within column = 10)

TEST ITEM	BEHAV	RECL	RECG	ORI	ORG	CONC	CALC	APRX	AGNOS	SPCH	SENS/MOT/RFLX	ITEM TOTAL
VARIABILITY (color/food/star)												
23 SENTENCE Artic geese / Greek									1			23
Fluency (ifs/Const)									1			
Init (I/He)									1			
24 COMPREHEN. Light/phone / Wind/door									1			24
25 NAMING (watch/arm/ color)									1			25
26 WORD GEN. (C) or (P)30sec N= / (G) or (H) N=									1			26
27 PROVERBS stitch cook / house minds fool swallow / hand penny wood pot				1								27
28 WRITING {Address} {Weather}				1					1			28
29 NAME (Name right) , sec / (Name left) , sec										1		29
30 TUNE (Copying) / (Generation)									1			30
31 RHYTHM COPYING									1			31
32 GENERAL KNOWLEDGE Lincoln JFK / Reagan Bush	1			1								32

200

33 VARIABILITY										33
34 VISUAL FIELDS include extinction test										34
35 VISUAL EXTINCTION TACTILE EXTINCTION L-R / R-L										35
36 2-PT DISCRIMINATION R / L										36
37 GRAPHESTHESIA each 1cm R / L										37
38 TIME PASSAGE										38
39 AGE vs D.O.B. min										39
40 SPACE ORIENTATION										40
41 OTHER(vision,hearing)										41
42 ADD-ON ** a. count b. same c. concept a b c d e										42

d.plantars

right ___ **PART B (FiNE) TOTAL**

left ___ **PART A (CORE) TOTAL**

e. next day **TOTAL**

END TIME : **SCORE**

VALIDITY SCORE :

| RECL | RECG | ORI | ORG | CONC | CALC | APRX | AGNOS | SPCH | SENS/MOT/RFLX | TESTED TOTAL |

TOTAL ___ Vis ___ Aud ___ Amot ___ Anx ___ Aggr ___ Loose ___ Lang ___ Illness ___ Intel ___ Drugs ___ Intv ___ Tree ___ Yes ___

VARIABILITY 1 Food ___ Color ___ Filmstar ___   Damage ___ Tested ___ Type ___

** 9,4,1 VER A   2 Food ___ Color ___ Filmstar ___   #25 COLOR

10,6,2 VER B   3 Food ___ Color ___ Filmstar ___   10/93

* Score normal if letter/seconds ratio is >3/2 for preferred hand and >3/4 for non-preferred hand.   ©VERNON M NEPPE

REVISED BRIEF PSYCHIATRIC RATING SCALE

Modified after Overall and Gorham; & Kay, Opler and Fiszbein[G,N,P]

NAME _____

AGE _____ HOSPITAL NUMBER _____

CODE _____ DIAGNOSIS _____ ADMIT DATE _____

DIRECTIONS : 0=not present 1=very mild 2= mild 3=moderate 4=moderately severe 5=severe 6=extremely severe (7=profound)

COLUMNS REFLECT CONVENTIONAL SCORING (2ND COLUMN) AND SCORING OF RATER-PATIENT DIFFERENCES (/ IN 1ST COLUMN)

	interv day		day interview day		BPRS	BPRS

RATER INITIALS

DATE

TIME

OVERALL CLINICAL IMPRESSION (rate items 1 to 18 only)

1. SOMATIC CONCERN--unrealistic bodily concern (P)[G1]
2. ANXIETY--fear, tension, concern, worry (P) [G2]
3. EMOTIONAL WITHDRAWAL--interview, interactions (R)[N2]
4. CONCEPTUAL DISORGANIZATION--thoughts, concerns (R;[P2]
5. GUILT FEELINGS--past behavior, remorse, shame (P)[G3]
6. TENSION--motor, nervousness, overactivity (R)[G4]
7. MANNERISMS & POSTURING--unnatural, bizarre (R)[G5]
8. GRANDIOSITY--exaggerated opinions, powers (P)[P5]
9. DEPRESSED MOOD--sorrow, sadness,pessimism (P,R)[G6]
10. HOSTILITY--verbal actions. animosity, disdain (R)[P7]
11. SUSPICIOUSNESS /PERSECUTION delusions,trust(R)[P6]
12. HALLUCINATORY BEHAVIOR perceptions (≤ 1 / week)(P,R)[P3]
13. MOTOR RETARDATION--speech, movement, tone (R) [G7]

14. UNCOOPERATIVENESS--guardedness, rejection (P,R) [G8]
15. UNUSUAL THOUGHT CONTENT--odd, bizarre, unusual (R)[G9]
16. BLUNTED AFFECT--reduced emotional tone (R)[N1]
17. EXCITATION agitation,hyperactivity,behavior(R)[P4]
18. SPONTANEITY, CONVERSATION FLOW reduction,apathy(R)[N6]
TOTAL BPRS SCORE (1-18)

19. CONCENTRATION--focus, sustain, change attention(P,R)[G11]
20. ORIENTATION--space, place, time (R)[G10]
21. PERPLEXITY--bewilderment, comprehension, ability to
cooperate, awareness (R)
TOTAL COP SCORE(19-21)
TOTAL RBPRS SCORE

NEW ITEMS ARE
CONCENTRATION AND PERPLEXITY

R REFLECTS RATER'S OPINION   LOW SCORE (RATER-PATIENT DIFF)
P REFLECTS PATIENT'S OPINION   FRUSTRATION RANK (R)-tolerance

proportion score =RBPRS/*items rated   PROPORTION SCORE 2signif dig
? rated 1 ; CR (COULDN'T RATE)=2
NR (NOT RATED) =2   --**validity**   VALIDITY

                                        First test Second test

frustration ranking is not formally part of RBPRS but an add-on item.

MEDICATION :

COMMENTS :G, N and P refer to General Psychopathology,Negative and Positive Symptoms in
the PANSS

©VERNON M NEPPE , NOVEMBER 1990 , SEATTLE

PROBLEM BEHAVIORS RATING SCALE (PBRS)   Code: _____   Rater Initials: __ __ __

Name : (first)_____ (mi)____(last)_____   Date : m ___/___/___ Hosp

( ) NURSING HOME	( ) INPATIENT	( ) AMBULATORY CLINIC	( ) IN HOME

SCORING: Circle problem behaviors based on direct observation of behaviors by you and coworkers only.
SEVERITY (in the past week): 0= within normal limits 1= severity mild and/or no intervention needed 2= severity moderate and/or intervention needed 3 = severity marked and/or urgent intervention needed U = Unknown ?= Uncertain

FREQUENCY: 0= no occurrences /within normal limits 1 = less than once weekly 2 = between one and six occurrences per week 3= at least once per day U= Unknown ?= Uncertain .

In the severity (**SEV**) and frequency (**FRQ**) column , enter the **highest ratings** obtained by *any* of the problem behaviors circled for that category . You may use the same or different symptoms for SEV and FRQ. Leave categories with 0 scores blank. Regard severity as the worst during the time period being measured usually the past week.

Example: Subject has three problem behaviors. Circle these three items. The greatest severity of any of these problem behaviors in the past week was moderate; the frequency was daily: Record **SEV score 2, FRQ score 3**

2	3	06 HALLUCINATIONS	Giggles talks to self Admits to : voices visions smells tastes sensations

SEV	FRQ	CATEGORY	PROBLEM BEHAVIORS
		01 APPEARANCE	Unkempt appearance Poor hygiene Drooling Poor care of own environment
		02 LEVEL OF AWARENESS	Poor attention Distractible Consciousness fluctuates Perplexed
		03 ORIENTATION	Disoriented to : time / place / person Loses way
		04 DAY-NIGHT INVERSION	Behavior worse at night Becomes confused at night
		05 THOUGHT FORM	Evades questions Content difficult to understand Illogical
		06 HALLUCINATIONS	Giggles talks to self Admits to : voices, visions, smells, tastes, sensations
		07 DELUSIONS	Others stealing Grandiose Persecutory Sexual Jealousy Other
		08 OBSESSIONS & PHOBIAS	Obsessional thoughts Compulsions Rituals Phobic behavior
		09 MEMORY	Needs reminding Forgetful Loses possessions

#	Category	Descriptors
10	COMMUNICATION	Loud noises Mute Has difficulty understanding Repeats words and phrases Screams Pronunciation difficult to understand
11	DAILY LIVING SKILLS	Difficulty with : combing hair, brushing teeth, dressing, writing
12	VISION PROBLEMS	Difficulty seeing Double or blurred vision
13	AUDITORY PROBLEMS	Hard of hearing
14	ANXIETY	Looks anxious Panic attacks
15	DEPRESSION	Weeping Crying Looks depressed
16	EXCITABILITY	Excitable Irritable Confrontative Euphoric Elated Shouting
17	LABILE MOOD	Moaning Variable mood (over minutes)
18	SELF -AWARENESS	Does not perceive self as ill Poor judgement
19	MOTIVATION/ENERGY	Does not complete simple tasks Lethargic Not motivated Unoccupied
20	GAIT	Stiff Slow Ataxic Shuffles Requires prostheses
21	INVOLUNTARY MOVEMENTS	Tics Tremor Mouth movements Other purposeless movements
22	AGITATION/RETARDATION	Restless Pacing Wandering Withdrawn Reclusive Catatonic Disrobing
23	SPHINCTER CONTROL	Urinary incontinence Fecal incontinence Fecal smearing Inappropriate voiding
24	POSITION DIFFICULTIES	Falls from bed/ chair / upright stance Requires physical restraints for safety
25	COMPLIANCE	Noncompliant with: medications, tasks, activities Won't attend groups Resistive
26	BEHAVIOR TO PROPERTY	Stealing Hoarding Smoking violations Destructive Hiding
27	SEXUAL BEHAVIOR	Sexually inappropriate touching: self , others. Exposing self. Sexual word usage.
28	BEHAVIOR TO OTHERS	Bothersome Intrusive Complaining Clinging /anxious attachment Suspicious
29	SLEEP BEHAVIOR	Sleeps too little Sleeps too much Difficulty falling asleep Day time sleepiness
30	EATING BEHAVIOR	Resists Eats non-food items Weight gain Weight loss Poor appetite
31	PAIN BEHAVIOR	Complains of pain Preoccupied by bodily symptoms
32	SUICIDAL BEHAVIOR	Suicide attempt Wishes to be dead Suicidal ideation Self-mutilation Requires physical restraints Requires close observation Evasive about suicide
33	DANGER TO OTHERS	Verbal abusiveness Angry Physically threatening Assaultive Throwing objects Fire-setting Requires close observation Requires physical restraints
	Total score per column	Maximum is 99. Minimum is 0.
	Total number of "U= unknown" ratings	
	Total number of "?= uncertain " ratings	

REFERENCES

Alves, W., Macciocchi, S. N., & Barth, J. T. (1993). Postconcussive symptoms after uncomplicated mild head injury. *Journal of Head Trauma Rehabilitation, 8*(3), 48–59.

Babikian, V. L., Wolfe, N., Linn, R., Knoefel, J. E., & Albert, M. L. (1990). Cognitive changes in patients with multiple cerebral infarcts. *Stroke, 21*(7), 1013–1018.

Binder, L. M. (1986). Persisting symptoms after mild head injury: A review of the postconcussive syndrome. *Journal of Clinical and Experimental Neuropsychology, 8*(4), 323–345.

Blumer, D., & Neppe, V. M. (in press). Atypical spells in the non-epileptic and psychopathology: A classification. In D. Blumer (Ed.), *Psychiatric aspects of epilepsy.* Washington, DC: APA Press.

Brown, S. J., Fann, J. R., & Grant, I. (1994). Postconcussional disorder: time to acknowledge a common source of neurobehavioral morbidity. *Journal of Neuropsychiatry and Clinical Neuroscience, 6*(1), 15–22.

Cohadon, F., Richer, E., & Castel, J. P. (1991). Head injuries: Incidence and outcome. *Journal of the Neurological Sciences, 103*, 27–31.

Colohan, A. R. T., Dacey, R. G., Alves, W. M., Rimel, R. W., & Jane, J. A. (1986). Neurologic and neurosurgical implications of mild head injury. *Journal of Head Trauma Rehabilitation, 1*(2), 13–21.

Davidoff, D. A., Kessler, H. R., Laibstain, D. F., & Mark, V. H. (1988). Neurobehavioral sequelae of minor head injury: A consideration of post-concussive syndrome versus post-traumatic stress. *Cognitive Rehabilitation, March/April,* 8–13.

Esselman, P. C., & Uomoto, J. M. (1995). Classification of the spectrum of mild traumatic brain injury. *Brain Injury, 9*(4), 417–424.

Ferrell, B. A., Ferrell, B. R., & Osterweil, D. (1990). Pain in the nursing home. *Journal of the American Geriatric Society, 38*(4), 409–414.

Folstein, M. F., Folstein, S. E., & McHugh, P. R. (1975). Mini-Mental State: A practical method for grading the cognitive state of patients for the clinician. *Journal of Psychiatric Research, 12*(3), 189–198.

Gagnon, M., Letenneur, L., Dartigues, J. F., Commenges, D., Orgogozo, J. M., Barberger, G. P., Alperovitch, A., Decamps, A., & Salamon, R. (1990). Validity of the Mini-Mental State examination as a screening instrument for cognitive impairment and dementia in French elderly community residents. *Neuroepidemiology, 9*(3), 143–150.

Galasko, D., Klauber, M. R., Hofstetter, C. R., Salmon, D. P., Lasker, B., & Thal, L. J. (1990). The Mini-Mental State Examination in the early diagnosis of Alzheimer's disease. *Archives of Neurology, 47*(1), 49–52.

Goethe, K. E., & Levin, H. S. (1984). Behavioral manifestations during the early and long-term stages of recovery after closed head injury. *Psychiatric Annals, 14*(7), 540–546.

Goodwin, G. T. (1989, 3rd quarter). Minor head injury: Are there persisting symptoms after recovery? *Institute Review,* p. 1.

Gouvier, W. D., Cubic, B., Jones, G., Brantley, P., & Cutlip, Q. (1992). Postconcussion symptoms and daily stress in normal and head injury college populations. *Archives of Clinical Neuropsychology, 7*, 193–211.

Gurland, B. J., Cote, L. J., Cross, P. S., & Toner, J. A. (1987). The assessment of cognitive function in the elderly. *Clinics in Geriatric Medicine, 3*(1), 53–63.

Kay, T., Harrington, D. E., Adams, R., Anderson, T., Berrol, S., Cicerone, K., Dahlberg, C., Gerber, D., Goka, R., Harley, P., Hilt, J., Horn, L., Lehmkuhl, D., & Malec, J. (1993). Definition of mild traumatic brain injury. *Journal of Head Trauma Rehabilitation, 8*(3), 86–87.

Kibby, M. Y., & Long, C. J. (1996). Minor head injury: Attempts at clarifying the confusion. *Brain Injury, 10*(3), 159–186.

Lowdon, I. M. R., Briggs, M., & Cockin, J. (1989). Post-concussion symptoms following minor head injury. *Injury, 20*, 193–194.

McAllister, T. W. (1992). Neuropsychiatric sequelae of head injuries. *Psychiatric Clinics of North America, 15*(2), 395–415.

Middleboe, T., Birket-Smith, M., Anderson, H., & Friis, M. L. (1992). Personality traits in patients with postconcussional sequelae. *Journal of Personality Disorders, 6*(3), 246–255.

Miller, L. (1992). Neuropsychology, personality, and substance abuse in the head injury case: Clinical and forensic issues. *International Journal of Law & Psychiatry, 15*(3), 303–316.

Naugle, R. I., & Kawczak, K. (1989). Limitations of the Mini-Mental State Examination. *Cleveland Clinic Journal of Medicine, 56*(3), 277–281.

Neppe, V. M. (1983a). *The psychology of déjà vu: Have I been here before?* Johannesburg: Witwatersrand University Press.

Neppe, V. M. (1983b). The olfactory hallucination in the psychic. In W. G. Roll, J. Beloff, & R. A. White (Eds.), *Research in parapsychology 1982* (pp. 234–237). Metuchen, NJ: Scarecrow Press.

Neppe, V. M. (1984a). The management of psychoses associated with complex partial seizures. In J. B. Carlile (Ed.), *Update on psychiatric management* (pp. 122–127). Durban: MASA.

Neppe, V. M. (1984b). Phenomenology and the temporal lobe. In W. G. Roll, J. Beloff, & R. A. White (Eds.), *Research in parapsychology 1983*. Metuchen, NJ: Scarecrow Press.

Neppe, V. M. (1999). *Cry the beloved mind: A voyage of hope.* Seattle, WA: Brainquest Press.

Neppe, V. M., & Blumer, D. (1998). *www.pni.org/neuropsychiatry/seizures/PND*.

Neppe, V., Chen, A., Davis, J. T., Sawchuk, K., & Geist, M. (1992). The application of the Screening Cerebral Assessment of Neppe (BROCAS SCAN) to a neuropsychiatric population. *Journal of Neuropsychiatry and Clinical Neuroscience, 4*(1), 85–94.

Neppe, V. M., & Tucker, G. J. (1988a). Modern perspectives on epilepsy in relation to psychiatry: Classification and evaluation. *Hospital and Community Psychiatry, 39*(3), 263–271.

Neppe, V. M., & Tucker, G. J. (1988b). Modern perspectives on epilepsy in relation to psychiatry: Behavioral disturbances of epilepsy. *Hospital and Community Psychiatry, 39*(4), 389–396.

Neppe, V. M., & Tucker, G. J. (1989). Atypical, unusual and cultural psychoses. In H. I. Kaplan & B. J. Sadock (Eds.), *Comprehensive textbook of psychiatry* (5th ed., pp. 842–852). Baltimore, MD: Williams & Wilkins.

Neppe, V. M., & Tucker, G. J. (1992). Neuropsychiatric aspects of seizure disorders. In S. C. Yudofsky & R. E. Hales (Eds.), *Textbook of neuropsychiatry* (pp. 397–426). Washington, DC: American Psychiatric Press.

Neppe, V. M., & Tucker, G. J. (1994). Neuropsychiatric aspects of epilepsy and atypical spells. In S. C. Yudofsky & R. E. Hales (Eds.), *Synopsis of textbook of neuropsychiatry* (pp. 397–426). Washington, DC: American Psychiatric Press.

Overall, J. C., & Gorham, D. P. (1962). The Brief Psychiatric Rating Scale. *Psychological Reports, 10,* 799–802.

Overall, J. E., & Beller, S. A. (1984). The Brief Psychiatric Rating Scale (BPRS) in geropsychiatric research: I. Factor structure on an inpatient unit. *Journal of Gerontology, 39*(2), 187–193.

Schwamm, L. H., Van Dyke, C., Kiernan, R. J., Merrin, E. L., & Mueller, J. (1987). The Neurobehavioral Cognitive Status Examination: Comparison with the Cognitive Capacity Screening Examination and the Mini-Mental State Examination in a neurosurgical population. *Annals of Internal Medicine, 107*(4), 486–491.

Thomsen, I. V. (1974). The patient with severe head injury and his family. *Scandinavian Journal of Rehabilitative Medicine, 6,* 180–183.

Tucker, G. J., & Neppe, V. M. (1988). Neurology and psychiatry. *General Hospital Psychiatry, 10*(1), 24–33.

Tucker, G. J., & Neppe, V. M. (1991). Neurologic and neuropsychiatric assessment of brain injury. In H. O. Doerr & A. S. Carlin (Eds.), *Forensic neuropsychology: Legal and scientific basis* (pp. 70–85). New York: Guilford Press.

Tucker, G. J., & Neppe, V. M. (1994). Seizures, 1. In J. M. Silver, S. C. Yudofsky, & R. E. Hales (Eds.), *Neuropsychiatry of traumatic brain injury* (pp. 513–532). Washington, DC: American Psychiatric Press.

11

Epilepsy Spectrum Disorder in the Context of Mild Traumatic Brain Injury

Richard J. Roberts
Veterans' Administration Medical Center, Iowa City, Iowa

We see what we look for. We look for what we know.

—Goethe

There is no area of clinical rehabilitation that better exemplifies this adage than MTBI.

—Nathan Zasler, MD

When we don't even believe that something is possible or that it exists, we fail to see it at all.

—Dorothy Otnow Lewis, MD

Within the past decade, neuropsychiatrists and neuropsychologists have focused increasing attention on a clinical syndrome that consists of the experiencing of multiple episodic phenomena reminiscent of partial seizure disorders; the experiencing of these episodic phenomena usually occurs in the context of marked affective lability and dysthymia (Neppe & Kaplan, 1988; Neppe & Tucker, 1994; Roberts et al., 1992; Roberts, Varney, Paulsen, & Richardson, 1990; Tucker, Price, Johnson, & McAllister, 1986; Verduyn, Hilt, Roberts, & Roberts, 1992). For the purposes of this chapter, such patients are referred to as manifesting *epilepsy spectrum disorder* (abbreviated ESD, as in Hines, Swan, Roberts, & Varney, 1995; Roberts et al., 1992), and the spell-like cognitive, affective, and psychosensory symptoms such patients manifest are described as *partial seizure-like*. Selection of the phrases *ESD* and *partial seizure-like* was guided by the dual goals of: (a) calling attention to the points of close similarity between the phenomenology of this syndrome and the phenomenology of conventionally accepted partial epileptic disorders (Daly, 1982; Devinsky & Luciano, 1988; ILAE, 1985), and (b) avoiding fruitless semantic debate (cf. Neppe & Tucker, 1994) as to whether such patients manifest a "true variant" of an established subtype of epilepsy, such as complex partial seizures (Neppe & Tucker, 1988).

The theses of this chapter are (a) that epilepsy spectrum disorder can and does occur following mild-to-moderate closed head trauma, and (b) that ESD is likely to prove to be a major factor contributing to unexpectedly poor clinical outcomes in the "miserable minority" who continue to manifest dysfunction following closed head trauma. Given that patients with ESD frequently obtain considerable benefit from treatment with anticonvulsant medications (Blumer, Heilbronn, & Himmelhoch, 1988; Hayes & Goldsmith, 1991; Neppe & Kaplan, 1988; Varney, Garvey, Campbell, Cook, & Roberts, 1993), it is important that clinicians who evaluate and treat patients with closed head injuries learn how to recognize cases of epilepsy spectrum disorder and how to intervene with such patients to improve long-term clinical outcomes. In order to facilitate these goals, subsequent sections of this chapter cover the following topics: Overview and Clinical Description of ESD, History of the Concept, Interviewing for Partial Seizure-Like Symptoms, The Role of Neuropsychological Assessment, Ancillary Neurodiagnostic Testing, Etiologic Considerations, Differential Diagnosis and Associated Features, and Treatment Considerations. The concluding section presents a brief, multiaxial schema for clinicians to guide the care and evaluation of dysfunctioning patients with mild TBI.

OVERVIEW AND CLINICAL DESCRIPTION OF ESD

Probably the best clinical description of ESD patients remains the seminal paper by Gary Tucker and his neuropsychiatric colleagues (1986) entitled Phenomenology of Temporal Lobe Dysfunction: A Link to Atypical Psychosis—A Series of Cases. In this article, these clinicians described 20 patients with the following core features: (a) multiple spells, (b) intense, episodic mood swings, (c) episodic cognitive dysfunction, (d) frequent suicidal ideation or attempts, (e) episodic psychosensory hallucinations, and (f) unusual nocturnal phenomena. In addition, these patients shared a number of associated characteristics. Nineteen had abnormal (but not necessarily clearly epileptiform) electroencephalograph (EEG) findings; the remaining patient was observed to display an automatism. Virtually all of the patients had been misdiagnosed as suffering from primary psychiatric disorders; however, when strict *DSM–III* criteria were applied, few actually met full diagnostic criteria. Most of these patients had poor responses to conventional psychotropic medications (such as antipsychotics, lithium, and tricyclics), which lower seizure threshold. Their clinical courses were atypical for most forms of psychosis because, in between intensely symptomatic episodes, there were intermittent periods of relatively "normal" functioning. Most importantly, significant clinical improvement was observed among these patients when they were treated with various anticonvulsants, even though most had extensive histories of being regarded as treatment-refractory. It was implied that such patients manifested a variant of complex partial seizures and that their symptoms reflected underlying electrophysiologic dysfunction, assumptions that Neppe and Tucker (1994) subsequently deemphasized. A major omission in the Tucker et al. 1986 report was that no information or speculation was included regarding the potential etiology of this protean but recognizable clinical syndrome.

From a neuropsychological perspective, Varney's research group independently confirmed the existence of patients similar to those described by Tucker and noted that many had sustained previous, mild to moderate closed head injuries (Roberts et al., 1992). Such patients were frequently misdiagnosed as having multiple, different, primary psychiatric disorders, often produced grossly abnormal and multiply elevated Minnesota Multiphasic Personality Inventory (MMPI) profiles, and frequently failed to perform within normal limits on a simple dichotic word listening task.

Following up on these observations, Verduyn and colleagues (1992) reported on 17 previously healthy individuals referred to a rehabilitation medicine practice following head trauma; these patients were noted to have developed multiple partial seizure-like symptoms subsequent to having sustained their well-documented, closed head injuries. Support for the assertion by Verduyn and colleagues that closed head injury was likely to be an etiologic factor in the onset of ESD came from large-scale questionnaire studies. In two separate questionnaire surveys of healthy, American college students, Roberts et al. (1990) found that history of head trauma with loss of consciousness was associated with the endorsement of a greater number of partial seizure-like symptoms. Using a similar questionnaire with a healthy, South American university students, Ardila and colleagues also demonstrated a significant, positive association between history of closed head trauma and endorsement of a greater breadth of partial seizure-like phenomena (Ardila, Nino, Pulido, Rivera, & Vanegas, 1993). Given evidence implicating mild to moderate traumatic brain injury (TBI) as a common cause of ESD, Hines and colleagues proposed a neurophysiological model that could explain how damage to inhibitory cells in the hippocampus could ultimately produce the wide range of symptomatology reported by ESD patients (Hines et al., 1995).

In addition to the research and clinical literature just described, several purely clinical descriptions of aspects of ESD deserve note. The case of "Jill Rasmussen" described in the popular press book *Seized* (LaPlante, 1993, p. 73) illustrates the complications of coping with ESD in daily life (although the patient's neuropsychologist and neurologist are quoted as viewing the patient as suffering from a variant of complex partial seizures). Another popular press account, *Robin's Story* (1981) by Carol Gino, realistically chronicled the problems and complications suffered by a young woman whose atypical electrophysiologic dysfunction is misdiagnosed as a severe, primary, psychiatric disturbance. A clinical case report by Veterans' Administration neuropsychologist Gerald Goldstein (1984) illustrated the complexities of making the diagnosis of ESD within the veteran population and the potential benefits to patient when an empirical trial of anticonvulsant medication is successful. More recently, Pincus and Lewis (cf. Lewis, 1998) noted that histories of cerebral damage with multiple episodic symptoms and "spells" are quite common in extremely violent young adults and teenage murderers.

HISTORY OF THE CONCEPT

Although the label *epilepsy spectrum disorder* is relatively new and not yet widely accepted, many of the spell-like episodic symptoms that are part of the syndrome were identified in the 19th century by early epileptologists such Hughlings Jackson (Daly, 1982) and Jean-Marie Charcot (Goetz, 1987). The following quote from Jackson's Lumelian lecture (1866) clearly indicates that he would have had little difficulty regarding the symptoms described by ESD patients as falling within the broad spectrum of the epilepsies:

> The word "epilepsy" should be degraded [i.e., expanded] and be used to imply the condition of nerve tissue in sudden and temporary loss of its function, whether that be loss of sight, loss of consciousness, or "running down of tension" which governs muscles. For it is not unlikely that the condition of nerve tissue is the same or similar ... when a patient loses sight for ... half a minute, or has a temporary loss of consciousness, or becomes unable to talk for a short time, or has a spasm on the hand, or the side of the face, or leg, or all three on one side. Probably, too, in cases in which a man all at once passes into a violent rage from no apparent cause, or into a state somewhat like somnambulism, in which he may walk a mile or two, or walk into a canal, or in which he takes off his boots in church, or undresses himself in the street, there is Epilepsy—using the new sense of the word—of some parts of the hemisphere. (p. 442)

Similarly, the neurologic historian Goetz (1987) described in detail a case of Charcot's who presented with bizarre ambulatory spells that were recognized by Charcot as fundamentally epileptic in nature. Charcot's patient, an otherwise healthy young man, experienced multiple episodes during which he suddenly became unaware of his surroundings, rambled around Paris and its outskirts, conversed, and had complex interactions with his fellow Parisians. For Charcot, the patient's normal functioning between spells suggested underlying epilepsy, and he treated the patient with bromides, which produced a favorable clinical response. Goetz commented:

> Charcot's suggestion that these events were epileptic was remarkable. Vaguely similar cases had been described, but always discussed in terms of post-ictal events or epileptic equivalents. . . . Sixty years later, in 1935, [S.A. Kinnear] Wilson proposed the term "psychic variant" to emphasize that these behaviors were not equivalent to epilepsy but were epilepsy itself in a distinct form that did not resemble tonic-clonic movements. (p. 1085)

Moving forward in time to the period between 1955 and 1975, psychiatrist Russell Monroe (1959, 1982) published extensively on the need for clinicians to focus on the episodic and paroxysmal phenomena displayed by atypical patients. Among other contributions, Monroe was responsible for developing and elaborating on the concepts of "atypical psychosis," "episodic dyscontrol," and "limbic ictus." He was also an advocate of using anticonvulsant medications with pharmacologically treatment-resistant patients and often theorized that the behavioral dysfunction of such patients reflected underlying electrophysiologic dysfunction in their brains.

Working independently of Monroe, a psychoanalyst named Jonas (1965) published a fascinating but seldom-cited monograph titled *Ictal and Subictal Neurosis*. This book summarized his observations on 102 patients who experienced multiple spells and odd symptoms with abrupt onset and limited duration. What initially stimulated Jonas's interest in such patients was observing firsthand the significant behavioral changes manifested by the son of a close friend a few months after that teenager had been briefly knocked unconscious during a basketball game. The following features characterized the patients in Jonas's sample: They reported multiple partial seizure-like symptoms, including intense and abrupt changes in affect; they were typically misdiagnosed, most often as malingerers, hysterics, psychopaths, or pseudoneurotic schizophrenics; they often responded positively to treatment with phenytoin (the major, effective anticonvulsant medication of that era); they were prone to have an excess of theta rhythm abnormalities on EEG; and many patients reported severe headaches or unusual cephalic sensations. Verbal psychotherapy was sometimes effective in promoting adjustment, but only after a reduction of symptoms had been produced by treatment with phenytoin. In addition, many of Jonas's patients acted like wary "burnt children" with regard to any proposed therapeutic endeavors on their behalf: "From the beginning, most of these patients were essentially distrustful and required considerable persuasion before accepting any medication. Their prevailing attitude was pessimistic and hopeless, as if they did not believe anything could help them" (p. vii). Although Jonas had intended to publish a second monograph on treatment and longer term outcome of his sample, none was forthcoming.

Two years prior to Tucker's 1986 case series, Goldstein (1984) published the case study of a veteran that was described in the previous section. Although forgoing debate as to whether his patient suffered some form of epilepsy, Goldstein emphasized the potential benefits of a well-reasoned, empirical trial of medications aimed at treating relevant target symptoms:

> In view of this combination of symptoms without definitive neurological documentation, the patient received a number of psychiatric diagnoses including hysterical neurosis—conversion type, passive-aggressive personality with hysterical features, and situational reaction with anxiety and depression. One examining neurologist explicitly stated that the patient had no neurological disease and was one of the 10–15% of normal people with abnormal EEGs. It is not our intention to declare that this patient actually did or did not have epilepsy.... The fact that ... the patient's symptoms were reduced by anticonvulsant and antimigraine medications may provide some organic basis for this disorder, but ... it is very hazardous to diagnose from drug response. (p. 70)

Two years after Tucker's case series was published, epileptologist Dietrich Blumer and colleagues reported on a series of 28 consecutive psychiatric patients who were "exemplary carbamazepine responders" (Blumer et al., 1988). Blumer described these patients as manifesting a temporal-lobe syndrome characterized by "atypical pleomorphic psychopathology," rapid mood swings, and subtle signs of central nervous system (CNS) impairment. Often there was a positive family history of epilepsy. According to these clinicians, "subtle seizures may be present and allow diagnosis of TLE [Temporal Lobe Epilepsy]; in the absence of any seizures, the disorders are identified as temporal lobe syndrome (TLS)" (p. 120).

There is considerable symptomatic and conceptual overlap between ESD and certain diagnostic categories in the currently accepted psychiatric nosology, DSM–IV (American Psychiatric Association, 1994). In particular, patients with ESD may meet many or many of the criteria for the following diagnoses: mood disorder due to general medical condition (*DSM–IV* Code 293.83); personality change due to general medical condition (310.1); and intermittent explosive disorder (312.34). Under Appendix B of *DSM–IV*, which covers Criterion Sets and Axes Provided for Further Study, many of the symptoms defining the category of postconcussional disorder (e.g., headache, excessive fatigue, vertigo, affective lability, etc.) clearly overlap with the phenomenologic complaints of ESD patients as discussed in the next section.

INTERVIEWING FOR PARTIAL SEIZURE-LIKE SYMPTOMS

During the past decade, a number of rating scales, interviews, and questionnaires have been developed that have potential relevance to epilepsy, partial seizures, temporal-lobe dysfunction, episodic symptoms, and ESD (Jampala, Atre-Vaidya, Taylor, Schrift, Srinivasaraghavan, & Sierles, 1992; Marakec & Persinger, 1990; Neppe, 1983; Neppe, Bowman, & Sawchuk, 1991; Persinger & Marakec, 1993; Reutens, 1992; Silberman, Post, Nurnberger, Theodore, & Boulenger, 1985; Teicher, Glod, Surrey, & Swett, 1993). However, because the Iowa Interview for Partial Seizure-like Symptoms (IIPSS) was developed expressly for the purpose of assessing for the presence of ESD (Roberts et al., 1990), this section focuses almost exclusively on the clinical use of the IIPSS.

The evolving item content of the IIPSS was drawn from the research literature on partial seizure symptoms (e.g., Devinsky & Luciano, 1991) and has been modified on several occasions based on using earlier versions with several hundred clinical patients who had sustained closed head trauma (and their collateral informants). The current version of the interview consists of 40 items and is reprinted in the Appendix following this chapter. To promote conceptual clarity, items have been grouped in the following rationally derived clusters: psychosensory symptoms, cognitive symptoms, affective symptoms, and nocturnal/sleep-related phenomena. The first three categories of symptoms are inadvertently highly similar to the subtyping of partial seizure symptoms advocated by Hughlings Jackson in the preceding century (Daly, 1982), With the IIPSS, the frequency of occurrence of 39 of the items is rated on a 7-point scale, ranging from 0 (never, or not in the past year) to 6 (more than once per day). The remaining item (i.e., progressive cognitive decline) is rated on a yes/no basis, with *yes* scored as a 6 and *no* scored as a 0. Typically, the scores from individual items are summed, and this total score is compared with normative standards from young adults with no history of head trauma, epilepsy, or other forms of neurological illness. Previously unpublished norms ($n = 115$) for the current 40-item version of the IIPSS are also presented in the Appendix. (It should be noted that the IIPSS is simply presented as a Medical Symptom Checklist when given to normal subjects for standardization; furthermore, when used in clinical practice, nothing is typically said to patients or family members about epilepsy or partial seizure disorders prior to covering the item content with them. Furthermore, the IIPSS is typically administered only after an open-ended interview has been completed.) On the 40-item version, a total score that exceeds the 95th percentile of this normative sample is generally regarded as clinically significant and, in the context of a history of prior closed head trauma, a cogent reason to suspect the presence of ESD. In addition to yielding the total score index, each of the 39 frequency-rated items in the interview has the 90th percentile for that given item connoted by a bold-faced number beneath the given item. This feature permits the interviewer to make a judgment at the time of the interview as to whether an individual item has been endorsed with a clinically significant frequency. Although there is some variation, in our experience a symptom that occurs at least three or four times per week is likely to be a clinically significant problem for the typical patient.

Between our research and Ardila's (Ardila et al., 1993), various versions of the IIPSS and similar instruments have been administered in questionnaire format to a total of several thousand control subjects. Previous studies with the IIPSS (Ardila et al., 1993; Roberts et al., 1990) have established the following findings with regard to the interview:

1. Asking people on a simple yes/no basis whether or not they have experienced a given symptom generally does not provide useful information, whereas asking about the frequency with which an individual has noticed a certain symptom does provide coherent information.

2. Partial seizure-like symptoms are reported by non-brain-injured, healthy, young adults, but they are *not* frequent.

3. It has proven feasible to use this semistructured interview clinically to identify ESD patients similar to those described in detail by Tucker and his colleagues (1986).

4. Among healthy volunteers, higher scores on earlier 30-item and 36-item versions of the IIPSS were significantly associated with history of head trauma, severe febrile illness, hypogeusia, and hyposmia.

5. Neither normal subjects nor clinical patients frequently endorsed nonepileptic foil items (e.g., episodic pain in the ear lobes), and hence these were dropped from the current version of the IIPSS.

It should be noted in passing that certain practitioners have criticized, directly or indirectly, the use of the IIPSS and similar patient-report instruments in evaluating the effects of suspected brain injuries (Rizzo & Tranel, 1996; Wong, Regennitter, & Barrios, 1994). In particular, Wong and her colleagues objected to the use of "poorly designed and leading questionnaires" that are viewed as suggesting to legitimate patients or even malingerers symptoms that they would not have complained about on their own initiative. In Wong's study where normal college students were instructed to malinger, their scores were somewhat elevated compared to uninstructed subjects; however, the mean score of the instructed malingerer group was nowhere near the mean scores of our various published, clinical samples with posttraumatic ESD.

Although such critical caveats are no doubt well intended, they minimize some of the complexities involved in interacting clinically with dysfunctional patients with mild TBI. In our experience, it is much more common for patients to underestimate the frequency with which their symptoms occur than to overestimate. This is particularly true for symptoms that are associated with compromised self-monitoring (e.g., brief confusional spells) or alteration of consciousness (e.g., memory lapses, unremembered actions and conversations) and for events that might be regarded as provoking shame after the fact (e.g., anger outbursts). In addition, many premorbidly normal individuals who develop ESD following head trauma are privately concerned that they may in fact be "going crazy" due to the plethora of involuntary symptoms and ego-dystonic aberrations that punctuate their conscious daily lives. In this regard, Jonas's (1965) observations (which clearly antedate the current, polarized, medicolegal climate surrounding brain injury litigation) concerning his patients' wariness and demoralization should be kept in mind. Additionally, we have observed that some stoic individuals (particularly combat-hardened veterans) may try to cope with their ESD symptoms by attempting to suppress their awareness of them in everyday life; such individuals tend to minimize the attention they pay to unwanted nuisances, such as episodic ringing in the ears or visual distortions. Once such individuals are asked about episodic symptoms by a concerned health care professional, they may track them more veridically and inform the clinician at a subsequent appointment that they had indeed underestimated the frequency of some symptoms; this pattern of improved symptom monitoring is not the same as "making up" symptoms that did not really exist in the first place, and it should not automatically be taken as prima facie proof that the patient is now lying or has been led into exaggerating symptom complaints by the interviewing clinician. Finally, ESD due to head trauma, particularly head trauma sustained in motor vehicle accidents, is likely to occur in the context of diminished executive function due to damage or dysfunction in the anterior portion of the brain due to direct impact or contrecoup. Such executive dysfunction may well interfere with a patient's capacity to recall all his or her symptoms or to relate symptoms in a coherent fashion to a health care professional, particularly if the professional is pressed for time. Thus, following a traditional open-ended interview in which the patients are given free rein to present their concerns, use of a semistructured interview can help to ensure that patients with executive dysfunction have not inadvertently failed to describe all relevant, troublesome, episodic phenomena to the clinician.

THE ROLE OF NEUROPSYCHOLOGICAL ASSESSMENT

The referral questions confronting the clinical neuropsychologist in the evaluation of ESD patients will vary depending on the circumstances surrounding the given referral. Based on our experience, clinical neuro-psychologists are often in the position of "discovering" (or detecting) and attempting to quantify and describe what is actually wrong with the mild to moderate TBI patient who has failed to recover. Because ESD has only recently been emphasized in the neuropsychiatric literature as a clinical entity in its own right, neuropsychologists almost never receive direct referrals that state "Please evaluate for ESD" as the explicit referral question. It is more likely that stated referral questions will involve memory loss, posttraumatic headaches, or episodic cognitive lapses if the patient has sought medical evaluation on his or her own initiative; on the other hand, anger outbursts, chronic dysthymia and suicidal ideation, or poor parenting are more common referral issues if a family member or signifi-cant other has compelled the patient to seek medical attention. In the event that the referral comes from an attorney rather than a health care professional, the referral question is likely to be more general, namely, "What, if anything, is wrong with this patient?" or "Does this patient show signs of a 'postconcussive syndrome'?" When referrals of patients with ESD emanate from vocational rehab specialists or employers, issues involving loss of cognitive efficiency, inconsistency in performance, mem-ory lapses, inability to function properly on the job site, excessive irrita-bility, and frequent absenteeism (most often due to chronic headaches) are likely to predominate. When a child with ESD is the identified patient, teachers and school psychologists are likely to express concern about inability to complete assignments, behavioral outbursts, atypical ADHD, stunted academic progress, and reduced reading comprehension. Geyde (1996) also called attention to the occurrrence of ESD-like symptoms in retarded individuals who engage in repeated, pointless, nonoperant aggression. In our experience, referrals from psychiatrists tend to be for treatment-refractory depression ("Is cognitive therapy indicated?") or pointless aggression ("Wife complains of verbal abuse, and patient is apparently genuinely remorseful"), whereas neurologists (especially those who are not disposed by formal training to view ESD patients as epileptic) will often refer for questions concerning atypical memory loss, persistent headaches, somatization, factitious disorder, or malingering. Generally, in such instances a given patient has complained of "too many" different symptoms (any one or two of which, in isolation, would be legitimately indicative of a simple partial seizure disorder) to appear credible to the neurologist or psychiatrist.

Regardless of the referral source and referral question, the utility of thorough history taking cannot be overemphasized (Fisher, 1982). With regard to ESD in the context of brain injury, the patient and his or her family may frequently fail to realize that there may be a causal connection between a past incident of head trauma and the patient's present suffering and distress. Therefore, it is important to establish whether or not (and also, at how many different times) the patient has sustained head trauma by interviewing the patient and ideally at least one well-informed collateral. At these early stages of the assessment process, it is best for the neuropsychologist to *refrain from impulsively assuming that a given episode of cranial trauma was clinically trivial* because: (a) the impact was too trivial, (b) there was no extended period of loss of consciousness, or (c) the patient's Glasgow Coma Scale was only in the range of 13 to 15. This temporary and voluntary "suspension of disbelief" on the part of the clinician seems warranted in the earliest stages of the neuropsychological exam, given that recent reviews have presented well-documented cases where seemingly minor motor vehicle impacts have exerted serious biomechanical forces on brain tissue (Liu, Chandran, Heath, & Unterharn-scheidt, 1984; Sweeney, 1992; Varney & Varney, 1995).

If the referral question, available medical documentation, patient interview data, and collateral interview raise suspicion of an ESD component to the patient's clinical presentation, the neuropsychologist should proceed with administering the IIPSS, or a similar instrument, following the customary, open-ended portion of the interview. If IIPSS responses are consistent with the presence of ESD, then formal neuropsychological assessment can be useful in attempting to support or refute that working clinical hypothesis. Here we wish to emphasize our personal preference for a flexible-battery, hypothesis-testing approach to assessment, one that permits the neuropsychologist to administer tests or directly observe patient behavior during the testing procedures, so that the qualitative features of performance, such as brief cognitive lapses and episodic word-finding problems, can be reliably noted. Even well-trained testing technicians may miss or discount relatively brief alterations in patient behavior if they do not have extensive experience observing and interacting with patients with posttraumatic ESD.

With regard to the formal testing portion of the neuropsych exam, it has often been remarked that no two instances of cranial trauma are exactly alike; therefore, test findings from ESD patients generally tend to be more variable than they are in focal stroke syndromes or following relatively discrete neurosurgical procedures. With regard to the most commonly administered types of tests, ESD patients with positive neuropsych findings will generally manifest mild to moderate problems with attention/concentration and may manifest difficulties with encoding and retrieval of information between short-term memory (STM) and long-term memory (LTM) stores. Also, in selected cases there may be some additional focal neuropsychological deficits attributable to gross structural lesions (ones that would usually be apparent on static neuroimaging studies such as computed tomography [CT] and magnetic resonance imaging [MRI]). The majority of patients who develop ESD following mechanical trauma also need to be tested and interviewed for signs and symptoms of frontal lobe dysfunction. Varney's Iowa Collateral Head Injury Interview is helpful in this regard, as well as formal testing of olfactory function (Varney & Menefee, 1993). Relatively less structured tasks such as Controlled Oral Word Association, Design Fluency (Varney et al., 1996), and the Tinker Toy task (Bayless, Roberts, & Varney, 1989) are also helpful in alerting the clinician to deficits in executive function that may interfere with treatment compliance and longer term outcome.

The single neurobehavioral test that has repeatedly proven to be highly sensitive to cognitive processing deficits associated with ESD is dichotic word listening (Roberts, Varney, Paulsen, & Richardson, 1990). In various studies, it has been demonstrated that 70% to 75% of patients with clinically significant symptoms of ESD fail simple dichotic word listening tasks. In fact, both bilateral and rather remarkable unilateral dichotic listening suppressions may occur that are comparable in size to those produced by patients with gross structural lesions due to stroke or tumor, which clearly sever primary auditory pathways (Damasio & Damasio, 1979). Furthermore, many ESD patients exhibit marked improvement in dichotic word listening performance when the episodic, partial seizure-like symptoms of ESD are successfully treated with anticonvulsant medications such as carbamazepine and valproic acid. Thus, periodic administration of dichotic word listening may help the clinician gauge the degree of improvement due to treatment with anticonvulsants.

An extensive discussion as to why dichotic listening has proven to be such an excellent neurobehavioral marker for ESD is beyond the scope of this chapter, and the interested reader is referred to a more detailed discussion of the clinical applications of dichotic tasks by Richardson and her colleagues (Richardson, Springer, Varney, Struchen, & Roberts, 1994). However, a few points deserve brief discussion. First, Roberts and colleagues have speculated elsewhere that dichotic listening performance deficits in untreated ESD patients are likely to reflect the adverse effects subclinical "neural noise" (cf. Hutt, 1972; Hutt & Fairweather, 1971) due to electrophysiological dysfunction in white matter (Richardson et al., 1994); in this regard, it is instructive to note that this sort of dichotic listening task is frequently failed by bona fide, neurologist-diagnosed epilepsy patients with conventional complex partial seizure disorders—even when such partial epileptics show no apparent structural lesions on CT or static MRI studies (Grote, Pierre-Louis, Smith, Roberts, & Varney, 1995; Lee et al., 1994). Second, dichotic listening is likely to be sensitive to momentary fluctuations in efficiency of cerebral functioning precisely because it requires patient to process a mild overload of auditory information in real time (unlike "static" neuropsychological measures such as an untimed verbal naming task). It is important to emphasize that the European concept of "transitory cognitive impairment" described in the epileptology literature seems quite relevant to understanding the cognitive problems experienced by ESD patients (Aarts, Binnie, Smit, & Wilkins, 1984; Binnie, Channon, & Marston, 1991; Shewmon & Erwin; 1989). As is true for their affective and behavioral symptoms, many of the cognitive deficits and complaints of ESD patients are highly variable and episodic in nature. Thus, within the same 3- to 4-hr testing session, cognitive efficiency may fluctuate extensively, and even rather severe deficits (e.g., gross anomia) may be transitory in nature, depending on electrophysiologically based oscillations in cerebral function. This also may help to explain in part why the mental efficiency and test performances of some head injury patients appear substantially different to different neuropsychological evaluators on different days. Lack of consistency in performance over time is occasionally presumed to constitute evidence of malingering or "psychological overlay" in TBI patients undergoing forensic evaluations; however, if ESD is a major part of the actual clinical for certain TBI patients, "unexpected" fluctuations over time or within testing sessions may actually be a legitimate characteristic of the patient's "best" performance. Before rejecting this notion out of hand, skeptics should consider the opinion of two giants of neurology. Henry Head (1926) wrote: "An inconsistent response is one of the most striking results produced by a lesion of the cerebral cortex" (p. 145). Decades later, Arthur Benton, the dean of American neuropsychology, emphasized a highly similar concept that he labeled "oscillation of function" (Benton, 1984). Thus, there are clear theoretical and observational precedents for brain-injured patients manifesting highly variable performance on cognitive tasks over time. There are also data from carefully time-locked electrophysiological studies (e.g., Shewmon & Erwin, 1989; Wieser, Hailermariam, Regard, & Landis, 1985) that demonstrate conclusively that brief disruptions of the electrical stability of restricted portions of the cerebrum can selectively impair specific cognitive performances without generalized cognitive dysfunction.

A final caveat with regard to formal psychological assessment of ESD patients deserves mention. Studies have demonstrated that the majority of ESD patients produce grossly abnormal, multiply elevated MMPI profiles with 7 or more of the 10 clinical scales elevated above the clinical cutoff of T-score = 69 (e.g., Roberts et al., 1989; Roberts, Gorman, Roecker, & Lee, 1993). (Although these earlier studies have not been replicated with the MMPI–2 to our knowledge, it seems likely that ESD patients would also produce extremely elevated profiles on this revision of the MMPI, given the extensive item overlap between the two instruments.) Such grossly elevated MMPI profiles appear to be highly sensitive to the neuropsychopathology of ESD, but are not specific for ESD and may be produced by other patient groups. Nevertheless, based on the available data, clinicians should avoid reflexively dismissing a patient who fits the ESD symptom profile as a somatizer, malingerer, or factitious exaggerator simply because the patient produces a bizarrely elevated MMPI profile. If the thesis underlying the present chapter is correct (namely, that ESD is frequently found in the "miserable minority" of mild TBI patients who do not recover as expected), then the most parsimonious way to account for the presence of a grossly elevated MMPI profiles is to consider the likelihood that polysymptomatic ESD patients veridically endorse a myriad of different types of symptoms on the MMPI. Elsewhere, other neurobehavioral experts have summarized additional reasons why the MMPI may have extremely limited utility in acutely ill neurologic populations (e.g., refer to chap. 13 in this volume).

ANCILLARY NEURODIAGNOSTIC TESTING

With regard to EEG evaluation, a fairly large-scale study of ESD patients estimated that roughly 10% of such patients generated interictal EEG findings that are read as "clearly epileptiform," and roughly 40% of these patients manifested some sort of EEG abnormality on standard EEG (Roberts et al., 1993). The yield of positive EEG findings is somewhat enhanced by using 24-hr ambulatory EEG protocols (provided that the entire protocol is reviewed and not just the epochs where a given patient has pressed the signal button). In any event, an extensive case report by Roberts and colleagues (Roberts, Manshadi, Bushnell, & Hines, 1995) demonstrated the fallacy of necessarily requiring positive EEG findings before one implements an empirical trial of treatment with anticonvulsants for the individual ESD patient.

Whether clearly epileptiform or nonspecific, EEG findings from ESD patients tend to be focal rather than diffuse. In addition to isolated frontotemporal spiking and spike-and-wave phenomena, ESD patients have been noted to demonstrate a surprisingly high frequency of theta bursts on EEG exams. Varney and colleagues described a selected series of patients with histories of mild-to-moderate closed head injury who manifested abnormal bursting in the 4–7 Hz range on either standard or 24-hr ambulatory EEG (Varney, Hines, Bailey, & Roberts, 1992). On an early 19-item forerunner of the IIPSS, the mean number of partial seizure-like symptoms endorsed by this theta burst sample with a clinically significant frequency was 15.3 (S.D. = 3.7). Roughly 76% of the sample performed defectively on dichotic word listening, despite manifesting relatively few cognitive deficits on other types of tasks.

Subsequently, there has been an unpublished conceptual replication of these findings in which endorsement of partial seizure-like symptoms of patients with theta bursts on EEG was contrasted with that of two matched comparison groups: patients with theta-delta slowing on EEG (but no bursting), and patients referred for EEG evaluation but found to have normal EEGs (Roberts & Varney, 1997). There were 38 subjects in the theta burst group and 30 subjects in both the normal EEG and theta-delta slowing comparison groups. The theta-delta slowing group was included to control for the presence of a clear electrophysiologic abnormality in roughly the same wavelength as the theta burst patients, but one that had no paroxysmal features. When medical records were exhaustively reviewed in this retrospective study, it was found that 55% of the theta burst patients had histories of at least mild to moderate closed head injury, versus 53% and 63% for the normal EEG and theta-delta slowing groups, respectively. Thus, all patients with theta bursting on EEG do not have histories of closed head injury; however, theta burst patients were significantly more likely than patients in the other two group to endorse the presence of episodic, partial seizure-like symptoms with clinically significant frequency. Furthermore, those 21/38 theta-burst patients who were found to have histories of closed head injury were even more likely to have complex partial seizure (CPS)-like phenomena described in their medical records, especially if they had sustained loss of consciousness due to head trauma. Similarly, seven theta-burst patients whose EEG tracings also showed evidence of isolated temporal lobe spiking had high rates of episodic phenomena reported in their medical records. Thus, the presence of theta bursts on EEG (with or without spiking) in the context of a preexisting closed head injury should alert the clinician to interview for the presence of ESD (cf. Bare, Burnstine, Fisher, & Lesser, 1994).

Clearly, more research is needed on the presumed, underlying electro-physiologic basis of ESD. However, the work of Wieser established that patients can suffer from clinically troublesome partial seizure phenomena without necessarily showing blatant abnormalities on traditional clinical EEG tracings. Similarly, Devinsky's group (Devinsky, Kelley, Porter, & Theodore, 1988) showed that simple partial seizure symptoms in well-di-agnosed epileptics seldom have obvious electrophysiological concomi-tants on standard surface EEG recordings. These observations have led some medical practitioners to debate the wisdom and expense of exhaus-tively pursuing the presence of an equivocal EEG abnormality prior to trying an empirical trial of one or another anticonvulsant when ESD is suspected after closed head injury (CHI) (Tierney & Fogel, 1995).

Although it is beyond the scope of this chapter to review the utility of functional imaging techniques in mild TBI patients with persistent neurobehavioral dysfunction, early observations suggest that positron emission tomography (PET) and neuroSPECT techniques may ultimately prove to have considerable practical utility in documenting the metabolic correlates of brain dysfunction in ESD patients following instances of closed head injury (e.g., Wu & Varney, 1998).

ETIOLOGIC CONSIDERATIONS

Delineation of the precise etiologic factors that can produce ESD has not been fully accomplished. Nevertheless, the reader should have deduced by now that the author's best hypothesis is that ESD is an environmentally acquired brain disorder and one presumably mediated by subtle electrical disturbances in the brain: a sort of "neural noise" capable of creating both positive/irritative and negative/deficit symptoms. It appears doubtful to us that many cases of ESD will prove to have a genetic basis or a learned or psychodynamic etiology. Because the concept of ESD has not yet been reified and included in *DSM–IV*, ICD-9, or most classificatory systems for epileptic syndromes, large-scale population study of various etiologic possibilities has not yet been proposed. What is offered in this section is largely speculative and is intended to promote discussion (rather than prematurely closing down discussion) on what causes this interesting syndrome.

At this very early juncture, the scant evidence available raises the possibility that the presumed brain dysfunction or neuronal damage underlying ESD may be traced to one or more of the following sites: (a) the hippocampus, (b) the brainstem, or (c) multiple scattered microfocal sites in cortex and white matter. It is also logically possible that dysfunc-tion or neuronal damage in some combination of these or other sites may prove necessary to precipitate full-blown ESD. As mentioned earlier, Hines and colleagues (Hines et al., 1995) postulated a neuroanatomical model in which damage to relatively few inhibitory pyramidal cell neurons in hippocampus could produce the myriad episodic symptoms found in ESD. For a more detailed explication of this hippocampal model, the interested reader is referred to that particular paper. With regard to the second possibility, Andy (1989) reported a detailed case of posttraumatic brain injury that conforms closely to the clinical description of ESD presented in this chapter. In this patient, stimulation from electrodes implanted in the brainstem greatly ameliorated the patient's CPS-like symptoms. Finally, with regard to the third possibility, Wu and Varney (1998) recently proposed that brain dysfunction in ESD following CHI may reflect the summative or interactive effects of multiple microfocal lesion at the juncture of white matter and various cortical regions, particularly in the anterior and mesial temporal lobe and occasionally the occipital lobe as well. The hypothesis is supported by the documentation of numerous small areas of increased metabolic activity found on the PET scans of a series of 16 clinical patients suffering from posttraumatic ESD. According to speculations by Wu and Varney, this clinical syndrome might constitute a sort of "multi-microfocal epilepsy" in which an ESD patient suffered the equivalent of several (or many) classic simple partial seizure-like spells emanating from different small regions of the individual patient's brain. The observation that cerebral malaria sufferers frequently develop ESD is also compatible with a multi-microfocal hypothesis in that this parasitic disease process can result in multiple pinhole hemorrhages in the brain (Varney, Roberts, Springer, Connell, & Wood, 1997). Obviously, a programmatic research effort employing multiple methodological approaches to studying brain function will be required to demonstrate conclusively the final neuroanatomical and/or neuroelectrical final common pathway(s) that underlie the multiform clinical presentation of ESD patients.

With regard to the medical factors or life events that precede the onset of diagnosable ESD in clinical practice, this chapter has focused largely on mechanical trauma to the head and brain as a frequent precursor of ESD. Head injuries of mild to moderate severity are likely to prove to be the most common etiology for ESD, particularly in heavily industrialized countries that rely on motor vehicles as the primary mode of transportation (Varney & Varney, 1995). ESD-like disturbances in more severely injured patients have also been observed in the postacute period of recovery (Barnhill & Gualtieri, 1989). In addition to trauma sustained in motor vehicle accidents, mechanical trauma due to falls, pedestrian and bicycle accidents, participation in contact sports and military combat (including concussion blasts from ordinance exploding at close range but not penetrating the body), penetrating missile wounds, the metabolic sequelae of severe body burns, electrocution, extended periods of hypoxia, the effects of severe febrile illnesses (i.e., in which the adult body temperature reaches 105°F or greater for extended periods of time), selected types of nervous system infections, and selected neurotoxic exposures are also likely to produce ESD. Indeed, Ardila's research demonstrated that in a tropical country, fever was more strongly related to the reporting episodic phenomena than head trauma (Ardila et al., 1993).

In particular, Varney and his associates recently focused attention on the postacute development of ESD in patients who have survived cerebral malaria (Richardson et al., 1994; Varney et al., 1997) and other forms of severe febrile illness while serving in the armed forces in Southeast Asia where falciparum malaria is endemic. For those who practice in Veterans' Administration (VA) facilities, it is worth noting that former American military personnel (particularly Vietnam combat veterans) with histories of closed head trauma or cerebral malaria in military service who present with histories of treatment-refractory depression or chronic posttraumatic stress disorder (PTSD) with dysphoria and rage outbursts (Richardson, Roberts, Hines, & Varney, 1989; Springer, Garvey, Varney, & Roberts, 1991) frequently manifest symptoms of ESD when specifically interviewed about episodic phenomena. The neurobehavioral dysfunction associated with the ESD of such veterans may readily confound and complicate the pharmacological and behavioral treatment of their affective and posttraumatic syndromes. Recently, the use of anticonvulsants was recommended in selected cases of PTSD (e.g., Lipper et al., 1986); it is possible that patients for whom anticonvulsant treatment is effective may concurrently suffer from ESD secondary to head trauma or some other cause. This would be a plausible and, in some ways, more parsimonious alternative to the hypothesis that the emotional stress of war itself somehow "kindles" the brain (Adamec, 1991; Kolb, 1987).

In summary, we suspect that mechanical forces applied to the head can produce subtle damage or dysfunction in one or in multiple loci in the brain and that the long-term effects of electrophysiologic dysfunction eventually result in the clinical manifestations of ESD. We also suspect that other processes that are capable of producing subtle brain injuries may result in clinically significant ESD, processes such as thermal trauma, anoxia, and some neurotoxic exposures. In order to be certain about the etiology (or etiologies) of ESD, large-scale prospective studies will undoubtedly be necessary. However, until ESD gains general acceptance as a recognizable neurobehavioral with significant implications for mental health practitioners, funding for such populations studies is not likely to be forthcoming from agencies that customarily fund traditional psychiatric or neurologic research proposals.

DIFFERENTIAL DIAGNOSTIC CONSIDERATIONS

The diagnosis of possible ESD following head trauma can be complicated by a variety of factors. Making this diagnosis correctly calls upon clinicians from various disciplines to think in complex ways about human behavior and brain dysfunction. Nevertheless, we have had great success in teaching well-intentioned health care professionals and open-minded graduate students to reliably make the sorts of distinctions described in this section. By far, the largest factors in learning to make the ESD diagnosis accurately are the open-mindedness and inquisitiveness of the clinician, rather than the intellectual demandingness of the diagnostic task itself. (To invoke the spirit of the three quotations at the very beginning of this chapter, the biggest obstacles to ESD patients receiving an accurate diagnosis seem to be that most clinicians either have not been trained to recognize the disorder or refuse to believe it exists, despite its repeated description in the neuropsychiatric literature.) ESD is best diagnosed using some sort of a structured interview such as the IIPSS, where the content of the interview is covered with both the patient and one or more knowledgeable, collateral informants. Spouses, parents, coworkers, children, teachers, vocational counselor, and caretakers can be invaluable sources of useful information.

Although there has been caustic debate over forensic practice between "believers" (who think that mild TBI can be selectively disabling) and "skeptics" (who think that the invariable outcome of mild TBI should be full psychosocial recovery) (cf. Fogel, Duffy, McNamara, & Salloway, 1992), family attorneys who spend extended periods of time listening to their clients and observing phenomena such as "blank spells" and episodic incoherent speech may also be useful sources of information, particularly if (a) there are no other collaterals and (b) the attorney has known the patient both before and after the head trauma. Ethical attorneys should want their clients to feel better, suffer less, and perform as well as possible on life tasks (just as fervently as ethical physicians or neuropsychologists want their patients to feel better) and should counsel their clients to comply with treatment if it is indicated. If the potential legal client with presumed ESD benefits from an empirical trial of anticonvulsant medication before that client's lawsuit is settled or adjudicated, this can provide face valid evidence that the particular head-injury litigant was actually hurt and responded to medical treatment. Put more bluntly, recovery prior to trial runs counter to the argument that all (or most) litigants in mild TBI cases seek to amplify, embellish, fabricate, or otherwise "hold on to" their meager complaints or symptoms, motivated consciously by overt greed or unconsciously by "secondary gain." In essence, if the patient is "cured before the verdict" (or at least improves substantially on a treatment regimen), this positive clinical response both benefits the patient's quality of life and strengthens the plaintiff's contention that he or she was indeed hurt in the first place. Thus, if ESD is suspected, the ethical attorney will not stand in the way of empirical medical and psychological treatment, but will facilitate development of a cooperative alliance between the often-dysfunctional and misunderstood patient/litigant and that patient's clinical caregivers.

Returning to the subject of differential diagnosis, the clinician needs to consider that, if our current theorizing is correct, then *ESD can coexist with almost any other psychiatric, neurobehavioral or medical condition.* Put another way, a vulnerable individual with preexisting schizophrenia, mental retardation, Grave's disease, or grand mal epilepsy could conceivably hit his or her head in a car accident, crack the windshield glass, lose consciousness briefly, and then develop symptoms of ESD over time. Obviously, the newly acquired symptoms of ESD would thus be embedded in the context of the patient's premorbid personality functioning, symptom complexes, preexisting phenomenology, conversational style of self-presentation, and legal status. Thus, a relatively thorough history taking and study of preexisting medical records is called for, and even more so in complex cases. In general, the evaluating clinician should be mindful of the need to tease apart: (a) the coexisting, non-ESD effects of closed head, (b) the symptoms of potentially comorbid psychiatric or psychological disorder (particularly affective disorder), and (c) the possibility of significant dissociative disorders (that can closely mimic many of the symptoms described by posttraumatic ESD patients) from the signs and symptoms of bona fide ESD.

When a person sustains a closed head injury that produces ESD, that same person is at risk for sustaining other deficits from that same closed head injury. Verduyn et al. (1992) previously noted that patients who experienced multiple partial seizure-like symptoms following head trauma were also prone to manifest hyposmia, parosmia, or partial anosmia and deficits on so-called "frontal-lobe tasks," in addition to providing real-world evidence of executive dysfunction in daily life (cf. chaps. 8 and 9, this volume). Thus, although the neuropathology underlying ESD and executive function deficits is likely to be different, patients with ESD due to apparent head trauma should also be routinely assessed for executive dysfunction, especially because executive function deficits often interfere with treatment outcome. Verduyn and his colleagues also noted that their head trauma patients could also show static neuropsychological deficits (e.g., poor nonverbal memory functioning, residual aphasia, etc.). Furthermore, patients may have had premorbid behavioral problems such as learning disabilities, poor impulse control, or substance abuse problems that can and do affect the clinical outcome of an instance of TBI.

Many patients with ESD also qualify for diagnoses of mood disorder, particularly treatment-refractory depression (Hayes & Goldsmith, 1991; Varney et al., 1993). Such patients have frequently failed to exhibit positive clinical responses to medications that lower seizure threshold, such as tricyclics and lithium, and may even have complained that they feel worse or have developed more symptoms on such drugs. Occasionally, patients with treatment-refractory anxiety disorders may also complain of multiple episodic symptoms and benefit from treatment with anticonvulsants when tricyclic medications have failed to produce the desired clinical relief. In patients with extended histories of failure to respond to conventional treatments for depression and anxiety, it is usually more productive to attempt to achieve maximal response to an anticonvulsant regimen and then to treat residual mood symptoms with a selective serotonin reuptake inhibitor (SSRI) or suitable antianxiety medication. Similarly, when patients with ESD and comorbid psychiatric or personality problems respond positively to an anticonvulsant regimen, they may become more amenable to psychological or behavioral therapies (e.g., treatment for coexisting PTSD from combat or a traffic accident) than they were prior to successful pharmacological treatment. To use an analogy, untreated ESD can act as an amplifier for other types of neuropsychiatric or psychological problems; once this amplifier is "turned down" with appropriate treatment, then progress can be made in dealing with the symptoms of other disorders or situational problems. In short, we are advocating that clinicians routinely assess the neuroelectric competence of the brain as if it were a completely separate "axis" in *DSM–IV*, or at least a distinct vector in determining clinical outcome following closed head injury.

One set of disorders that may mimic the clinical presentation of ESD, in our clinical experience, is extreme dissociative disorders (Roberts, 1998). Dissociative patients without ESD may actually endorse many of the phenomenological symptoms of ESD on a dissociative basis rather than on a neuroelectric basis. Although some experts such as Ross (Ross et al., 1989) have stated that the differentiation of dissociative identity disorder (DID) from classic partial seizure disorders is fairly clear, our experience is that under certain circumstances it can be somewhat difficult to distinguish the symptom reporting that characterizes ESD from the phenomenology of certain dissociating patients. The real-world differentiation of ESD from pathological dissociation is further complicated by the observation that dissociation and proneness to seizure symptoms may co-occur with a nonnegligible frequency. Thus, for example, a radical change in behavior following a head injury could conceivably destabilize the electrical organization of the brain and be interpreted as a retraumatization of a previously traumatized and highly dissociative individual. Although careful history taking (Steinberg, Cichetti, Buchanan, Hall, & Rounsaville, 1993) and painstaking electrophysiological assessment can pay dividends in extremely complex situations where there is suspicion of symptoms of both ESD and pathological dissociation, in hopelessly involved cases it may prove necessary to institute a carefully monitored trial of anticonvulsant therapy and observe the outcome very closely. Fortunately for the clinician, however, the majority of cases referred for neurobehavioral assessment following closed head injury probably do not also entail the sort of catastrophic sexual abuse, torture, and neglect generally required developmentally to produce a full-blown dissociative disorder (Allen, 1995).

No section on differential diagnosis and mild TBI would be complete without some reference to the current malingering controversy. Our belief is that for every truly factitious or malingering patient that presents in the context of a lawsuit, there are likely to be scores of bona fide ESD patients that are lost in the morass of the medical, mental health and rehabilitation systems; these individuals often go untreated, or have their problems ignored, discounted, or misinterpreted. Ultimately, our contribution to the malingering controversy is deceptively simple: *Regardless of the etiology of the various types of dysfunctional behavior patients may display following an apparent closed head injury, the clinician's task is to assist the patient in attempting to reduce the degree of documented dysfunction whenever this is possible. Evaluating and treating the patient should be accomplished in a manner that respects the patient, acknowledges the patient's and family's rights to have input in clinical decision making, and that preserves the practitioner's professional integrity.* We regard this dictum as being equally applicable to dealing with malingerers (who generally have adopted self-defeating and nonproductive life strategies), patients who suffer from emotionally based PTSD, ESD patients, or those who must cope with the effects of documented cortical atrophy (i.e., a patient that all parties would agree is "genuinely" brain-damaged). In each instance, the clinician should attempt to recommend "what's best" for the individual patient, explain the complexities of the case to concerned parties in comprehensible language, have a reasoned rationale for choosing "what's best" based on the clinical and research literature, and be willing to say "I don't know" when the clinician genuinely doesn't know something. In addition, clinicians should remain open to and tolerant of dissenting clinical opinions in areas where new information and concepts are becoming available on almost a monthly basis. Only by maintaining a civilized dialogue will active interventionists and more conservative practitioners eventually resolve current differences of opinion regarding "best practices" for patients who do not recover premorbid function following mild TBI.

TREATMENT CONSIDERATIONS

As neuropsychologists, it is not our intention to practice medicine in this chapter, but rather to report on the impressions we have gleaned from observing knowledgeable physicians who have treated the target symptoms of ESD. For detailed information regarding the dosing of individual medications and potential side effects, the reader who desires greater depth of coverage is referred to the physician-authored chapters in this volume and other pertinent reviews of pharmacological intervention following mild TBI. However, the neuropsychologist bears partial responsibility for monitoring and reporting on the perceived effects of pharmacological treatment, as does any member of an interdisciplinary care team. These caveats aside, it should be apparent from the material in this chapter that the author believes that anticonvulsant therapy should be a primary consideration if one suspects the presence of ESD following closed head injury.

As Fogel pointed out (Fogel et al., 1992), neurologists and other physicians who deal with the brain-injured differ as to how aggressively interventionist they are in the use of medications versus how conservative they are with a class of drugs, many of which can have significant side effects. Current enthusiasm for the use of anticonvulsants is captured by the following quotation from Tierney and Fogel (1995):

> Antiepileptic drugs are used in patients with TBI (1) to treat seizures, (2) to stabilize mood or control impulsive behavior, and (3) to treat paroxysmal posttraumatic symptoms that are not clearly epileptic, such as sudden-onset headaches, dizzy spells, or anxiety attacks. Carbamazepine and valproate ... are the agents most prescribed by psychiatrists. (pp. 337–338)

Similarly precedent for using such agents to treat ESD can be found in the writings of prominent neuropsychiatrists Neppe and Tucker (1994):

> In our experience, many of these patients respond well to carbamazepine (Tegretol, particularly), phenytoin (Dilantin), or valproate (Depakene/Depakote). This may or may not imply that these patients have seizurelike episodes. (p. 416)

Alternatively, the caution advocated in a recent, comprehensive volume edited by Rizzo and Tranel (1996) represents a more conservative point of view:

> *Primum non noscere*—that is first of all, do no harm. Do not treat with medicines of unproven efficacy for which there are no clear indications because the side effects outweigh the benefits. For example, avoid anticonvulsants in patients without seizures. (p. 15)

Thus, although papers describing ESD and treatment of ESD were available to contributors to Rizzo and Tranel's (1996) edited book entitled *Head Injury and Postconcussive Syndrome*, one finds no overt mention of ESD as a potential contributor to postconcussive neurobehavioral dysfunction in this tome and little enthusiasm for clinical intervention with anticonvulsants, except in patients with traditional, classical seizure disorders. Clearly, the focus of the present chapter, and indeed the present volume, represents an interventionist approach to treating persistently dysfunctioning patients following mild TBI. However, in the interests of fairness, it is important to acknowledge and present the viewpoints of therapeutic moderates and skeptics. In the words of Hachinski (cited in Fogel et al., 1992), "Without therapeutic enthusiasm there would be no innovation, and without skepticism there would be no proof" (p. 459).

For those therapeutically aggressive clinicians seeking to reduce symptoms of ESD, we would agree with Tierney and Fogel (1995) that carbamazepine and valproate are most likely the first-line medications for treating posttraumatic, episodic, or paroxsymal phenomena. Both drugs have been demonstrated repeatedly to be effective treatment for controlling classic partial seizure disorders. There are some data in the neuropharmacology literature that suggest that carbamazepine may be a better choice when episodic rage outbursts are a prominent part of the posttraumatic clinical picture, whereas valproate may have somewhat greater anxiolytic effects. In our experience, both medications may alleviate some or all of the associated dysphoria and episodic depressive spells reported by many ESD patients. If residual depressive symptoms remain after the treating physician believes maximum therapeutic benefit has been reached with a trial of a single anticonvulsant, treatment of the residual depressive symptomatology with an SSRI or Trazodone may be considered. As described earlier, use of tricyclics, lithium, and antipsychotic medications should generally be avoided in the drug treatment of ESD patients (unless deemed absolutely necessary) because these medications generally lower seizure threshold. Just as residual affective symptoms may require additional psychopharmacological intervention, residual or persistent symptoms of headache, head pain, and cephalic auras or illusions may well require additional treatment beyond just anticonvulsants. The interested reader is referred to chapter 17 by Hines in this volume.

In the event that a given patient cannot tolerate the side effects of either carbamazepine or valproate or does not experience symptomatic relief from either drug, second-line therapeutic considerations include phenytoin and gabapentin. Most patients who are treated with phenytoin do not achieve as broad-based symptom relief as those who respond well to carbamazepine or valproate; however, we concur with the early observations of Jonas (1965) that the degree of symptom relief that can be obtained with phenytoin is still worthy of considering the use of this drug, which usually has primary application in the treatment of generalized epilepsies. Early indications suggest that gabapentin (i.e., Neurontin), a newer anticonvulsant medication, may have less potency to reduce the frequency and severity of the cognitive and sensory symptoms of ESD than the recommended first line anticonvulsants, but may contribute significantly to ameliorating the posttraumatic mood symptoms associated with the syndrome. One practitioner who has used Neurontin to treat posttraumatic spells humorously remarked on its "neuro-thymic" effects in certain TBI patients. If all else fails, some degree of symptom relief may be achieved by using a relatively longer acting benzodiazepine such as clonazepam (i.e., Klonopin), which also reduces seizure threshold.

With regard to drug combinations, the physicians who have managed our ESD patients most effectively have generally found that monotherapy with a single anticonvulsant is preferable to polypharmacy, whenever possible. Occasionally, a given ESD patient will respond better to a regimen involving more than one anticonvulsant medication, especially in those circumstances where ESD coexists with a generalized seizure disorder within a single patient. With regard to dosage levels, these same physicians have generally found that anticonvulsants are effective for treating ESD at the same dosage levels that are commonly recommended for using these agents to treat classic complex partial seizure disorders. However, some patients may exhibit an excellent clinical response at lower doses than are generally needed to treat classic partial seizure disorders. Obviously, the lower the dose required to produce maximal response, the better, given that most anticonvulsants are capable of producing serious side effects, particularly at higher dosage levels. A valuable reference for the intricacies of using anticonvulsant medications is the volume edited by Levy, Mattson, and Meldrum (1995) entitled *Antiepileptic Drugs* (4th ed.).

With regard to the rate at which target symptoms improve in successfully treated patients, there are no hard and fast rules, merely sketchy guidelines. In our experience, it is the psychosensory symptoms of ESD that tend to remit first, followed by the affective symptoms, and often headache. Unfortunately, the cognitive, mnemonic, and information-processing symptoms of ESD tend to be the slowest to respond and are more refractory to full resolution. We do not feel that there are sufficient data to be able to predict on an individual case-by-case basis the extent of recovery possible for each patient treated. The attitude of the treating practitioner should be characterized by cautious optimism and full disclosure of potential risks, given that no double-blind study of drug treatment in ESD patients has yet been published, to the best of our knowledge. Generally, there is somewhat more reason to be therapeutically optimistic in ESD cases caused by severe febrile illnesses, such as cerebral malaria, because postfever patients are somewhat less prone to suffer the sorts of associated executive dysfunction deficits associated with blunt trauma compared to posttraumatic ESD patients.

We have observed physicians deal with a number of events having to do with drug response and patient compliance that have considerable significance for practice in the real world. The following 10 points are presented so that other practitioners can be sensitive to these issues without having to learn about them "the hard way":

1. When a previously well-treated ESD patient complains of symptom breakthrough (or, alternatively, the spouse complains), compliance failure should strongly be suspected; this is especially true if the patient has been demonstrated to manifest problems with posttraumatic executive dysfunction (e.g., poor judgment, absentminded, etc.). Usually the best alternative is to place a responsible individual in charge of the patient's medication compliance to determine if the positive response can be reinstated with consistent dosing of medications.

2. When some patients have been effectively treated for an extended period, they may abruptly take themselves off their medication regimens precisely because they now "feel good" and have forgotten or suppressed how poorly they felt prior to treatment. Sometimes the patient himself or herself will present with this confession, and sometimes a spouse or other significant collateral will insist that the patient return for treatment once the noncompliance has become known. Occasionally, some patients with ESD symptoms can be weaned off anticonvulsants after a few months or a year (cf. Neppe & Kaplan, 1988); however, many patients may require longer treatment before tapering or reduction in dosage levels or blood levels is considered.

3. Some practitioners with whom we have worked believe that stable blood levels are more easily maintained when Tegretol is prescribed, rather than generic carbamazepine.

4. Families or spouses will occasionally become more distressed when a patient's clinically salient ESD symptoms are brought under good control with anticonvulsants because of his or her inertia, lack of spontaneity, or social inappropriateness due to coexisting damage or dysfunction in the frontal lobes. Prior to successful treatment of the ESD symptoms, families may actually display more compassion for the dysfunctional mild TBI individual because use it is apparent to them that the patient is really "ill" and suffering a great deal. Paradoxically, once the salient episodic symptoms have been brought under better control, the family may begin to recognize the full scope of the patient's comorbid executive dysfunction and become less sympathetic, more easily irritated by thoughtless behavior, or horrified at the residual behavioral inertia (e.g., "He looks like my dad, but he doesn't do anything but sit on the couch any more"). When this happens, various family members may need their own individual and family support sessions from a savvy counselor

or therapist, and referral to a local chapter of the National Head Injury Association may pay great dividends.

5. Depending on the extent to which episodes of rage and explosive dyscontrol (Elliott, 1992; Lewis, 1998) are part of the clinical picture, practitioners working with ESD patients may have the same sort of responsibilities to ensure that family members will not suffer from the abusive effects of interpersonal violence as do family therapists working with people who batter. The safety of family members from emotional and physical abuse due to witnessing or being assaulted during a rage attack should always be assessed.

6. Even if the patient's ESD symptoms were caused by an etiology other than CHI (e.g., febrile illness), patients need to be warned repeatedly about taking precautions lest they sustain subsequent head trauma (i.e., seatbelt use, wearing helmets during biking, quitting rough contact sports, etc.) and need to avoid exposure to potential neurotoxins (e.g., compounds used in car restoration, organic solvents, farm chemicals, carbon monoxide, etc.). Obviously, patients with ESD who are still exposed to neurotoxic chemicals should be removed from the site of the exposure immediately; such cases may experience a reduction in symptoms when they are no longer exposed to toxins and do not tend to exhibit as positive a clinical reponse to anticonvulsant therapy as to ESD patients with other presume etiologies. Although much research work remains to be done, it seems likely the cerebral cell loss associated with the "neuropathology of everyday life" in industrialized societies is likely to be additive or interactive in producing subtle electrophysiological dysfunction.

7. Tegretol may lose some of its potency if it is stored in a highly humid environment, so patients and families should be advised that it is best not stored in the bathroom or any other humid area.

8. Clinicians should be advised that carbamazepine can lower the potency of certain birth control pills, leaving the adolescent or young woman with ESD vulnerable to an unwanted or at least unanticipated pregnancy. (Levy, Mattson, & Meldrum, 1995)

9. A previously positive and stable drug response may evaporate when a patient develops a fever from any cause (e.g., a cold virus) or contracts stomach flu with vomiting and diarrhea that interfere with the absorption of the particular anticonvulsant medications.

10. Similarly, in extremely hot weather (above 90°F), patients who have previously exhibited positive response to Tegretol may abruptly show poorer treatment response due to excessive consumption of liquids, dehydration associated with excessive sweating, or electrolyte imbalance; workers who necessarily must spend extended periods outside in the heat (e.g., roofers, farmers, construction workers) may be especially vulnerable to this transient complication of treatment.

A PROPOSED SCHEMA TO GUIDE CARE
OF THE MILD TBI PATIENT

It is only within the past decade that mainstream psychiatric thought has clearly endorsed including the problems faced by dysfunctioning TBI patients in the formal psychiatric nomenclature. In the words of Grant and colleagues (Brown, Fann, & Grant, 1994):

> We argue that there is sufficient research to indicate that postconcussional symptoms occur and that they tend to have a predictable configuration. It is necessary to recognize the existence of "Postconcussional Disorder" in our nosology in order to provide more prompt diagnosis and management and to facilitate scholarly communication and research regarding this important neurobehavioral disorder. (p. 16)

From the preceding material in this chapter, the reader should have rightfully concluded that the authors believe that unrecognized ESD can play a major part in many cases of "postconcussional disorder" with poor recovery (i.e., Ruff's "miserable minority"; Ruff, Camenzulis, & Mueller, 1996).

Although formal recognition of the postconcussional syndrome is helpful to medicine and society in that it calls attention to the plight of the brain-injured, we believe (in accordance with Verduyn et al.) that clinicians are better off looking at mild TBI patient problems on a number of different axes. In the words of Verduyn and colleagues (1992):

> Rather than clumping the plethora of symptoms and complaints described by such patients and their families under the broad rubric of "post-concussional syndrome," clinicians can produce significant improvement by evaluating and treating (if possible) the following components of the patient's presentation: (a) partial seizure-like phenomena; (b) residual mood symptoms; (c) headache problems; (d) static cognitive deficits (e.g., poor nonverbal memory); and (e) frontal lobe dysfunction. . . . In addition, there is generally a significant need for patient education and extensive consultation with family members, employers, school personnel, attorneys, and insurance carriers regarding the nature of a given patient's problems and long-term prognosis. (p. 255)

The sort of well-intentioned "team effort" needed to provide optimal care for dysfunctioning mild TBI patients is very similar to the ideal approach to managing epilepsy described in detail by Devinsky (1994). However, even optimal care from a collaborative and therapeutically aggressive team of health care professionals does not necessarily translate into full recovery of premorbid levels of social, vocational, or academic functioning for all members of the "miserable minority."

Although the proposition that ESD is a recognizable and treatable neurobehavioral disorder may strike some conservative readers as premature or speculative, the material reviewed in this chapter does lead to a number of testable hypotheses that can be tested by clinical and experimental research in the laboratories of other investigators. Hopefully, if there is compelling reason to revise this chapter in the next 5 to 10 years, the impact of new studies will have led to more precise, formal diagnostic criteria for making the ESD diagnosis and generally agreed-on clinical treatment algorithms. In the meantime, the analysis presented in this chapter may influence some practitioners to interview more aggressively for posttraumatic episodic phenomena, to confirm their hunches regarding the presence of ESD by seeking EEG evaluation and neuropsychological testing with dichotic listening, and to consider empirical treatment of ESD when they sincerely believe that the patient stands to benefit.

If subsequent clinical observations and research do not support the broad outline of ESD that has been presented in this chapter, the lives of the brain-injured and their loved ones will hopefully benefit from the development of new and better conceptualizations of persistent dysfunction following mild TBI.

APPENDIX
Iowa Interview for Partial Seizure-like Symptoms
(IIPSS 40-item version)

ID NUMBER: _____   DATE: _____

INTERVIEWER: _____   TOTAL SCORE: _____

Numeric Response Frequencies
0 never, or not in the past year
1 two or three times in the past year
2 at least once a month
3 at least once a week
4 several times a week
5 once a day
6 more than once a day

SENSORY SYMPTOMS

1. OLFACTORY ILLUSIONS: Do you sometimes smell things which other people can't smell, such as feces, urine, rot, body odor, or smoke?

0   never, or not in the past year
1   two or three times in the past year
2   at least once a month
3   at least once a week
4   several times a week
5   once a day
6   more than once a day

Be sure in responding to this that the smells you reports have no apparent cause (e.g., smelling kitty litter when you don't have a cat).
0 1 2 3 4 5 6 _____

2. GUSTATORY ILLUSIONS: Do you sometimes have a bad taste in your mouth, such as a metallic taste, that comes and goes for no reason?
0 1 2 3 4 5 6 _____

3. ILLUSIONS OF MOVEMENT: Do you sometimes sense movement in your peripheral vision, but when you turn to look you cannot see anything there?
0 1 2 3 4 5 6 _____

4. VISUAL ILLUSIONS: Do you sometimes see things in your peripheral vision, such as stars, bugs, snakes, worms, or threads?
0 1 2 3 4 5 6 _____

5. ILLUSIONS OF SHADOWY CREATURES: DO you sometimes see mice or cockroaches run across the floor, but when you turn to look, you do not see them?
0 1 2 3 4 5 6 _____

6. HAPTIC ILLUSIONS: Do you sometimes feel as though bugs are crawling on you, or that something is brushing up against your skin, such as a cobweb?
0 1 2 3 4 5 6 _____

7. EPISODIC NUMBNESS: Do you sometimes go numb in a part of your body for no apparent reason?
0 1 2 3 4 5 6 _____

8. EPISODIC TINNITUS: Do you sometimes get a ringing, buzzing, rushing, or tapping noise in your ears that comes and goes for no reason?
0 1 2 3 4 5 6 _____

> 0 never, or not in the past year
> 1 two or three times in the past year
> 2 at least once a month
> 3 at least once a week
> 4 several times a week
> 5 once a day
> 6 more than once a day

9. AUDITORY ILLUSIONS: Do you sometimes answer the telephone only to find that it had not actually been ringing?
0 **1** 2 3 4 5 6 _____

10. SICK HEADACHES: Do you sometimes get severe headaches that are so bad you become nauseated or want to throw up?
0 1 **2** 3 4 5 6 _____

11. EPISODIC CEPHALIC PAIN: Do you sometimes get a pain in your head that you would not classify as a headache?
0 1 **2 3** 4 5 6 _____

12. ILLUSION OF URINARY URGENCY: Do you sometimes have marked urinary urgency, but fail to produce any urine when going to the bathroom?
0 1 2 3 4 5 6 _____

13. MICROPSIA: Are there times when objects appear to be much smaller or much further away from you than they really are?
0 1 2 3 4 5 6 _____

14. MACROPSIA: Are there times when objects seem much larger or closer to you than they really are?
0 1 **2** 3 4 5 6 _____

15. EPISODIC DIZZINESS: Are there times when you become dizzy for no apparent reason?
0 1 **2 3** 4 5 6 _____

16. EPISODIC VERTIGO: Are there times when the room seems as though it is spinning around you for no particular reason?
0 1 **2 3** 4 5 6 _____

17. EPIGASTRIC SENSATION: Are there times when it feels like your stomach or internal organs are rising up into your chest?
0 1 2 3 4 5 6 _____

0 never, or not in the past year
1 two or three times in the past year
2 at least once a month
3 at least once a week
4 several times a week
5 once a day
6 more than once a day

COGNITIVE SYMPTOMS

18. SPEECH PROBLEMS: Do you sometimes have trouble with the pronunciation of words with the effect that you appear a bit intoxicated even though you are not?
0 1 2 3 4 5 6 _____

19. WORD-FINDING LAPSES: Is it a common problems of yours that you will suddenly have trouble thinking of words you should know and were able to say moments before?
0 1 2 3 4 5 6 _____

20. SPEAKING JARGON: Do you sometimes find that you have uttered a sentence that doesn't make any sense and involves words other than those you wished to say?
0 1 2 3 4 5 6 _____

21. CONFUSIONAL SPELLS: Do you sometimes become quite suddenly and intensely confused or perplexed and then have the feeling pass in a few minutes?
0 1 2 3 4 5 6 _____

22. ENVIRONMENTAL DISTORTION: Do you sometimes have an overwhelming feeling that things are weird, strange, or wrong, sort of like entering the "twilight zone?"
0 1 2 3 4 5 6 _____

23. JAMAIS VU: Do you sometimes feel that familiar places or persons are somehow not familiar or the way they should be?
0 1 2 3 4 5 6 _____

24. DEJA VU: Do you sometimes get the feeling that you have experienced something or been someplace before, even though you know you have not?
0 1 2 3 4 5 6 _____

      0 never, or not in the past year
      1 two or three times in the past year
      2 at least once a month
      3 at least once a week
      4 several times a week
      5 once a day
      6 more than once a day

25. MEMORY GAPS: Do you have clear cut gaps in your memory during which you cannot remember anything that happened over a period of five minutes?
0 1 2 3 4 5 6 _____

26. DISCONTINUOUS TV VIEWING: Do you sometimes find that you have missed major sections of TV shows you have been watching, like someone has spliced out a section of a movie?
0 1 2 3 4 5 6 _____

27. AUTOMATIC DRIVING: Have you ever found yourself driving without remembering how you got there or where you were going?
0 1 2 3 4 5 6 _____

28. UNRECALLED BEHAVIORS: Do people often tell you about things you have said or done for which you have no memory at all?
0 1 2 3 4 5 6 _____

29. VISUAL FIXATION: Do you have spells where you become sort of hypnotized by a bright or shiny object?
0 1 2 3 4 5 6 _____

30. STARING SPELLS: Do people often tell you that there are times when you are staring and have a blank look on your face?
0 1 2 3 4 5 6 _____

31. MENTAL DECLINE: Do you feel that your memory or concentration is getting substantially worse every year?
NO **YES** (0 = NO, 6 = YES) _____

32. LOSS OF CONSCIOUSNESS: Do you sometimes lose consciousness or just black out?
0 1 2 3 4 5 6 _____

0   never, or not in the past year
1   two or three times in the past year
2   at least once a month
3   at least once a week
4   several times a week
5   once a day
6   more than once a day

AFFECTIVE SYMPTOMS

33. DYSPHORIC SPELLS: Do you sometimes become abruptly more depressed than you were a few minutes or seconds earlier with no apparent reason?
0 1 2 3 4 5 6 _____

34. PANIC/ANXIETY SPELLS: Are you often inclined to panic or become very anxious for no reason?
0 1 2 3 4 5 6 _____

35. TEMPER OUTBURSTS: Do you sometimes become extremely and intensely angry for no reason?
0 1 2 3 4 5 6 _____

36. UNRECALLED ANGER: Do people tell you that you have become very angry and you do not remember doing so?
0 1 2 3 4 5 6 _____

NOCTURNAL PHENOMENA

37. PARASOMNIA: Do you walk and/or talk in your sleep such that you are capable of interacting with people (even incoherently), performing complex activity (possibly odd), or are capable of doing things that are sufficiently complex and purposeful that another person would think you were awake?
0 1 2 3 4 5 6 _____

38. IRRESISTIBLE SLEEPINESS: Do you sometimes feel an irresistible urge to sleep during the day and then sleep so soundly that no one can arouse you?
0 1 2 3 4 5 6 _____

0   never, or not in the past year
1   two or three times in the past year
2   at least once a month
3   at least once a week
4   several times a week
5   once a day
6   more than once a day

39. NOCTURNAL SWEATING: Do you sometimes wake up to realize that you have been sweating so much that the bed sheets are soaked?
0 1 2 3 4 5 6 _____

40. NIGHTMARES WITH NOCTURNAL INSOMNIA: Do you have vivid nightmares followed by abrupt awakening and insomnia lasting at least one hour?
0 1 2 3 4 5 6 _____

Note: The boldfaced numeric response frequency under each item corresponds to the 90th percentile cutoff for that item in the healthy, young adult population.

*   *   *

Normative Data for the 40-item version of the IIPSS

Total Score	n	Percentile
>70	1	—
60–69	2	99th
50–59	4	97th
40–49	9	94th
30–39	10	87th
20–29	27	77th
10–19	38	54th
0–9	24	21st

Notes: Total N = 115.
95th percentile cutoff for the normal population is a Total Score of 55.

REFERENCES

Aarts, J. H. P., Binnie, C. D., Smit, A. M., & Wilkins, A. J. (1984). Selective cognitive impairment during focal and generalized epileptiform EEG activity. *Brain, 107*, 293–307.
Adamec, R. E. (1990). Does kindling model anything clinically relevant? *Biological Psychiatry, 27*, 249–279.

American Psychiatric Association. (1994). *Diagnostic and statisical manual of mental disorders* (4th ed.). Washington, DC: American Psychiatric Press.

Allen, J. G. (1995). *Coping with trauma: A guide to self-understanding*. Washington, DC: American Psychiatric Press.

Andy, O. J. (1989). Post concussion syndrome: Brainstem seizures—A case report. *Clinical Electroencephalography, 20*, 24–34.

Ardila, A., Nino, C. R., Pulido, E., Rivera, D. B., & Vanegas, C. J. (1993). Episodic psychic symptoms in the general population. *Epilepsia, 34*, 133–140.

Barnhill, L. J., & Gualtieri, C. T. (1989). Two cases of late-onset psychosis after head injury. *Neuropsychiatry, Neuropsychology, and Behavioral Neurology, 2*, 211–217.

Bare, M. A., Burnstine, T. H., Fisher, R. S., & Lesser, R. P. (1994). Electroencephalographic changes during simple partial seizures. *Epilepsia, 35*, 715–720.

Bayless, J. B., Roberts, R., & Varney, N. R. (1989). Tinker Toy performance of patients with closed head trauma. *Journal of Clinical and Experimental Neuropsycyhology, 11*, 913–917.

Benton, A. R. (1984). Neuropsychological assessment. In H. I. Kaplan & B. J. Sadock (Eds.), *Comprehensive textbook of psychiatry* (3rd ed., Vol. 1, pp. 520–529). Baltimore, MD: Williams & Wilkins.

Binnie, C. D., Channon, S., & Marston, D. L. (1991). In D. B. Smith, D. M. Treiman, & M. R. Trimble (Eds.), *Advances in neurology, Vol. 55: Neurobehavioral problems in epilepsy* (pp. 152–168). New York: Raven Press.

Blumer, D., Heilbronn, M., & Himmelhoch, J. (1988). Indications for carbamazepine in mental illness: Atypical psychiatric disorder or temporal lobe syndrome? *Comprehensive Psychiatry, 29*, 108–122.

Brown, S. J., Fann, J. R., & Grant, I. (1994). Postconcussional disorder: Time to acknowledge a common source of neurobehavioral morbidity. *Journal of Neuropsychiatry and Clinical Neurosciences, 6*, 15–22.

Daly, D. D. (1982). Complex partial seizures. In J. Laidlaw & A. Richens (Eds.), *A textbook of epilepsy* (pp. 131–146). Edinburgh: Churchill Livingstone.

Damasio, A. R., & Damasio, H. (1979). "Paradoxic" ear extinction in dichotic listening: Possible anatomic significance. *Neurology, 29*, 644–653.

Devinsky, O. (1994). *A guide to understanding and living with epilepsy*. Philadelphia: F. A. Davis.

Devinsky, O., Kelley, K., Porter, R. J., & Theodore, W. H. (1988). Clinical and electrographic features of simple partial seizures. *Neurology, 38*, 1347–1352.

Devinsky, O., & Luciano, D. (1991). Psychic phenomena in partial seizures. *Seminars in Neurology, 11*, 100–109.

Elliott, F. A. (1992). Violence—The neurologic contribution: An overview. *Archives of Neurology, 49*, 595–603.

Fisher, C. M. (1982). Fisher's rules. *Archives of Neurology, 39*, 389–390.

Fogel, B., Duffy, J., McNamara, M. E., & Salloway, S. (1992). Skeptics and enthusiasts in neuropsychiatry. *Journal of Neuropsychiatry, 4*, 458–462.

Geyde, A. (1996). A nonconvulsive ictal signs checklist. *Habilitative Mental Healthcare Newsletter, 15*, 71–80.

Gino, C. (1981). *Robin's story*. New York: Bantam.

Goetz, C. C. (1987). Charcot at the Salpetriere: Ambulatory automatisms. *Neurology, 37*, 1084–1088.

Goldstein, G. C. (1984). Neuropsychological assessment of psychiatric patients. In G. Goldstein (Ed.), *Advances in clinical neuropsychology* (Vol. 1, pp. 59–75). New York: Plenum Press.

Grote, C., Pierre-Louis, S., Smith, M., Roberts, R., & Varney, N. (1995). Significance of unilateral ear extinction on the dichotic listening test. *Journal of Clinical and Experimental Neuropsychology, 17*, 1–8.

Hayes, S., & Goldsmith, B. K. (1991). Psychosensory symptomatology in anticonvulsant-responsive psychiatric illness. *Annals of Clinical Psychiatry, 29*, 108–122.

Head, H. (1926). *Aphasia and kindred disorders of speech.* Cambridge: Cambridge University Press.

Hines, M., Swan, C., Roberts, R. J., & Varney, N. R. (1995). Characteristics of and mechanisms of epilepsy spectrum disorder: An explanatory model. *Applied Neuropsychology, 2*, 1–6.

Hutt, S. J. (1972). Experimental analysis of brain activity and behavior in children with "minor" seizures. *Epilepsia, 13*, 520–534.

Hutt, S. J., & Fairweather, H. (1971). Spike-wave paroxysms and information-processing. *Proceedings of the Royal Society of Medicine, 64*, 918–919.

International League Against Epilepsy. (1985). Proposal for classification of epilepsies amd epileptic syndromes. *Epilepsia, 26*, 268–278.

Jackson, J. H. (1866). Clinical remarks on cases of temporary loss of speech and/or power of expression and on epilepsies. *Medical Times Gazette, 1*, 442–443.

Jampala, V. C., Atre-Vaidya, N., Taylor, M. A., Schrift, M. J., Srinivasaraghavan, J., & Sierles, F. S. (1992). A profile of psychomotor symptoms (POPS) in psychiatric patients. *Neuropsychiatry, Neuropsychology, and Behavioral Neurology, 5*, 15–19.

Jonas, A. D. (1965). *Ictal and subictal neurosis.* Springfield, IL: C. C. Thomas.

Kolb, L. C. (1987). A neuropsychological hypothesis explaining posttraumatic stress disorders. *American Journal of Psychiatry, 144*, 989–995.

LaPlante, E. (1993). *Seized.* New York: Harper Collins.

Lee, G. Loring, W., Varney, N. R., Roberts, R., Newell, J., Martin, J., Smith, J., King, D., Meador, K., & Murro, A. (1994). Do dichotic listening asymmetries predict side of temporal lobe seizure onset? *Epilepsy Research, 19*, 153–160.

Levy, R. H., Mattson, R. H., & Meldrum, B. S. (1995). *Antiepileptic drugs* (4th ed.). New York: Raven Press.

Lewis, D. O. (1998). *Guilty by reason of insanity.* New York: Fawcett Columbine.

Lipper, S., Davidson, J. R. T., Grady, T. A., Edinger, J. D., Hammett, E. B., Mahoney, S. L., & Cavenar, J. O. (1986). Preliminary study of carbamazepine in post-traumatic stress disorder. *Psychosomatics, 27*, 849–854.

Liu, Y. K., Chandran, K. B., Heath, R. G., & Unterharnscheidt, F. (1984). Subcortical EEG changes in rhesus monkeys following experimental hyperextension-hyperflexion (whiplash). *Spine, 9*, 329–338.

Makarec, K., & Persinger, M. A. (1990). Electroencephalographic validation of a temporal lobe signs inventory in a normal population. *Journal of Research in Personality, 34*, 323–327.

Monroe, R. R. (1959). Episodic behavior disorder—Schizophrenia or epilepsy. *Archives of General Psychiatry, 1*, 205–214.

Monroe, R. R. (1982). Limbic ictus and atypical psychosis. *Journal of Nervous and Mental Disorders, 170*, 711–716.

Neppe, V. N. (1983). Temporal lobe symptomatology in subjective paranormal experients. *Journal of the American Society of Psychic Research, 77*, 1–30.

Neppe, V. N., Bowman, B. R., & Sawchuck, K. S. L. J. (1991). Carbamazepine for atypical psychosis with episodic hostility: A preliminary study. *Journal of Nervous and Mental Disease, 179*, 439–441.

Neppe, V. N., & Kaplan, C. (1988). Short-term treatment of atypical spells with carbamazepine. *Clinical Neuropharmacology, 11*, 287–289.

Neppe, V. N., & Tucker, G. J. (1988). Modern perspectives on epilepsy in relation to psychiatry. *Hospital and Community Psychiatry, 39*, 389–396.

Neppe, V. N., & Tucker, G. J. (1994). Neuropsychiatric aspects of seizure disorders. In S. Yudofsky & S. Silver, *The American Psychiatric Press textbook of neuropsychiatry* (pp. 397–425). Washington, DC: American Psychiatric Press.

Persinger, M. A., & Marakec, K. (1993). Complex partial epileptic signs as a continuum from normals to epileptics: Normative data and clinical populations. *Journal of Clinical Psychology, 49,* 33–45.

Reutens, D. C. (1992). Validation of a questionnaire for clinical seizure diagnosis. *Epilepsia, 33,* 1065–1071.

Richardson, E., Roberts, R. J., Hines, M. E., & Varney, N. R. (1989). Long term sequelae of malaria in Vietnam veterans. *VA Practitioner, 2,* 51–60.

Richardson, E., Springer, J., Varney, N. R., Struchen, M., & Roberts, R. (1994). Dichotic listening in the clinic: New neuropsychological applications. *Clinical Neuropsychologist, 8,* 416–429.

Rizzo, M., & Tranel, D. (1996). *Head injury and postconcussive syndrome.* New York: Churchill Livingstone.

Roberts, M. A., Manshadi, F. F., Bushnell, D. L., & Hines, M. E. (1995). Neurobehavioral dysfunction following mild traumatic brain injury in childhood: A case report with positive findings on PET. *Brain Injury, 9,* 427–436.

Roberts, R. J. (1998). *Unexplained cognitive deterioration in mid-life.* Unpublished data presented to the annual meeting of the Midwest Neuropsychology Group, Milwaukee, WI.

Roberts, R. J., Gorman, L. L., Lee, G. P., Hines, M. E., Richardson, E. D., Riggle, T. A., & Varney, N. R. (1992). The phenomenology of multiple partial seizure-like symptoms without stereotyped spells: An epilepsy spectrum disorder? *Epilepsy Research, 13,* 167–177.

Roberts, R. J., Gorman, L. L., Roecker, C., & Lee, G. P. (1993, February). *A comparision of MMPI profiles of complex partial seizure patient and patients endorsing multiple seizure-like complaints.* Poster presentation at the 21st annual meeting of the International Neuropsychological Society, Galveston, TX (abstr.).

Roberts, R. J., Paulsen, J. S., Marchman, J. N., & Varney, N. R. (1989). MMPI profiles of patients who endorse multiple partial seizure symptoms. *Neuropsychology, 2,* 183–198.

Roberts, R. J., & Varney, N. R. (1997). *Theta bursts redux.* Unpublished paper presented at the annual meeting of the Midwest Neuropsychology Group, Madison, WI.

Roberts, R. J., Varney, N. R., Hulbert, J. R., Paulsen, J. S., Richardson, E. D., Springer, J. A., Smith-Shepherd, J., Swan, C. S., Legrand, J. A., Harvey, J. H., Struchen, M. A., & Hines, M. E. (1990). The neuropathology of everyday life: The frequency of partial seizure symptoms among normals. *Neuropsychology, 4,* 65–86.

Roberts, R. J., Varney, N. R., Paulsen, J. S., & Richardson, E. D. (1990). Dichotic listening and complex partial seizures. *Journal of Clinical and Experimental Neuropsychology, 12,* 448–458.

Ross, C. A., Heber, S., Anderson, G., Norton, G. R., Anderson, B. A., del Campo, M., & Pillay, N. (1989). Differentiating multiple personality disorder and complex partial seizures. *General Hospital Psychiatry, 11,* 54–58.

Ruff, R. M., Camenzuli, L., & Mueller, J. (1996). Miserable minority: Emotional risk factors that influence the outcome of a mild traumatic brain injury. *Brain Injury, 10,* 551–565.

Shewmon, D. A., & Erwin, R. J. (1989). Transient impairment of visual perception induced by single interictal occipital spikes. *Journal of Clinical and Experimental Neuropsychology, 11,* 657–691.

Silberman, E. K., Post, R. M., Nurnberger, J., Theodore, W., & Boulenger, J. (1985). Transient sensory, cognitive, and affective phenomena in affective illness: A comparison with complex partial epilepsy. *British Journal of Psychiatry, 146,* 81–89.

Springer, J. A., Garvey, M. J., Varney, N. R., & Roberts, R. J. (1991). Dichotic listening failure in dysphoric neuropsychiatric patients who endorse multiple seizure-like symptoms. *Journal of Nervous and Mental Disease, 179,* 459–467.

Steinberg, M., Cichetti, D., Buchanan, J., Hall, P., & Rounsaville, B. (1993). Clinical assessment of dissociative symptoms and disorders: The structured clinical interview for DSM–IV dissociative disorders (SCID-D). *Dissociation, 6,* 3–15.

Sweeney, J. E. (1992). Non-impact brain injury: Grounds for clinical study of neuropsychological effects of acceleration forces. *Clinical Neuropsychologist, 6,* 443–457.

Teicher, M. H., Glod, C. A., Surrey, J., & Swett, C. (1993). Early childhood abuse and limbic system ratings in adult psychiatric outpatients. *Journal of Neuropsychiatry, 5,* 301–306.

Tierney, J. G., & Fogel, B. S. (1995). Neuropsychiatric sequelae of mild traumatic brain injury. In A. Stoudamire & B. S. Fogel (Eds.), *Medical-psychiatric practice* (Vol. 3, pp. 307–380). Washington, DC: American Psychiatric Press.

Tucker, G. J., Price, T. R. P., Johnson, V. B., & McAllister, T. (1986). Phenomenology of temporal lobe dysfunction: A link to atypical psychosis—A series of cases. *Journal of Nervous and Mental Disease, 174,* 348–356.

Varney, N. R., Garvey, M., Campbell, D., Cook, B., & Roberts, R. (1993). Identification of treatment-resistant depressives who respond favorably to carbamazepine. *Annals of Clinical Psychiatry, 5,* 117–122.

Varney, N. R., Hines, M. E., Bailey, C., & Roberts, R. J. (1992). Neuropsychiatric correlates of theta bursts in patients with closed head injury. *Brain Injury, 6,* 449–508.

Varney, N. R., & Menefee, L. (1993). Psychosocial and executive deficits following closed head injury: Implications for orbital frontal cortex. *Journal of Head Trauma Rehabilitation, 8,* 32–44.

Varney, N. R., Struchen, M., Hanson, T., Franzen, K., Connell, S., & Roberts, R. (1996). Design fluency among normals and patients with closed head injury. *Archives of Clinical Neuropsychology, 11,* 345–351.

Varney, N. R., Roberts, R. J., Springer, J., Connell, S. K., & Wood, P. (1997). Neuropsychiatric sequelae of cerebral malaria in Vietnam veterans. *Journal of Nervous and Mental Disease, 185,* 695–703.

Varney, N. R., & Varney, R. N. (1995). Brain injury without head injury: Some physics of automobile collisions with particular reference to brain injuries occurring without physical head trauma. *Applied Neuropsychology, 2,* 47–62.

Verduyn, W. H., Hilt, J., Roberts, M. A., & Roberts, R. J. (1992). Multiple partial seizure-like symptoms following "minor" closed head injury. *Brain Injury, 6,* 245–260.

Wieser, H. G., Hailermariam, M., Regard, M., & Landis, T. (1985). Unilateral limbic epileptic status activity: Stereo EEG, behavioral, and cognitive data. *Epilepsia, 26,* 19–29.

Wong, J. L., Regennitter, R. P., & Barrios, F. (1994). Base rate and simulated symptoms of mild head injury among normals. *Archives of Clinical Neuropsychology, 9,* 411–425.

Wu, J., & Varney, N. R. (1998, August). *Quantitative PET findings in premorbidly high functioning patients with mild head injury.* Unpublished presentation at the annual convention of the American Psychological Association, San Franscisco, CA.

Malingering Traumatic Brain Injury: Current Issues and Caveats in Assessment and Classification

Jill S. Hayes
Louisiana State University School of Medicine, New Orleans

Robin C. Hilsabeck
William Drew Gouvier
Louisiana State University

An estimated 2 million individuals seek medical attention every year as the result of a closed head injury (Kraus & Sorenson, 1994). Because accidents (e.g., falls, motor vehicle accidents) account for approximately 50% of all head traumas, it is not surprising that many patients present not only for evaluation and treatment but also to a personal injury attorney for possible assistance in securing financial compensation. Given today's litigious society, opportunity, motive, and lack of consequences for frivolous lawsuits provide an impetus for malingering. The lure of millions of dollars awarded by the courts for lost cognitive abilities may lead litigants to "enhance" deficits related to their injuries. Of course, for genuine impairments, large awards are not unreasonable. For example, West and Knowles (1991) reported that for midcareer males without a college education who are unable to return to work, loss of earnings alone typically exceeds half a million dollars. As a result of these various factors, and coupled with the observation that brain injuries are a nonobvious cause of disability (Gouvier, Steiner, Jackson, Schlater, & Rain, 1991), closed head injury is the most common neuropsychological syndrome feigned (Haines & Norris, 1995).

According to Youngjohn (1995), some attorneys feel it would be "legal malpractice" not to coach their client on psychological testing prior to evaluation. In fact, in a survey of 70 practicing attorneys, 80% reported believing they should inform their clients about psychological testing, and half believed they should educate the plaintiff about symptom validity scales (Wetter & Corrigan, 1995). Furthermore, manuals are published on preparing the mildly head-injured plaintiff for litigation, on how to be awarded social security disability, and on how to obtain 100% service-connected disability for mental health impairment (Taylor, Harp, & Elliott, 1992). Given the results of analogue research on the effects of coaching (Lamb, Berry, Wetter, & Baer, 1994; Martin, Bolter, Todd, Gouvier, & Niccolls, 1993; Martin, Gouvier, Todd, Bolter, & Niccolls, 1992), clinicians must be cognizant of the possibility that litigants may be provided information about specific psychological and neuropsychological tests. This rehearsal by litigants not only compromises the results of neuropsychological testing, but also may lead to inappropriate evaluations, unnecessary services, increased monetary settlements, and favorable verdicts.

Accordingly, assessment of malingering is a challenge for neuropsychologists. A naive clinician may believe he or she can definitively identify malingering. Given the *DSM-IV* definition of malingering as the "intentional production of false or grossly exaggerated physical or psychological symptoms, motivated by external incentives such as avoiding military conscription or duty, avoiding work, obtaining financial compensation, evading criminal prosecution, obtaining drugs, or securing better living conditions" (American Psychiatric Association, 1994, p. 360), one can see how easily a clinician may err in his or her judgment. Experienced clinicians know malingering is more complex. In the neuropsychological arena, a clinician must distinguish among symptoms with organic causation, functional causation, and conscious, deliberate causation, and then make an attribution about the degree to which each of these vectors contribute to the overall clinical presentation. In this chapter, we discuss the definition of malingering, detection strategies using both existing neuropsychological measures and those designed specifically for malingering detection, the importance of base rate analysis in determining the validity and effectiveness of detection measures, pitfalls of misclassification, and issues for further consideration.

DEFINITION OF MALINGERING

As noted by Rogers (1990; Rogers, Sewell, & Goldstein, 1994), malingering may be considered an adaptive behavior. An individual may view an evaluation as possibly damaging, and therefore malinger for fear of losing out on something important if he or she performs in an honest and forthright manner. Consequently, an individual may malinger in one of two ways. The first is by exaggerating or producing false psychiatric or neurologic symptoms (e.g., hallucinations, memory impairment). The second is by denying or downplaying psychiatric symptomatology. Price

(1995) identified these two types of malingering as simulation and dissimulation, respectively.

Use of the term *malingering* in the literature has been inconsistent. Some authors (e.g., Pope, Butcher, & Seelen, 1993) assert dissimulation is feigning nonexistent problems or exaggerating real difficulties. Others feel the opposite, that dissimulation is intentional downplaying of psychological difficulties (Graham, Watts, & Timbrook, 1991; Harvey & Sipprelle, 1976; Hayes et al., 1998). In an effort to establish uniformity, for the remainder of the chapter, we use the term *simulation* to refer to "faking bad" to mimic or exaggerate psychological or neuropsychological deficits in order to appear impaired, and the term *dissimulation* to refer to "faking good" in order to appear psychologically healthy or fit. Because simulation is more often associated with closed head injury, it is our focus in the following pages.

Simulation

Simulation may be viewed on a continuum. The easiest simulator to identify is an individual with no real neuropsychological deficits who blatantly falsifies difficulties in obvious ways (e.g., cannot remember his or her name, can recall words but not recognize them, cannot repeat one number). This individual is relatively rare in clinical practice, though most clinicians have interviewed at least one (Williams, 1998). Price (1995) termed this form of malingering "symptom invention."

On the other end of the continuum is the simulator who has experienced neuropsychological deficits that have either resolved or continue to a lesser degree. This simulator has been referred to as an "opportunistic malingerer" (Price, 1995). This individual likely exaggerates his or her deficits, rather than blatantly falsifying them. Correct classification may be further complicated by selective exaggeration of only one or two complaints (e.g., memory difficulties). These persons are difficult to identify because they can produce a more accurate deficit profile based on prior subjective experiences. Their subjective experiences of cognitive impairments combined with factual information from attorneys, doctors, and other patients help refine their presentations. This may be thought of as a shaping process in which the simulator's behavior is shaped with every contact with health care and legal professionals after experiencing an injury. Additionally, the individual may have been involved in more than one lawsuit, given several depositions, and undergone many independent medical evaluations. All of these experiences contribute to a learning history that makes discrimination of the simulator from the truly impaired individual a formidable and often frustrating task.

Prevalence

Although the prevalence of simulating cognitive deficits is unknown, preliminary estimates range from 15% to 64% depending on the population studied. For example, 18% of Social Security Administration disability claimants (Guilmette, Sparadeo, Whelihan, & Buongiorno, 1994), 47% of workers' compensation applicants (Youngjohn, 1991), 33% of mildly head-injured individuals (Binder, 1993b; Binder & Willis, 1991) and 60% to 64% of personal injury litigants (Greiffenstein, Baker, & Gola, 1994; Heaton, Smith, Lehman, & Vogt, 1978) have been reported to involve some aspect of simulation. Trueblood and Schmidt (1993; Trueblood, 1994) identified approximately 15% of consecutive outpatients at a private neuropsychological practice as probable malingerers based on two criteria: (a) scoring below chance on a forced-choice procedure or (b) improbably poor neuropsychological test performance (e.g., zero on Grip Strength). Their base rate is noteworthy because it is based on objective criteria for simulating and encompasses all referrals to a neuropsychology clinic, making their findings more generalizable to the average clinician's patient population.

SIMULATION DETECTION STRATEGIES

Evidence of simulation may occur during any phase of an evaluation, including data collection, interview, or testing. All of these components should be examined carefully by the neuropsychologist prior to forming an opinion about the existence of simulation.

Background Information

Prior to the evaluation, a thorough investigation includes obtaining pre-injury records (e.g., school, employment, police/accident/arrest, medical) to help ascertain premorbid levels of functioning. Note that a release of information sent to the primary data source may yield some information, but complete records often are not provided. For example, when requesting academic records, a separate file may be kept by the school counselor. It is important to specify on the request form all sources of information sought, including transcripts, standardized test scores, psychological testing and treatment, and behavioral data. Another common example occurs when requesting employment data. Separate records may exist in the Human Resources Office. Furthermore, when requesting medical records, specify the need for complete records (e.g., all nurses' notes, all evaluations in every department). Otherwise, all one may receive would be the discharge summary, which is usually lacking in qualitative information.

In addition, a separate request to the emergency medical service provider may be required.

Not only do preinjury records provide historical facts, they also provide qualitative information about the character of the patient (Price, 1995). For example, does the individual have external incentives for simulation? Does he or she have a history of bankruptcy or financial strain? Does the individual or a family member have a history of litigation? Is his or her employment history continuous or fragmented? or Does the individual have a history consistent with a possible personality disorder?

Behavioral Observations

Important information may be obtained from the clinical interview and behavioral observations. The simulator's approach to the evaluation may range from outrageous confidence in the examiner's ability (i.e., "I know you are the only one who can understand my problems") to frank aggression or physical threat if the simulator's "deficits" are not confirmed by the examiner. The simulator may try to take control of the interview and behave or endorse items in a bizarre manner in an attempt to convince the clinician of his or her "deficits." Similarly, the simulator may try to manipulate the examiner in an ingenuous manner by answering vaguely, speaking slowly, hesitating frequently, asking for questions to be repeated, arriving late for an appointment, canceling at the last minute, or refusing to complete certain tasks or the entire evaluation due to pain or psychological and / or cognitive deficits. The simulator may seek to present his or her preinjury medical and psychological profile as unrealistically healthy, when in fact records indicate otherwise. With regard to prior treatment efficacy, the simulator may indicate prior treatment did not work, and he or she "knows" other treatments will be of no benefit or too inconvenient (Price, 1995).

Lack of internal consistency among test behaviors and responses over the course of a lengthy evaluation often alerts the clinician to the possibility of simulation—the patient's responses do not make "neuropsychological sense" (Franzen, Iverson, & McCracken, 1990). Specific presentation anomalies may include an improbable number of symptoms, extreme symptom severity, ridiculous symptoms (e.g., fingernails itching), appearance of symptoms during the interview that were not evident prior to the evaluation (e.g., inability to write their name during testing, but ability to sign the consent form or legal documents), and complaints inconsistent with the usual course of any recognized mental disorder. Our personal favorite is the simulator who has a vague recollection of important personal information (e.g., prior psychiatric history), but has a photographic memory of events and symptoms related to the injury and presents these difficulties in an exaggerated and dramatic manner (i.e., anterograde amnesia less severe than retrograde amnesia). Another possible indicator suggested by Schacter (1986) is that simulators may underestimate their abilities to recall information even with the aid of powerful cues.

In addition to behavioral observations during the interview, behavior during testing can be revealing. Simulators may provide "near misses" in responses to questions (e.g., how many weeks are there in a year—50; Bash & Alpert, 1980), and they may fail tasks even severely impaired individuals can pass (floor effect—e.g., unable to repeat the number "six"; Rogers, Harrell, & Liff, 1993). Incorrect answers to easy items as opposed to harder items have been reported as well (Rogers, Harrell, & Liff, 1993). Simulation detection by this technique has been termed the "performance curve strategy" by Goldstein (1945). Another example of the performance curve strategy is failing to show primacy effects in learning new information (Wiggins & Brandt, 1988). Neuropsychological tests such the Paced Auditory Serial Addition Test (PASAT; Gronwall & Wrightson, 1974), the Test of Nonverbal Intelligence (TONI; Brown, Sherbenou, & Johnsen, 1982), and Raven's Progressive Matrices (RPM; Raven, 1960; Raven, Court, & Raven, 1976) have been studied in this regard (Frederick & Foster, 1991; Gudjonsson & Shackleton, 1986; Strauss, Spellacy, Hunter, & Berry, 1994).

To our knowledge, only two researchers have reported results on how individuals said they would emulate cognitive deficits (Goebel, 1983; Iverson, 1995). After speaking with 141 normal and brain-impaired analogue simulators, Goebel (1983) found 36% reported they would slow their performance or look confused, 30% indicated they would give the wrong answer, and 14% stated they would show motor incoordination. Other strategies reported by 2% or less included feigning memory impairment, ignoring stimuli, changing emotional states, and stuttering. Still, 92% of Goebel's participants said they could have faked better, and 10% indicated not faking at all. Reasons related by the participants for their less than optimal faking performances were unfamiliarity with the tasks, lack of preparation to fake the tasks, the tests were too easy to fake, they got too involved in the tests to fake, or the presence of the examiner discouraged faking.

More recently, Iverson (1995) asked undergraduates, community volunteers, psychiatric inpatients, and inmates from a minimum security prison how they would feign a memory deficit. Results were divided into two major categories: behavior prior to the evaluation, and behavior during the evaluation. These results are summarized in Table 12.1.

Aberrant Profiles on Neuropsychological Tests

Some clinicians consider improbably poor performances on neuropsychological measures indicative of simulation. Research in this area is desirable for three reasons:

TABLE 12.1
Self-Reported Strategies for Faking Memory Impairment

	Frequency in Total Sample (n = 160)
Behavior prior to seeing the psychologist	
• Spend time convincing yourself that you really do have memory problems	6
• Confuse appointment times or miss appointments	6
• Plan carefully and stick to your story	4
• Rely on prompts to remember daily routines	3
• Research memory loss	3
Behavior during interview or testing	
(a) Type of memory complaints	
• Fake total amnesia	26
• Fake partial amnesia: Forget most events before and after accident; forget people's names; forget things from past	19
• Forget day-to-day things: Friends' phone numbers, appointments, chores, errands	6
(b) Overt and covert testing behavior	
• "Go blank"—completely forget material presented	16
• Ask examiner to repeat questions; get directions confused	11
• "Space off," don't pay attention, poor concentration	10
• Act confused	8
• Slow response times, frequent hesitation	5
• Random responding	5
• Bizarre responding	4
• Confabulate	4
• Pretend testing is too hard and you cannot continue	3
• Forget things from earlier in the interview or from the beginning of testing	3
• Could not think of other strategies for faking memory impairment	49

Note. From Iverson (1995). Adapted with permission.

1. These tests are given anyway; therefore, administration is cost-effective and time-efficient.

2. These tests are not easily recognized as simulation measures.

3. Simulation of performance patterns of truly impaired individuals is more difficult.

With this goal in mind, Rawling and colleagues (1992, 1993; Rawling & Brooks, 1990; Rawling & Coffey, 1994) developed the Simulation Index (SI). The SI is derived from a qualitative analysis of errors made on the Wechsler Adult Intelligence Scale–Revised (WAIS–R; Wechsler, 1981) and the Wechsler Memory Scale (WMS; Wechsler, 1945, 1974). It was recently revised (SI–R) to incorporate the revised version of the WMS (WMS–R; Wechsler, 1987). The analysis identifies and weights 15 error types or signs occurring frequently in a simulation group, and 5 additional error types occurring frequently in a head-injured group. The error scores are summed to produce the index score. A validation study of the SI–R by Milanovich, Axelrod, and Millis (1996) suggested over one-third of the mixed clinical sample were falsely classified as simulators. These authors recommended raising the cutoff score to decrease Type II errors. Continued investigation of this index is required before its clinical utility can be established.

More recently, Reitan and Wolfson (1996, 1997) developed a Retest Consistency Index based on serial testing sessions using six measures: WAIS–R Comprehension, Picture Arrangement, and Digit Symbol, the Category Test (Reitan & Wolfson, 1993), Part B of the Trail Making Test (TMT; Reitan & Wolfson, 1993), and the Tactual Performance Test-Localization (TPT-Loc; Reitan & Wolfson, 1993). Calculation of the index involves two steps: (a) transformation of the difference scores from two test administrations to scaled scores and (b) summing the scaled scores. Reitan and Wolfson reported that 90% of a litigating sample scored 17 or higher, whereas 95% of nonlitigants scored 16 or less. Although the nonlitigating sample was more severely impaired on objective measures (e.g., neurologic evidence of injury), the authors appear to equate litigating status with simulation. Future research should include identified simulators to assess the validity of the Retest Consistency Index.

Additional performance patterns on neuropsychological tests that have been reported to differentiate simulators from truly impaired individuals include:

- Digit Span Backward greater than Digit Span Forward (Binder & Willis, 1991; Iverson & Franzen, 1996).
- Difference score of WAIS–R Vocabulary minus Digit Span age-corrected scaled scores (Mittenberg, Theroux-Fichera, Zielinski, & Heilbronner, 1995).
- Recognition memory worse than free recall on tests such as the California Verbal Learning Test (CVLT; Delis, Kramer, Kaplan, & Ober, 1987), Memory Assessment Scales (MAS; Williams, 1991), Rey Auditory Verbal Learning Test (RAVLT; Rey, 1964), and WMS–R (Beetar & Williams, 1995; Binder, Villaneuva, Howieson, & Moore, 1993; Iverson & Franzen, 1996; Millis, Putnam, Adams, & Ricker, 1995; Trueblood, 1994).
- Failing to show primacy/recency effects on list learning (Wiggins & Brandt, 1988).
- General Memory Index greater than the Attention/Concentration Index on the WMS–R (Mittenberg, Azrin, Millsaps, & Heilbronner, 1993).

- Low number of total words recalled over five learning trials and low long delayed cued recall on the CVLT (Millis et al., 1995).
- Performing below chance levels on forced-choice format tasks such as the Auditory Discrimination Test (Hall & Pritchard, 1996; Language Research Association, 1958) Recognition Memory Test (RMT; Warrington, 1984), RAVLT, Seashore Rhythm Test (SRT; Reitan & Wolfson, 1993), and the TONI (Frederick & Foster, 1991; Frederick, Sarfaty, Johnston, & Powel, 1994; Gfeller, Cradock, & Falkenhain, 1994; Millis, 1992; Millis & Putnam, 1994; Trueblood & Schmidt, 1993) See Larrabee (in press) for cutoff values on commonly used memory tests (e.g., RMT, CVLT, RAVLT).
- More distortion errors and less perseveration errors on the Benton Visual Retention Test (BVRT; Sivan, 1992; Benton & Spreen, 1961).

Although much research has been conducted on these test performance patterns and measures, it is unclear in many studies whether these signs are valid and effective predictors of simulation. Many researchers report only results of discriminant function analyses, which tend to capitalize on chance error (Williams, 1998). Cutoff scores are often not provided, and cross-validation on clinical populations is often lacking. Although the findings of discriminant analysis classification studies are potentially interesting, this research may be of little utility to practicing neuropsychologists because specific cutoff scores are not typically provided. For instance, how many points greater does the WMS–R General Memory Index need to be than the Attention/Concentration Index in order for it to be a valid and effective indicator of simulation?

To answer questions such as this, information about a given measure's cutting score(s), sensitivity, specificity, and false positive and false negative error rates is necessary (Bar-Hillel, 1980; Duncan & Snow, 1987; Willis, 1984). *Sensitivity* refers to correct identification of simulators by the measure, whereas *specificity* refers to the measure's ability to correctly classify nonsimulators. A false positive or Type I error occurs when the measure suggests an individual is simulating when he or she is not, and a false negative or Type II error results when the individual is a simulator but the measure does not identify the individual as such. If a test is a valid indicator, then sensitivity divided by the false positive error rate will be numerically greater than the false negative error rate divided by specificity. To determine the effectiveness of a measure (superiority of classification over base rate alone), knowledge of the base rate (i.e., number of simulators divided by the total population) is necessary. In order for a measure to be effective at identifying simulation, the base rate must be greater than the measure's false positive plus false negative error rates (cf. Faust & Nurcombe, 1989; Gouvier, Hayes, & Smiroldo, 1998). If the measure's combined error rate is greater than the base rate, use of the base rate information alone is more accurate, overall.

Validity and effectiveness of current neuropsychological measures were calculated for studies reporting sensitivity, specificity, false positive and false negative error rates, and cutoff scores and are summarized in Table 12.2. The determination of effectiveness of these simulation measures (and those appearing in Table 12.3) was based on the Trueblood and Schmidt (1993; Trueblood, 1994) base rate estimate of 15% of consecutive outpatient referrals to a neuropsychological private practice. Unfortunately, a comprehensive review of the literature in which existing neuropsychological measures are used for simulation detection (Beetar & Williams, 1995; Bernard, 1990; Bernard & Fowler, 1990; Bernard, Houston, & Natoli, 1993; Bernard, McGrath, & Houston, 1996; Bruhn & Reed, 1975; Goebel, 1983; Hayward, Hall, Hunt, & Zubrick, 1987; Heaton et al., 1978; Hunt & Older, 1943; King, Klebe, & Davis, 1996; Mensch & Woods, 1986; Mittenberg et al., 1993; Mittenberg, Rothoic, Russell, & Heilbronner, 1996; Palmer, Boone, Allman, & Castro, 1995; Pollaczek, 1952; Reitan & Wolfson, 1996, 1997; Tenhula & Sweet, 1996) revealed only two studies reporting the necessary data (Trueblood, 1994; Trueblood & Schmidt, 1993).

Trueblood and Schmidt (1993) administered a battery of neuropsychological tests to 106 consecutive outpatients. Sixteen individuals were identified as probable simulators (i.e., forced-choice testing below chance and/or improbably poor neuropsychological test performance) and were matched with 16 control participants for age, gender, and education. Measures administered included the Halstead–Reitan Neuropsychological Battery (Reitan & Wolfson, 1993), WAIS–R, Wide Range Achievement Test–Revised (WRAT–R; Jastak & Wilkinson, 1984), WMS, Continuous Visual Memory Test (CVMT; Trahan & Larrabee, 1988), and the CVLT. Of 14 possible simulation indicators suggested by prior research, only 7 successfully identified the probable simulators in their sample. Using similar measures, Trueblood (1994) compared the qualitative and quantitative neuropsychological test performances of 22 probable simulators with 22 matched control participants (one probable simulator was his own control) and identified only nine variables that successfully discriminated between the two groups. As Table 12.2 indicates, all identified indicators from both studies were valid; however, none were effective. None of these indicators would be effective identifiers of simulation when the base rate for simulation is less than 19% to 26% or greater than 74% to 81%. Most of these indicators have the potential to be effective only when the base rate for simulation falls into the narrowly truncated range of approximately 40% to 60%. Therefore, superior classification accuracy would occur using base rate information alone, but of course, no simulators would be identified.

TABLE 12.2

Validity and Effectiveness of Simulation Detection Using Existing Neuropsychological Measures

Population	Tests	Cut-Off Scores	Sensitivity	Specificity	False Positive Error Rate	False Negative Error Rate	Valid?	Effective?
Trueblood and Schmidt (1993) Consecutive outpatients with potential secondary gain, n = 16 probable malingerers, n = 16 matched controls	SSP Errors	>17	63%	94%	6%	37%	Yes	No
	GNDS	>44	63%	100%	0%	37%	Yes	No
	DS-ACSS	<7	69%	94%	6%	31%	Yes	No
	FTNB Ttl errs	>5	63%	94%	6%	37%	Yes	No
	FA Ttl errs	>3	63%	94%	6%	37%	Yes	No
	SRT errors	>8	56%	100%	0%	44%	Yes	No
	CVLT-RM	<13	56%	100%	0%	44%	Yes	No
	Total indicators	>2	81%	100%	0%	19%	Yes	No
Trueblood (1994) Consecutive outpatients with potential secondary gain, n = 22 probable malingerers, n = 22 matched controls	DS-ACSS	<7	77%	86%	14%	23%	Yes	No
	Voc-ACSS	<7	36%	95%	5%	64%	Yes	No
	PC-ACSS	<7	41%	95%	5%	59%	Yes	No
	DSy-ACSS	<5	27%	100%	0%	73%	Yes	No
	Barona-IQ	>18	45%	100%	0%	55%	Yes	No
	WAIS-R Indic.	>1	64%	95%	5%	36%	Yes	No
	CVLT-TWR	<48	80%	95%	5%	20%	Yes	No
	CVLT-RM	<13	75%	91%	9%	25%	Yes	No
	CVLT Indic.	>0	90%	91%	9%	10%	Yes	No

Note. SSP Errors = Speech Sounds Perception Test Errors; GNDS = General Neuropsychological Deficits Scale; DS-ACSS = Digit Span Age-Corrected Scaled Score; FTNB Ttl errs = Finger Tip Number Writing Total Errors; FA Ttl errs = Finger Agnosia Total Errors; SRT errors = Seashore Rhythm Test Errors; CVLT-RM = California Verbal Learning Test Recognition Memory; Total indicators = number of tests in the simulation range; Voc-ACSS = Vocabulary Age Corrected Scaled Score; PC-ACSS = Picture Completion Age Corrected Scaled Score; DSy = Digit Symbol Age Corrected Scaled Score; Barona-IQ = Barona Index minus obtained WAIS-R IQ; Wais-R Indic. = number of WAIS-R subtests in the simulation range; CVLT-TWR = California Verbal Learning Test Total Words Recalled; CVLT Indic. = number of California Verbal Learning Test indicators in the simulation range.

TABLE 12.3

Validity and Effectiveness of Measures Designed to Detect Dissimulation

	Population	Tests	Cutoff Scores	Sensitivity	Specificity	False Positive Error Rate	False Negative Error Rate	Valid?	Effective?
Iverson and Franzen (1996)	Undergraduates (n = 20), psychiatric inpatients (n = 20), memory-disordered patients (n = 20). Within subjects analogue design with undergraduates and psychiatric inpatients	Wiggins & Brandt Autobiographical Interview—total missed of 17 questions	>3	77.5%s	100%	0%	22.5%	Yes	No
Arnett, Hammeke, and Schwartz (1995)	Study One Undergraduate simulators (n = 49), neurologically impaired patients (n = 34)	Memory for Fifteen Items Test	<3 rows correct	63%	74%	26%	37%	Yes	No
			<9 items correct	61%	76%	24%	39%	Yes	No
			<8 items correct	59%	82%	18%	41%	Yes	No
			<2 rows correct	47%	97%	3%	53%		
	Study Two: Simulating medical students (n = 25), neurologically impaired patients (n = 25)		<3 rows correct	76%	80%	20%	24%		
			<9 items correct	72%	84%	16%	28%		
			<8 items correct	68%	84%	16%	32%		
			<2 rows correct	64%	96%	4%	36%		
Greiffenstein, Baker, and Gola (1996). Griffin, Glassmire, Henderson, and McCann (in press)	Severe TBI patients (n = 55), probable malingerers (n = 90). Undergraduates (n = 63) and clinical subjects (n = 21)	Memory for Fifteen Items Test Rey II	<10	64%	78%	22%	36%	Yes	No
Iverson and Franzen (1996)	Undergraduates (n = 20), psychiatric inpatients (n = 20), memory-disordered patients (n = 20). Within subjects analogue design with undergraduates and psychiatric inpatients	Memory for Sixteen Items Test	>8 Omissions	23%	100%	0%	77%	Yes	No
			>6 Omissions	33%	98%	2%	67%	Yes	No
			<6 Total correct	40%	100%	0%	60%	Yes	No

Study	Sample	Test	Cutoff criteria						
Guilmette, Hart, and Guiliano (1993)	Brain-damaged subjects (n = 18), undergraduate simulators (n = 29), undergraduate controls (n = 20) Psychiatric group omitted because data not reported	Hiscock Forced Choice Procedure (72 total points)	<66 (more than six errors)	90%	100%	0%	10%	Yes	Yes
Guilmette, Hart, Guiliano, and Leininger (1994)	Brain-damaged subjects (n = 20), psychiatric inpatients (n = 20), undergraduate simulators (n = 20)	Abbreviated Hiscock Forced Choice Procedure (36 total points)	<33 items correct (more than four errors)	85%	97.5%	2.5%	15%	Yes	No
Slick, Hopp, Strauss, and Spellacy (1996)	Undergraduate controls (n = 95), undergraduate simulators (n = 43), compensation-seeking patients (n = 206), non-compensation-seeking patients (n = 32)	Victoria Symptom Validity Test (48 items) Compensation seeking patients were omitted because their simulation status was unknown.	Scores of less than 16 on the easy and/or hard items Questionable and malingering classifications were collapsed to calculate the following data	81%	100%	0%	29%	Yes	No
Greiffenstein, Baker, and Gola (1994)	Traumatic brain injury patients (n = 33), patients with persistent postconcussive syndrome (n = 30), probable malingerers (n = 43)	Portland Digit Recognition Test	<59 correct <64 correct TBI and persisting postconcussive patient data were averaged	65% 75%	91% 79%	9% 21%	35% 25%	Yes Yes	No No
Rose, Hall, and Szalda-Petree (1995)	Uncoached undergraduate simulators (n = 30), coached undergraduate simulators (n = 30), closed head injury patients (n = 30), community control subjects (n = 30)	Portland Digit Recognition Test–Computerized Version Sensitivity and specificity rates not reported for community control subjects	<40 correct	64%	89%	11%	36%	Yes	No

(Continued)

TABLE 12.3
(Continued)

	Population	Tests	Cutoff Scores	Sensitivity	Specificity	False Positive Error Rate	False Negative Error Rate	Valid?	Effective?
Iverson, Franzen, and McCracken (1994)	Psychiatric inpatients (n = 60), community volunteer controls (n = 60), memory-impaired patients (n = 60). Within subjects analogue design with undergraduates and psychiatric inpatients	21-Item Test	<9 <12	38% 70%	100% 96%	0% 4%	62% 30%	Yes Yes	No No
Iverson, Franzen, and McCracken (1991)	Undergraduate controls (n = 20), undergraduate simulators (n = 20), memory-impaired patients (n = 20)	21-Item Test	<5 on free recall <3 on free recall <13 on recog.	75% 35% 100%	72.5% 92.5% 97.5%	27.5% 7.5% 2.5%	25% 65% 0%	Yes Yes Yes	No No Yes
Hilsabeck, LeCompte, Zuppardo, and Mitchell (1997)	Undergraduate controls (n = 72), undergraduate simulators (n = 58), severe TBI memory-impaired patients (n = 2)	Word Completion Memory Test	<9 on recog. R <9 or Inclusion <15	65% 93%	100% 100%	0% 0%	35% 7%	Yes Yes	No Yes
Greiffenstein, Baker, and Gola (1996)	Severe TBI patients (n = 55), probable malingerers (n = 90)	Rey Word Recognition List	<6 correct <5 (total correct minus false positives)	80% 72%	93% 84%	7% 16%	20% 28%	Yes Yes	No No
Greiffenstein, Baker, and Gola (1994)	Traumatic brain injury patients (n = 33), patients with persistent postconcussive syndrome (n = 30), probable malingerers (n = 43)	Rey Word Recognition List	<7 correct <5 correct TBI and persisting postconcussive patient data were averaged	60% 83%	90% 80%	10% 20%	40% 17%	Yes Yes	No No

A Catalog of Simulation Detection Tests

Although performance patterns on existing neuropsychological tests may successfully discriminate between analogue simulators and truly impaired individuals, tests specifically designed to detect simulation (i.e., domain-specific tests) have been found to be more successful (Greiffenstein, Gola, & Baker, 1995; Hiscock, Branham, & Hiscock, 1994). Domain-specific tests fall into one of four categories based on their underlying principles: (a) floor effect, (b) symptom validity/forced-choice testing, (c) response bias/response inconsistency, and (d) priming/implicit memory. When possible, cutoff scores, sensitivity, specificity, and false positive and false negative error rates from representative studies are summarized in Table 12.3. In addition, validity and effectiveness (using the hypothetical base rate estimate for simulation of 15%) of each measure are presented.

Floor Effect

As noted earlier, the floor effect refers to performing worse on a measure than a very severely impaired individual would. Simulation detection measures in this category include the Autobiographical Interview (Wiggins & Brandt, 1988), the Memory for Fifteen Items Test (MFIT; Rey, 1941, 1964; Lezak, 1995), the Memorization of Sixteen Items Test (MSIT; Paul, Franzen, Cohen, & Fremouw, 1992), and the Rey Word Recognition List (WRL; Lezak, 1983).

Autobiographical Interview. This interview consists of 12 questions about an individual's personal history and recent daily events (Wiggins & Brandt, 1988). Four amnesic individuals were compared to analogue simulators and control participants in the original study. For the 12 questions, one amnesic failed to recall her social security number, one failed to recall what she had for dinner the previous night, and two failed to recall the experimenter's name on the second day. Therefore, out of 48 possible answers across participants, only four errors were made by the amnesics (8% failure rate). In contrast, the analogue simulators' failure rates on every question ranged from 10% (i.e., recognizing the experimenter's name given four choices) to 48% (i.e., remembering their social security number). Iverson and Franzen (1996) modified the Autobiographical Interview by including questions from the Information subtest of the WMS–R (total = 17 questions) and obtained results consistent with the original authors.

Memory for Fifteen Items Test (MFIT). On the MFIT, the individual is asked to view an array of 15 items for 10 sec. The stimulus is then withdrawn and the individual is asked to reproduce the items from memory. The procedure assumes the simulator will view the MFIT as a difficult test of memory, reproducing few of the 15 items. Several scoring methods involving both qualitative and quantitative analyses have been proposed, but none have been universally accepted. Suggested scoring methods have included number of correct rows, number of correct items, and spatial location (Arnett, Hammeke, & Schwartz, 1995; Bernard & Fowler, 1990; Davidson, Suffield, Orenczuk, Nantau, & Mandel, 1991; Goldberg & Miller, 1986; Griffin, Normington, & Glassmire, 1996; Hays, Emmons, & Lawson, 1993; Lee, Loring, & Martin, 1992; Lezak, 1995; Schretlen, Brandt, Krafft, & Van Gorp, 1991). Much research has examined the validity of the MFIT as a simulation detection test, with a growing consensus that it is likely to detect only a minority of unsophisticated simulators because it is either too easy or too obvious to be faked (DiCarlo, Gfeller, & Drury, 1996; Goebel, 1989; Haines & Norris, 1995; Millis & Kier, 1995).

Griffin, Glassmire, Henderson, and McCann (1997) redesigned the MFIT with four goals in mind:

1. To increase the discriminability between simulators and cognitively impaired individuals and between simulators and persons with psychiatric illnesses.
2. To improve face validity by increasing the level of difficulty.
3. To standardize the instructions.
4. To offer a simple scoring system utilizing both quantitative and qualitative analyses of responses.

Their revised version is termed the Rey II, and the authors suggested using this version over the MFIT because of better classification rates.

Memory for Sixteen Items Test (MSIT). In this modified version of the MFIT, Paul et al. (1992) eliminated the geometric figures and added a fourth item to each of the remaining four rows (e.g., A B C D). Three cutting scores can be derived from the MSIT:

1. Number of correct items in their proper locations.
2. Number of omissions.
3. Number of original items reproduced more than once plus the number of confabulated items (i.e., additions or intrusions).

Unfortunately, little research exists on the utility of this measure (Franzen & Martin, 1996; Iverson & Franzen, 1996).

Word Recognition List (WRL). The WRL (Lezak, 1983) consists of a study phase (i.e., the patient is read 15 words aloud) and a recognition phase (i.e., the patient is asked to circle the 15 study words out of 30 total words). Simulation is suggested when the individual has a low total correct score and/or a low total correct minus false positive score. Although this test has existed for many years, little research exists with regard to its discriminant power (Greiffenstein, Baker, & Gola, 1994, 1996).

Symptom Validity/Forced-Choice Tests

Although Brady and Lind (1961) were the first researchers to introduce symptom validity testing when their patient with hysterical blindness demonstrated worse than chance levels of performance, Pankratz and colleagues (1979, 1983; Binder & Pankratz, 1987; Pankratz, Fausti, & Peed, 1975) popularized this technique as an effective means of detecting simulation of cognitive impairments. Symptom validity/forced-choice measures are based on a binomial distribution (Rogers, Harrell, & Liff, 1993). Using a binomial distribution, if a patient is given a choice between A or B on a 100-item test, that person would be expected to score within the range of 50 ± 8 by chance alone (Frederick & Foster, 1991). If he or she scores below 42, then simulation is likely at the 95% confidence level, as the response protocol would suggest he or she was able to consistently discern the correct answer and give the incorrect one (Rogers, Harrell, & Liff, 1993). Cutoff scores can be computed to estimate the probability of simulation in tests of shorter or greater length by reference to the binomial distribution and normal probability curve.

An advantage of symptom validity testing is that it can be adapted to any measure where a two-alternative format is possible. Frederick, Carter, and Powel (1995) reported using this type of paradigm with three patients. Based on "forgotten" interview data, these researchers developed an individualized forced-choice questioning procedure to detect simulation. They recommended using greater than 25 items to decrease Type I and Type II errors. The primary disadvantages of a forced-choice procedure are that very few simulators score below chance on these measures (Rogers, Harrell, & Liff, 1993), administration time can be lengthy if many trials are needed (e.g., up to 60 min), and little information about cognitive ability is added (Haines & Norris, 1995).

Hiscock Forced Choice Procedure (HFCP). The HFCP (Hiscock & Hiscock, 1989), also known as the Digit Memory Test (DMT), was developed to improve on the simple methodology suggested by Binder and Pankratz (i.e., asking the patient to specify whether a black pen or yellow pencil was presented over 100 trials; Binder & Pankratz, 1987).

Hiscock and Hiscock (1989) substituted five-digit numbers as the target stimuli in order to make the task appear more difficult, and they varied the length of interval between stimulus presentation and response (e.g., 5 sec, 10 sec). Research has been conducted with various populations, including patients with severe but static cerebral dysfunction and memory-disordered patients (Guilmette, Hart, & Giuliano, 1993; Guilmette, Hart, Giuliano, & Leininger, 1994; Guilmette, Sparadeo, Whelihan, & Buongiorno, 1994; Prigatano & Amin, 1993) and with consonants rather than numbers (i.e., Malingered Memory Deficit Test; Bickart, Mayer, & Connell, 1991). Overall, this research indicates the HFCP can reliably discriminate between simulators and nonsimulators.

Victoria Symptom Validity Test (VSVT). This modification of the HFCP reduced the number of items from 72 to 48 (three trials of 16) and included both easy (i.e., no overlap in digits between foil and target) and difficult items (i.e., foil has same numbers as the target but two digits are transposed; Slick, Hopp, Strauss, Hunter, & Pinch, 1994; Slick, Hopp, Strauss, & Spellacy, 1996). It is assumed that easy items will be answered correctly more often than hard items when an individual is answering honestly. Slick and colleagues (1996) reported that performance on the VSVT is relatively unaffected by level of cognitive functioning, but little research exists regarding this measure.

Portland Digit Recognition Test (PDRT). Initially, Binder (1990) reported the PDRT consisted of 108 trials (i.e., six blocks of 18 items), but later Binder and Willis (1991) presented validity data on a 72-item version (four blocks of 18 items). The initial 36 items are considered easy items, and the remaining 36 are reported to be hard items. Although the PDRT is similar to the HFCP, it changed the length of the retention intervals, and the task of counting backward between stimulus presentation and response was added. Binder and colleagues hypothesized that these changes would increase the sensitivity of the forced-choice procedure, thereby identifying more simulators. Baker, Hanley, Jackson, Kimmance, and Slade (1993) supported this assertion when a similar distracter task aided in differentiating performances of head-injured individuals and simulating participants. Initial validity data appear promising (Binder, 1992, 1993a, 1993b, 1993c; Peck, Mitchell, Baber, & Blumberg, 1996), and the PDRT has been successfully converted into a computerized version (PDRT–C; Rose, Hall, & Szalda-Petree, 1995). Using the PDRT–C, Rose et al. (1995) found response latency added incremental validity in the detection of analogue simulators. Additional advantages of using a computerized version are the decreased face validity of the test, the ability to randomize item difficulty, and reduced personnel time for administration and scoring (Haines & Norris, 1995).

Multi-Digit Memory Test (MDMT). Prior to the development of the PDRT–C, Niccolls and Bolter (1991) offered a computerized version of symptom validity testing modeled after the HFCP. These researchers recognized the advantages of a computerized format for recording response latencies and convenience of administration and scoring. The MDMT retention intervals between stimulus presentation (i.e., three sets of 24 trials) and response are 2, 7, and 15 sec, respectively. Although the MDMT discriminates between analogue simulators and closed head injury patients (Martin et al., 1992, 1993), future research using probable simulators is needed to evaluate this test's validity and effectiveness.

21-Item Test. This forced-choice procedure, which is a derivative of Brandt, Rubinsky, and Lassen's (1985) 20-item word list, uses two 21-item word lists (Iverson, Franzen, & McCracken, 1991). Each word list contains seven rhyming words, seven semantically similar words, and seven semantically unrelated words. The individual is initially read either word list, and then is asked to recall as many words from the list as possible. Finally, he or she is read word pairs (i.e., one word from the original list and one from the alternate list) and is asked to choose the target from the original list. Research suggests this is a promising simulation detection measure (Iverson & Franzen, 1996; Iverson, Franzen, & McCracken, 1991, 1994).

Test of Memory Malingering (TOMM). Rees and colleagues (Gansler, Tombaugh, Petterson-Moczynski, & Rees, 1995; Rees, 1996; Rees & Tombaugh, 1996) developed and validated the TOMM for the detection of simulated memory impairment. This test consists of two learning trials, each composed of a study and test phase. During the study phase, the patient is shown 50 line-drawn pictures for 3 sec. Next, the patient is shown the target stimuli paired with a line drawing not previously shown (i.e., distracter) and is asked which drawing was seen before. Feedback is given after each response, and a delayed retention trial is administered in the same manner after a 20-min delay. Researchers indicate this measure is robust to age, education, and neurological impairment, reporting that 94% of all nondemented patients and 99.9% of cognitively intact community residents were correctly classified (Tombaugh et al., 1996). Still, future research using a clinical population of suspected simulators is essential to establish the validity and effectiveness of this proposed measure.

Response Bias/Response Inconsistency

The underlying principle behind the Dot Counting Test (DCT; Rey, 1941), the Forced-Choice Test of Nonverbal Ability (FCTNA; Frederick & Foster, 1991; Frederick et al., 1994), and the Minnesota Multiphasic Personality Inventory–2 (MMPI–2; Butcher, Dahlstrom, Graham, Tellegen, & Kaemmer, 1989) validity scales (i.e., L, F, K, TRIN, VRIN, Fb, Ds-r2, Fp) is response bias and/or response inconsistency. It is hypothesized that a simulator may answer in a random or inconsistent manner, signaling the clinician to the possibility of incomplete effort, noncompliance, and/or simulation.

Dot Counting Test (DCT). In this simulation detection measure, the individual is asked to count sets of ungrouped and grouped dots. It is assumed he or she should take longer to count the ungrouped dots relative to the grouped dots, with time increasing as the number of dots increases (Binks, Gouvier, & Waters, 1997; Franzen & Martin, 1996; Greiffenstein et al., 1994; Paul et al., 1992). Although several variables have been investigated to determine which is the best indicator of simulation (e.g., total time for ungrouped dots minus total time for grouped dots, sum of instances in which grouped count times exceeded the corresponding ungrouped times), Binks et al. (1997) found the best discriminator between simulators and a mixed patient group was the total number of incorrect responses across both grouped and ungrouped trials. Similarly, Paul et al. (1992) reported the best discriminator as the number of correct responses across all trials.

Forced-Choice Test of Nonverbal Ability (FCTNA). The FCTNA was developed by Frederick and Foster (1991) to address concerns about the limitations of symptom validity testing. These authors supposed that the easy versus hard item dichotomy could be more effectively utilized if these items were randomized rather than presented in an ascending order of difficulty (easy to hard). They asserted that randomization of item presentation makes it more difficult to identify easy and hard items, leading to inconsistent performances across item difficulty. To maximize the likelihood of detecting inconsistent responding, the FCTNA has two 50-item versions so performances can be compared across versions. Therefore, the FCTNA has a total of 100 items.

The FCTNA yields three indicators: (a) slope, (b) consistency ratio (CR), and (c) the product of the two (slope*CR). The slope is the performance curve from least to most difficult test item. The CR is the ratio of number of equivalent item pairs in which both items are answered correctly to the total test score divided by two. CRs of .50 or less are considered indicative of simulation. Frederick et al. (1994) found a negative slope was characteristic of the performances of cognitively impaired persons and normals, whereas a near-zero slope was more representative of simulation. Research to date suggests that the slope*CR indicator is the most sensitive measure of response bias (Frederick & Foster, 1991; Frederick et al., 1994).

Minnesota Multiphasic Personality Inventory–2 (MMPI–2). Although many investigators have examined the influence of simulation on MMPI and MMPI–2 responses (Austin, 1992; Bagby, Buis, & Nicholson, 1995; Bagby, Rogers, & Buis, 1994; Berry, Baer, & Harris, 1991; Berry et al., 1992; Berry, Wetter, Baer, Widiger, Sumpter, Reynolds, & Hallam, 1991; Brophy, 1995; Cassisi & Workman, 1992; Cernovsky, 1989; DuAlba & Scott, 1993; Fox, Gerson, & Lees-Haley, 1995; Gillis, Rogers, & Dickens, 1990; Graham et al., 1991; Grossman, Haywood, Ostrov, Wasyliw, & Cavanaugh, 1990; Grossman, Haywood, & Wasyliw, 1992; Grossman & Wasyliw, 1988; Hawk & Cornell, 1989; Heilbrun, Bennett, White, & Kelly, 1990; Hsu, Santelli, & Hsu, 1989; Hyer, Fallon, Harrison, & Boudewyns, 1987; Iverson, Franzen, & Hammond, 1995; Lees-Haley, 1991, 1992; Lees-Haley & Fox, 1990; Paolo & Ryan, 1992; Pensa, Dorfman, Gold, & Schneider, 1996; Perconte & Goreczny, 1990; Rogers, Bagby, & Chakraborty, 1993; Rogers, Sewell, & Salekin, 1994; Roman, Tuley, Villaneuva, & Mitchell, 1990; Smith & Frueh, 1996; Timbrook, Graham, Keiller, & Watts, 1993; Viglione, Fals-Stewart, & Moxham, 1995; Walters, 1988; Walters, White, & Greene, 1988; Wasyliw, Grossman, Haywood, & Cavanaugh, 1988; Weed, Ben-Porath, & Butcher, 1990; Wetter, Baer, Berry, Smith, & Larsen, 1992; Wetzler & Marlowe, 1990; Woychyshyn, McElheran, & Romney, 1992), relatively little research exists with regard to simulation of closed head injury symptoms and MMPI–2 responses. In part, this may be due to interpretative concerns when using the MMPI–2 with a neurologically compromised population. For example, Mittenberg, Tremont, and Rayls (1996) suggested that impairments in intelligence, memory, attention, and concentration may lead to validity scale elevations, and Gass and colleagues (Gass, 1991, 1992; Gass, Russell, & Hamilton, 1990) found closed head injury patients had elevated T-scores on scales 1, 2, 3, 7, and 8 compared to normals.

In spite of these potential limitations, investigation of simulation of cognitive impairments on the MMPI–2 is important, given that the MMPI–2 is often administered in neuropsychological evaluations (Lees-Haley, Smith, Williams, & Dunn, 1996). With this in mind, Lamb et al. (1994) studied the effects of two types of information (i.e., information about the validity scales and/or closed injury sequelae) on ability to simulate on the MMPI–2. They found that both types of information influenced responses of analogue simulators and control participants but in different ways. Participants given information about CHI symptoms had inflated scores on Scales F, 2, and 6, whereas participants with knowledge of the validity scales had deflated scores on both the validity and clinical scales. Based on these data, they concluded that coaching influences MMPI–2 test results. Wetter and Deitsch (1996) investigated if individuals instructed to fake closed head injury symptoms on the MMPI–2 could respond consistently across serial test administrations. They found that analogue simulators could feign these symptoms in a reliable manner. Berry et al. (1995) compared MMPI–2 responses of analogue simulators, compensation-seeking closed head injury patients, non-compensation-seeking closed head injury patients, and normals. Results indicated the first two groups scored significantly higher on Scales F, Fb, F-K, and Ds2 and significantly lower on Scale K than the latter two groups. As noted by Berry and colleagues, however, compensation-seeking closed head injury patients are not necessarily simulating but may be overreporting their symptoms due to real distress. Unfortunately, there is no way to discern which interpretation of the data is correct. Another important finding of their study was that the VRIN scale was insensitive to overreporting of closed head injury symptoms. Accordingly, the authors suggested when the VRIN score is elevated, confusion or random responding is highly likely, although replication of this finding is desirable.

Priming/Implicit Memory Tests. Research using implicit memory or priming tasks (Roediger & Blaxton, 1987; Schacter, 1987; Tulving & Schacter, 1990) also shows promise in the detection of simulation. On implicit memory tasks, participants are not told they will be tested on their recall of presented material, whereas on explicit memory tasks, participants are specifically told their memory for the material will be tested. In contrast to performance on explicit memory tasks, amnestic and demented patients often perform within normal limits on tests of implicit memory (Cermak, Talbot, Chandler, & Wolbarst, 1985; Graf, Squire, & Mandler, 1984; Shiamamura, 1986). Common implicit memory tasks include word-stem completion, word-fragment completion, and picture-fragment completion (Java, 1994; Lynch, 1994; Roediger, 1990; Schacter, 1987; Searleman & Herrmann, 1994).

Wiggins and Brandt (1988) were the first to investigate the ability of an implicit memory task (i.e., word-stem completion) to detect simulation. Their results suggested the task was unsuccessful in discriminating analogue simulators from amnesics and control participants. However, Horton, Smith, Barghout, and Connolly (1992) changed the instructions given to participants and found significant differences between simulators and nonsimulators. Their results suggested further study of implicit memory tasks for the detection of simulation was warranted.

In two recent studies, Davis and colleagues (Davis, King, Bloodworth, Spring, & Klebe, 1997; Davis, King, Klebe, Bajszar, Bloodworth, & Wallick, 1997) implemented two implicit memory tests (i.e., word-stem completion and classification of dot patterns) to detect simulation. Using a discriminant function analysis, the authors reported correct classification of 92% of control participants and 73% of analogue simulators with the word-stem completion task (Davis, King, Klebe, Bajszar, Bloodworth, & Wallick, 1997). In the second study using the dot pattern task (Davis, King, Blood-worth, Spring, & Klebe, 1997), a memory-impaired group was included, and discriminant function classification rates were 80% for control participants, 65% for analogue simulators, and 80% for memory-impaired patients.

Hilsabeck, LeCompte, Zuppardo, and Mitchell (1997) developed the Word Completion Memory Test (WCMT) to detect sophisticated attempts at simulating memory impairments. The WCMT consists of two subtests: Inclusion and Exclusion. On the Inclusion subtest, participants are asked to copy and rate the pleasantness of 30 common words. Then they are given 30 word stems and are asked to complete the word stems with words from the list they just saw. On the Exclusion subtest, after copying and rating the pleasantness of 30 different common words, participants are asked to complete a new set of 30 word stems with words that were not from the list they just saw. Three scores are computed:

1. The "I" score (number of word stems completed with words from the Inclusion subtest study list).
2. The "E" score (number of word stems completed with words from the Exclusion subtest study list).
3. The "R" score ("I" score minus "E" score).

Initial data appear promising (see Table 12.3), and additional validation studies are in progress.

Multiple Measures for Simulation Detection

Most of the studies just described use either existing neuropsychological measures or domain-specific simulation tests to aid in the detection of feigning. Although domain-specific simulation measures have been found to be more sensitive to feigning than neuropsychological tests (Greiffenstein et al., 1995; Hiscock et al., 1994), most neuropsychologists rely on a battery approach for assessment of functioning. Therefore, we recommend future research focus on exploring the classification accuracy of multiple detection strategies as previously suggested by Rogers, Harrell, and Liff (1993). An industrious researcher would follow the model offered by Trueblood and Schmidt (1993) in providing not only cutoff scores and sensitivity and specificity rates for individual tests, but also for a combination of indicators. For example, what are the sensitivity and specificity rates of WAIS–R Digit Span age-corrected scaled scores less than 7, PDRT scores less than 64, and Speech-Sounds Perception Test (SSPT; Reitan & Wolfson, 1993) errors greater than 17? What does a common simulation "profile" look like? Although this line of research may be neglected due to lack of uniformity in test batteries administered by neuropsychologists (Rogers, Harrell, & Liff, 1993), if a simulation "profile" can be identified, this information may help the clinician tailor the test battery when potential for secondary gain is involved.

INCREASING VALIDITY OF SIMULATION DETECTION

The validity of simulation detection measures is compromised by four primary factors, which are discussed next:

- Poor psychometric research.
- Variable group membership.
- Limited generalizability of analogue research.
- Differential vulnerability of measures.

Poor Psychometric Research

Simulation detection research has failed to adequately address basic test construction principles. Based on our review of the literature, no researchers have provided data on the reliability (e.g., test–retest, internal consistency) of these simulation measures. Although several validity studies have been conducted, many are based on small sample sizes with circumscribed groups, and only one study has examined convergent and divergent validity (Slick et al., 1996). As stated in previous sections, sensitivity and specificity data, as well as cutoff scores, are imperative to assist clinicians in test selection and interpretation of findings, and authors simply must begin consistently reporting their base rate estimates for simulation whenever they publish research in this area.

Variable Group Membership

Support for simulation detection measures has been compromised by the wide variability of the samples used in validation studies. Although various impaired groups often may have overlapping cognitive difficulties, they do not necessarily share equivalent cognitive deficits and therefore should not be directly compared without great trepidation. This same criticism applies to the composition of simulation groups. Detailed reports of inclusion and exclusion criteria for group membership will allow neuropsychologists to make more useful comparisons across studies and to their own patient population. Other research is limited by comparing litigating and nonlitigating groups. Although interesting, these studies are limited because involvement in litigation does not always equal simulation. Differences between these groups may be attributable to other factors, such as more severe cognitive impairments and/or psychological distress.

To address these concerns, Greiffenstein et al. (1994) and Trueblood and Schmidt (1993) provided guidelines for inclusion of probable or suspected simulators in a clinical sample. These researchers operationally defined membership status, allowing replication and generalization of their findings. As noted by Haines and Norris (1995), advantages of using probable simulators from a clinical population are the presence of known motivation to simulate, motivation to avoid detection, and experience with the traumatic event. Another consideration for selection of validation samples concerns characteristics of control participants. Most simulation research uses a sample of convenience (e.g., college undergraduates) as the comparison group. It is likely that there are significant differences between the convenience sample and persons most likely to sustain a head injury. Future research should endeavor to match head-injured individuals with persons showing risk factors for head injury (e.g., substance abuse, low socioeconomic status [SES], low education, risk-taking behaviors). Using these individuals as control participants may help tease out variability in performances due to premorbid factors.

Limited Generalizability of Analogue Research

The generalizability of analogue research is limited because analogue study participants suffer a lack of motivation, knowledge, and personal experience with the traumatic event. However, results of a recent study by Hayes, Martin, and Gouvier (1995) indicated college students with a history of mild head injury and knowledge of head injury sequelae were not able to simulate more effectively than college students without this experience and knowledge. This finding suggests that motivational factors may be the primary limitations of analogue research. The advantage of an analogue design is the base rate for simulation is fixed by the experimenter. Because this is an important element for establishing validity and effectiveness of simulation detection measures, the analogue design is a useful tool. Therefore, the challenge is to increase the generalizability of analogue research.

One method researchers have used to increase the external validity of analogue research is to coach analogue simulators. Unfortunately, investigators thus far have failed to develop a systematic method of coaching prohibiting comparisons of results across studies. Coaching paradigms range from participants reading a paragraph or scenario to participants attending a seminar on symptoms experienced by individuals with closed head injury, and these are typically one-time only sessions. Because litigants have both the incentive and motivation to "perfect their performances," a more structured and in-depth coaching process may be necessary to help the analogue simulator more adequately mimic sequelae of closed head injury. This method should not be viewed as a "one-shot deal," but as a continual shaping process ecologically closer to the one that occurs in the real world, with multiple examinations, independent medical evaluations, and depositions. Lamb et al. (1994) offered a methodology more closely approximating a shaping process. These researchers provided participants information about symptoms of head injury and the validity scales of the MMPI–2. Subsequently, mastery of the material was ensured before administration of the MMPI–2.

Another way to help determine the generalizability of analogue data is to compare performances of coached and suspected simulators on neuropsychological and domain specific measures. Moreover, following the lead of Goebel (1989) and Rogers (1988), implementation of postexperiment questionnaires inquiring about performance strategies, compliance with simulation and test instructions, possible incentives that would increase motivation to feign, and information needed to effectively simulate deficits associated with closed head injury would be useful for providing exclusionary criteria and future directions for research.

Differential Vulnerability of Measures

The neuropsychologist must be aware of those measures more susceptible to simulation. Research has suggested self-report measures are more vulnerable to faking than objective measures (Martin, Hayes, & Gouvier, 1996). However, although self-report measures such as the Iowa Inventory for Partial Seizure Like Symptoms and the Post Concussion Symptom Questionnaire are vulnerable to simulation, Wong, Regennitter, and Barrios (1994) showed that although overendorsement of seizure-like symptoms by analogue simulators was significantly different from control participants, it fell substantially below the level of seizure endorsement among criterion patients. We recommend that clinicians use the information provided on sensitivity and specificity rates in Tables 12.2 and 12.3 to aid in test selection and interpretation for simulation detection.

PITFALLS OF MISCLASSIFICATION

Classical testing theory begins with the tenet that any observed score represents an individual's true score plus an additional error score associated with various threats to the internal and external validity of the test device. If error occurs in every observation, the discernment of truth becomes more difficult. Closer examination of common errors occurring in neuropsychological diagnosis may allow the clinician to manage the problem with ever-present error more effectively.

Type I and Type II errors hold profound significance for the entire diagnostic endeavor. These considerations apply in the traditional domain of diagnosing psychopathology or neuropsychopathology against a background of normalcy, but they apply equally well when diagnosing simulation (normalcy masquerading as pseudopathology) against a background of psychopathology or neuropsychopathology. In the traditional clinical endeavor, a Type I error may result in an individual being stigmatized with a wrong label and receiving inappropriate treatment, whereas a Type II error results in an individual in need of service slipping through the cracks. However, the typical clinical setting is fraught with built-in redundancies that make these outcomes less likely. For example, response to treatment is monitored in the Type I patient and continued presentation of symptom complaints is noted in the Type II patient; deviations from the expected course in either case would lead to further inquiry and more careful diagnostic evaluation. This is not the case in simulation diagnoses.

Simulation diagnoses are frequently made outside the contact of routine care and monitoring, and thus the safeguard redundancies just noted are not likely to be present. The costs of misclassification in simulation diagnoses remain weighty, however. Although a Type II error allows for the successful perpetration of fraud and resultant costs to a third-party payer, the moral consequences of a Type I error may be even higher, and force one to ask the rhetorical question, what is the dollar value of an honest person's reputation? Not only is his or her reputation at stake, but also the potential loss of just compensation and needed services for a real injury made trivial by the incorrect simulation diagnosis.

Given a test with known error rates, the base rate of the condition being diagnosed determines whether or not that test will be an effective adjunct to diagnosis of the condition (i.e., adds useful signal). When base rates are less than the test's combined error rate, relying on the test for diagnosis adds noise rather than signal to the diagnostic process, and overall accuracy declines relative to diagnosis based on base rates alone. In a very real sense, this causes the truth value of a psychologist's testimony to vary as a joint function of the error rates of the tests and the base rates of simulation. Well-intended psychologists could swear to tell the truth, the whole truth, and nothing but the truth, but wrongfully malign an honest patient because of his or her lack of knowledge about these relationships. It is imperative for psychologists who take the oath to be aware of base rates for symptom complaints and test failures among

normal individuals, as well as among individuals with known pathologies. Only by factoring these considerations into their clinical judgment
can psychologists minimize the occasions in which they honestly testify
to their belief in erroneous conclusions that cannot be supported in the
light of base-rate analysis.

ISSUES FOR FURTHER CONSIDERATION

In an area in which the basics of reliability, validity, and effectiveness of
diagnostic instruments are just now being established, there are clearly
many future fields that need plowing. This section presents some important issues in the detection of simulation that need to be addressed before
our abilities to detect feigning can be on an equal level with our other
neuropsychological diagnostic skills.

First is the question of premorbid functioning. There is a wealth of
literature regarding techniques for estimating premorbid intellectual
abilities (e.g., Barona, Reynolds, & Chastain, 1984) in order to provide an
index against which to judge the extent of neurocognitive losses. Sadly,
20 years after Wilson et al. (1978) presented their technique for estimating
premorbid intelligence, their caveat "that the use of these equations be
restricted to research applications such as the matching of neurologically-
impaired subjects along measures of estimated premorbid IQ" (p. 174)
still applies. Although researchers have undertaken many of the challenges put forth by Wilson and colleagues (1978) and advanced the status
of premorbid IQ by studying various groups of patients and different
techniques, such as implementing a current performance procedure (i.e.,
National Adult Reading Test; Nelson, 1982) and combining a current
performance measure with demographic-based information (Friedberg &
Gouvier, 1996), much further work needs to be accomplished. Until the
issue of accurately estimating premorbid abilities is adequately addressed,
our ability to identify simulation will be limited.

The intrinsic unreliability of symptom self-report is well known. Nonetheless, that unreliability is a topic worthy of study in its own right, and
if demonstrated to be consistent may allow for data correction strategies
that permit accurate appraisal of self-report data. For example, Hilsabeck,
Gouvier, and Bolter (1997) found self-report of neuropsychological symptoms is influenced by current perceptions of change in physical and
emotional status. More specifically, pre- and postinjury symptom ratings
were generated by participants who had experienced high or low levels
of significant life stress not involving significant physical injury and
participants who had suffered a closed head injury or back injury. Back-
injured participants reported current symptom reports on par with the

uninjured groups, but markedly deflated preinjury symptom reports, reflecting their perceptions of having gone from "being wonderful" to being "just ok." Clearly, physical injury to the body is a factor that contributes to a rose-colored bias in retrospective self-report. Even more telling are the data from the head-injured group, whose physical injuries to their bodies directly affected their organs of adaptation (i.e., their brains). These participants showed preinjury symptom ratings that were "just lovely," like their back-injured counterparts, but their current symptom ratings were significantly elevated above and beyond those of the other three groups, reflecting their perceptions that things had gone from "extra lovely" to "just awful," and that their current lots in life were even more unhappy than that of their back-injured counterparts. It should be noted that none of these head-injured participants was involved in litigation or had any chance of financial or tangible secondary gain to encourage their illness behaviors.

These findings are in direct contrast to and contradict the conclusions of Lees-Haley, Williams, and English (1996), who reported a comparison of litigating (i.e., primarily closed head injury participants) and nonlitigating (and not closed head injury patients) participants who had not been subjected to physical injury but instead were seeking routine "treatment for a wide range of common ailments and persons scheduled for annual physicals" (p. 813). Lees-Haley and colleagues concluded that memory bias of the sort that Hilsabeck, Gouvier, and Bolter (1997) identified in their head-injured and back-injured group was due to the variable of litigation, but the influence of the key variable in the Hilsabeck et al. study, the impact of organic/physical injury versus mere psychosocial distress, was not systematically controlled.

The preceding paragraph exemplifies how under some circumstances, it is "normal" to report a perfectly rosy path in the face of present difficulties, whereas in other similar circumstances, challenges faced in the past and present are not perceived to be much different from each other. This forces the question, just what does it mean to be normal? Reitan and Wolfson (1994) observed that neuropsychologists continually struggle with what "normal" is. Paradoxically, if we could get 100% accurate in identifying normal individuals, we would never wrongly label an honest individual again. True, some malingerers would slip through (Type II errors), but this occurs already. Duncan and Snow (1987) observed that "thirty years after Meehl and Rosen (1955, p. 194) demonstrated the importance of base rates, we can reaffirm their statement that 'base rates are virtually never reported' " (p. 369). This statement is just as true today as it was then, and "our ignorance of base rates is nothing more subtle than our failure to compute them" (Meehl & Rosen, 1955, p. 213). Redoubled efforts to define normalcy would go a long way toward returning psychologists to the moral high ground in this thorny area of simulation detection and diagnosis.

The question of normalcy must be answered on three fronts. In terms of symptom self-report, obviously in some circumstances it is normal to complain, and in others, it is not. Clearer elucidation of the environmental, encephalic, and interoceptive variables that determine these responses are called for. The second front is in terms of the "normalcy" of test performance. Authors have suggested that certain patterns of score discrepancies might reflect simulation. For example, Mittenberg et al. (1995) offered WAIS–R Vocabulary minus Digit Span as one potentially sensitive indicator. It should be noted, however, that these WAIS–R subtests load on separate factors, and thus may largely represent independent functions. Perhaps a more theory-driven approach would involve looking for anomalous patterns of score discrepancies within factors, rather than across factors.

Nonetheless, for simulation detectors to win the battle on this psychometric front, some suggest it will be necessary to compile voluminous demographically corrected tables describing the significance of score discrepancies on a myriad of tests and standard psychological batteries.

Rogers, Bagby, and Dickens (1992) provided a model for the evaluation of simulation in a psychiatric population. Their Structured Interview of Reported Symptoms (SIRS) has several subdomains whose raw scores are transferred into simulation classification categories (i.e., definite malingering, probable malingering, indeterminate malingering, and honest). In their manual, Rogers et al. provided classification accuracy data based on certain profiles of scores (e.g., 100% chance the individual is a malingerer, one definite; 100% chance the individual is a malingerer, four probable). Ultimately, a SIRS-type algorithm will need to be developed, relating the probability of simulation to the proportion of pathognomic or questionable signs drawn from comparisons with these tables. In real life, this is a heroic undertaking, but unlikely to ever occur as tables will need to provide adjustments for all known contributors to brain function variance (e.g., childhood developmental history, substance use, medical history, participation in sports, traumatic events) and even then won't be able to account for the residual individual variation. A more economical approach would entail developing norms for specific populations to aid in the determination of normal versus impaired performances. For example, Airy-Eggertsen, Selby, and Laver (1996) compared mean scores of 39 neuropsychological measures in criminal and noncriminal populations. The criminal sample scored significantly lower on 32 of the 39 measures, suggesting the need to expand norms to avoid misclassification in a criminal population.

Third, and most promising, are efforts to use electrophysiological measures for the identification of normalcy. Although initial results are no more promising than currently available strategies, it is expected that with further refinement and development, procedures such as evoked potential analysis, qualitative electroencephalograph (EEG), and functional neuroimaging may hold promise in the reliable identification of normal brain functioning and therefore simulation (Rosenfeld, Sweet, Chuang, Ellwanger, & Song, 1996).

As stated previously, using multiple measures for simulation detection is necessary, for no one test will consistently cut it. Current approaches that rely on the inclusion of a single, easily coached and rather self-evident forced-choice measure may allow for the occasional identification of an obvious simulator, but one can only wonder how many simulators slip by undetected. Further compounding this problem is the danger that a Type I error on this single test may result in an honest individual being punished as a liar and a fraud. Almost 40 years ago, Campbell and Fiske (1959) recognized the foolishness of such practice, and we have warmly embraced their multitrait, multimethod guidelines when assessing for psychopathology. Why should we hold our standards for the assessment of simulation any lower? It is incumbent on neuropsychologists to take charge and lay out a multitrait, multimethod protocol for identifying simulated neuropsychological deficits.

Every year, if not every day, we have to wage our salvation upon some prophesy based upon imperfect knowledge.

—Oliver Wendell Holmes

REFERENCES

Airy-Eggertsen, A. S., Selby, M. A., & Laver, G. D. (1996, October). *Comparison of neuropsychological performance in forensic and non-forensic populations*. Paper presented at the annual meeting of the National Academy of Neuropsychology, New Orleans, LA.

American Psychiatric Association. (1994). *Diagnostic and statistical manual of mental disorders* (4th ed.). Washington, DC: Author.

Arnett, P. A., Hammeke, T. A., & Schwartz, L. (1995). Quantitative and qualitative performance on Rey's 15-Item Test in neurological patients and dissimulators. *Clinical Neuropsychologist, 9*(1), 17–26.

Austin, J. S. (1992). The detection of fake good and fake bad on the MMPI-2. *Educational and Psychological Measurement, 52*(3), 669–674.

Bagby, R., Buis, T., & Nicholson, R. A. (1995). Relative effectiveness of the standard validity scales in detecting fake-bad and fake-good responding: Replication and extension. *Psychological Assessment, 7*(1), 84–92.

Bagby, R. M., Rogers, R., & Buis, T. (1994). Detecting malingered and defensive responding on the MMPI-2 in a forensic inpatient sample. *Journal of Personality Assessment, 62*(2), 191–203.

Baker, G. A., Hanley, J. R., Jackson, H. F., Kimmance, S., & Slade, P. (1993). Detecting the faking of amnesia: Performance differences between simulators and patients with memory impairment. *Journal of Clinical and Experimental Neuropsychology, 15*(5), 668–684.

Bar-Hillel, M. (1980). The base-rate fallacy in probability judgments. *Acta Psychologica, 44,* 211–233.

Barona, A., Reynolds, C. R., & Chastain, R. (1984). A demographically based index of premorbid intelligence for the WAIS–R. *Journal of Consulting and Clinical Psychology, 52,* 885–887.

Bash, I., & Alpert, M. (1980). The determination of malingering. *Annals of the New York Academy of Sciences, 347,* 36–99.

Beetar, J. T., & Williams, J. M. (1995). Malingering response styles on the Memory Assessment Scales and symptom validity tests. *Archives of Clinical Neuropsychology, 10*(1), 57-72.

Benton, A., & Spreen, O. (1961). Visual memory test: The simulation of mental competence. *Archives of General Psychiatry, 4,* 79–83.

Bernard, L. C. (1990). Prospects for faking believable memory deficits on neuropsychological tests and the use of incentives in simulation research. *Journal of Clinical and Experimental Neuropsychology, 12*(5), 715–728.

Bernard, L. C., & Fowler, W. (1990). Assessing the validity of memory complaints: Performance of brain-damaged and normal individuals on Rey's task to detect malingering. *Journal of Clinical Psychology, 46,* 432–436.

Bernard, L. C., Houston, W., & Natoli, L. (1993). Malingering on neuropsychological memory tests: Potential objective indicators. *Journal of Clinical Psychology, 49*(1), 45–53.

Bernard, L. C., McGrath, M. J., & Houston, W. (1996). The differential effects of simulating malingering, closed head injury, and other CNS pathology on the Wisconsin Card Sorting Test: Support for the "pattern of performance" hypothesis. *Archives of Clinical Neuropsychology, 11*(3), 231–245.

Berry, D. T. R., Baer, R. A., & Harris, M. J. (1991). Detection of malingering on the MMPI: A meta-analysis. *Clinical Psychology Review, 11,* 585–598.

Berry, D. T. R., Wetter, M. W., Baer, R. A., Larsen, L., Clark, C., & Monroe, K. (1992). MMPI-2 random responding indices: Validation using a self-report methodology. *Psychological Assessment, 4*(3), 340–345.

Berry, D. T. W., Wetter, M. W., Baer, R. A., Widiger, T. A., Sumpter, J. C., Reynolds, S. K., & Hallam, R. A. (1991). Detection of random responding on the MMPI-2: Utility of F, Back F, and VRIN scales. *Psychological Assessment: A Journal of Consulting and Clinical Psychology, 3*(3), 418–423.

Berry, D. T. R., Wetter, M. W., Baer, R. A., Youngjohn, J. R., Gass, C. S., Lamb, D. G., Franzen, M. D., MacInnes, W. D., & Buchholz, D. (1995). Overreporting of closed-head injury symptoms on the MMPI-2. *Psychological Assessment, 7*(4), 517–523.

Bickart, W. T., Mayer, R. G., & Connell, D. K. (1991). The symptom validity technique as a measure of feigned short-term memory deficit. *American Journal of Forensic Psychology, 2,* 3–11.

Binder, L. M. (1990). Malingering following minor head trauma. *Clinical Neuropsychologist, 4*(1), 25–36.

Binder, L. M. (1992). Malingering detected by forced choice testing of memory and tactile sensation: A case report. *Archives of Clinical Neuropsychology, 7,* 155-163.

Binder, L. M. (1993a). An abbreviated form of the Portland Digit Recognition Test. *Clinical Neuropsychologist, 7*(1), 104–107.

Binder, L. M. (1993b). Assessment of malingering after mild head trauma with the Portland Digit Recognition Test. *Journal of Clinical and Experimental Neuropsychology, 15*(2), 170–182.

Binder, L. M. (1993c). Assessment of malingering after mild head trauma with the Portland Digit Recognition Test: Erratum. *Journal of Clinical and Experimental Neuropsychology, 15,* 852.

Binder, L. M., & Pankratz, L. (1987). Neuropsychological evidence of a factitious memory complaint. *Journal of Clinical and Experimental Neuropsychology, 9*(2), 161–171.

Binder, L. M., Villaneuva, M. R., Howieson, D., & Moore, R. T. (1993). The Rey AVLT recognition task measures motivational impairment after mild head trauma. *Archives of Clinical Neuropsychology, 8*, 137–147.

Binder, L. M., & Willis, S. C. (1991). Assessment of motivation after financially compensable minor head trauma. *Psychological Assessment: A Journal of Consulting and Clinical Psychology, 3*(2), 175–181.

Binks, P. G., Gouvier, W. D., & Waters, W. F. (1997). Malingering detection with the Dot Counting Test. *Archives of Clinical Neuropsychology, 12*(1), 41–46.

Brady, J. P., & Lind, D. L. (1961). Experimental analysis of hysterical blindness. *Archives of General Psychiatry, 4*, 331–339.

Brandt, J., Rubinsky, E., & Lassen, G. (1985). Uncovering malingered amnesia. *Annals of the New York Academy of Sciences, 44*, 502–503.

Brown, L., Sherbenou, R. J., & Johnsen, S. K. (1982). *Test of nonverbal intelligence: A language-free measure of cognitive ability.* Austin, TX: Pro-Ed.

Brophy, A. L. (1995). Gough's F-K Dissimulation Index on the MMPI-2. *Psychological Reports, 76*, 158.

Bruhn, A. R., & Reed, M. R. (1975). Simulation of brain damage on the Bender–Gestalt test by college subjects. *Journal of Personality Assessment, 39*, 244–255.

Butcher, J., Dahlstrom, W., Graham, J., Tellegen, A., & Kaemmer, B. (1989). *Minnesota Multiphasic Personality Inventory-2 (MMPI-2): Manual for administration and scoring.* Minneapolis, MN: University of Minnesota Press.

Campbell, D., & Fiske, D. (1959). Convergent and discriminant validation by the multi-trait–multi-method matrix. *Psychological Bulletin, 54*, 81–105.

Cassisi, J. E., & Workman, D. E. (1992). The detection of malingering and deception with a short form of the MMPI-2 based on the L, F, and K Scales. *Journal of Clinical Psychology, 48*(1), 54–58.

Cermack, L., Talbot, N., Chandler, K., & Wolbarst, L. (1985). The perceptual priming phenomenon in amnesia. *Neuropsychologia, 23*(5), 615–622.

Cernovsky, Z. Z. (1989). Another case of pseudonormal MMPI Validity (F) Scale Score. *Psychological Reports, 65*, 450.

Davidson, H., Suffield B., Orenczuk, S., Nantau, K., & Mandel, A. (1991, February). *Screening for malingering using the Memory for Fifteen Items Test (MFIT).* Poster presented at the International Neuropsychological Society, Nineteenth Annual Meeting, San Antonio, TX.

Davis, H. P., King, J. H., Bloodworth, M. R., Spring, A., & Klebe, K. J. (1997). The detection of simulated malingering using a computerized category classification test. *Archives of Clinical Neuropsychology, 12*(3), 191–198.

Davis, H. P., King, J. H., Klebe, K. J., Bajszar, G., Jr., Bloodworth, M. R., & Wallick, S. L. (1997). The detection of simulated malingering using a computerized priming test. *Archives of Clinical Neuropsychology, 12*(2), 145–153.

Delis, D. C., Kramer, J. H., Kaplan, E., & Ober, B. A. (1987). *California Verbal Learning Test: Adult version.* San Antonio, TX: Psychological Corporation.

DiCarlo, M. A., Gfeller, J. D., & Drury, J. A. (1996, October). *Assessing feigned cognitive impairment with Rey's 14-Item Memory Test: Is this task easy or what?* Poster presented at the Annual Meeting of the National Academy of Neuropsychology, New Orleans, LA.

DuAlba, L., & Scott, R. L. (1993). Somatization and malingering for workers' compensation applicants: A cross-cultural MMPI study. *Journal of Clinical Psychology, 49*(6), 913–917.

Duncan, D., & Snow, W. (1987). Base rates in neuropsychology. *Profession Psychology: Research and Practice, 18*(4), 368–370.

Faust, D., & Nurcombe, B. (1989). Improving the accuracy of clinical judgement. *Psychiatry, 52*, 197–208.

Fox, D. D., Gerson, A., & Lees-Haley, P. R. (1995). Interrelationship of MMPI–2 validity scales in personal injury claims. *Journal of Clinical Psychology, 51*(1), 42–47.

Franzen, M. D., Iverson, G. L., & McCracken, L. M. (1990). The detection of malingering in neuropsychological assessment. *Neuropsychology Review, 1*(3), 247–279.

Franzen, M. D., & Martin, N. (1996). Do people with knowledge fake better? *Applied Neuropsychology, 3,* 82–85.

Frederick, R. I., Carter, M., & Powel, J. (1995). Adapting symptom validity testing to evaluate suspicious complaints of amnesia in medicolegal evaluations. *Bulletin of the American Academy of Psychiatry and the Law, 23*(2), 231–237.

Frederick, R. I., & Foster, H. G., Jr. (1991). Multiple measures of malingering on a forced-choice test of cognitive ability. *Psychological Assessment: A Journal of Consulting and Clinical Psychology, 3*(4), 596–602.

Frederick, R. I., Sarfaty, S. D., Johnston, D., & Powel, J. (1994). Validation of a detector of response bias on a forced-choice test of nonverbal ability. *Neuropsychology, 8*(1), 118–125.

Friedberg, S. C., & Gouvier, W. D. (1996). Estimation of premorbid intelligence: A combined demographic and psychometric approach. *Archives of Clinical Neuropsychology, 11,* 5. (Abstract).

Gansler, D., Tombaugh, T. N., Petterson-Moczynski, N. P., & Rees, L. M. (1995, October). *Test of memory and malingering (TOMM): Initial validation in a traumatic injury cohort.* Poster presented at the Annual Meeting of the National Academy of Neuropsychology, San Francisco, CA.

Gass, C. S. (1991). MMPI–2 interpretation and closed head injury: A correction factor. *Psychological Assessment: A Journal of Consulting and Clinical Psychology, 3*(1), 27–31.

Gass, C. S. (1992). MMPI–2 interpretation of patients with cerebrovascular disease: A correction factor. *Archives of Clinical Neuropsychology, 7,* 17–27.

Gass, C. S., Russell, E. W., & Hamilton, R. A. (1990). Accuracy of MMPI-based inferences regarding memory and concentration in closed head trauma patients. *Psychological Assessment, 2,* 175–178.

Gfeller, J. D., Cradock, M. M., & Falkenhain, M. A. (1994, November). *Detecting feigned neuropsychological impairment with the Seashore Rhythm Test.* Poster presented at the Annual Conference of the National Academy of Neuropsychology, Orlando, FL.

Gillis, J. R., Rogers, R., & Dickens, S. E. (1990). The detection of faking bad response styles on the MMPI. *Canadian Journal of Behavioural Science, 22*(4), 408–416.

Goebel, R. A. (1983). Detection of faking on the Halstead–Reitan Neuropsychological Test Battery. *Journal of Clinical Psychology, 39*(5), 731–742.

Goldberg, J. O., & Miller, H. R. (1986). Performance of psychiatric inpatients and intellectually deficient individuals on a task that assesses the validity of memory complaints. *Journal of Clinical Psychology, 42,* 792–795.

Goldstein, H. (1945). A malingering key for mental tests. *Psychological Bulletin, 42,* 104–118.

Gouvier, W. D., Hayes, J. S., & Smiroldo, B. B. (1998). The significance of base rates, test sensitivity, test specificity, and subjects' knowledge of symptoms in assessing TBI sequelae and malingering. In C. Reynolds (Ed.), *Detection of malingering in head injury litigation* (pp. 55–79). New York: Plenum Press.

Gouvier, W. D., Steiner, D. D., Jackson, W. T., Schlater, D., & Rain, J. S. (1991). Employment discrimination against handicapped job candidates: An analog study of the effects of neurological causation, visibility of handicap, and public contact. *Rehabilitation Psychology, 36,* 121–129.

Graf, P., Squire, L., & Mandler, G. (1984). The information that amnesic patients do not forget. *Journal of Experimental Psychology: Learning, Memory and Cognition, 10*(1), 164–178.

Graham, J. R., Watts, D., & Timbrook, R. E. (1991). Detecting fake-good and fake-bad MMPI–2 profiles. *Journal of Personality Assessment, 57*(2), 264–277.

Greiffenstein, M. F., Baker, W. J., & Gola, T. (1994). Validation of malingered amnesia measures with a large clinical sample. *Psychological Assessment*, 6(3), 218–224.

Greiffenstein, M. F., Baker, W. J., & Gola, T. (1996). Comparison of multiple scoring methods for Rey's Malingered Amnesia Measures. *Archives of Clinical Neuropsychology*, 11(4), 283–293.

Greiffenstin, M. F., Gola, T., & Baker, W. J. (1995). MMPI–2 validity scales versus domain specific measures in detection of factitious traumatic brain injury. *Clinical Neuropsychologist*, 9(3), 230–240.

Griffin, G. A. E., Glassmire, D. M., Henderson, E. A., & McCann, C. L. (1997). Rey II: Redesigning the Rey screening test of malingering. *Journal of Clinical Psychology*, 53(7), 757–766.

Griffin, G. A., Normington, J., & Glassmire, D. (1996). Qualitative dimensions in scoring the Rey Visual memory Test of Malingering. *Psychological Assessment*, 8(4), 383–387.

Gronwall, D. M. A., & Wrightson, P. (1974). Delayed recovery of intellectual function after minor head injury. *Lancet*, ii, 995–997.

Grossman, L. S., Haywood, T. W., Ostrov, E., Wasyliw, O., & Cavanaugh, J. L., Jr. (1990). Sensitivity of MMPI validity scales to motivational factors in psychological evaluations of police officers. *Journal of Personality Assessment*, 55(3&4), 549–561.

Grossman, L. S., Haywood, T. W., & Wasyliw, O. E. (1992). The evaluation of truthfulness in alleged sex offenders' self-reports: 16PF and MMPI validity scales. *Journal of Personality Assessment*, 59(2), 264–275.

Grossman, L. S., & Wasyliw, O. E. (1988). A psychometric study of stereotypes: Assessment of malingering in a criminal forensic group. *Journal of Personality Assessment*, 52(3), 549–563.

Gudjonsson, G. H., & Shackleton, H. (1986). The pattern of scores on Raven's Matrices during "faking bad" and "non faking" performance. *British Journal of Clinical Psychology*, 25, 35–41.

Guilmette, T. J., Hart, K. J., & Giuliano, A. J. (1993). Malingering detection: The use of a forced-choice method in identifying organic versus simulated memory impairment. *Clinical Neuropsychologist*, 7(1), 59–69.

Guilmette, T. J., Hart, K. J., Giuliano, A. J., & Leininger, B. E. (1994). Detecting simulated memory impairment: Comparison of the Rey Fifteen-Item Test and the Hiscock Forced-Choice Procedure. *Clinical Neuropsychologist*, 8(3), 283–294.

Guilmette, T. J., Sparadeo, F. R., Whelihan, W., & Buongiorno, G. (1994). Validity of neuropsychological test results in disability evaluations. *Perceptual and Motor Skills*, 78, 1179–1186.

Haines, M. E., & Norris, M. P. (1995). Detecting the malingering of cognitive deficits: An update. *Neuropsychology Review*, 5(2), 125–148.

Hall, H. V., & Pritchard, D. A. (1996). *Detecting malingering and deception*. Delray Beach, FL: St. Lucie Press.

Harvey, M., & Sipprelle, C. (1976). Demand characteristic effects on the subtle and obvious scales of the MMPI. *Journal of Personality Assessment*, 40, 539–544.

Hawk, G. L., & Cornell, D. G. (1989). MMPI profiles of malingerers diagnosed in pretrial forensic evaluations. *Journal of Clinical Psychology*, 45(4), 673–678.

Hayes, J. S., Hilsabeck, R. C., Bentz, B. B., Diefenbach, G., Powers, D. A., Smiroldo, B. B., & Witt, J. (1998). The Assessment of Dissimulation Scale (ADS): A new test to detect "faking good" (abstr.). *Archives of Clinical Neuropsychology*, 13, 27. (Abstract)

Hayes, J. S., Martin, R., & Gouvier, W. D. (1995). Influence of prior knowledge and experience on the ability to feign mild head injury symptoms in head-injured and non-head-injured college students. *Applied Neuropsychology*, 2, 63–66.

Hays, J. R., Emmons, J., & Lawson, K. A. (1993). Psychiatric norms for the Rey 15-Item Visual Memory Test. *Perceptual and Motor Skills*, 76, 1331–1334.

Hayward, L., Hall, W., Hunt, M., & Zubrick, S. R. (1987). Can localized brain impairment be simulated on neuropsychological test profiles? *Australian and New Zealand Journal of Psychiatry, 21*, 87–93.

Heaton, R. K., Smith, H. H., Jr., Lehman, R. A. W., & Vogt, A. T. (1978). Prospects for faking believable deficits on neuropsychological testing. *Journal of Consulting and Clinical Psychology, 46*(5), 892–900.

Heilbrun, K., Bennett, W. S., White, A. J., & Kelly, J. (1990). A MMPI-based empirical model of malingering and deception. *Behavioral Sciences and the Law, 8*, 45–53.

Hilsabeck, R. C., Gouvier, W. D., & Bolter, J. F. (1997). *Reconstructive memory processes in recall of neuropsychological symptomatology.* Manuscript submitted for publication.

Hilsabeck, R. C., LeCompte, D. C., Zuppardo, M. C., & Mitchell, M. M. (1997). *The Word Completion Memory Test (WCMT): A test to detect sophisticated malingerers.* Manuscript submitted for publication.

Hiscock, C. K., Branham, J. D., & Hiscock, M. (1994). Detection of feigned cognitive impairment: The two-alternative forced-choice method compared with selected conventional tests. *Journal of Psychopathology and Behavioral Assessment, 16*(2), 95–110.

Hiscock, M., & Hiscock, C. K. (1989). Refining the forced-choice method for the detection of malingering. *Journal of Clinical and Experimental Neuropsychology, 11*(6), 967–974.

Horton, K. D., Smith, S. A., Barghout, N. K., & Connolly, D. A. (1992). The use of indirect memory tests to assess malingered amnesia: A study of metamemory. *Journal of Experimental Psychology: General, 121*(3), 326–351.

Hsu, L. M., Santelli, J., & Hsu, J. R. (1989). Faking detection validity and incremental validity of response latencies to MMPI subtle and obvious items. *Journal of Personality Assessment, 53*(2), 278–295.

Hunt, W. A., & Older, H. J. (1943). Detection of malingering through psychometric tests. *Naval Medical Bulletin, 41*, 1318–1323.

Hyer, L., Fallon, J. H., Jr., Harrison, W. R., & Boudewyns, P. A. (1987). MMPI overreporting by Vietnam combat veterans. *Journal of Clinical Psychology, 43*(1), 79–83.

Iverson, G. L. (1995). Qualitative aspects of malingered memory deficits. *Brain Injury, 9*(1), 35–40.

Iverson, G. L., & Franzen, M. D. (1996). Using multiple objective memory procedures to detect simulated malingering. *Journal of Clinical and Experimental Neuropsychology, 18*(1), 38–51.

Iverson, G. L., Franzen, M. D., & Hammond, J. A. (1995). Examination of inmates' ability to malinger on the MMPI-2. *Psychological Assessment, 7*(1), 118–121.

Iverson, G. L., Franzen, M. D., & McCracken, L. M. (1994). Application of a forced-choice memory procedure designed to detect experimental malingering. *Archives of Clinical Neuropsychology, 9*(5), 437–450.

Iverson, G. L., Franzen, M. D., & McCracken, L. M. (1991). Evaluation of an objective assessment technique for the detection of malingered memory deficits. *Law and Human Behavior, 15*(6), 667–676.

Jastak, S., & Wilkinson, G. S. (1984). *Wide Range Achievement Test–Revised.* Wilmington, DE: Jastak Assessment Systems.

Java, R. (1994). States of awareness following word stem completion. *European Journal of Cognitive Psychology, 6*(1), 77–92.

King, J. H., Klebe, K. J., & Davis, H. P. (1996, October). *The effects of coaching on detecting simulators of a memory deficit on three tests of episodic memory, two tests of semantic memory, and two tests of nondeclarative memory.* Poster session presented at the annual meeting of the National Academy of Neuropsychology, New Orleans, LA.

Kraus, J. F., & Sorenson, S. B. (1994). Epidemiology. In J. M. Silver, S. C. Yudofsky, & R. E. Hales (Eds.), *Neuropsychiatry of traumatic brain injury* (pp. 3–41). Washington, DC: American Psychiatric Press.

Lamb, D. G., Berry, D. T. R., Wetter, M. W., & Baer, R. A. (1994). Effects of two types of information on malingering of closed head injury on the MMPI–2: An analog investigation. *Psychological Assessment, 6*(1), 8–13.

Language Research Association. (1958). *The Auditory Discrimination Test*. Chicago: Author.

Larrabee, G. J. (in press). On modifying recognition memory tests for detection of malingering. *Neuropsychology*.

Lee, G. P., Loring, D. W., & Martin, R. C. (1992). Rey's 15-Item Memory Test for the detection of malingering: Normative observations on patients with neurological disorders. *Psychological Assessment, 4*(1), 43–46.

Lees-Haley, P. R. (1991). Ego strength denial on the MMPI–2 as a clue to simulation of personal injury in vocational neuropsychological and emotional distress evaluations. *Perceptual and Motor Skills, 72*, 815–819.

Lees-Haley, P. R. (1992). Efficacy of MMPI–2 validity scales and MCMI–II modifier scales for detecting spurious PTSD claims: F, F–K, Fake Bad Scale, Ego Strength, Subtle-Obvious subscales, DIS, and DEB. *Journal of Clinical Psychology, 48*(5), 681–689.

Lees-Haley, P. R., & Fox, D. D. (1990). MMPI Subtle-Obvious Scales and malingering: Clinical versus simulated scores. *Psychological Reports, 66*, 907–911.

Lees-Haley, P. R., Smith, H. H., Williams, C. W., & Dunn, J. T. (1996). Forensic neuropsychological test usage: An empirical survey. *Archives of Clinical Neuropsychology, 11*, 45–51.

Lees-Haley, P. R., Williams, C. W., & English, L. T. (1996). Response bias in self-reported history of plaintiffs compared with nonlitigating patients. *Psychological Reports, 79*, 811–818.

Lezak, M. (1983). *Neuropsychological assessment* (2nd ed.). New York: Oxford University Press.

Lezak, M. (1995). *Neuropsychological assessment* (3rd ed.). New York: Oxford University Press.

Lynch, W. (1994). Software update. *Journal of Head Trauma Rehabilitation, 9*(2), 104–108.

Martin, R. C., Bolter, J. F., Todd, M. E., Gouvier, W. D., & Niccolls, R. (1993). Effects of sophistication and motivation on the detection of malingered memory performance using a computerized forced-choice task. *Journal of Clinical and Experimental Neuropsychology, 15*(6), 867–880.

Martin, R. C., Gouvier, W. D., Todd, M. E., Bolter, J. F., & Niccolls, R. (1992). Effects of task instruction on malingered memory performance. *Forensic Reports, 5*(4), 393–397.

Martin, R. C., Hayes, J. S., & Gouvier, W. D. (1996). Differential vulnerability between postconcussion self-report and objective malingering tests in identifying simulated mild head injury. *Journal of Clinical and Experimental Neuropsychology, 18*(2), 265–275.

Meehl, P., & Rosen, A. (1955). Antecedent probability and the efficiency of psychometric signs, patterns, or cutting scores. *Psychological Bulletin, 52*, 194–216.

Mensch, A. J., & Woods, D. J. (1986). Patterns of feigning brain damage on the LNNB. *International Journal of Clinical Neuropsychology, 8*(2), 59–63.

Milanovich, J. R., Axelrod, B. N., & Millis, S. R. (1996). Validation of the Simulation Index–Revised with a mixed clinical population. *Archives of Clinical Neuropsychology, 11*(1), 53–59.

Millis, S. R. (1992). The Recognition Memory Test in the detection of malingered and exaggerated memory deficits. *Clinical Neuropsychologist, 6*, 406–414.

Millis, S. R., & Kier, S. (1995). Limitations of the Rey Fifteen-Item Test in the detection of malingering. *Clinical Neuropsychologist, 9*(3), 241–244.

Millis, S. R., & Putnam, S. H. (1994). The Recognition Memory Test in the assessment of memory impairment after financially compensable mild head injury: A replication. *Perceptual and Motor Skills, 79*, 384–386.

Millis, S. R., Putnam, S. H., Adams, K. M., & Ricker, J. H. (1995). The California Verbal Learning Test in the detection of incomplete effort in neuropsychological evaluation. *Psychological Assessment, 7*(4), 463–471.

Mittenberg, W., Azrin, R., Millsaps, C., & Heilbronner, R. (1993). Identification of malingered head injury on the Wechsler Memory Scale–Revised. *Psychological Assessment, 5*(1), 34–40.

Mittenberg, W., Rothoic, A., Russell, E., & Heilbronner, R. (1996). Identification of malingered head injury on the Halstead–Reitan Battery. *Archives of Clinical Neuropsychology, 11*(4), 271–281.

Mittenberg, W., Theroux-Fichera, S., Zielinski, R. E., & Heilbronner, R. L. (1995). Identification of malingered head injury on the Wechsler Adult Intelligence Scale–Revised. *Professional Psychology: Research and Practice, 26*(5), 491–498.

Mittenberg, W., Tremont, G., & Rayls, K. R. (1996). Impact of cognitive function on MMPI-2 validity in neurologically impaired patients. *Assessment, 3*(2), 157–163.

Nelson, H. E. (1982). *National Adult Reading Test (NART): Test manual.* Windsor, UK: NFER Nelson.

Niccolls, R., & Bolter, J. F. (1991). *Multi-Digit Memory Test.* San Luis Obispo, CA: Wang Neuropsychological Laboratories.

Palmer, B. W., Boone, K. B., Allman, L., & Castro, D. B. (1995). Co-occurrence of brain lesions and cognitive deficit exaggeration. *Clinical Neuropsychologist, 9*(1), 68–73.

Pankratz, L. (1979). Symptom validity testing and symptom retraining: Procedures for the assessment and treatment of functional sensory deficits. *Journal of Consulting and Clinical Psychology, 47,* 409–410.

Pankratz, L. (1983). A new technique for the assessment and modification of feigned memory deficit. *Perceptual and Motor Skills, 57,* 367–372.

Pankratz, L., Fausti, S. A., & Peed, S. (1975). A forced-choice technique to evaluate deafness in the hysterical or malingering patient. *Journal of Consulting and Clinical Psychology, 43,* 421–422.

Paolo, A. M., & Ryan, J. J. (1992). Detection of random response sets on the MMPI-2. *Psychotherapy in Private Practice, 11*(4), 1–8.

Paul, D. S., Franzen, M. D., Cohen, S. H., & Fremouw, W. (1992). An investigation into the reliability and validity of two tests used in the detection of dissimulation. *International Journal of Clinical Neuropsychology, 14,* 1–9.

Peck, E. A., Mitchell, S. A., Baber, C., & Blumberg, J. (1996, October). *The use of the Portland Digit Recognition Test in the medicolegal assessment of head injury patients.* Paper presented at the annual meeting of the National Academy of Neuropsychology, New Orleans, LA.

Pensa, R., Dorfman, W. I., Gold, S. N., & Schneider, B. (1996). Detection of malingered psychosis with the MMPI-2. *Psychotherapy in Private Practice, 14*(4), 47–63.

Perconte, S. T., & Goreczny, A. J. (1990). Failure to detect fabricated posttraumatic stress disorder with the use of the MMPI in clinical population. *American Journal of Psychiatry, 147*(8), 1057–1060.

Pollaczek, P. P. (1952). A study of malingering on the CUS abbreviated intelligence scale. *Journal of Consulting Psychology, 8,* 77–81.

Pope, K., Butcher, J., & Seelen, J. (1993). *The MMPI, MMPI-2 and MMPI-A in court: A practical guide for expert witnesses and attorneys.* Washington, DC: American Psychological Association.

Price, J. R. (1995, November). *Identification of malingering and symptom exaggeration.* Workshop presented at the fifteenth annual conference of the National Academy of Neuropsychology, San Francisco, CA.

Prigatano, G. P., & Amin, K. (1993). Digit Memory Test: Unequivocal cerebral dysfunction and suspected malingering. *Journal of Clinical and Experimental Neuropsychology, 15*(4), 537–546.

Raven, J. C. (1960). *Guide to the Standard Progressive Matrices.* London: H. K. Lewis.

Raven, J. C., Court, J. H., & Raven, J. (1976). *Revised manual for Raven's Progressive Matrices.* London: H. K. Lewis.

Rawling, P. J. (1992). The simulation index: A reliability study. *Brain Injury, 6*(4), 381–383.

Rawling, P. J. (1993). *Simulation Index–Revised manual*. Balgowiah, Australia: Rawling & Associates.

Rawling, P. J., & Brooks, D. N. (1990). Simulation Index: A method for detecting factitious errors on the WAIS–R and WMS. *Neuropsychology, 4*, 223–228.

Rawling, P. J., & Coffey, G. L. (1994). The Simulation Index: A single case study. *Australian Psychologist, 29*(1), 38–40.

Rees, L. M. (1996). *A test of memory malingering: A simulation study and clinical validation*. Unpublished PhD dissertation, Carleton University, Ottawa, Ontario.

Rees, L. M., & Tombaugh, T. N. (1996, October). *Validation of the Test of Memory Malingering (TOMM) using a simulation paradigm*. Poster presented at the Annual Meeting of the International Neuropsychological Society, Chicago.

Reitan, R. M., & Wolfson, D. (1993). *The Halstead–Reitan Neuropsychological Test Battery: Theory and clinical interpretation* (2nd ed.). Tucson, AZ: Neuropsychology Press.

Reitan, R. M., & Wolfson, D. (1994, November). *Practical approaches to puzzling problems in neuropsychology using the Halstead–Reitan Battery*. Workshop presented at the 14th annual meeting of the National Academy of Neuropsychology, Orlando, FL.

Reitan, R. M., & Wolfson, D. (1996). The question of validity of neuropsychological test scores among head-injured litigants: Development of a Dissimulation Index. *Archives of Clinical Neuropsychology, 11*(7), 573–580.

Reitan, R. M., & Wolfson, D. (1997). Consistency of neuropsychological test scores of head-injured subjects involved in litigation compared with head-injured subjects not involved in litigation: Development of the Retest Consistency Index. *Clinical Neuropsychologist, 11*(1), 69–76.

Rey, A. (1941). L'Examen psychologie dans les cas d'encepalopathie traumatique. [Psychological examination of cases of brain damage]. *Archives de Psychologie, 28*(112), 286–340.

Rey, A. (1964). *L'Examen clinique en psychologie*. [The clinical examination in psychology]. Paris: Presses Universitaires de France.

Roediger, H. (1990). Implicit memory: Retention without remembering. *American Psychologist, 45*(9), 1043–1056.

Roediger, H., III, & Blaxton, T. (1987). Effects of varying modality, surface features, and retention interval on priming in word-fragment completion. *Memory & Cognition, 15*(5), 379–388.

Rogers, R. (1988). *Clinical assessment of malingering and deception*. New York: Guilford Press.

Rogers, R. (1990). Models of feigned mental illness. *Professional Psychology: Research and Practice, 21*, 182–188.

Rogers, R., Bagby, R. M., & Chakraborty, D. (1993). Feigning schizophrenic disorders on the MMPI–2: Detection of coached simulators. *Journal of Personality Assessment, 60*(2), 215–226.

Rogers, R., Bagby, R. M., & Dickens, S. E. (1992). *Structured interview of reported symptoms (SIRS) and professional manual*. Odessa, FL: Psychological Assessment Resources, Inc.

Rogers, R., Harrell, E. H., & Liff, C. D. (1993). Feigning neuropsychological impairment: A critical review of methodological and clinical considerations. *Clinical Psychology Review, 13*, 255–274.

Rogers, R., Sewell, K. W., & Goldstein, A. M. (1994). Explanatory models of malingering: A prototypical analysis. *Law and Human Behavior, 18*(5), 543–552.

Rogers, R., Sewell, K. W., & Salekin, R. T. (1994). A meta-analysis of malingering on the MMPI–2. *Psychological Assessment, 1*(3), 227–237.

Roman, D. D., Tuley, M. R., Villaneuva, M. R., & Mitchell, W. E. (1990). Evaluating MMPI validity in a forensic psychiatric population: Distinguishing between malingering and genuine psychopathology. *Criminal Justice and Behavior, 17*(2), 186–198.

Rose, F. E., Hall, S., & Szalda-Petree, A. D. (1995). Portland Digit Recognition Test–Computerized: Measuring response latency improves the detection of malingering. *Clinical Neuropsychologist, 9*(2), 124–134.

Rosenfeld, J. P., Sweet, J. J., Chuang, J., Ellwanger, J., & Song, L. (1996). Detection of simulated malingering using forced choice recognition enhanced with event-related potential recording. *Clinical Neuropsychologist, 10*(2), 163–179.

Schacter, D. L. (1986). Feeling-of-knowing ratings distinguish between genuine and simulated forgetting. *Journal of Experimental Psychology: Learning, Memory, and Cognition, 12*, 30–41.

Schacter, D. L. (1987). Implicit memory: History and current status. *Journal of Experimental Psychology: Learning, Memory and Cognition, 13*(3), 501–518.

Schretlen, D., Brandt, J., Krafft, L., & Van Gorp, W. (1991). Some caveats in using the Rey 15-Item Memory Test to detect malingered amnesia. *Psychological Assessment: A Journal of Consulting and Clinical Psychology, 3*(4), 667–672.

Searleman, A., & Herrmann, D. (1994). *Memory from a broader perspective.* New York: McGraw-Hill.

Shiamamura, A. (1986). Priming effects in amnesia: Evidence for a dissociable memory function. *Quarterly Journal of Experimental Psychology, 38A*, 619–644.

Sivan, A. B. (1992). *Benton Visual Retention Test* (5th ed.). San Antonio, TX: Psychological Corporation.

Slick, D., Hopp, G., Strauss, E., Hunter, M., & Pinch, D. (1994). Detecting dissimulation: Profiles of simulated malingerers, traumatic brain-injury patients, and normal controls on a revised version of Hiscock and Hiscock's Forced Choice Memory Test. *Journal of Clinical and Experimental Neuropsychology, 16*(3), 472–481.

Slick, D. J., Hopp, G., Strauss, E., & Spellacy, F. J. (1996). Victoria Symptom Validity Test: Efficiency for detecting feigned memory impairment and relationship to neuropsychological tests and MMPI-2 Validity Scales. *Journal of Clinical and Experimental Neuropsychology, 18*(6), 911–922.

Smith, D. W., & Frueh, B. C. (1996). Compensation seeking, comorbidity, and apparent exaggeration of PTSD symptoms among Vietnam combat veterans. *Psychological Assessment, 8*(1), 3–6.

Strauss, E., Spellacy, F., Hunter, M., & Berry, T. (1994). Assessing believable deficits on measures of attention and information processing capacity. *Archives of Clinical Neuropsychology, 9*, 483–490.

Taylor, J. S., Harp, J. H., & Elliott, T. (1992). Preparing the plaintiff in the mild brain injury case. *Trial Diplomacy Journal, 15*, 65–72.

Tenhula, W. N., & Sweet, J. J. (1996). Double cross-validation of the Booklet Category Test in detecting malingered traumatic brain injury. *Clinical Neuropsychologist, 10*(1), 104–116.

Timbrook, R. E., Graham, J. R., Keiller, S. W., & Watts, D. (1993). Comparison of the Wiener–Harmon Subtle–Obvious Scales and the standard validity scales in detecting valid and invalid MMPI-2 profiles. *Psychological Assessment, 5*(1), 53–61.

Tombaugh, T. N., White, R. F., Cyrus, P., Krengle, M., Rose, F. E., & Fernandes, L. (1996, October). *Validation of the Test for Memory Malingering (TOMM) with cognitively intact and neurological impaired subjects.* Poster presented at the 16th Annual Meeting of the National Academy of Neuropsychology, New Orleans, LA.

Trahan, D. E., & Larrabee, G. J. (1988). *Continuous Visual Memory Test.* Odessa, FL: Psychological Assessment Resources.

Trueblood, W. (1994). Qualitative and quantitative characteristics of malingered and other invalid WAIS–R and clinical memory data. *Journal of Clinical and Experimental Neuropsychology, 16*(4), 597–607.

Trueblood, W., & Schmidt, M. (1993). Malingering and other validity considerations in the neuropsychological evaluation of mild head injury. *Journal of Clinical and Experimental Neuropsychology, 15*(4), 578–590.

Tulving, E., & Schacter, D. (1990). Priming and human memory systems. *Science, 247*, 301–306.

Viglione, D. J., Jr., Fals-Stewart, W., & Moxham, E. (1995). Maximizing internal and external validity in MMPI malingering research: A study of a military population. *Journal of Personality Assessment, 65*(3), 502–513.

Walters, G. D. (1988). Assessing dissimulation and denial on the MMPI in a sample of maximum security, male inmates. *Journal of Personality Assessment, 52*(3), 465–474.

Walters, G. D., White, T. W., & Greene, R. L. (1988). Use of the MMPI to identify malingering and exaggeration of psychiatric symptomatology in male prison inmates. *Journal of Consulting and Clinical Psychology, 56*(1), 111–117.

Warrington, E. K. (1984). *Recognition Memory Test: Manual.* Berkshire: UK: NFER-Nelson.

Wasyliw, O. E., Grossman, L. S., Haywood, T. W., & Cavanaugh, J., Jr. (1988). The detection of malingering in criminal forensic groups: MMPI validity scales. *Journal of Personality Assessment, 52*(2), 321–333.

Wechsler, D. (1945). A standardized memory scale for clinical use. *Journal of Psychology, 19,* 87–95.

Wechsler, D. (1974). *Wechsler Memory Scale manual.* San Antonio, TX: Psychological Corporation.

Wechsler, D. (1981). *The Wechsler Adult Intelligence Scale–Revised manual.* New York: Psychological Corporation.

Wechsler, D. (1987). *Wechsler Memory Scale–Revised manual.* San Antonio, TX: Psychological Corporation.

Weed, N. C., Ben-Porath, Y. S., & Butcher, J. N. (1990). Failure of Wiener and Harmon Minnesota Multiphasic Personality Inventory (MMPI) Subtle scales as personality descriptors and as validity indicators. *Psychological Assessment: A Journal of Consulting and Clinical Psychology, 2*(3), 281–285.

West, M. A., & Knowles, D. (1991). Estimating cost of care and economic loss of brain injury. In H. O. Doerr & A. S. Carlin (Eds.), *Forensic neuropsychology: Legal and scientific bases* (pp. 214–227). New York: Guilford Press.

Wetter, M. W., Baer, R. A., Berry, D. T. R., Smith, G. T., & Larsen, L. H. (1992). Sensitivity of MMPI-2 validity scales to random responding and malingering. *Psychological Assessment, 4*(3), 369–374.

Wetter, M. W., & Corrigan, S. K. (1995). Providing information to clients about psychological tests: A survey of attorneys' and law students' attitudes. *Professional Psychology: Research and Practice, 26*(5), 474–477.

Wetter, M. W., & Deitsch, S. E. (1996). Faking specific disorders and temporal response consistency on the MMPI-2. *Psychological Assessment, 8*(1), 39–47.

Wetzler, S., & Marlowe, D. (1990). "Faking bad" on the MMPI, MMPI-2, and Millon–II. *Psychological Reports, 67,* 1117–1118.

Wiggins, E. C., & Brandt, J. (1988). The detection of simulated amnesia. *Law and Human Behavior, 12*(1), 57–78.

Williams, J. M. (1991). *Memory Assessment Scales professional manual.* Odessa, FL: Psychological Assessment Resources.

Williams, J. M. (1998). The malingering of memory disorder. In C. Reynolds (Ed.), *Detection of malingering in head injury litigation* (pp. 105–132). New York: Plenum Press.

Willis, W. (1984). Reanalysis of an actuarial approach to neuropsychological diagnosis in consideration of base rates. *Journal of Consulting and Clinical Psychology, 52*(4), 567–569.

Wilson, R., Rosenbaum, G., Brown, G., Rourke, D., Whitman, D., & Grisell, J. (1978). An index of premorbid intelligence. *Journal of Consulting and Clinical Psychology, 46,* 1544–1555.

Wong, J. L., Regennitter, R. P., & Barrios, F. (1994). Base rate and simulated symptoms of mild head injury among normals. *Archives of Clinical Neuropsychology, 9,* 411–425.

Woychyshyn, C. A., McElheran, W. G., & Romney, D. M. (1992). MMPI validity measures: A comparative study of original with alternative indices. *Journal of Personality Assessment, 58*(1), 138–148.

Youngjohn, J. R. (1991). Malingering of neuropsychological impairment: An assessment strategy. *A Journal for the Expert Witness, the Trial Attorney, the Trial Judge, 4,* 29–32.

Youngjohn, J. R. (1995). Confirmed attorney coaching prior to neuropsychological evaluation. *Assessment, 2*(3), 279–283.

13

Use of the MMPI with Mild Closed Head Injury

Lloyd I. Cripe
Private Practice, Seattle, Washington

> *Do not believe in anything simply because you have heard it. Do not believe in anything simply because it is spoken and rumored by many. Do not believe in anything merely on the authority of your teachers and written in your religious books. Do not believe in traditions because they have been handed down for many generations. But after observation and analysis, when you find that anything agrees with reason and is conducive to the good and benefit of one and all, then accept it and live up to it.*
>
> —Buddha

The Minnesota Multiphasic Personality Inventory (MMPI) is frequently used in the neuropsychological assessment of mild head injured persons. The motivation for this use is the hope that the combination of the neuropsychological tests and the MMPI will help with questions of differential diagnosis and ferret out the complex interaction of neurologic and psychiatric disorders.

Table 13.1 presents the neuropsychological and MMPI test data of a 36-year-old male mild head injured patient 2 years following injury. He has 11.5 years of formal education. Do the tests indicate a brain-based disorder? Do the tests indicate the presence of a psychiatric disorder? Do the tests indicate that either a brain disorder or a psychiatric disorder is the dominant cause of whatever problems he is experiencing? To what extent are "emotional factors" or some type of psychological reaction contributing to his real-world problems? Are there premorbid personality factors complicating his current problems? Is poor motivation or even

TABLE 13.1
Test Data of a Mild Head Injured Patient

Neuropsychological		MMPI	
WAIS–R FSIQ	91	?	10
WAIS–R VIQ	96	L	76
WAIS–R PIQ	86	F	73
Digit Symbol	7	K	64
Halstead Index	0.4	1	113
Dodrill Index	10/16 (63%)	2	120
SDMT Written	49	3	111
SDMT Oral	48	4	79
WMS Stories	13/3	5	61
WMS Visual	3/2	6	70
REY AVLT Trial V	9	7	81
Consonant Trigram	12, 8, 7	8	96
PASAT Mean	4.96	9	58
Pritchard Memory	76%	0	56
Dot Count Group	23	C.N.S. Items	63
Dot Count Ungroup	32	CRIMAX	Neuro

malingering contributing to whatever weak performances he manifests on the neuropsychological tests? These are questions that frequently challenge clinicians working with mild head injured persons.

This chapter explores the use of the MMPI with mild head injury patients. What are the challenges using this test instrument with this patient group? How useful is it to unravel the questions of differential diagnosis, determining the presence or absence of psychiatric disorder, emotional factors, and motivation problems? How can the test be best used to understand the person and help with treatment interventions? These are the basic questions that are addressed. [Note: In this chapter, the terms *MMPI* and *MMPI–2* are collapsed into the single term *MMPI* unless specified otherwise.]

WHAT DO WE KNOW ABOUT THE MMPI PROFILES OF MILD HEAD INJURED PERSONS?

> *A great many people think they are thinking when they are merely rearranging their prejudices.*
>
> —William James

We all know and agree that mild closed head injury occurs and can have neurobehavioral effects. Practicing neuropsychologists observe patients at various stages of recovery from mild head injuries. We know that the majority of these patients appear to have good recoveries within several months with no obvious significant permanent brain impairment.

We know that there are mild head injured patients with persistent problems that do not have good recoveries (Cicerone & Kalmar, 1995). About 10%–12% of patients with mild head injuries have poor outcomes. There is considerable disagreement and speculation among physicians and neuropsychologists regarding the causes of the persistent problems in mild head injured persons. Some think that these persons are frankly brain injured. Others think that the patients with persistent problems are having psychological reactions driven by some combination of preinjury and litigation factors. Some think there is a mix of brain impairment and psychological factors. In medical-legal situations, polarizations exist between plaintiff-oriented experts claiming frank brain damage and defense-oriented experts claiming psychological factors and manipulation. Speculative opinions abound regarding the cause of these prolonged problems, but exact causes of these poor outcomes are basically unknown.

Kay (1991) and Kay, Newman, Cavallo, Ezrachi, and Resnick (1992) presented a useful model of functional disability after mild traumatic brain injury that argues for an interaction of brain-based deficits and complex psychosocial interactions that eventually account for the persistent dysfunction.

Cripe (1996b) discussed the challenges in neuropsychological assessment of the mild head injured person. He suggested that our limited knowledge base, misconceptions, biases, the fact of multiple disorders with overlapping symptoms, and the limited assessment technology all pose significant challenges and potential pitfalls for accurately diagnosing and understanding mild head injured patients. Our ignorance and biases seem to fuel the controversies, driving us to act more from biased opinion of what we think we know, rather than from a position of what we really do know.

We know that mild head injury patients as a group generate elevated MMPI profiles, especially on Scales 1, 2, 3, 7, and 8. Table 13.2 summarizes the demographic and MMPI data of 236 (101 females, 135 males) taken from the author's clinical practice. Figure 13.1 presents the group MMPI profile. The mean age, education, and WAIS–R FSIQ are 40.36 years, 12.68 years, and 102.41, respectively. The mean time from injury to evaluation was 2.36 years. All of these patients were involved in personal injury litigation. Mild head injury was defined as any injury to the head with between 0 and 30 min of loss of consciousness and the development of reported cognitive changes. Many of the cases involved cervical strain injuries and the development of acute and then chronic pain problems following injury.

This group profile has elevations on Scales 1, 2, 3, 7, and 8. This profile configuration is similar to other reported groups of mild head injury

TABLE 13.2
Demographics and MMPI Scales of 236 Mild Closed
Head Injury Patients (101 Females and 135 Males)

Variable	Mean	SD	Minimum	Maximum
Age	40.36	13.71	16.00	77.00
Education	12.68	3.28	0.00	20.00
WAIS–R FSIQ	102.41	13.08	70.00	142.00
?	1.70	4.09	0.00	26.00
L	52.16	7.28	36.00	80.00
F	59.93	10.54	42.00	113.00
K	55.61	9.28	33.00	81.00
1	75.15	14.69	36.00	113.00
2	76.05	15.60	42.00	120.00
3	74.07	12.15	45.00	111.00
4	64.25	10.95	36.00	97.00
5	54.53	11.08	26.00	88.00
6	61.06	11.07	35.00	97.00
7	68.13	13.25	39.00	103.00
8	71.92	14.54	43.00	119.00
9	58.02	11.23	33.00	93.00
0	55.95	10.13	27.00	80.00
C.N.S. Items	37.46	14.43	5.00	73.00

Note. Observe elevation of Scales 1, 2, 3, 7, and 8.

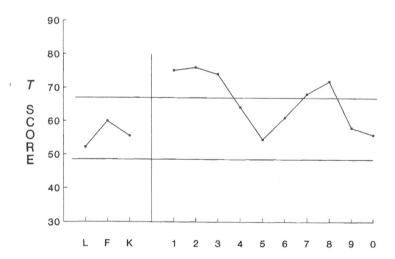

FIG. 13.1. Group MMPI profile of 236 mild head injured persons.

patients, with only the elevations varying somewhat from sample to sample (Berry et al., 1995; Cattelani, Gugliotta, Maravita, & Mazzucchi, 1996; Cicerone & Kalmar, 1995; Diamond, Barth, & Zilmer, 1988; Leininger, Kreutzer, & Hill, 1991; Suhr, Tanel, Wefel, & Barrash, 1997; Youngjohn, Davis, & Wolf, 1997; Youngjohn, Burrows, & Erdal, 1995). Based on these findings, it is safe to assume that as a group, mild head injured patients with persistent problems consistently generate MMPI profiles with relative elevations on Scales 1, 2, 3, 7, and 8. They do not as a group match the normal MMPI reference group.

We also know that the group MMPI profiles of persons with mild closed head injuries tend to be more elevated than those of severe closed head injured persons (Berry et al., 1995; Leininger et al., 1991; Suhr et al., 1997; Youngjohn et al., 1997). This finding has recently been called by Youngjohn et al. (1997) a "paradoxical severity effect." This term stems from the "dose-response" idea that if all head injury can be conceptualized as the same entity on a continuum from mild to severe, then higher elevations on the MMPI scales from the mild head injury patients appear to be a paradox. However, a mild head injury and a severe head injury may be different entities with different pathophysiologies. Additionally, as discussed later in this chapter, it is a misconception to believe that increased elevations on the MMPI necessarily mean more of a symptom or trait.

We know that the detection of malingering in mild head injury patients cannot be reliably done with the MMPI. A number of studies have investigated the potential of the MMPI to discriminate symptom overelaboration, poor test-taking motivation, malingering, and the effects of litigation in mild head injured persons and injured persons in general (Berry et al., 1995; Fordyce, Roueche, & Prigatano, 1983; Greiffenstein, Gola, & Baker, 1995; Lees-Haley, 1997; Slick, Hopp, Strauss, & Spellacy, 1996; Suhr et al., 1997; Youngjohn et al., 1997). The research results are mixed and yield little clinical usefulness. There are probably many factors contributing to these results (Faust, 1995; Zielinski, 1994). The definitions are variable and muddled. The criterion groups are difficult to define. It is difficult to find true malingering subjects for research. The overall conceptualization of the research often lacks an appreciation of the complexity involved. The detection of malingering is probably more complex than currently conceptualized and requires the consideration of many other factors than a single test instrument like the MMPI.

WHAT DO WE KNOW ABOUT THE MMPI
AND NEUROLOGIC PATIENTS?

To a mouse, cheese is cheese, and that is why mouse traps work.
—Wendell Johnson

We know that neurologic patients as a group elevate on Scales 1, 2, 3, 7, and 8 (Alfano, Finlayson, Stearns, & Nielson, 1990; Cripe, 1996a; Dikmen & Reitan, 1977; Gass, 1991a). We also know that some neuropathologies elevate more than others. For example, multiple sclerosis patients as a group tend to have very high elevations on these scales (Marsh, Hirsch, & Leung, 1982; Matthews, Cleeland, & Hopper, 1970; Meyerink, Reitan, & Selz, 1988; Mueller & Girace, 1988).

We also know that many other medical patient groups have elevations on these scales (Osborne, 1985; Schwartz & Krupp, 1971; Spergel, Ehrlich, & Glass, 1978). Pain and headache patients often generate MMPI profiles with elevations on these scales (Love & Peck, 1987; Miller & Kraus, 1990; Ziegler & Paolo, 1995).

The basic reason that neurologic patients elevate on Scales 1, 2, 3, 7, and 8 is that the inventory is loaded with many items that can be endorsed by a neurologic patient because of their neurologic disorders and the resulting real-world problems rather than necessarily due to psychiatric disorders, "emotional factors," or maladjustment.

Using an empirical key approach, Cripe (1996a) identified 85 items on the MMPI (see Appendix A) and 111 items on the MMPI–2 (see Appendix B) that are potentially endorsed by a neurologic patient because of their neurobehavioral problems. These items are called the C.N.S. items (Cripe Neurologic Symptom items). The items are subdivided into 17 symptom subgroups (e.g., Attention/Mental Control, Memory, Sensory, etc.). When neurologic patients endorse these items, due to their neurologic problems, Scales 1, 2, 3, 7, and 8 are elevated because the C.N.S. items load heavily on these scales.

In essence, a neurologic patient may elevate on these scales because of their neurologic symptoms, and not necessarily because of a psychiatric disorder. They may not be somatizing, depressed, or maladjusted in any manner, although the profile can easily be misconstrued as indicating that there are "emotional factors" or a psychiatric disturbance on board.

Because so many different medical and psychiatric patient groups will generate elevations on these scales for different reasons, it is not possible to simply look at the clinical scales of an MMPI profile and determine the patient's group membership. Cripe, Maxwell, and Hill (1995) studied a large sample of normal, neurologic, chronic pain (with and without surgery), and outpatient psychiatric groups to see if clinical or research scales could actually differentiate the groups. They found that although all the patient groups are easily distinguished from the normal reference group, it was not possible to correctly classify the patient groups either clinically or with multiple discriminate function analysis using the basic clinical or research scales alone or in combination. A discriminant function analysis using the C.N.S. items and subgroupings demonstrated promise in correctly classifying the groups with a 78% overall accuracy.

We also know that there is virtually no correlation between performance on the MMPI and performance on neuropsychological tests (Gass, 1991b, 1996; Gass & Ansley, 1994; Gass, Burda, Starkey, & Dominguez, 1992; Gass & Daniel, 1990; Gass, Russell, & Hamilton, 1990; Gass & Russell, 1986). For example, there is no useful correlation between Scale 2 (depression) of the MMPI and neuropsychological tests of attention and memory. This lack of correlation between the MMPI scales and neuropsychological tests is troubling if one assumes that the MMPI is in fact measuring depression and we also assume that depression can or does have some adverse effect on attention and memory. If one holds these assumptions, this lack of correlation seriously challenges the notion that emotional factors necessarily affect performance on neuropsychological tests (Reitan & Wolfson, 1997). The lack of correlation is probably related to the structure of the MMPI questions and how well they tap into the details of neuropsychological impairments, and the difference between self-report of problems (with the constraints of the MMPI), and performance on specific neuropsychological tasks.

PROBLEMS USING THE MMPI WITH NEUROLOGIC PATIENTS

> *It's not what we don't know, but what we know that ain't so that gets us into trouble.*
>
> —Will Rogers

The basic problem in trying to do differential diagnosis with the MMPI to rule in or out neurologic versus pain versus depression versus somatization versus "emotional factors" is the fact that all of these and other conditions can have similar symptoms that result in endorsing similar items that produce elevations on Scales 1, 2, 3, 7, and 8 for different reasons. This confounds research conceptualization, implementation, and interpretation. If there was one invariant reason or disorder that caused an MMPI scale to elevate, then a simple straightforward unbending cookbook interpretation could be made with each patient who elevates on that scale. Elevations on the scales would invariantly mean the presence of psychopathology or "emotional factors." If a person from any patient group elevated on the scales in question, it would be indicative of the presence of a psychological abnormality and its associated psychiatric disorder. Unfortunately, it's not that simple. For example, a person might respond *true* to an item that asks for a *true* or *false* response to the statement

"My memory seems to be all right" for different reasons, depending on what type of disorder is causing the symptom. Regardless, the endorsement will elevate several MMPI scales, giving the illusion that whatever diagnostic label is attached to the scales is the driving cause for the endorsement.

Cripe (1996a, 1996b) discussed several underlying beliefs and misconceptions that misguide clinicians' thinking. One misconception is the belief that the MMPI measures general emotional adjustment in neurologic patients. No adequate validation research has been done to demonstrate this. The concept has been driven by a logic that assumes elevations on the MMPI are probably linked to maladjustment.

The thinking follows these lines. If some persons elevate on a scale for reasons of maladjustment, for example, Scale 1, then anyone who elevates on that scale is maladjusted. The common assumption would be that the person has a somatizing maladjustment. Another line of reasoning says that if the reference group is well adjusted, then anyone who deviates from that group is maladjusted. The MMPI is seen as a sort of general barometer of life adjustment. Therefore, if psychiatric patients elevate on the MMPI, and if neurologic patients elevate on the MMPI, then both groups are elevating for the same reasons and must be maladjusted. Such reasoning could only be true if there was only one invariant reason why an elevation on the MMPI would occur. It also overlooks the fact that 30% of normal controls elevate on one or more MMPI scales.

Another misconception is that when a scale elevates more and more, the elevation indicates more and more of a particular trait or mental state. For example, a T-score of 50 on Scale 2 means no depression, a T-score of 70 means the presence of some mild depression, a T-score of 90 means a lot more depression, a T-score of 100 means more severe depression, and so on. How this idea was germinated and then grew in clinical psychology is not clearly known.

The scales do not really measure unitary traits or states. The scales were never psychometrically designed to represent a continuum of a particular trait. The scales are best thought of as discriminators of group membership. As a scale elevates, it means that the person performing on that scale is looking less and less like the reference group. It is an indicator of the probability that the person does or does not belong to the reference group. In other words, a T-score of 100 on Scale 2 is a strong probability statement that the person doesn't belong to the reference group. If there were only one other group on the planet that behaved that way on that particular MMPI scale, then the probability would be very high that if they don't belong to the reference group, then they must exclusively belong to a second group of persons labeled "depressed." The clinician would be able to say with great certainty that the patient belongs to the group of persons with a depressed state of mind, but would not be able to say anything about the degree of depression. The issue of degree of group membership has become confused with the issue of the degree or amount of a symptom. A study of the items making up the scales reveals that the items are not particularly scaled to the general scale headings (e.g., Hypochondriasis, Depression, etc.), and the items are not Likert scales. Additionally, the validation research discriminating groups from normals is replete with validation criterion problems and limited in scope. It is fairly easy to discriminate deviations from the normal reference group, but very difficult to discriminate deviations that distinguish multiple groups. Multiple discrimination of clinical groups is commonly expected in clinical practice, but the application of the MMPI is usually based on a single group comparison.

PROBLEMS USING THE MMPI AS A MEASURE OF PERSONALITY AND EMOTIONS

> *Although everyone experiences emotions, emotion cannot be easily defined, and it is difficult to measure something that cannot be defined.*
> —Kenneth Heilman

Another potential use of the MMPI in the study of neurologic patients is the study of personality and emotions. Neurologic disorders from either disease or trauma always interact with a person's psychological style or personality. The disorder may have direct effects on the control and expression of personality or emotion, or there can be indirect effects of various reactions to the disorder and the resulting problems.

To best understand how a person is adjusting to his or her neurologic condition, and to determine if there is maladjustment, it is important to understand the person's longstanding personality traits. For example, a person with obsessive-complusive personality traits may have a reaction to acquired neuropsychological problems quite different from that of a person with hysteroid personality traits. The need to understand personality style and the different reactions to neurologic injury has been discussed by Ruff, Mueller, and Jurica (1996) and Kay (1992), but is unfortunately not very well researched by neuropsychologists.

Trying to use the MMPI to understand either direct organic changes in personality and emotion or the person's longstanding personality traits and reactions is extremely limited (Cripe, 1997). The test will not do the expected job of understanding such complicated matters. The instrument was not developed from personality theory or research. The matter of assessing personality and emotions in neurologic patients is much more complicated than attaching a single self-report inventory to a battery of neuropsychological tests. It requires a comprehensive assessment process approach rather than reliance on a single test. Cripe (1997) discussed guidelines for the assessment of personality in the brain-impaired patient. The reader is referred to this writing for a deeper understanding of the challenges and ideas on how to best deal with this complicated matter.

THE SAFEST ASSUMPTION

> *Knowledge is the small part of ignorance that we arrange and classify.*
> —Ambrose Gwinett Bierce

Because of the problems with item content, the discrimination of patient groups, the lack of validation of maladjustment, the meaning of scale elevations, and many other psychometric issues (Helmes & Reddon, 1993), the use of the MMPI with neurologic patients is precarious. Frankly, it will not do all the things that neuropsychologists hope it can do. Because of the problems, Cripe (1996a) concluded:

> The safest and most logical assumption to make if a medical or neurologic patient elevates on scales 1, 2, 3, 7 or 8 is that the patient has some awareness of his/her problems and is reporting the problems within the limitations and constrictions of the MMPI item pool. Patients simply see themselves as having difficulties related to their medical problems and are trying to communicate this awareness. The fact that they are aware of problems does not necessarily indicate that they are distraught about the problems or emotionally maladjusted. Nor does the awareness of problems necessarily validate the medical reality of the reported symptoms. Although awareness is a necessary condition for reporting symptoms, it is not a necessary or sufficient condition for declaring maladjustment or for determining the presence or absence of a medical disorder. While the possibility exists that patients are having difficulty in adapting to the problems, the elevations on the MMPI scales are potentially affected by the neurobehavioral symptoms, and cannot discriminate this disturbance.
>
> Another complication with interpreting MMPI profiles is the fact that some neurologic patients are not aware of their symptoms and can generate flat profiles which falsely give the illusion that they are problem free and well adjusted. To conclude that a flat MMPI profile with such a person is evidence of a good adjustment can be misleading.
>
> There currently is no way that a clinician can determine, on the basis of an MMPI inspection alone, that a neurologic patient is particularly distraught, distressed, or emotionally maladjusted or well adjusted. All that can be reasonably and safely concluded is that neurologic patients who

elevate on the MMPI are aware of symptoms and are reporting them within the confines of the MMPI questions. (p. 101)

PROBLEMS IN USING THE MMPI WITH MILD HEAD INJURED PATIENTS

> *What we observe is not nature itself, but nature exposed to our method of questioning.*
> —Werner Heisenberg

Mild head injured persons are a patient group with several potential problems that include slowed rate of information processing, impaired complex attention, impaired short-term memory, impaired control of emotions, pain syndromes, psychological distress, and environmental stress. It is hoped that the use of the MMPI in the assessment will help with the differential diagnosis of organic versus functional disorders, unmask variants of poor test-taking effort, exaggeration, or malingering, and help understand personality and emotion factors. Given the limitations of the MMPI with neurologic patients as discussed earlier, the MMPI is probably poorly suited to fulfill these hopes.

Neuropsychologists are asking too much of the MMPI as a diagnostic instrument with this patient group. The false hope that the instrument can do the expected job complicates research and clinical activities.

If researchers or clinicians approach their studies with the idea that the MMPI performance of neurologic patients is not affected by item content and assume that the elevations from these patients on the various scales are invariantly indicative of emotional or psychiatric problems, their conclusions will be guided by misconception. It is common in neuropsychological research of neurologic patients to see elevations on group MMPI profiles interpreted as indicating the presence of emotional, personality, psychiatric, or adjustment problems with no other validating information.

If clinicians approach the study of an individual with the idea that MMPI elevations are invariantly linked to problems with emotions, personality, psychiatric disorder, or adjustment problems, their interpretation of the test results will be skewed in the direction of attaching "emotional factors" as a cause. This will be further magnified in cases where the neuropsychological disorder is milder in manifestation and where the etiologies are less certain. If the neuropsychological test results are mild in presentation, and the MMPI profile is significantly elevated, the conclusion will be that some emotional problem such as a psychiatric disorder accounts for the complaints and the mild neurobehavioral problems noted on the neuropsychological tests. There is a tendency to overidentify psychiatric disorder.

It is very common in mild head injury cases with prolonged problems to observe the following: The patient has complaints of problems with low energy, concentration, forgetfulness, pain, headaches, emotional re-activeness, and mild depression. With appropriate testing and careful analysis, neuropsychological test results often indicate subtle to mild problems with rate of information processing, complex attention process-ing, and short-term memory. The MMPI often indicates significant eleva-tions on Scales 1, 2, 3, and possibly 7 and 8. The typical interpretation of the findings is that the person is doing quite well neuropsychologically, but has significant emotional reactions and problems that account for the complaints and the mild findings on the neuropsychological tests. If the MMPI profile is highly elevated, the tendency is to raise the question of somatization and possible conscious or unconscious motivation problems. Of course, if the examiner has a priori beliefs that mild head injured persons cannot and should not have prolonged problems, any mild prob-lems found on neuropsychological tests will be attributed to personality issues, psychiatric disturbance, or manipulation for financial gain. The MMPI is interpreted to bolster this idea and explain away the neuropsy-chological findings. These conclusions about the test results are misguided by the erroneous test and patient assumptions held by the examiners prior to conducting the individual or group study.

Think about these complicating factors: The types of problems the patients are experiencing and reporting are guaranteed to effect and elevate the MMPI Scales 1, 2, 3, 7, and 8. The types of neurobehavioral problems experienced are by nature milder and manifest on neuropsy-chological measures in subtle ways. There is no correlation between MMPI scales and neuropsychological tests. The MMPI as commonly used cannot discriminate neurologic versus psychiatric versus pain versus psychiatric patients. The MMPI is replete with items that can be endorsed for reason of neurologic disorder. The test is not able to assess the complexities of emotions and personality. All of the problems in using the MMPI with neurologic patients are present, but further complicated by the complex and illusive nature of mild closed head injury.

These are fertile conditions for misinterpretation and misunderstand-ing. It is a veritable minefield of interpretation hazzards. Only the exam-iner armed with a clear understanding of the potential traps will avoid a chain reaction of inaccurate destructive conclusions.

THE BEST ALTERNATIVE

We should be careful to get out of an experience only the wisdom that is in it—and stop there; lest we be like the cat that sits down on a hot stove-lid.

> *She will never sit down on a hot stove-lid again, and that is well; but also*
> *she will never sit down on a cold one anymore.*
>
> —Mark Twain

Given all these potential problems using the MMPI with neurologic patients, and mild head injured persons in particular, what can be done to avoid misuse and misunderstanding?

Some advocate that items be identified and subtracted out of the MMPI profile before proceeding on with a traditional clinical interpretation (Alfano, Paniak, & Finlayson, 1993; Alfano, Neilson, Paniak, & Finlayson, 1992; Gass & Russell, 1991; Gass & Wald, 1997). This approach is precarious. The identification of items that will discriminate groups is subject to criterion validation problems, and there will be considerable variability in selected groups from different studies. The clinical need is to separate multiple groups, not just demonstrate differences between the mild head injured and another single group. The items that are identified usually represent overlapping symptoms found in all the patient groups involved in the diagnostic differential. More importantly, the subtraction of items from the MMPI makes it a different instrument. It requires considerable research to validate the "new" MMPI to see if it can in fact discriminate whatever it is hoped that it will discriminate. This has not been done. Additionally, this subtraction approach does not appreciate the deeper problems and complexities involved with the use of the MMPI and neurologic patients as discussed above. Attempting to tease out psychiatric problems, conduct differential diagnosis, and determine maladjustment is much more complicated than these researchers have assumed.

The best alternative is to realize the complexities and problems in using this single instrument and don't rely so heavily upon it. A more comprehensive diagnostic process is needed to do the job of assessing a person's adjustment, personality, emotions, motivations, and the presence or absence of a psychiatric disorder (Cripe, 1997). The MMPI alone is best viewed as the person's attempt to communicate their problems within the constraints of a structured self-report inventory. We can best use this information to understand their perceived problems and develop treatment interventions.

GUIDELINES

> *Anyone can make the simple complicated. Creativity is making the*
> *complicated simple.*
>
> —Charles Mingus

Given the problems and challenges in using the MMPI with mild head injured patients, the following brief guidelines are suggested. Further suggestions are available in the author's previous writings (Cripe, 1989, 1996a, 1996b, 1997).

- Be fully aware of the problems and challenges in using this instrument with this patient group.
- Do not rely heavily on this or any other single test to study the complexities of a person's adjustment, personality or psychiatric status. If you want to understand these matters, use a comprehensive evaluation process that considers many sources of information (Cripe, 1997).
- Consider using newer technology. The MMPI was conceptualized over 50 years ago based on the ideas about mental disorders of that era. Recent revisions have not tackled the underlying assumptions nor resolved many of the inherent psychometric problems (Helmes & Reddon, 1993). The more recently developed Personality Assessment Inventory–Revised (PAI-R) by Morey (1991) is conceptually and psychometrically sound and seems to deliver more accurate clinical information (White, 1996), even though it too has many items that can be endorsed by neurologic patients because of neurologic disorder and will affect some of the scales. The SOM and DEP scales of the PAI-R are particularly impacted by mild head injury symptoms.
- If the MMPI is used, view it simply as a tool to understand the person's perception of their problems.
- When interpreting the MMPI results, use an item analysis approach rather than a scale analysis approach.
- Carefully consider the C.N.S. items and their subgroupings to best understand problem areas.
- Consider how the overall MMPI profile has been affected and elevated by the endorsement of C.N.S. items.
- Do not subtract out items and then proceed with a traditional clinical interpretation of the profile.
- Do not use cookbook or computer-generated interpretations with neurologic patients in general and especially with this patient group. They just are not appropriate.
- Be conservative in reporting and writing the MMPI findings.
- Recognize the limits of our technology and accept the fact that ultimately the study and understanding of such complicated phenomenon is a subjective matter that has to rely on a broad range of qualitative and quantitative information from many sources (Cripe, 1996c). Even the best tests are subjectively interpreted, even if the interpretive statements are housed in a computer program file.

A CASE EXAMPLE

We see what we look for. We look for what we know.

—Goethe

We don't see things as they are, we see things as we are.

—Anais Nin

The case data presented in Table 13.1 are used as an example for applying the recommended guidelines.

The MMPI validity scales are elevated on scales L and F. Six of the clinical scales are above a T score of 70, with Scales 1, 2, 3, and 8 very highly elevated. It is tempting to quickly conclude that whoever generated this profile must be very disturbed, suffering from a somatoform disorder, and maybe exaggerating symptoms or even malingering. The neuropsychological test data in Table 13.1 suggest poor performance on neurobehavioral measures, but given the MMPI profile, are these poor test performances related to a psychological condition? Obviously, such thoughts are driven by old habits and have to be resisted in light of the problems we have discussed about using the MMPI with this patient group.

The safest general conclusion at this point in the analysis of the MMPI performance is that the patient sees himself as having a variety of problems and it is highly improbable that he belongs to the reference group. However, this alone does not reveal in what other group membership he may reside.

Although there are 10 "cannot say" items, and Scales L and F are elevated, an analysis of test taking validity using Greene's approach (1991) suggests that the test is valid and further analysis is warranted.

A closer analysis of the MMPI items shows that the patient endorsed 63 C.N.S. items. This is a higher number of items than the mean of 38 (see Table 13.1) and a range of 5 to 73 items found in a large group of mild head injured persons. Table 13.3 is the list of C.N.S. subgroups and the actual items endorsed. The patient sees himself as having a variety of physical and mental problems that are potentially associated with neurologic disorders. The types of problems endorsed are seen in persons with prolonged physical and cognitive problems following mild head injuries.

Figure 13.2 presents the patient's MMPI profile with and without the C.N.S. items. It is obvious that his overall profile was significantly affected by these items. This provides a useful illustration of the effect of the patient's endorsement of these items on the profile, but as discussed earlier, it is not advisable to try to interpret the profile with the C.N.S. items subtracted.

Regarding group membership, there is no way to clinically look at the patient's MMPI profile and determine to which patient group he most

TABLE 13.3
Case Example 63 C.N.S. Items by Subgroups

Number	Response	Item
AM (Attention/Mental Control), 8 of 9 items endorsed		
32.	T	I find it hard to keep my mind on a task or job.
46.	F	My judgment is better than it ever was.
168.	T	There is something wrong with my mind.
182.	T	I am afraid of losing my mind.
328.	T	I find it hard to keep my mind on a task or job.
335.	T	I cannot keep my mind on one thing.
356.	T	I have more trouble concentrating than others seem to have.
374.	T	At periods my mind seems to work more slowly than usual.
LA (Appetite), 1 of 2 items endorsed		
155.	F	I am neither gaining or losing weight.
FE (Fatigue/Energy) 3 of 5 items endorsed		
163.	F	I do not tire quickly.
272.	F	At times I am full of energy.
544.	T	I feel tired a good deal of the time.
HE (Health), 3 of 3 items endorsed		
51.	F	I am in just as good physical health as most of my friends.
153.	F	During the past few years I have been well most of the time.
160.	F	I have never felt better in my life than I do now.
HD (Headaches), 4 of 5 items endorsed		
44.	T	Much of the time my head seems to hurt all over.
114.	T	Often I feel as if there were a tight band about my head.
116.	T	The top of my head sometimes feels tender.
190.	F	I have very few headaches.
IC (Incontinence), 1 of 1 item endorsed		
462.	F	I have had no difficulty starting or holding my urine.
ME (Memory), 3 of 3 endorsed		
178.	F	My memory seems to be all right.
342.	T	I forget right away what people say to me.
560.	T	I am greatly bothered by forgetting where I put things.
MT (Motor), 4 of 6 items endorsed		
103.	F	I have little or no trouble with my muscles twitching or jumping.
186.	T	I frequently notice my hands shakes when I try to do something.
187.	F	My hands have not become clumsy or awkward.
330.	F	I have never been paralyzed or had any unusual weakness of any of my muscles.
PN (Pain), 1 of 2 items endorsed		
243.	F	I have few or no pains.
SB (Seizures/Blank Episodes), 4 of 5 items endorsed		
154.	F	I have never had a fit or convulsion.
156.	T	I have had periods in which I carried on activities without knowing later what I had been doing.
174.	F	I have never had a fainting spell.
251.	T	I have had blank spells in which my activities were interrupted and I did not know what was going on around me.

(Continued)

TABLE 13.3
(Continued)

Number	Response	Item
SE (Sensory), 10 of 15 items endorsed		
47.	T	Once a week or oftener I feel suddenly hot all over, without apparent cause.
185.	F	My hearing is apparently as good as that of most people.
188.	F	I can read a long while without tiring my eyes.
214.	F	I have never had any breaking out on my skin that has worried me.
273.	T	I have numbness in one or more regions of my skin.
274.	F	My eyesight is as good as it has been for years.
281.	F	I do not often notice my ears ringing or buzzing.
334.	T	Peculiar odors come to me at times.
496.	F	I have never seen things doubled (that is, an object never looks like two objects to me without my being able to make it look like one object).
508.	F	I believe my sense of smell is as good as other people's.
SX (Sexual), 3 of 4 items endorsed		
20.	F	My sex life is satisfactory.
179.	T	I am worried about sex matters.
310.	F	My sex life is satisfactory.
SD (Sleep Disturbance), 4 of 5 items endorsed		
3.	F	I wake up fresh and rested most mornings.
5.	T	I am easily awakened by noise.
43.	T	My sleep is fitful and disturbed.
152.	F	Most nights I go to sleep without thoughts or ideas bothering me.
SL (Speech/Language), 2 of 3 items endorsed		
119.	F	My speech is the same as always (not faster or slower, or slurring; no hoarseness).
159.	T	I cannot understand what I read as well as I used to.
VN (Vertigo/Nausea), 4 of 4 items endorsed		
23.	T	I am troubled by attacks of nausea and vomiting.
175.	F	I seldom or never have dizzy spells.
192.	F	I have had no difficulty in keeping my balance in walking.
288.	T	I am troubled by attacks of nausea and vomiting.
VO (Vocational), 1 of 1 item endorsed		
9.	F	I am about as able to work as I ever was.

probably belongs. The high Scales 1, 2, 3, 7, and 8 profile can be found in many patient groups (e.g., various medical, neurologic, pain, psychiatric-somatoform, psychiatric reaction, malingering). A multivariate discriminant function analysis developed by Cripe et al. (1995), the CRIMAX, predicts that the patient's MMPI performance is best classified as belonging to a neurologic patient group as compared to a normal, neurologic, pain, outpatient psychiatric crisis, and random responder groups. The function has an overall 78% correct classification rate.

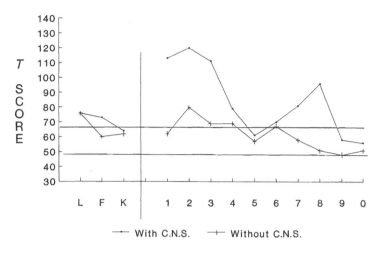

FIG. 13.2. Patient MMPI profiles with and without C.N.S. items.

Based on this analysis, the following description of the patient's MMPI could be appropriately written as part of a more comprehensive evaluation report:

> Mr. Smith produces a valid MMPI profile with high elevations on Scales 1, 2, 3, 7, and 8. He sees himself as having a variety of physical and mental problems and is concerned about them. He endorsed 63 C.N.S. items (Cripe Neurologic Symptom items). The C.N.S. items are items on the MMPI potentially endorsed by a neurologic patient because of their neurologic symptoms. These items can elevate Scales 1, 2, 3, and 8 for reasons other than psychiatric symptoms. His profile was obviously affected by the endorsement of the C.N.S. items. He sees himself as having problems in many areas to include: attention/mental control, emotional control, fatigue, general health, headaches, memory, motor, sensory, pain, seizure/blank episodes, sleep, sex, and vertigo/nausea. This type of profile is clearly not seen in normal functioning persons. It can be seen in a variety of medical, neurologic and psychiatric conditions. It is somewhat unusually elevated for patients with mild head injuries, but can be found in this group. A discriminant function analysis (CRIMAX) of Mr. Smith's MMPI variables classified him as most probably belonging to a neurologic patient group. This function classifies with a 78% overall accuracy whether a patient's MMPI performance best fits a random, normal, neurologic, pain, or outpatient psychiatric group. Further clinical information is necessary to determine the most appropriate diagnosis of Mr. Smith's reported problems.

Note that this interpretation does not use statements from cookbooks or computer interpretations. It does not go beyond the limits of what the instrument can realistically do with this complicated patient group. Keep in mind that this is just a statement about the patient's MMPI and doesn't represent the complete final conclusions and understanding that would be discussed in a comprehensive neuropsychological report.

CONCLUSION

> *If you do not understand a man you cannot crush him. And if you do understand him, very probably you will not.*
>
> —G. K. Chesterton

The hope that the MMPI can be attached to a battery of neuropsychological tests and adequately perform differential diagnosis of neurologic and psychiatric disorders, assess the complexities of personality, emotions, and motivation, and determine overall life adaptation, in a complicated phenomenon like mild closed head injury, is a false hope based on many misconceptions. A single test with all the problems discussed cannot hope to fulfill these expectations. However, the test can be used with other information to better understand the patient's perception of their problems.

Over the course of 25 years, the author's professional journey has encountered over 500 cases of mild closed head injury. The author listened and studied the patients as open-mindedly and carefully as possible. Most of the persons observed are in the 10+% group of mild head injured persons with persistent problems. The observations indicate many similarities in their stories and problems. They initially thought their problems would quickly go away after a reasonable recovery time, but the problems didn't. They experienced persistent cognitive problems mostly involving poor concentration and forgetfulness. These cognitive problems either developed early or evolved over a period of weeks and months following injury. They often noticed the problems most on return to work or school demands. They have problems with decreased energies and with emotional reactiveness. Many experienced initial acute pains and then chronic pain, mostly involving the head, neck and back. Their activity levels were diminished. The majority were basically normally adapted persons prior to injury, and it is difficult to blame their problems on some preexisting medical or psychiatric condition. Their personal and vocational roles were often adversely affected by their problems. Many were employed, but others were not gainfully employed. Many were financially stressed due to decreased occupational ability and treatment costs. A few appeared to be experiencing extreme somatoform reactions. Even fewer appeared to be frank malingers. Most experienced confusing medical diagnosis, management, and treatment. Most were involved in personal injury litigation because their injuries occurred as victims of accidents and they live in

North America, where there is a constitutional right to pursue compensation when wronged by others.

Many of these patients initially received good medical screening to rule out severe injury requiring intensive medical intervention. Treatments and management after the initial screening varied. Some were well managed, but most were not. Some patients initially received adequate funding from insurance carriers, but the funds were cut off after several months of persistent problems. The persons were left to their own resources for any further help. Often, they could not afford further care. Many were understandably demoralized and frustrated about their problems and situation. Some were very angry at being harmed for no fault of their own and then left to their own to deal with pain and suffering.

In the course of their medical and legal encounters, most of these patients have been administered an MMPI. Frequently the interpretations of the test were made without consideration of the issues discussed in this chapter. The interpretations were often insulting to the patients. The test conclusions were often poorly conceptualized and driven by misconceptions that were insensitive to the complex problems these patients were truly experiencing. In some cases the interpretations in the context of the medical-legal arena were outright pejorative, taking the form of a sort of "character assassination" blaming whatever handy post hoc factor(s) for the person's acquired problems. In effect, little to no understanding occurred, insult was added to injury, and no practical interventions were given.

Because mild head injury sequelae are complicated, the exact causes are somewhat mysterious, our knowledge base is incomplete, and our technology is limited, there is a need to approach the study of these cases with openness and a full awareness of the strengths and limitations of our methods. Our basic goal as scientist-clinicians should be to understand these patients and the problems they are experiencing with the hope that this leads to useful interventions and outcomes. We must avoid consciously or unconsciously compounding their problems. Mild closed head injured persons with persistent complications are real people from all walks of life struggling with significant problems. As suffering human beings, they deserve better than to be caught in the cross fire of our controversies and misconceptions.

When assessing these persons, we should be armed with the best science available, but not fool ourselves into believing that our science is complete. We need to see these persons as *unique individuals* and not *group means*. We must never forget that whether or not we believe or disbelieve in single case studies, our next patient will be one. Out best is to understand. At minimum, we should "do no harm."

85 Cripe Neurologic Symptom (C.N.S.)
Items for the MMPI (Group Form)

Attention/Mental Control (AM), 9 items: 32.T, 46.F, 134.T, 168.T, 182.T, 328.T, 335.T, 356.T, 374.T.
Appetite (LA), 2 items: 155.F, 424.T.
Emotional Control (EC), 12 items: 22.T, 75.T, 105.T, 129.T, 158.T, 234.F, 242.F, 326.T, 336.T, 337.T, 399.F, 468.T.
Fatigue/Energy (FE), 5 items: 163.F, 189.T, 272.F, 505.T, 544.T.
Health (HE), 3 items: 51.F, 153.F, 160.F.
Headaches (HD), 5 items: 44.T, 108.T, 114.T, 161.T, 190.F.
Incontinence (IC), 1 item: 462.F.
Memory (ME), 3 items: 178.F, 342.T, 560.T.
Motor (MT), 6 items: 103.F, 186.T, 187.F, 330.F, 405.F, 540,F.
Pain (PN), 2 items: 243.F, 68.F.
Seizures/Blank Episodes (SB), 5 items: 154.F, 156.T, 174.F, 194.T, 251.T.
Sensory (SE), 15 items: 7.F, 47.T, 62.T, 184.T, 185.F, 118.F, 214.F, 273.T, 274.F, 281.F, 334.T, 341.T, 496.F, 508.F, 541.T.
Sexual (SX), 4 items: 20.F, 179.T, 310.F, 519.T.
Sleep Disturbance (SD), 5 items: 3.F, 5.T, 43.T, 152.F, 211.T.
Speech/Language (SL), 3 items: 119.F, 159.T, 332.T.
Vertigo/Nausea (VN), 4 items: 23.T, 175.F, 192.F, 288.T.
Vocational (VO), 1 item: 9.F.

Note. An item is given 1 raw score point if endorsed in the direction indicated.

111 Cripe Neurologic Symptom (C.N.S.) Items for the MMPI-2

Attention/Mental Control (AM), 7 items: 31.T, 122.T, 299.T, 325.T, 341.T, 475.T, 525.T.
Biobehavioral (BB), 6 items: 12.F, 20.F, 143.F, 166.T, 208.F, 253.T.
Emotional/Behavior Control (EB), 22 items: 23.T, 37.T, 38.T, 93.T, 102.T, 116.T, 146.T, 213.T, 223.F, 226.T, 233.T, 271.T, 301.T, 302.T, 372.F, 389.T, 400.T, 405.F, 430.T, 469.T, 513.T, 564.F.
Fatigue/Energy (FE), 6 items: 152.F, 175.T, 330.F, 366.T, 464.T, 561.F.
General Cognitive (GC), 10 items: 32.T, 43.F, 109.F, 135.T, 170.T, 180.T, 206.F, 309.T, 482.T, 491.T.
Headache (HD), 6 items: 40.T, 57.F, 97.T, 101.T, 149.T, 176.F.
Health (HE), 4 items: 33.F, 45.F, 141.F, 148.F.
Memory (ME), 5 items: 165.F, 308.T, 472.T, 533.T, 565.T.
Motor (MT), 6 items: 91.F, 172.T, 177.F, 295.F, 404.F, 476.T.
Pain (PN), 2 items: 47.F, 224.F.
Seizure/Blank Episodes (SB), 5 items: 142.F, 159.F, 168.T, 182.T, 229.T.
Sleep Disturbance (SD), 6 items: 3.F, 5.T, 39.T, 140.F, 258.T, 293.T.
Sensory (SE), 13 items: 8.F, 44.T, 53.T, 173.F, 194.F, 198.T, 204.F, 247.T, 249.F, 252.T, 255.F, 298.T, 307.T.
Speech/Language (SL), 3 items: 106.F, 147.T, 296.T.
Social (SO), 5 items: 83.F, 86.F, 367.T, 480.T, 507.T.
Vertigo/Nausea (VN), 3 items: 18.T, 164.F, 179.F.
Vocational (VO), 2 items: 10.F, 517.T.

Note. An item is given 1 raw score point if endorsed in the direction indicated.

REFERENCES

Alfano, D., Paniak, C., & Finlayson, M. (1993). The MMPI and closed head injury: A neurocorrective approach. *Neuropsychiatry, Neuropsychology, & Behavioral Neurology, 6*(2), 111–116.

Alfano, D., Neilson, P., Paniak, C., & Finlayson, M. (1992). The MMPI and closed-head injury. *Clinical Neuropsychologist, 6*(2), 134–142.

Alfano, D. P., Finlayson, M. A. J., Stearns, G. M., & Nielson, P. M. (1990). The MMPI and neurologic dysfunction: Profile configuration and analysis. *Clinical Neuropsychologist, 4*(1), 69–79.

Berry, D. T., Wetter, M. W., Baer, R. A., Gass, C. S., Franzen, M. D., Youngjohn, J. R., Lamb, D. G., & MacInnes, W. D. (1995). Overreporting of closed-head injury symptoms on the MMPI-2. *Psychological Assessment, 7*(4), 517–523.

Cattelani, R., Gugliotta, R., Maravita, A., & Mazzucchi, A. (1996). Post-concussive syndrome: paraclinical signs, subjective symptoms, cognitive functions and MMPI profiles. *Brain Injury, 10*(3), 187–195.

Cicerone, K. D., & Kalmar, K. (1997). Does premorbid depression influence post-concussive symptoms and neuropsychological functioning? *Brain Injury, 11*(9), 643–648.

Cicerone, K. D., & Kalmar, K. (1995). Persistent postconcussion syndrome: The structure of subjective complaints after mild traumatic brain injury. *Journal of Head Trauma Rehabilitation, 10,* 1–17.

Cripe, L. I. (1989). Neuropsychological and psychosocial assessment of the brain-injured person: Clinical concepts and guidelines. *Rehabilitation Psychology, 34*(2), 93–100.

Cripe, L. I. (1996a). The mmpi in neuropsychological assessment: a murky measure. *Applied Neuropsychology, 3,* 4, 97–103.

Cripe, L. I. (1996b). The role of neuropsychology in mild traumatic brain injury: Diagnosis verses misdiagnosis. *i.e. Magazine, 3,* 3.

Cripe, L. I. (1996c). The ecological validity of executive function testing. In R. J. Sbordone & C. J. Long (Eds.), *Ecological validity of neuropsychological assessment* (pp. 171–202). Delray Beach, FL: GR Press & Lucie Press.

Cripe, L. I. (1997). Personality assessment of brain-impaired patients. In M. Maruish (Ed.), *Theoretical foundations of clinical neuropsychology for clinical practitioners* (pp. 119–142). Hillsdale, NJ: Lawrence Erlbaum Associates.

Cripe, L. I., Maxwell, J. K., & Hill, E. L. (1995). Multivariate discriminant function analysis of neurologic, pain, and psychiatric patients with the MMPI. *Journal of Clinical Psychology, 51,* 258–268.

Diamond, R., Barth, J. T., & Zilmer, E. A. (1988). Emotional correlates of mild closed head trauma: The role of the MMPI. *The International Journal of Clinical Neuropsychology, 1*(1), 35–40.

Dikmen, S., & Reitan, R. (1977). MMPI correlates of adaptive ability deficits in patients with brain lesions. *Journal of Nervous & Mental Disease, 165*(4), 247–254.

Faust, D. (1995). The detection of deception. *Neurology Clinics, 13*(2), 255–265.

Fordyce, D. J., Roueche, J. R., & Prigatano, G. P. (1983). Enhanced emotional reactions in chronic head trauma patients. *Journal of Neurology, Neurosurgery, and Psychiatry, 46,* 620–624.

Gass, C. (1991a). MMPI-2 interpretation and closed head injury: A correction factor. *Psychological Assessment: A Journal of Consulting and Clinical Psychology, 3,* 27–31.

Gass, C. (1991b). Emotional variables and neuropsychological test performance. *Journal of Clinical Psychology, 47*(1), 100–104.

Gass, C. (1996). MMPI-2 variables in attention and memory test performance. *Psychological Assessment, 8*(2), 135–138.

Gass, C., & Ansely, J. (1994). MMPI correlates of poststroke neurobehavioral deficits. *Archives of Clinical Neuropsychology, 9*(5), 461–469.

Gass, C., Burda, P., Starkey, T., & Dominguez, F. (1992). MMPI interpretation of psychiatric inpatients: Caution in making inferences about concentration and memory. *Journal of Clinical Psychology, 48*(4), 493–499.

Gass, C., & Daniel, S. (1990). Emotional impact on Trail Making Test performance. *Psychological Reports, 67*(2), 435–438.

Gass, C., & Russell, E. (1986). Differential impact of brain damage and depression on memory test performance. *Journal of Consulting & Clinical Psychology, 54*(2), 261–263.

Gass, C., & Russell, E. (1991). MMPI profiles of closed head trauma patients: Impact of neurologic complaints. *Journal of Clinical Psychology, 47*(2), 253–260.

Gass, C., Russell, E., & Hamilton, R. (1990). Accuracy of MMPI-based inferences regarding memory and concentration in closed-head-trauma patients. *Psychological Assessment, 2*(2), 175–178.

Gass, C., & Wald, H. (1997). MMPI–2 interpretation and closed-head trauma: Cross-validation of a correction factor. *Archives of Clinical Neuropsychology, 12*(3), 199–205.

Greene, R. L. (1991). *The MMPI-2/MMPI: An interpretive manual.* Boston: Allyn and Bacon.

Greiffenstein, M., Gola, T., & Baker, J. (1995). MMPI-2 validity scales versus domain specific measures in detection of factitious traumatic brain injury. *Clinical Neuropsychologist, 9*(3), 230–240.

Helmes, E., & Reddon, J. (1993). A perspective on developments in assessing psychopathology: A critical review of the MMPI and MMPI-2. *Psychological Bulletin, 113*(3), 453–471.

Kay, T. (1992). Neuropsychological diagnosis: Disentangling the multiple determinants of functional disability after mild traumatic brain injury. In L. Horn & N. Zasler (Eds.), *Rehabilitation of post-concussive disorders: Physical medicine and rehabilitation state of the art reviews* (pp. 109–127). Philadelphia: Hanley and Belfus.

Kay, T., Newman, B., Cavallo, M., Ezrachi, O., & Resnick, M. (1992). Toward a neuropsychological model of functional disability after mild traumatic brain injury. *Neuropsychology, 6*, 371–384.

Lees-Haley, P. (1997). MMPI–2 base rates for 492 personal injury plaintiffs: Implications and challenges for forensic assessment. *Journal of Clinical Psychology, 53*(7), 745–755.

Leininger, B. E., Kreutzer, J. S., & Hill, M. R. (1991). Comparison of minor and severe head injury emotional sequelae using the MMPI. *Brain Injury, 5*(2), 199–205.

Love, A., & Peck, C. (1987). The MMPI and psychological factors in chronic low back pain: A review. *Pain, 28*(1), 1–12.

Marsh, G., Hirsch, S., & Leung, G. (1982). Use and misuse of the MMPI in multiple sclerosis. *Psychological Reports, 51*(3, Pt 2), 1127–1134.

Matthews, C., Cleeland, C., & Hopper, C. (1970). Neuropsychological patterns in multiple sclerosis. *Diseases of the Nervous System, 31*(3), 161–170.

Meyerink, L, Reitan, R., & Selz, M. (1988). The validity of the MMPI with multiple sclerosis patients. *Journal of Clinical Psychology, 44*(5), 764–769.

Miller, T., & Kraus, R. (1990). An overview of chronic pain. *Hospital & Community Psychiatry, 41*(4), 433–440.

Morey, L. C. (1991). *Personality Assessment Inventory: Professional manual.* Odessa, FL: Psychological Assessment Resources.

Mueller, S., & Girace, M. (1988). Use and misuse of the MMPI, a reconsideration. *Psychological Reports, 63*(2), 483–491.

Osborne, D. (1985). The MMPI in medical practice. *Psychiatric Annals, 15*(9), 534–541.

Reitan, R., & Wolfson, D. (1997). Emotional disturbances and their interaction with neuropsychological deficits. *Neuropsychology Review, 7*(1), 3–19.

Ruff, R., Mueller, J., & Jurica, P. (1996). Estimating premorbid functioning levels after traumatic brain injury. *Neurorehabilitation, 7*, 39–53.

Schwartz, M., & Krupp, N. (1971). The MMPI "conversion V" among 50,000 medical patients: A study of incidence, criteria, and profile elevation. *Journal of Clinical Psychology, 27*(1), 89–95.

Slick, D., Hopp, G., Strauss, E., & Spellacy, F. (1996). Victoria Symptom Validity Test: Efficiency for detecting feigned memory impairment and relationship to neuropsychological tests and MMPI–2 validity scales. *Journal of Clinical & Experimental Neuropsychology, 18*(6), 911–922.

Spergel, P., Ehrlich, G., & Glass, D. (1978). The rheumatoid arthritic personality: A psychodiagnostic myth. *Psychosomatics, 19*(2), 79–86.

Suhr, J., Tranel, D., Wefel, J., & Barrash, J. (1997). Memory performance after head injury: contributions of malingering, litigation status, psychological factors, and medication use. *Journal of Clinical and Experimental Neuropsychology, 19*(4), 500–514.

White, J. (1996). Review of the Personality Assessment Inventory: A new psychological test for clinical and forensic assessment. *Australian Psychologist, 31*(1), 38–40.

Youngjohn, J. R., Burrows, L., & Erdal, K. (1995). Brain damage or compensation neurosis? The controversial post-concussion syndrome. *Clinical Neuropsychologist, 9*(2), 112–123.

Youngjohn, J. R., Davis, D., & Wolf, I. (1997). Head injury and the MMPI–2: Paradoxical severity effects. *Psychological Assessment, 9*(3), 177–184.

Ziegler, D., & Paolo, A. (1995). Headache symptoms and psychological profile of headache-prone individual: A comparison of clinic patients and controls. *Archives of Neurology, 52*(6), 602–606.

Zielinski, J. (1994). Malingering and defensiveness in the neuropsychological assessment of mild traumatic brain injury. *Clinical Psychology: Science & Practice, 1*(2), 169–184.

Postconcussional Disorder: Background to DSM–IV and Future Considerations

Ronald M. Ruff
University of California, San Francisco

Igor Grant
University of California, San Diego

This chapter is written for two reasons. In the first section, we attempt to shed some light on why the postconcussive disorder was introduced for the first time in the *Diagnostic and Statistical Manual of Mental Disorders*, 4th ed. (*DSM–IV*). The second section addresses a number of issues for consideration in refining the diagnostic criteria for a future *DSM–V*.

PSYCHIATRY'S NOSOLOGY FOR THE POSTCONCUSSIVE DISORDER

At the time when *DSM–IV* was first printed in May 1994, two standardized definitions were available in the literature for the diagnosis of mild traumatic brain injury (MTBI). Two decades earlier, Teasdale and Jennett (1974) introduced the Glasgow Coma Scale, which has been widely used by neurosurgeons. The American Congress of Rehabilitation Medicine (1993) formed a committee that introduced an alternate definition for MTBI. For a more detailed discussion of these definitions, see chapter 7. What led to the psychiatrists establishing yet another definition?

In 1993, a position paper was authored by Brown, Fann, and Grant entitled Postconcussional Disorder: Time to Acknowledge a Common Source of Neurobehavioral Morbidity. This paper relied on a MEDLINE search to examine the research on MTBI conducted between 1986 and 1993. This included a review of the epidemiology, definitions applied, and research findings. The authors concluded that "there are serious consequences to the lack of a proper diagnostic category from postconcussional disorder" (p. 15). The first consequence, according to the authors, was the difficulty of communication among clinicians due to a lack of adequate characterization; second, they emphasized that diagnostic frameworks persist that perpetuated the myth that "milder brain injuries basically are due to many patients exaggerating their complaints because they may be 'hysterical' or because they may be malingerers." Thus, Brown, Fann, and Grant were the first to propose that *DSM–IV* should contain a specific diagnostic category of "Postconcussional Disorder." They concluded their article with specific diagnostic recommendations, which are contained in Table 14.1.

The framework for these criteria is based on three clusters of symptoms: the *somatic* cluster, which can include headaches, fatigue, dizziness (vertigo) and visual or hearing impairments; a *cognitive* cluster, which may be comprised of concentration and memory problems; and an *affective* cluster, which can include irritability, anxiety, and depression. Brown et al. explicitly acknowledged that under A, the criteria selected were arbitrary. However, the authors attempted to find a balance between a "momentary, fleeting loss of consciousness with short amnesia" that might be difficult to

TABLE 14.1
Diagnostic Recommendations for
Postconcussional Disorder (Brown et al., 1993)

A. History of head injury that includes at least two of the following:
   1. Loss of consciousness for 5 min or less.
   2. Posttraumatic amnesia of 12 hr or more.
   3. Onset of seizures (posttraumatic epilepsy) within 6 months of head injury.
B. Current symptoms (these must either be new symptoms or substantially worsening preexisting symptoms) to include:
   1. At least the following two cognitive difficulties:
      a. Learning or memory (recall).
      b. Concentration.
   2. At least three of the following affective or vegetative symptoms:
      a. Easy fatigability.
      b. Insomnia or sleep/wake cycle disturbances.
      c. Headache (substantially worse than before the injury).
      d. Vertigo/dizziness.
      e. Irritability and/or aggression on little or no provocation.
      f. Anxiety, depression, or lability of affect.
      g. Personality change (examples: social or sexual inappropriateness, childlike behavior).
      h. Asponteneity/apathy.
C. Symptoms are associated with a significant difficulty with maintaining premorbid occupational or academic performance, or with a decline in social, occupational, or academic performance.

diagnose reliably and risks Type I errors, and on the other hand missing a significant concussive event through further excessive restrictions (Type II error). Thus, a criteria was set at greater than 5 min of loss of consciousness, and greater than 12 hr of posttraumatic amnesia. Criterion B lists the cognitive, somatic, and affective residua that must be new or significantly increased subsequent to the MTBI. Finally, Criterion C identifies symptoms that must produce some social-occupational disability. Brown, Fann, and Grant concluded their paper by stating the following:

> We argue that there is sufficient research to indicate that postconcussional symptoms occur and that they tend to have a predictable configuration. It is necessary to recognize the existence of "postconcussional disorder" in our nosology in order to provide more prompt diagnosis and management, and to facilitate scholarly communication and research regarding this important neurobehavioral disorder. (p. 21)

All of the opinions just expressed were those of the authors, and were not identical to those established by the American Psychiatric Association task force for *DSM–IV*. Indeed, there was some debate as to whether a postconcussional disorder should be included, because it may encourage litigation or potential misuse. However, this argument was overcome by pointing out that the focus of *DSM* is on classifying patients in a scholarly fashion, and that in doing so this does not enhance or by itself invite misuse or litigation. In the hands of the task force, some changes were made to the criteria outlined in Table 14.1, and the final criteria established by *DSM–IV* are presented in Table 14.2. If one carefully reviews the task force's work, one finds the following changes:

• Criterion A was reduced to a history of head trauma caused by significant cerebral concussion. Specific time parameters for both loss of consciousness and posttraumatic amnesia were no longer firmly stated, yet the manifestation of both remained as criteria. However, in the text a definite threshhold was suggested, and they stated that

for example, should include:
1. a period of unconsciousness lasting more than 5 minutes
2. a period of posttraumatic amnesia that lasts more than 12 hours after the closed head injury, or
3. new onset of seizures (or marked worsening of pre-existing seizure disorder) that occurs within the first six months after a closed head injury.

It was, however, recognized that the onset of seizures is less common.
• Under Criterion B, the cognitive symptoms need to be established based on "evidence from neuropsychological testing or quantified

TABLE 14.2
Research Criteria for Postconcussional Disorder

A. A history of head trauma that has caused significant cerebral concussion. *Note:* The manifestations of concussion include loss of consciousness, posttraumatic amnesia, and, less commonly, posttraumatic onset of seizures. The specific method of defining this criterion needs to be established by further research.

B. Evidence from neuropsychological testing or quantified cognitive assessment of difficulty in attention (concentrating, shifting focus of attention, performing simultaneous cognitive tasks) or memory (learning or recalling information).

C. Three (or more) of the following occur shortly after the trauma and last at least 3 months:
   1. Becoming fatigued easily.
   2. Disordered sleep.
   3. Headache.
   4. Vertigo or dizziness.
   5. Irritability or aggression on little or no provocation.
   6. Anxiety, depression, or affective lability.
   7. Changes in personality (e.g., social or sexual inappropriateness).
   8. Apathy or lack of spontaneity.

D. The symptoms in Criteria B and C have their onset following head trauma or else represent a substantial worsening of preexisting symptoms.

E. The disturbance causes significant impairment in social or occupational functioning and represents a significant decline from a previous level of functioning. In school-age children, the impairment may be manifested by a significant worsening in school or academic performance dating from the trauma.

F. The symptoms do not meet criteria for Dementia Due to Head Trauma and are not better accounted for by another mental disorder (e.g., Amnestic Disorder Due to Head Trauma, Personality Change Due to Head Trauma).

cognitive assessment." The emphasis for the cognitive evaluation remains on attention and memory.

• Under Criterion C, both the somatic and the cognitive issues were maintained with slight changes in wording. An important change that was added was that three or more of the symptoms have to persist for *at least* 3 months.

• Criterion D emphasizes that the symptoms should have their onset following the head trauma, or must represent a substantial worsening of existing symptoms.

• Criterion E is basically similar to Criterion C of Table 14.1.

• Finally, Criterion F was added to review the symptoms and ascertain whether they are not better accounted for by another mental disorder, such as dementia due to head trauma, amnestic disorder due to head trauma, or personality change due to head trauma.

Although these criteria were finally selected, the task force continued to disagree, and the question was raised as to whether the diagnosis for a postconcussive disorder should be established as its own diagnostic category. A compromise was reached that the present diagnosis should first be introduced as a research criterion. All along, the task force considered input from recognized experts, and it also received a number of unsolicited letters. In order to give the reader a flavor of some of the issues that were raised, allow us to quote a few passages from these letters without identifying the authors:

• "Your review of minor head injuries does not distinguish between general outcome vs. outcome in those with complicated recoveries (i.e., early findings in all head injuries vs. persistent difficulties in a fraction of the bigger group). If you are focusing on the fraction of those with complicated recoveries, your review of the literature presents a much more settled picture of the etiology of postconcussional disorder than I believe to be the case. Although people have reported persistent neuropsychological and pathological findings, these types of impairments have not been related to the complaints designated as postconcussional disorders. Furthermore, some of the studies you reference have had difficulties documenting that their findings are head injury related rather than related to pre-existing conditions."

• "I think one of the major issues . . . has to do with the actual time course of the symptoms. . . . In my clinical experience, patients who have suffered a true concussion often show substantial improvements within 3–6 months . . . in contrast, those patients in whom I am convinced there is significant psychiatric overlay and/or are exaggerating their symptoms often state that as much as one to two years after their injuries, some symptoms worsen with the passage of time, rather than getting better."

• "I have often been discouraged with the *DSM–III* classification of neuropsychological impairment . . . for example, the notion of an organic personality syndrome existing in the absence of cognitive impairment, I think is not based on empirical evidence. I have never seen a patient who has affective disturbances who does not also have some associated cognitive disturbance."

• "The postconcussion syndrome is a widespread disorder, with primarily psychiatric symptoms. It is frequently ignored by neurologists who want hard data on which to base their diagnosis. The syndrome has drawn the attention of neuropsychologists who are limited in the tools with which they assess such patients, and of course are markedly limited in their ability to appropriately treat the postconcussion syndrome patient, who usually has many other associated posttraumatic conditions."

• "While I certainly appreciate the need to avoid Type I error, I, too feel that the seizure criteria [are] too restrictive, and may lead to Type II errors. Perhaps replacing [these] criteria with an item using the Glasgow Coma Scale would be more appropriate. This brings up the fundamental question regarding the definition of postconcussional disorder: Should the diagnosis be restricted to only those who have suffered a 'mild traumatic brain injury' or should it encompass all patients with a 'significant' brain injury?"

• "It is important to point out that in the paper from Harvey Levin (The Multigroup Study) that many patients, even though they have appeared to have returned to normal within three months, did not. Normal is simply defined as being within two standard deviations of the mean, and not in terms of prior test results."

• "One of the questions is whether we should accept a further category in which the patient's symptoms are mild, but for example there is an abnormality on CT or MRI vs. patients who do not have positive neuroimaging."

• "Furthermore, it is important to point out that in patients with normal MRI and CT scans, there are a small group of patients, perhaps 10–15%, who have persistent deficits. In a recent PET study by Ron Ruff, abnormalities were demonstrated in patients who were complaining of symptomatology even though they have normal structural imaging studies."

• "Many mild head injured patients with postconcussional symptoms have less than a five minute loss of consciousness, and in fact some cannot document any loss of consciousness. For this reason, the definition of 'concussion' has, in a practical sense, been changing over the years to include a 'change' in consciousness or loss of consciousness. For this reason, I would suggest that you consider (1) changing loss of consciousness for five minutes or more to 'loss or change of consciousness for five minutes or more.' This would allow us to include a significant number of patients who describe a dazed condition or amnesia for many minutes following the accident when there are concomitant reports from others at the scene of the accident who state that the individual was conscious and talking and carrying out activities."

• "The Riml, et al. and Barth, et al. studies, although including patients with up to 20 minutes of unconsciousness, generally evaluated patients with two minutes or less of unconsciousness. The animal studies by Gennerali, I believe, all used two minutes of unconsciousness as a criteria for mild head injury."

• "Posttraumatic amnesia of 12 hours minimum also appears excessive. ... Many of my mild head injury patients who suffer significant postconcussive symptoms report several hours of posttraumatic amnesia, many of which exceed 12 hours. There are others, however, who may report 5–6 hours of true posttraumatic amnesia, yet nonetheless experience significant long term cognitive and emotional deficits. I realize that strict criteria are undoubtedly required here, yet I believe some of the head injury symptoms suggested in Section A could also easily apply to moderate head injury."

ISSUES THAT NEED TO BE SORTED OUT FOR *DSM–V*

Let us raise the key issues that will need to be addressed in order for us to reach a more refined nosology in the future.

What Should Be the Cutoffs for Loss of Consciousness and Posttraumatic Amnesia?

Setting loss of consciousness (LOC), for example, at 5 min or more is recognized as arbitrary. However, for clinicians these arbitrary cutoffs present tremendous hurdles. For example, what is the clinician to do if there is a definite LOC, yet the duration is unknown? It should be noted that in the three-center study (Levin et al., 1987), the authors found that approximately 50% of the 155 patients were unable to quantify the length of their LOC. This is comparable to our clinical experience, because many patients are simply unable to estimate the LOC in exact numbers of minutes. Frequently, MTBI patients are alone at the time of the injury, and even if there are bystanders, these individuals may not have the wherewithal to give a more reliable time estimate of LOC. Moreover, LOC is frequently buried within a posttraumatic amnestic period (PTA). How is the patient going to remember the length of unconsciousness, if the memory for hours after the trauma is gone? The constraints for establishing the duration of PTA are the same as for LOC. How do you remember what you don't remember? Besides, what would be the neuronal mechanism for encoding this information? If we do not come to terms with these limitations for the quantifications of LOC and PTA, we miss the real challenges that diagnosticians face.

Before addressing a potential solution, let us raise one more issue. The literature on MTBI has established that an actual *loss* of consciousness is not the essential criterion for a concussion, but rather the *change or alteration* of consciousness. Thus, it has become generally recognized that a concussion can result subsequent to an altered sense of consciousness (Kay, Newman, Cavallo, Ezrachi, & Resnick, 1992; Ruff et al., 1994). The diagnostic criteria established by the American Congress of Rehabilitation Medicine have incorporated this into their definition. Therefore, the question that will remain pertinent in the future is not whether there was a

TABLE 14.3
Types of MTBI

	Type I	Type II	Type III
LOC	Altered state or transient loss	Definite loss with time unknown or <5 min	Loss 5–30 min
PTA	1–60 sec	60 sec–12 hr	> 12 h
Neurological symptoms	One or more	One or more	One or more

3-, 5-, or 10-min loss of consciousness, but rather, was there an alteration or change of consciousness? However, the question remains whether, for example, an individual who sustains an altered sense of consciousness for a few seconds followed by a few minutes of PTA has the same recovery and outcome as an individual who has a 20-min LOC with over 12 hr of PTA. The literature will have to address this issue, and thus a research diagnosis is called for that will encourage such comparisons. For this reason, we propose (as outlined earlier in chapter 7) that instead of one arbitrary cutoff we consider three types of MTBI (see Table 14.3). Type I corresponds with the more lenient criteria set forth by the American Congress of Rehabilitation Medicine, and Type III represents the more conservative criteria that were selected for *DSM–IV*. Type II bridges these two. Future research may allow us to separate these different types into clinically meaningful categories. Moreover, such a subdivision is superior to having discrepant definitions for the various disciplines.

Is a Concussion the Same as a Postconcussive Disorder?

The simple answer is, of course, no. Both the Glasgow Coma Scale (GCS) and the definition of the American Congress of Rehabilitation Medicine (ACRM) provide the diagnostic criteria for a concussion, whereas *DSM–IV* has established a definition for the postconcussive disorder that can only be diagnosed 3 months postinjury. Once again, this leaves the clinician in a difficult position. How do I diagnose a patient who has had a concussion and presents with significant deficits 2 months after the injury? No doubt, the 3 months represents an arbitrary cutoff, but for the clinician a more fluid and continuous definition would be beneficial. Does it make sense to diagnose a concussion according to either the GCS score or the ACRM criteria, and then 3 months later use a different definition? We think not! The definitions for a concussion and a postconcussive disorder need to be aligned. The term *postconcussional disorder* should refer to the sequelae that follow a concussion. The literature suggests that most MTBI patients present with residuals during the first month, whereas a minority (10%–20%) of these patients present with more chronic difficulties even after 1 year (McLean et al., 1983; Rutherford, Merrett, & McDonald, 1978). Therefore, it may make sense to separate these postconcussive disorders into the following three time parameters: symptom presentation during the first month as *acute*, problems that persist between the first month and 12 months as *subacute*, and *chronic* for a postconcussive disorder that prevails past 1 year. These time parameters would allow us to distinguish the majority of MTBI patients who make a good recovery from the minority with a poor recovery even 1 year posttrauma, that is, the Miserable Minority.

In summary, the entry criteria for a *concussion* should be as follows:

A. History of a mild traumatic brain injury that includes at least one of the following:
   1. Loss or alteration of consciousness; alteration cannot be caused by emotional reaction to trauma.
   2. Posttraumatic amnesia.
   3. Focal neurological deficit.
B. *Postconcussive disorders* refer to somatic, cognitive, and emotional residua that should be classified as follows:
   1. Acute: lasting up to 1 month postinjury.
   2. Subacute: duration greater than 1 month and less than 12 months.
   3. Chronic: greater than 1 year.

What Role Do Preinjury Functioning Levels Play?

DSM–IV Criteria C and D list the typical symptoms that should either have their onset following the brain trauma or else represent a substantial worsening of preexisting symptoms. Thus, it becomes essential that the clinician establish and estimate premorbid functioning levels.

In the literature, preexisting personality types have been identified as making individuals more vulnerable to TBIs (Kay et al., 1993; Ruff, Mueller, & Jurica, 1996). Indeed, premorbid emotional problems are often cited as being the main factor for a poor outcome (Karzmark, Hall, & Englander, 1995). Moreover, preexisting neurological factors can also play a role; prior brain injuries, alcohol abuse, or other neurological illnesses render individuals more vulnerable to the cell loss from a cerebral concussion (Annegers, Grabow, Kurland, & Laws, 1980). If we are to learn why a minority of MTBI patients suffer from chronic postconcussive disorders, it is essential that preexisting vulnerabilities are carefully determined. Age also appears to play a role, in that individuals generally over the age of 40 years have a poorer outcome than those who are younger (Vollmer et al., 1991). For a summary on how preinjury functioning levels can be evaluated, see Ruff, Camenzuli, and Mueller (1996).

What Role Do Comorbid Features Play?

In the literature, it has been pointed out that a concussion frequently coexists with neck injuries, back pain, and even vestibular injuries (Alexander, 1995). Any or all of these can lead to pain. Thus, it is critical that not only the somatic, physical, and emotional residua be clearly delineated, but also that the interaction of residua within and between these areas be examined. For example, a sleep-cycle disturbance can lead to fatigue, which can, in turn, interfere with attention. Kay et al. (1993) eloquently described dysfunctional loops that can persist and even become self-sustaining. Thus, explanations and models need to be evaluated, which would allow us to understand interactions among comorbid features.

Do We Need a Postaccident Disorder?

The preceding recommendations would essentially lead to less stringent criteria for the concussive events, and thus avoid Type II errors. However, in doing so the risk of Type I errors has been increased. Thus, for individuals who present a chronic postconcussive disorder (i.e., over 1 year in duration) and who have been diagnosed with a very mild concussion (e.g., Type I; see Table 14.3), the question should be raised as to whether indeed these difficulties are directly related to the concussion per se. An alternate diagnosis is called for if the symptom presentation can be attributed to comorbid features or explained by premorbid symptoms. However, within these cases it is frequently difficult to ascertain whether the posttraumatic symptoms result primarily from a cerebral concussion, as opposed to an interaction of physical, cognitive, and emotional symptoms that have formed a self-sustaining cluster that was triggered by the accident. Perhaps a new category needs to be developed to capture those individuals whose symptoms are caused by the accident but are not principally attributable to brain damage. The diagnosis of a posttraumatic stress disorder does not apply to many of these patients, because they have no memory of the accident itself (due to LOC or PTA), and thus do not meet the criteria of being traumatized by the accident itself.

REFERENCES

Alexander, M. P. (1995). Mild traumatic brain injury: Pathophysiology, natural history, and clinical management. *Neurology, 45,* 1253–1250.

American Congress of Rehabilitation Medicine. (1993). Definition of mild traumatic brain injury. *Journal of Head Trauma Rehabilitation, 8*(3), 86–87.

Annegers, J. F., Grabow, J. D., Kurland, L. T., & Laws, E. R. (1980). The incidence, causes, and secular trends of head trauma in Olmsed County, Minnesota 1935–1974. *Neurology, 30*, 912–919.

Brown, S. J., Fann, J. R., & Grant, I. (1993). Postconcussional Disorder: Time to acknowledge a common source of neurobehavioral morbidity. *Journal of Neuropsychiatry and Clinical Neurosciences, 6*, 15–22.

Karzmark, P., Hall, K., & Englander, J. (1995). Late-onset post-concussion symptoms after mild brain injury: The role of premorbid, injury-related, environmental and personality factors. *Brain Injury, 9*(1), 21–26.

Kay, T., Newman, B., Cavallo, M., Ezrachi, O., & Resnick, M. (1992). Toward a neuropsychological model of functional disability after mild traumatic brain injury. *Neuropsychology, 6*, 371–384.

Levin, H., Mattis, S., Ruff, R. M., Eisenberg, H. M., Marshall, L. F., Tabaddor, K., High, W. M., & Frankowski, R. F. (1987). Neurobehavioral outcome following minor head injury: a three-center study. *Journal of Neurosurgery, 66*, 234–243.

McLean, A., Temkin, N. R., Dikmen, S., & Wyler, A. R. (1983). The behavioral sequelae of head injury. *Journal of Clinical Neuropsychology, 5*, 361–376.

Ruff, R. M., Crouch, J. A., Tröster, A. I., Buchsbaum, M. S., Lottenberg, S., Somers, L. M., & Marshall, L. F. (1994). Selected cases of poor outcome following minor brain trauma: Comparing neuropsychological and positron emission tomography assessment. *Brain Injury, 8*, 297–308.

Ruff, R. M., Camenzuli, L. F., & Mueller, J. (1996). Miserable Minority: Emotional risk factors that influence the outcome of a mild traumatic brain injury. *Brain Injury, 10*, 551–565.

Ruff, R. M., Mueller, J., & Jurica, P. (1996). Estimation of premorbid functioning after traumatic brain injury. *NeuroRehabilitation, 7*, 39–53.

Rutherford, W. H., Merrett, J. D., & McDonald, J. R. (1978). Symptoms at one year following concussion from minor head injuries. *Injury, 10*, 255–230.

Teasdale, G., & Jennett, B. (1974). Assessment of coma and impaired consciousness: A practical scale. *Lancet, 2*, 81–84.

Vollmer, D. G., Torner, J. C., Jane, J. A., Sadovnik, B., Charlebois, D., Eisenberg, H. M., Foulkes, M. A., Marmarou, A., & Marshall, L. F. (1991). Age and outcome following traumatic coma: Why do older patients fare worse? *Journal of Neurosurgery Report on the Traumatic Coma Data Bank, 75*, 37–49.

Current Controversies
in Mild Head Injury: Scientific
and Methodologic Considerations

Glenn J. Larrabee
Sarasota Memorial Hospital
and
Center for Neuropsychological Studies,
University of Florida

In 1986, Binder reviewed the existing literature on mild head injury (MHI) and concluded that brain damage *sometimes* (his emphasis) could occur as a direct result of MHI. Binder also noted that persistent postconcussion symptoms (PCS) may be maintained by multiple mechanisms, including psychogenic factors, brain injury, and effects of physical trauma not involving the brain (e.g., injury to the neck).

Since Binder's (1986) review, there is an increasing body of research demonstrating that most persons have a good outcome following a single MHI (Dikmen, McLean, & Tempkin, 1986; Levin et al., 1987; Newcombe, Rabbitt, & Briggs, 1994). In the most comprehensive study to date, Dikmen, Machamer, Winn, and Temkin (1995) found that head injury (HI) subjects who took up to 1 hr to follow a doctor's commands following injury (some of whom had computed tomography [CT] abnormalities) did not differ from non-HI orthopedically injured control subjects when examined at 1 year posttrauma.

Binder, Rohling, and Larrabee (1997) conducted a meta-analysis based on data from eight MHI studies (including Dikmen et al., 1995). *Meta-analysis* refers to a variety of procedures that allow aggregation of individual study effect sizes, for subsequent statistical analysis (Rosenthal, 1991). A common technique is to compute effect sizes as the distance between control and experimental (e.g., MHI) sample means in standard deviation units, which can be based on the control group standard deviation, d, or on g, the pooled standard deviation of both groups (Glass, McGaw, & Smith, 1981; Rosenthal, 1991).

The meta-analysis conducted by Binder et al. (1997) comprised 11 samples totaling 314 MHI, and 308 control subjects. Average effect sizes, weighted for sample size, were quite small, with a mean d of .12 ($p < .03$), and a mean g of .07 ($p < .12$). Effect sizes of this magnitude are equivalent to a 2-point change in WAIS–R Full Scale IQ (Wechsler, 1981) or WMS–R (Wechsler, 1987) General Memory Index, which is less than the measurement error of these indices. Analyzed by neuropsychological domain (e.g., attention, memory), only the domain of attention yielded a significant effect size, with a mean d of .20 and a mean g of .17. These effect sizes are equivalent to a 3-point change in WMS–R (Wechsler, 1987) Attention Concentration, again, less than the measurement error of this index. Utilizing a variety of estimating procedures, Binder et al. determined a 5% prevalence of chronic neuropsychological impairment following mild MHI. Employing a predictive value analysis (Baldessarini, Finklestein, & Arana, 1983), Binder et al. demonstrated that neuropsychological assessment was likely to have positive predictive value less than 50%, indicating that clinicians would be more likely to be correct when not diagnosing brain injury than when diagnosing brain injury in cases with chronic disability after MHI.

In a review article accompanying the Binder et al. (1997) meta-analysis, Binder (1997) reviewed 17 studies covering 2,660 MHI subjects, and found that approximately 14% had long-term work disability (2 months to 5 years follow-up). Seven percent to 8% of subjects remained symptomatic on a long-term basis. Considering the meta-analytic data, symptom base rates, and nonneurologic psychosocial factors, Binder suggested that the association between MHI and cognitive deficits, symptoms, and disability may not be causal. Consequently, he argued for a careful differential diagnosis of the MHI patient, in which alternative medical and psychiatric explanations for persistent PCS were considered. Although Binder cautioned against complete dismissal of a neurologic basis to persistent PCS, he noted there was little evidence for neurological causation of most persistent complaints.

Others have argued for a close association between MHI and persistent PCS, and contend that persistent PCS is primarily a neurophysiological disturbance, rather than a psychological response to injury (Szymanski & Linn, 1992). Some have argued for study of "nonimpact" brain injury (Sweeney, 1992), and Varney and Varney (1995) proposed a kinematic model, derived from physics, to estimate g forces in a particular accident in which the subject has not sustained direct trauma to the head. Others have investigated clinic patients with MHI who have persistent complaints following their injury, and demonstrated reduced performance relative to control subjects (Guilmette & Rasile, 1995; Leininger, Gramling, Farrell, Kreutzer, & Peck, 1990).

Ruff (chap. 7, this volume) notes that up to 10% to 20% of the MHI population has a poor outcome, identifying this group as the "Miserable Minority." Ruff calls for a multifactorial approach to evaluating each case, similar, in some respects, to Binder's (1997) suggestions for careful differential diagnosis. Similar views are expressed by Malec (chap. 2, this volume), who notes that 20% to 40% of MHI subjects have residual long-term symptoms or disability. Malec also recommends intensive differential diagnosis, including consideration of malingering. Both Ruff and Malec call for more detailed grading of the severity of MHI than is currently available (e.g., Glasgow Coma Scale [GCS] of 13–15), and encourage research directed at the early identification of those at risk for persistent PCS.

What are the reasons for the apparent differences, on the one hand, between the empirical findings of Dikmen et al. (1995) and Binder et al. (1997) documenting little evidence for persistent deficits, versus the empirical data reported by Guilmette and Rasile (1995) and Leininger et al. (1990)? How can the positions taken by Sweeney (1992) and Szymanski and Linn (1992), suggesting the potential for a neurological basis to persisting complaints in MHI patients, be reconciled with the fact that the Dikmen et al. (1995) MHI subjects, some of whom lost consciousness for up to 1 hr and had CT abnormalities, made full recovery at 1 year? Are these different results due to failure of large-scale investigations such as Dikmen et al. (1995) or Binder et al. (1997) to consider important subgroups of MHI (Ruff's "Miserable Minority"), or are the differences the result of Leininger et al. (1990) or Guilmette and Rasile (1995) studying nonrepresentative, skewed or biased samples?

Differences in research methodology may explain these differing results (Alexander, 1995; Dikmen & Levin, 1993; Stuss, 1995). The majority of the investigations of MHI have focused on neuropsychological methodologies, which rely heavily on symptomatic complaints and neuropsychological test performance. These methods can be quite sensitive to the presence of brain dysfunction, but also can be affected by non-brain-injury psychological and motivational factors that reduce specificity (i.e., result in high false positive errors).

FACTORS RELATED TO SYMPTOMATIC COMPLAINT

There is increasing evidence of a poor association between symptomatic complaint and actual neuropsychological performance in clinical samples. Denial or minimization of deficits (anosognosia) is seen in traumatic brain injury (Prigatano & Altman, 1990; Prigatano, Altman, & O'Brien, 1990); nontraumatic focal left- and right-hemisphere disease (Prigatano, 1996); and Alzheimer-type dementia (Feher, Larrabee, Sudilovsky, & Crook, 1994; Feher, Mahurin, Inbody, Crook, & Pirozzolo, 1991). There is a poor association between the memory complaints of depressed patients and their actual performance (Williams, Little, Scates, & Blockman, 1987). Memory self-assessments by normal healthy elderly are more closely associated with affective distress (Larrabee & Levin, 1986; Larrabee, West, & Crook, 1991) or with degree of somatization (Hanninen et al., 1994) than they are with actual memory test performance.

There is a also a lack of specificity of so-called "postconcussive" symptoms for MHI. Dikmen et al. (1986) were the first to demonstrate the nonspecificity of PCS. Only 3 of 12 symptoms (bothered by noise, insomnia, and memory difficulties) discriminated MHI from controls at 1 month, with no significant MHI/control differences at 1 year posttrauma. Lees-Haley and Brown (1993) found high endorsement rates for PCS-type complaints in outpatients, without history of central nervous system (CNS) disease, being seen in a family practice office (e.g., 62% endorsed "headaches"; 38% endorsed "irritability"; 26% endorsed "difficulty concentrating"). Lees-Haley and Brown (1993) also found that 170 personal injury claimants filing claims for emotional distress or industrial stress, who had no claim for neuropsychological impairment or history of CNS trauma, showed even higher rates of PCS-type symptoms (e.g., 88% had "headaches"; 77% "irritability"; 78% had "difficulty concentrating").

Putnam and Millis (1994) reported similar data in their analysis of MMPI–2 item endorsement by the test normative sample. Forty percent of females and 37% of males complained of forgetting where they left things, and 67% of females and 65% of males endorsed the item "at periods my mind seems to work more slowly than usual" (Butcher, Dahlstrom, Graham, Tellegen, & Kaemmer, 1989). Finally, Mittenberg, Digiulio, Perrin, and Bass (1992) demonstrated that noninjured subjects asked to imagine they sustained a MHI endorsed the same symptom items as were endorsed by actual head trauma patients, suggesting that expectation may play a role in generating PCS.

Altogether these data indicate the inadvisability of selecting for research MHI subjects on the basis of continuing symptomatic complaint. Underscoring this recommendation is the possibility that some MHI patients may be malingering and exaggerating their symptomatic complaints (see chap. 12 by Hayes, Hilsabeck, & Gouvier, this volume). Malingering can take one of three forms including (a) exaggeration or fabrication of symptomatic complaints, (b) deliberately poor performance on cognitive tasks, or (c) both (a) and (b) combined. Regarding symptomatic complaint, the MMPI/MMPI–2 standard validity scales are sensitive to exaggerated psychopathology (Berry et al., 1995; Heaton, Smith, Lehman, & Vogt, 1978), but may miss exaggerated, nonpsychotic, posttraumatic, and emotional and physical symptomatology that is detected by the Fake Bad Scale (FBS) published by Lees-Haley and colleagues (Lees-Haley, English, & Glenn, 1991; Lees-Haley, 1992; also see Larrabee, 1998).

NEUROLOGIC AND NONNEUROLOGIC EFFECTS ON NEUROPSYCHOLOGICAL TEST PERFORMANCE

Motivational effects can also be a factor on neuropsychological testing. Hayes, Hilsabeck, and Gouvier (chap. 12, this volume) discuss several different approaches to evaluation of malingering in detail. I presented (Larrabee, 1990, 1992, 1997) a four-part model for analyzing consistency of test performance, including analysis of consistency between and within test domains, consistency with known neurobehavioral patterns such as amnesia and dementia, consistency of performance with injury severity, and consistency of test performance with a patient's behavior. Although I intended this model for analyzing the data of an individual case, the model can be applied to analysis of research data; in particular the analysis of performance in relation to injury severity.

Financial incentive is a powerful motivator. Rohling, Binder, and Langhinrichsen-Rohling (1995) reported a significant effect size of nearly one-half standard deviation, 0.48, for chronic pain, and Binder and Rohling (1996) reported a very similar financial incentive effect size for head trauma, 0.47, with the largest financial incentive effect sizes seen in MHI. Other data pertinent to the potential nonspecificity of neuropsychological test performance for MHI include the effect size of 0.67 associated with hypertension (Binder et al., 1997; Waldstein, Manuck, Ryan, & Muldoon, 1991).

The already mentioned financial incentive effect sizes can be compared to the well-documented "dose effect" of head trauma—that is, the association of more pronounced long-term impairment with greater initial severity of trauma (Levin, Benton, & Grossman, 1982). Dikmen et al. (1995) presented data on the largest cohort of subjects covering the greatest severity range, with the most comprehensive assessment, best selected control groups, and a minimal 1 year attrition rate. Binder et al. (1997) computed effect sizes based on g (the pooled standard deviation of control and head trauma severity groups) for the Dikmen et al. subjects, with "time to follow commands" the severity indicator. These effect sizes, as a function of injury, were: less than 1 hr, 0.02; 1–24 hr, 0.23; 2–5 days, 0.45; 6–13 days, 0.69; 14–28 days, 1.33; and 29 days or more, 2.30. As I noted (Larrabee, 1997), the effect size for the Leininger et al. (1990) MHI cases, half of whom did not lose consciousness, was 0.57, equivalent to the effect size of the Dikmen et al. group experiencing between 1 to 2 weeks of coma.

A similar comparison can be made for the data reported by Guilmette and Rasile (1995). The effect size, g, for this study was -1.10, more than one standard deviation. Hence, the performance of the Guilmette and Rasile MHI group, none of whom had loss of consciousness over 30 min or posttraumatic amnesia (PTA) beyond 24 hr, yielded an effect size equivalent to that produced by the Dikmen et al. (1995) group with 2 to 4 weeks of coma. Because Guilmette and Rasile specifically studied verbal memory, the effect size from their study can also be compared to the effect size for the Verbal Selective Reminding Test in the Dikmen et al. (1995) research. Again, the Guilmette and Rasile value of 1.10 falls closest to the Selective Reminding effect size of 1.25, characterizing the Dikmen et al. group that sustained between 2 and 4 weeks of coma.

Hence, the Leininger et al. (1990) and Guilmette and Rasile (1995) MHI subjects, chosen on the basis of persisting complaint, produced effect sizes equivalent to subjects who experienced between 1 and 4 weeks of coma. An inconsistency of this magnitude suggests that factors other than head trauma may be responsible for the poor performance of these subjects. Both Leininger et al. (1990) and Guilmette and Rasile (1995) considered the possibility of motivational factors. Leininger et al. analyzed their subjects on the basis of who was pursuing litigation. Only one of eight differences was significant, and failed to reach significance after Bonferroni correction; however, the sample sizes were quite small and were unequal (MHI in litigation = 39; nonlitigating = 14).

Guilmette and Rasile (1995) tested all MHI subjects in litigation for presence of malingering on a forced-choice symptom validity procedure, and all exceeded a predetermined performance cutoff for malingering. These authors did not experimentally or statistically match MHI with controls on level of performance on the forced choice procedure. Hence, they were unable to control for more subtle motivational effects that may have been present.

The preceding analysis of effect sizes, comparing "symptomatic" subjects (Guilmette & Rasile, 1995; Leininger et al., 1990) with subjects studied prospectively (Dikmen et al., 1995), raises questions about the specificity of neuropsychological test scores to persistent deficits in MHI. The following sections consider factors that may predispose a MHI patient to persistent deficits, followed by consideration of future research on MHI.

FACTORS POTENTIALLY RELATED TO PERSISTENT DEFICITS FOLLOWING MILD TBI

Certain injury variables may predispose a MHI patient to more prolonged recovery and/or to persistent problems on a neurologic basis. Certain subject variables may predispose a particular patient to more prolonged symptomatology on a psychological basis.

Injury Variables

For a small percentage of subjects, persistency of deficit may be related to neurologic factors. Levin, Williams, Eisenberg, High, and Guinto (1992) found that some patients who had previously demonstrated MRI abnormalities following mild to moderate head injury could have continuing reduction in neuropsychological performance despite radiologic disappearance of the lesion. They speculated that this could represent persisting abnormality, and recommended that metabolic imaging might prove useful in clarifying the pathophysiologic basis of the persisting sequelae.

Wilson, Teasdale, Hadley, Wiedmann, and Lang (1993) found that some persons could sustain brief loss of consciousness, yet suffer posttraumatic amnesia (PTA) of more than 1 week. Duration of coma correlated at .83 with initial GCS; however, coma duration only correlated .50 with duration of PTA. Patients with coma over 6 hr demonstrated a greater concordance of coma duration with duration of PTA; however, eight patients in coma for less than 6 hr had PTA of over 1 week. Three of these eight had only brief loss of consciousness. These data indicate that both GCS and duration of PTA should be used to rank trauma severity, because some head trauma that appears to be "mild" by GCS may actually have suffered more severe injury, as indicated by a period of protracted PTA.

The presence of preexisting MHI is believed by some to result in longer recovery time from subsequent MHI (Gronwall, 1989; Gronwall & Wrightson, 1975). This would be consistent with the hypothesis that repetitive MHI may have a cumulative effect. In contrast, Bijur, Haslum, and Golding (1996) did not find evidence for cumulative effect of MHI, comparing children with one, two, or three MHIs with non-head-injured orthopedic trauma controls. Bijur et al. interpreted their data as suggesting that cognitive deficits associated with multiple MHI are secondary to social and personal factors related to multiple injuries, rather than resulting from damage to the head.

If multiple MHI may have a cumulative effect, then a single MHI might cause a reduction in what Satz (1993) has termed "brain reserve capacity." Support for presence of reduced cerebral reserve, apparent under increased physiological stress, is provided by Ewing, McCarthy, Gronwall, and Wrightson (1980), who found evidence for persisting cognitive deficits in apparently recovered MHI subjects who were subjected to hypoxic stress. An hypothesis of reduced cerebral reserve is contradicted, however, by data reported by Alterman, Goldstein, Shelly, and Bober (1985), who found no significant neuropsychological performance differences between alcoholic subjects with and without history of MHI. The findings of Alterman et al. (1985) are supported by Dikmen, Donovan, Loberg, Machamer, and Tempkin (1993), who found no significant interactions

between alcohol use and head trauma severity in relationship to neuropsychological outcome. Also arguing against reduced cerebral reserve are
data reported by Bornstein et al. (1993), who found no significant differences between HIV positive subjects with and without history of MHI.

Subject Variables

Age may also predispose to longer recovery and to greater potential for
persistent deficits following mild to moderate head injury. Goldstein et
al. (1994) found that 22 older patients (mean age 67.8 years), examined
within 7 months of having sustained a mild ($n = 6$) or moderate ($n = 16$)
head trauma, produced significantly lower neuropsychological performances relative to demographically similar control subjects. Goldstein et
al. (1994) recommended additional research on long-term outcome of
mild/moderate head injury in the aged, including evaluation of potential
for increased risk of Alzheimer-type dementia (AD).

Subsequently, Goldstein et al. (1996) compared the neuropsychological
performance of 14 older adults with mild ($n = 2$) and moderate ($n = 12$)
HI, with the performance of 14 patients suffering the early stages of AD,
and with that of 14 demographically matched controls. The HI subjects
and AD subjects did not differ significantly from one another on the
Mini-Mental State (MMSE), with mean scores of 25.4 and 23.5, respectively. Both patient groups performed significantly less well than the
controls. HI patients showed better overall memory performance than
AD patients, and demonstrated better semantic relative to phonemic
fluency performance, a pattern not evident in AD.

These data reported by Goldstein et al. (1994, 1996), are suggestive of
potential for greater morbidity in older subjects suffering MHI. Additional
research is needed, however, to evaluate long-term residual effects in mild
versus moderate MHI. Both of the Goldstein et al. investigations combined
mild and moderate head injury in one group, and the groups were heavily
weighted with more severely injured patients (i.e., 73% of the Goldstein
et al., 1994, subjects had moderate MHI, and 86% of the Goldstein et al.,
1996, subjects had moderate MHI). Also, the majority of subjects were
examined in the subacute stages of recovery; for example, 19 of the 22
subjects in Goldstein et al. (1994) were studied within 3 months of injury,
and the 14 HI subjects in Goldstein et al. (1996) were tested an average
of 31 days postinjury. Hence, the Goldstein et al. (1994, 1996) investigations do not provide evidence on the relationship of increased age to
long-term persistence of deficits following MHI.

Binder (1997) extensively reviewed a variety of neurologic and nonneurologic factors related to differential diagnosis of the effects of MHI.
This review considered several nonneurologic factors related to symp-

tomatic complaint and neuropsychological test performance, including the presence of premorbid psychosocial dysfunction, occupational and educational status, premorbid learning disability, personal and family history of alcoholism, depression, anxiety, somatoform disorder, and malingering. In particular, Binder emphasized the nonspecificity of both symptomatic complaint and neuropsychological test performance, a point also made in this chapter.

Two papers reviewed by Binder are particularly illuminating. Fenton, McClelland, Montgomery, MacFlynn, and Rutherford (1993) found that MHI patients had more frequent adverse life events than case controls in the year preceding their injury. Patients with persistent PCS had more chronic social difficulties than those with MHI who had fully recovered, and persistent PCS was more likely in older, female subjects. Fenton et al. concluded that the emergence and persistence of PCS are associated with social adversity before the accident, and that although young males are at greatest risk of MHI, older women are at greater risk for persistent PCS.

Alexander (1992) studied HI patients grouped as mild (length of coma less than 15 min; length of PTA less than 24 hr) versus moderate to severe (length of coma greater than 15 min; duration of PTA greater than 24 hr). The mild group had no genuine neurologic abnormalities on motor examination; however, 26% of the mild also had unequivocally feigned deficits (not seen at all in the severe cases). Mild cases showed significantly greater depression and headache, compared to severely injured patients.

Other investigators have emphasized the role of somatization in maintenance of PCS. Mittenberg et al. (1992) draw directly from the literature on somatization and proposed a model whereby mild TBI patients reattribute benign emotional, physiological, and memory symptoms to their injury, with symptom expectancies biasing selective attention to internal states, interacting with autonomic/emotional responses. Putnam and Millis (1994) drew a parallel between the self-directed selective attention suggested by Mittenberg et al. (1992) and the self-directed selective attention to bodily sensations in persons with elevated bodily concerns (see Watson & Pennebaker, 1989), arguing that persistent PCS is best conceptualized as a type of somatoform disorder.

Based on their earlier research on expectation effects and PCS in MHI, Mittenberg and colleagues (Mittenberg, Tremont, Zielinski, Fichera, & Rayls, 1996) reported a successful cognitive behavioral treatment program for PCS. This program involved a detailed treatment manual intended to support reattribution of symptoms to selective attention, transient responses to stress, and anxiety-arousing or depressive self-statements, rather than to brain injury. Additionally, it was emphasized that the goal of treatment was not to render patients "asymptomatic," because the symptoms normally occur with a certain frequency in noninjured persons (cf. Lees-Haley & Brown, 1993; Mittenberg et al., 1992; Putnam & Millis, 1994). This treatment program resulted in shorter average symptom duration, and significantly fewer symptoms at 6 months posttrauma for treated versus nontreated MHI subjects.

The somatization explanation of persistent PCS offered by Mittenberg et al. (1992) and Putnam and Millis (1994) is compelling, and renders PCS amenable to treatment, as demonstrated by Mittenberg et al. (1996). The somatization explanation of PCS also illustrates the significant negative iatrogenic potential of misdiagnosing a MHI patient with "brain damage," when symptoms and test performance can be accounted for by nonneurologic factors.

FUTURE RESEARCH

The Binder et al. (1997) finding of a 5% prevalence of neuropsychological impairment, Binder's (1997) empirical estimate of 7% to 8% persisting symptoms and work disability of 14%, Ruff's estimate (chap. 7, this volume) of 10% to 20% with persisting complaints (the "Miserable Minority"), and Malec's (chap. 2, this volume) estimate of 20% to 40% of MHI with persistent complaints support continued research on the outcome of MHI. The nonspecificity of both symptoms and test performance demonstrated in the current chapter underscores the need for well-controlled research designs.

The optimal research design should follow MHI subjects prospectively, from the time of their injury, as well as follow an orthopedic trauma control group. In this fashion, MHI and controls should be generally equivalent on every aspect (e.g., preinjury demographic and socioeconomic factors related to trauma; experience of physical trauma requiring hospitalization; pain; psychological reaction to trauma; proportion of the sample in litigation), with the exception of presence/absence of head injury. To date, the only investigation of adults that has met these criteria, with the additional benefit of limited attrition on long-term follow-up, is the Dikmen et al. (1995) outcome study. Absence of persisting effect of MHI has also been reported for children, contrasting MHI with non-head-injured orthopedic trauma controls (Asarnow et al., 1995).

In addition to conducting in-depth neuropsychological evaluation, measures of personality and motivational status should be included. The work of Fenton et al. (1993) demonstrates the need to obtain detailed preinjury psychosocial assessment, a point emphasized by Binder (1997) in his recent review paper; in other words, greater attention must be paid to the effects of nonneurologic variables on the production and maintenance of chronic complaints following MHI.

Studies that evaluate persons with persistent complaints only, who have not been followed prospectively, run the risk of studying a skewed, nonrepresentative sample. This was illustrated in this chapter by comparison of the effect sizes for the Leininger et al. (1990) and Guilmette and Rasile (1995) investigations, with effect sizes for the full spectrum of head trauma severity reported by Dikmen et al. (1995). Thus, there is no clearly apparent logical or scientific rationale to account for why the Leininger et al. (1990) MHI subjects, half of whom did not even lose consciousness, or the Guilmette and Rasile (1995) MHI patients, who had less than 30 min loss of consciousness, should perform at a level similar to the Dikmen et al. (1995) subjects who had experienced 1 to 2 or 2 to 4 weeks of coma.

Consequently, it is better to study Ruff's "miserable minority" in the context of prospective follow-up, as a true subset of the majority of MHI patients who show good recovery. This subset could be identified via predetermined objective criteria (e.g., greater than one *SD* below control mean performance) or through a posteriori cluster analysis of the total MHI sample at 1-year follow-up.

Any investigator wishing to study symptomatic MHI subjects in a clinical investigation should follow the same strategy as suggested for prospective investigation: use of orthopedic trauma controls, matched on demographic factors. In addition, it is essential that nonprospective research on symptomatic MHI match the performance of control and MHI patients on tasks such as the Portland Digit Recognition Test (Binder & Willis, 1991), to control for the effects of motivation on neuropsychological outcome measures. It is not sufficient to exclude subjects whose performance falls below preestablished cutoffs for malingering, because the MHI group may still contain subjects with suboptimal motivation of subclinical severity. Use of orthopedic trauma controls would also provide some control for effects of chronic pain, a variable related to chronic complaints and to test performance in MHI (Alexander, 1992; Taylor, Cox, & Mailis, 1996; Uomoto & Esselman, 1993). Indeed, Taylor et al. (1996) found no group differences on the Paced Auditory Serial Addition Test (PASAT) or Consonant Trigrams when whiplash patients without direct trauma to the head or loss of consciousness were compared to moderate/severe TBI, or to patients with chronic pain syndrome without history of head injury. These findings bear directly on the viability of the construct of "whiplash brain damage" (cf. Sweeney, 1992).

Redefining Severity of MHI

The papers by Levin et al. (1992) and Wilson et al. (1993) illustrate that for some patients, persistent PCS may be related to neurological variables. The Wilson et al. paper underscores the value of using both GCS and duration of PTA in classifying trauma severity. The Levin et al. paper demonstrates the value of early MRI, and highlights the need for concomitant functional neuroimaging studies such as positron emission tomography (PET) or single-photon emission computed tomography (SPECT).

Actually, one could legitimately argue that we are missing more accurate identification of MHI persons at risk for persistent PCS, because of inadequate characterization of initial severity, and/or because of inadequate measurement of outcome.

Ruff (chap. 7, this volume) proposes subclassifying MHI by severity as Type I (altered state or transient loss of consciousness; PTA 1–60 sec; one or more neurological symptoms); Type II (definite loss of consciousness of unknown duration or less than 5 min; PTA of 60 sec to 12 hr; one or more neurological symptoms); and Type III (loss of consciousness 5–30 min; PTA greater than 12 hr; one or more neurological symptoms). Malec (chap. 2, this volume) discusses the American Academy of Neurology criteria for grading severity of sports concussion with and without loss of consciousness.

Subdividing MHI by severity is also supported by Culotta, Sementilli, Gerold, and Watts (1996), who found greater need for neurosurgical intervention, more computed tomography (CT) scan abnormalities, and increased incidence of skull fractures in patients with Glasgow Coma Scale (GCS) of 13, compared to GCS of 14. Patients with GCS of 14 had greater morbidity than patients with GCS of 15. Culotta et al. recommended segregating MHI subjects with GCS of 15 from those with scores of 14 and 13.

Varney and Varney (1995; also see chap. 3 by R. Varney and Roberts, this volume) have proposed a novel means of grading severity of head trauma by estimating, via a kinematic formula, the acceleration experienced by the occupants of motor vehicles (and their heads) during collisions. None of the cases reported by Varney and Varney (1995) suffered direct head-contact trauma, but all suffered neurologic and/or neuropsychological injuries typical of patients with closed head trauma. Case 1 of their series sustained an estimated acceleration between 67 g and 101 g, followed by a brief loss of consciousness, 24 hr of severe confusion and disorientation (she did not recognize her husband or family members), 5 days of PTA, and had CT evidence of a parenchymal hemorrhage in the anterior right temporal lobe. Although this case would be best characterized as a moderate MHI, given the CT findings and duration of PTA, most of the cases reported by Varney and Varney would fall in the category of MHI.

Thus, refining means of estimating severity of MHI may be helpful in identifying patients at risk for persistent deficits; however, it is important that any proposed schema for grading MHI demonstrate a "dose effect."

That is, MHI patients with Ruff's (chap. 7, this volume) Type I injury should perform better on neuropsychological tests and have fewer chronic PCS than patients with Type II injury, who should show better outcome than those with Type III. Employing the Varney and Varney schema, there should be a negative correlation between estimated g force and neuropsychological performance, and a positive correlation between g force and acute posttraumatic symptomatology. Moreover, the g force estimates should increase across the full range of head trauma severity (i.e., mild, moderate and severe), demonstrate stronger correlations with depth and extent of neuroradiologically defined lesions than are currently demonstrated with GCS (Levin et al., 1988), and have stronger correlations with neuropsychological tests than demonstrated between neuropsychological tests and time to follow commands (Dikmen et al., 1995).

Novel Measures of Outcome in MHI

Technologically enhanced measures of electrophysiologic activity such as signal-averaged, fast-Fourier-transformed electroencephalograph (EEG) (quantitative or QEEG), and functional neuroimaging such as single-photon emission computed tomography (SPECT; Holman & Devous, 1992), have been considered as measures of outcome in MHI. These new methodologies are of particular interest because they can provide measures of actual neurophysiological function and intuitively should be less affected by the motivational state of the patient (i.e., they should be more "objective").

QEEG abnormalities have been identified in MHI patients 3–10 days posttrauma (Tebano et al., 1988) and, on average, 8 days posttrauma (Thatcher, Walker, Gerson, & Geisler, 1989). These initial findings, in the acute stages of recovery, are of interest; however, neither set of investigators correlated QEEG findings with neuropsychological measures of memory and information processing, which also would have been expected to show abnormalities at 1 week post MHI. Hence, the incremental validity of QEEG over established neuropsychological procedures cannot be evaluated.

Thatcher et al. (1989) reported an impressive 94.8% correct hit rate for discriminating 83 normal from 264 MHI patients. They provided additional cross-validations of the QEEG discriminant function, but the cross-validations are incomplete. The first cross-validation used the same controls, with a new sample of MHI, rather than independent control and experimental subjects. The second cross-validation utilized 144 outpatients ranging from 6 to 624 days posttrauma, with no control subjects, and obtained an 87.5% hit rate (*note*: without a control group, identifying all cases as MHI would have resulted in a 100% hit rate). The third cross-validation included 70 MHI and 4 normals, resulting in 95.2% accuracy (note: with the imbalance in experimental and control group sizes, merely identifying all subjects as MHI would have resulted in a 94.6% hit rate).

SPECT has been demonstrated to be more sensitive to residual focal lesions in severe head trauma than CT scan and magnetic resonance imaging (MRI), either alone or in combination (Gray, Ichise, Chung, Kirsh, & Franks, 1992; Newton et al., 1992). SPECT showed a "dose effect" in a prospective investigation of mild and moderate HI (Jacobs, Put, Ingels, & Bossuyt, 1994). Moderate HI patients showed more SPECT abnormalities (60% of patients) than mild HI patients (36% of patients), with both groups studied a maximum of 4 weeks posttrauma. Initial SPECT abnormalities were predictive of continuing symptoms at 3-month follow-up for mild and moderate HI. Mild to moderate HI patients with initially normal SPECT had better outcome at 3-month follow-up, for a predictive value of 97% for a favorable outcome.

These results show the potential value of SPECT and QEEG; however, much additional research is needed to establish these techniques as routine procedures sensitive to the effect of MHI. First, any new technology for measuring brain function should demonstrate the characteristic "dose effect" of poorer function associated with more severe initial injury, at a level equal to or superior to that established for neuropsychological tests (Dikman et al., 1995; Levin et al., 1982). Second, novel functional neuroimaging procedures should also correlate in a meaningful manner with established neuropsychological measures (following adjustment for relevant demographic factors)—in particular, tests of memory and information processing—in groups of patients representing the full spectrum of severity of MHI, with follow-up over 1 year posttrauma, to evaluate chronic effects. Finally, novel neuroimaging and neurophysiologic measures must show specificity for MHI—that is, show results that discriminate MHI from other conditions known to affect neuropsychological test performance, including attention deficit disorder, learning disability, depression, anxiety and other primary psychiatric disturbance, personal and/or family history of alcohol abuse, and any other condition known to have potential for alteration of neurobehavioral processes.

The problem of poor specificity is precisely the reason why major professional groups have not recommended the routine clinical or forensic use of QEEG, positron emission tomography (PET), and SPECT in mild MHI (American Academy of Neurology, 1989, 1996, 1997; Society of Nuclear Medicine Brain Imaging Council, 1996). In this vein, Deutsch (1992), in a review of the frontal cerebral blood flow literature, concluded that reduction of frontal lobe physiological activity was frequently secondary to an altered pattern of mental activity, rather than representative of pathology in the frontal lobes. In normal subjects engaged in demanding cognitive tasks requiring vigilance, directed attention, set shifting, and decision making, frontal blood flow typically increases. During passive stimulation, with no particular task demand or stimulus induced mental activity, Deutsch noted a drop in frontal blood flow. It is intriguing to consider how these cerebral blood flow data may reflect nonneurologic attentional and motivational activity, and correlate with other neuroimaging methodologies focusing on level of frontal lobe activity in MHI.

CONCLUSIONS

This chapter provides a scientific and methodological critique of research on MHI. Although sufficient data exist to justify continued research on the effects of MHI, particularly focusing on the "Miserable Minority" who have persisting complaints, careful attention is required to experimental design, control of neurologic and nonneurologic factors, and issues of sensitivity and specificity. In closing, we must keep in mind Stuss's caution, in an editorial accompanying Alexander's (1995) review of MHI, that "everything must make sense" (Stuss, 1995, p. 1251).

ACKNOWLEDGMENTS

The author gratefully acknowledges Dr. Laurence M. Binder for his review of this chapter, and the assistance of Susan M. Towers, Kristin Kravitz and the Medical Library of Sarasota Memorial Hospital in its preparation.

REFERENCES

Alexander, M. P. (1992). Neuropsychiatric correlates of persistent postconcussive syndrome. *Journal of Head Trauma Rehabilitation, 7*, 60–69.

Alexander, M. P. (1995). Mild traumatic brain injury: Pathophysiology, natural history, and clinical management. *Neurology, 45*, 1253–1260.

Alterman, A. I., Goldstein, G., Shelly, C., & Bober, B. (1985). The impact of mild head injury on neuropsychological capacity in chronic alcoholics. *International Journal of Neuroscience, 28*, 155–162.

American Academy of Neurology, Therapeutics and Technology Assessment Subcommittee. (1989). Assessment: EEG brain mapping. *Neurology, 39*, 1100–1102.

American Academy of Neurology, Therapeutics and Technology Assessment Subcommittee. (1996). Assessment of brain SPECT. *Neurology, 46*, 278–285.

American Academy of Neurology, Therapeutics and Technology Subcommittee. (1997). Assessment of digital EEG, quantitative EEG, and EEG brain mapping: Report of the

American Academy of Neurology and the American Clinical Neurophysiology Society. *Neurology, 49*, 277–292.

Asarnow, R. F., Satz, P., Light, R., Zaucha, K., Lewis, R., & McCleary, C. (1995). The UCLA study of mild closed head injury in children and adolescents. In S. H. Broman & M. E. Michel (Eds.), *Traumatic head injury in children* (pp. 117–146). New York: Oxford University Press.

Baldessarini, R. J., Finklestein, S., & Arana, G. W. (1983). The predictive power of diagnostic tests and the effects of prevalence of illness. *Archives of General Psychiatry, 40*, 569–573.

Berry, D. T. R., Wetter, M. W., Baer, R. A., Youngjohn, J. R., Gass, C. S., Lamb, D. G., Franzen, M. D., MacInnes, W. D., & Bucholz, D. (1995). Overreporting of closed head injury symptoms on the MMPI-2. *Psychological Assessment, 7*, 517–523.

Bijur, P. E., Haslum, M., & Golding, J. (1996). Cognitive outcome of multiple mild head injuries in children. *Developmental and Behavioral Pediatrics, 17*, 143–148.

Binder, L. M. (1986). Persisting symptoms after mild head injury. A review of the postconcussive syndrome. *Journal of Clinical and Experiemental Neuropsychology, 8*, 323–346.

Binder, L. M. (1997). A review of mild head trauma. Part II: Clinical implications. *Journal of Clinical and Experimental Neuropsychology, 19*, 432–457.

Binder, L. M., & Rohling, M. L. (1996). Money matters: A meta-analytic review of the effects of financial incentives on recovery after closed head injury. *American Journal of Psychiatry, 153*, 5–8.

Binder, L. M., Rohling, M. L., & Larrabee, G. J. (1997). A review of mild head trauma. Part I: Meta-analytic review of neuropsychological studies. *Journal of Clinical and Experimental Neuropsychology, 19*, 421–431.

Binder, L. M., & Willis, S. C. (1991). Assessment of motivation after financially compensable minor head trauma. *Psychological Assessment, 3*, 175–181.

Bornstein, R. A., Podraza, A. M., Para, M. F., Whitacre, C. C., Fass, R. J., Rice, R. R., & Nasrallah, H. A. (1993). Effect of minor head injury on neuropsychological performance in asymptomatic HIV-1 infection. *Neuropsychology, 7*, 228–234.

Butcher, J. N., Dahlstrom, W. G., Graham, J. R., Tellegen, A., & Kaemmer, B. (1989). *Minnesota Multiphasic Personality Inventory-2 (MMPI-2): Manual for administration and scoring.* Minneapolis: University of Minnesota Press.

Culotta, V. P., Sementilli, M. E., Gerold, K., & Watts, C. C. (1996). Clinicopathological heterogeneity in the classification of mild head injury. *Neurosurgery, 38*, 245–250.

Deutsch, G. (1992). The nonspecificity of frontal dysfunction in disease and altered states: Cortical blood flow evidence. *Neuropsychiatry, Neuropsychology, and Behavioral Neurology, 5*, 301–307.

Dikmen, S. S., Donovan, D. M., Loberg, T., Machamer, J. E., & Temkin, N. R. (1993). Alcohol use and its effects on neuropsychological outcome in head injury. *Neuropsychology, 7*, 296–305.

Dikmen, S. S., & Levin, H. S. (1993). Methodological issues in the study of mild head injury. *Journal of Head Trauma Rehabilitation, 8*, 30–37.

Dikmen, S. S., Machamer, J. E., Winn, H. R., & Temkin, N. R. (1995). Neuropsychological outcome at 1-year post head injury. *Neuropsychology, 9*, 80–90.

Dikmen, S. S., McLean, A., & Temkin, N. (1986). Neuropsychological and psychosocial consequences of minor head injury. *Journal of Neurology, Neurosurgery, and Psychiatry, 49*, 1227–1232.

Ewing, R., McCarthy, C., Gronwall, D., & Wrightson, P. (1980). Persisting effects of minor head injury observable during hypoxic stress. *Journal of Clinical Neuropsychology, 2*, 147–155.

Feher, E. P., Larrabee, G. J., Sudilovsky, A., & Crook, T. H. (1994). Memory self-report in Alzheimer's disease and in age-associated memory impairment. *Journal of Geriatric Psychiatry and Neurology, 7*, 58–65.

Feher, E. P., Mahurin, R. K., Inbody, S. B., Crook, T. H., & Pirozzolo, F. J. (1991). Anosognosia in Alzheimer's disease. *Neuropsychiatry, Neuropsychology, and Behavioral Neurology, 4,* 136–146.

Fenton, G., McClelland, R., Montgomery, A., MacFlynn, G., & Rutherford, W. (1993). The postconcussional syndrome: Social antecedents and psychological sequelae. *British Journal of Psychiatry, 162,* 493–497.

Glass, G. V., McGaw, B., & Smith, M. L. (1981). *Meta-analysis in social research.* Newbury Park: Sage.

Goldstein, F. C., Levin, H. S., Presley, R. M., Searcy, J., Colohan, A. R. T., Eisenberg, H. M., Jann, B., & Bertolino-Kusnerik, L. (1994). Neurobehavioral consequences of closed head injury in older adults. *Journal of Neurology, Neurosurgery and Psychiatry, 57,* 961–966.

Goldstein, F. C., Levin, H. S., Roberts, V. J., Goldman, W. P., Kalechstein, A. S., Winslow, M., & Goldstein, S. J. (1996). Neuropsychological effects of closed head injury in older adults: A comparison with Alzheimer's disease. *Neuropsychology, 10,* 147–154.

Gray, B. G., Ichise, M., Chung, D. G., Kirsh, J. C., & Franks, W. (1992). Technetium-99*m*-HMPAO SPECT in the evaluation of patients with a remote history of traumatic brain injury: A comparison with x-ray computed tomography. *Journal of Nuclear Medicine, 33,* 52–58.

Gronwall, D. (1989). Cumulative and persisting effects of concussion on attention and cognition. In H. S. Levin, H. M. Eisenberg, & A. L. Benton (Eds.), *Mild head injury* (pp. 153–162). New York: Oxford University Press.

Gronwall, D., & Wrightson, P. (1975). Cumulative effect of concussion. *Lancet, 2,* 995–997.

Guilmette, T. J., & Rasile, D. (1995). Sensitivity, specificity and diagnostic accuracy of three verbal memory measures in the assessment of mild brain injury. *Neuropsychology, 9,* 338–344.

Hanninen, T., Reinikainen, K. J., Helkala, E.-L., Koivisto, K., Mykkaren, L., Laakso, M., Pyorala, K., & Riekkinen, P. J. (1994). Subjective memory complaints and personality traits in normal elderly subjects. *Journal of the American Geriatric Society, 42,* 1–4.

Heaton, R. K., Smith, H. H., Jr., Lehman, R. A., & Vogt, A. J. (1978). Prospects for faking believable deficits on neuropsychological testing. *Journal of Consulting and Clinical Psychology, 46,* 892–900.

Holman, B. L., & Devous, M. D. (1992). Functional brain SPECT: The emergence of a powerful clinical method. *Journal of Nuclear Medicine, 33,* 1888–1904.

Jacobs, A., Put, E., Ingels, M., & Bossuyt, A. (1994). Prospective evaluation of technetium-99*m*-HMPAO SPECT in mild and moderate traumatic brain injury. *Journal of Nuclear Medicine, 35,* 942–947.

Larrabee, G. J. (1990). Cautions in the use of neuropsychological evaluation in legal settings. *Neuropsychology, 4,* 239–247.

Larrabee, G. J. (1992). Interpretive strategies for evaluation of neuropsychological data in legal settings. *Forensic Reports, 5,* 257–264.

Larrabee, G. J. (1997). Neuropsychological outcome, post concussion symptoms and forensic considerations in mild closed head injury. *Seminars in Clinical Neuropsychiatry, 2,* 196–206.

Larrabee, G. J. (1998). Somatic malingering on the MMPI and MMPI-2 in personal injury litigants. *The Clinical Neuropsychologist, 12,* 179–188.

Larrabee, G. J., & Levin, H. S. (1986). Memory self-ratings and objective test performance in a normal elderly sample. *Journal of Clinical and Experimental Neuropsychology, 8,* 275–284.

Larrabee, G. J., West, R. L., & Crook, T. H. (1991). The association of memory complaint with everyday memory performance. *Journal of Clinical and Experimental Neuropsychology, 13,* 484–496.

Lees-Haley, P. R. (1992). Efficacy of MMPI-2 validity scales and MCMI-II modifier scales for detecting spurious PTSD claims: F, F-K, Fake Bad Scale, Ego Strength, Subtle-Obvious Subscales, Dis, and DEB. *Journal of Clinical Psychology, 48,* 681–688.

Lees-Haley, P. R., & Brown, R. S. (1993). Neuropsychological complaint base rates of 170 personal injury claimants. *Archives of Clinical Neuropsychology, 8,* 203–209.

Lees-Haley, P., English, L. T., & Glenn, W. J. (1991). A fake bad scale on the MMPI-2 for personal injury claimants. *Psychological Reports, 68,* 203–210.

Leininger, B. E. Gramling, S. E., Farrell, A. D., Kreutzer, J. S., & Peck, E. A. (1990). Neuropsychological deficits in symptomatic minor head injury patients after concussion and mild concussion. *Journal of Neurology, Neurosurgery, and Psychiatry, 53,* 293–296.

Levin, H. S., Benton, A. L., & Grossman, R. G. (1982). *Neurobehavioral consequences of closed head injury.* New York: Oxford University Press.

Levin, H. S., Mattis, S., Ruff, R. M., Eisenberg, H. M., Marshall, L. F., Tabaddor, K., High, W. M., Jr., & Frankowski, R. F. (1987). Neurobehavioral outcome of minor head injury: A three center study. *Journal of Neurosurgery, 66,* 234–243.

Levin, H. S., Williams, D., Crofford, M. J., High, W. M., Eisenberg, H. M., Amparo, E. G., Guinto, F. C., Kalisky, Z., Handel, S. F., & Goldman, A. M. (1988). Relationship of depth of brain lesions to consciousness and outcome after closed head injury. *Journal of Neurosurgery, 69,* 861–866.

Levin, H. S., Williams, D. H., Eisenberg, H. M., High, W. M., & Guinto, F. C. (1992). Serial MRI and neurobehavioral findings after mild to moderate closed head injury. *Journal of Neurology, Neurosurgery and Psychiatry, 55,* 255–262.

Mittenberg, W., DiGuilio, D. V., Perrin, S., & Bass, A. E. (1992). Symptoms following mild head injury: Expectation as aetiology. *Journal of Neurology, Neurosurgery, and Psychiatry, 55,* 200–204.

Mittenberg, W., Tremont, G., Zielinski, R. F., Fichera, S., & Rayls, K. R. (1996). Cognitive behavioral prevention of post-concussion syndrome. *Archives of Clinical Neuropsychology, 11,* 139–145.

Newcombe, F., Rabbitt, P., & Briggs, M. (1994). Minor head injury: Pathophysiological or iatrogenic sequelae? *Journal of Neurology, Neurosurgery, and Psychiatry, 57,* 709–716.

Newton, M. R., Greenwood, R. J., Britton, K. E., Charlesworth, M., Nimmon, C. C., Carroll, M. J., & Dolke, G. (1992). A study comparing SPECT with CT and MRI after closed head injury. *Journal of Neurology, Neurosurgery, and Psychiatry, 55,* 92–94.

Prigatano, G. P. (1996). Behavioral limitations TBI patients tend to underestimate: A replication and extension to patients with lateralized cerebral dysfunction. *Clinical Neuropsychologist, 10,* 191–201.

Prigatano, G. P., & Altman, I. M. (1990). Impaired awareness of behavioral limitations after traumatic brain injury. *Archives of Physical Medicine and Rehabilitation, 71,* 1058–1064.

Prigatano, G. P., Altman, I. M., & O'Brien, K. P. (1990). Behavioral limitations that brain injured patients tend to underestimate. *Clinical Neuropsychologist, 4,* 163–176.

Putnam, S. H., & Millis, S. R. (1994). Psychosocial factors in the development and maintenance of chronic somatic and functional symptoms following mild traumatic brain injury. *Advances in Medical Psychotherapy, 7,* 1–22.

Rohling, M. L., Binder, L. M., & Langhinrichsen-Rohling, J. (1995). Money matters: A meta-analytic review of the association between financial compensation and the experience and treatment of chronic pain. *Health Psychology, 14,* 537–547.

Rosenthal, R. (1991). *Meta-analytic procedures for social research* (rev. ed). Beverly Hills, CA: Sage.

Satz, P. (1993). Brain reserve capacity on symptom onset after brain injury: A formulation and review of evidence for threshold therapy. *Neuropsychology, 7,* 273–295.

Society of Nuclear Medicine Brain Imaging Council. (1996). Ethical clinical practice of functional brain imaging. *Journal of Nuclear Medicine, 37,* 1256–1259.

Stuss, D. T. (1995). A sensible approach to mild traumatic brain injury. *Neurology, 45,* 1251–1252.

Sweeney, J. E. (1992). Non-impact brain injury: Grounds for clinical study of the neuropsychological effects of acceleration forces. *Clinical Neuropsychologist*, 6, 443–457.

Szymanski, H. V., & Linn, R. (1992). A review of the post-concussion syndrome. *International Journal of Psychiatry in Medicine*, 22, 357–375.

Taylor, A. E., Cox, C. A., & Mailis, A. (1996). Persistent neuropsychological deficits following whiplash: Evidence for chronic mild traumatic brain injury? *Archives of Physical Medicine and Rehabilitation*, 77, 529–535.

Tebano, M. T., Cameroni, M., Gallozzi, G., Loizzo, A., Palazzino, G., Pezzini, G., & Ricci, G. F. (1988). EEG spectral analysis after minor head injury in man. *Electroencephalography and Clinical Neurophysiology*, 70, 185–189.

Thatcher, R. W., Walker, R. A., Gerson, I., & Geisler, F. H. (1989). EEG discriminant analysis of mild head trauma. *Electroencephalography and Clinical Neurophysiology*, 73, 94–106.

Uomoto, J. M., & Esselman, P. C. (1993). Traumatic brain injury and chronic pain: differential types and rates by head injury severity. *Archives of Physical Medicine and Rehabilitation*, 74, 61–64.

Varney, N. R., & Varney, R. N. (1995). Brain injury without head injury. Some physics of automobile collisions with particular reference to brain injuries occurring without physical head trauma. *Applied Neuropsychology*, 2, 47–62.

Waldstein, S. R., Manuck, S. B., Ryan, C. M., & Muldoon, M. F. (1991). Neuropsychological correlates of hypertension: Review and methodologic considerations. *Psychological Bulletin*, 110, 451–468.

Watson, D., & Pennebaker, J. W. (1989). Health complaints, stress, and distress: Exploring the central role of negative affectivity. *Psychological Review*, 96, 234–254.

Wechsler, D. (1981). *Wechsler Adult Intelligence Scale-Revised. Manual.* San Antonio, TX: Psychological Corporation.

Wechsler, D. (1987). *Wechsler Memory Scale-Revised. Manual.* San Antonio, TX: Psychological Corporation.

Williams, J. M., Little, M. M., Scates, S., & Blockman, N. (1987). Memory complaints and abilities among depressed older adults. *Journal of Consulting and Clinical Psychology*, 55, 595–598.

Wilson, J. T., Teasdale, G. M., Hadley, D. M., Wiedman, K. D., & Lang, D. (1993). Post-traumatic amnesia: Still a valuable yardstick. *Journal of Neurology, Neurosurgery, and Psychiatry*, 56, 198–201.

16

Mild Brain Injury and Mood Disorders: Causal Connections, Assessment, and Treatment

Thomas W. McAllister
Laura A. Flashman
Dartmouth Medical School,
Lebanon, New Hampshire

The epidemiology, neurological evaluation, and neuropsychological assessment of mild traumatic brain injury (MTBI) have recently gained the attention of both researchers and clinicians. The evaluation and treatment of emotional sequelae have received less attention (O'Hara, 1988). Many individuals with MTBI sustain minimal or no loss of consciousness, and therefore receive minimal (or no) medical follow-up or education (Kraus & Nourjah, 1988). As a result, they receive little if any information about possible sequelae following their injury, and do not know why they are experiencing cognitive, physical, and/or emotional problems. This lack of information often results in "unexplainable" symptoms that may cause emotional distress, confusion, and the inaccurate perception that a person is "going crazy." Even following a brief emergency room visit or neurological/neuropsychological screening, evidence of MTBI may be overlooked, and individuals may be told prematurely that all of their symptoms will clear. This prognosis may lead individuals to have unrealistic expectations about recovery, readiness to return to work, and ability to resume responsibilities. When they do return to work, they may be faced with family members, employers, and coworkers who are confused about the presentation of new "odd" behaviors, emotional displays, and lapses of memory. Failure to understand the cause of these behaviors can lead to misinterpretation of the symptoms as being due to malingering or laziness, resulting in the isolation of patients with MTBI from much-needed support.

Individuals with MTBI typically survive the trauma with relatively intact intellect, self-awareness, language, and sensory-motor skills. This relatively intact cognition allows for greater awareness of specific cognitive losses, physical changes, and emotional distress. With this insight, stress and worry may be much more intense and rapid in onset than for persons with more severe injury. Further, there may be an exacerbation of emotional symptomatology, as patients whose injuries are overlooked initially may experience a critical delay in diagnosis and subsequent referral for appropriate treatment.

Mood disorders are a common complication of mild traumatic brain injury. It is common to explain this observation by invoking reactive or psychological mechanisms, "wouldn't you be depressed if . . . ?" However, it is more likely that there is a complex interaction between the profile of brain injury (location and type), the interval between the injury and the onset of the mood symptoms, the genetic vulnerabilities of the individual, and the meaning of the sequelae to a given individual (McAllister & Price, 1990).

It is important to place this observation in a larger context. Expression and regulation of mood are commonly disordered following moderate and severe traumatic brain injury as well as MTBI (McAllister, 1992a). In fact, this is true of virtually all disorders of the central nervous system (CNS) (McAllister & Price, 1990). Because the CNS insult in patients with MTBI is often less obvious, there is a tendency to discount the severity of their symptoms (whether it be cognitive or affective) on the one hand, or attribute all of their symptoms to psychiatric mechanisms on the other hand. When viewed against the backdrop of the increased rate of mood disorders associated with cerebrovascular disease, the dementias, epilepsy, as well as moderate and severe traumatic brain injury, the high frequency of mood disorders associated with MTBI is less surprising.

RELATIONSHIP TO PREMORBID
CHARACTERISTICS OF AT-RISK POPULATION

It is also important to consider the at-risk population for traumatic brain injury. MTBI occurs much more commonly in males than in females, and predominantly in the second and third decades of life (Department of Health and Human Services, 1989; Kraus & Nourjah, 1988, 1989). Patients with MTBI are much more likely to have had a previous traumatic brain injury and have rates of probable learning disabilities predating the MTBI approaching 50% in some studies (Dicker, 1992; Silver & McAllister, 1997). Roughly 50% of traumatic brain injuries involve the use of alcohol. Thirty percent to 60% of the patients in these accidents are intoxicated at the time of the injury. The majority of these individuals have alcohol abuse or dependence syndromes (Sparadeo, Strauss, & Barth, 1990). Personality styles characterized by impulsive, hyperactive, and risk-taking traits are more common in traumatic brain injured patients (McAllister, 1992a; Rutter, Chadwick & Shaffer, 1983; Silver, Yudofsky, & Hales, 1987). Fenton, McClelland, Montgomery, MacFlynn, & Rutherford (1993) reported a significantly higher incidence of "life events" among those receiving MTBI in the 12 months before the accident than in a group of controls matched for age, gender, and social class. These life events included ill health, job and school changes, and relationship issues. Various medical, psychiatric, and psychosocial difficulties are reportedly more common in the families of children who suffer a traumatic brain injury than in controls (Brown & Davidson, 1978; Rutter et al., 1983). Thus any discussion of the occurrence and etiology of mood disorders in the traumatic brain injury population, whether mild or severe, must take into account these issues.

DEPRESSION IN NEUROLOGICAL DISORDERS

Much of the work exploring the relationship between brain injury or illness and subsequent changes in mood regulation comes from studies of poststroke depression (see Starkstein & Robinson, 1992, for overview) but appears generalizable to other brain disorders (McAllister & Price, 1990) and in particular to traumatic brain injury (Robinson, Boston, Starkstein, & Price, 1988; Starkstein, Boston, & Robinson, 1988; Starkstein et al., 1990). It is instructive to review this literature, as it can inform our understanding about mood disorders in the context of mild traumatic brain injury.

Although it was initially assumed that poststroke depression was a psychological response to the associated disability (Fisher, 1961; Ullman & Gruen, 1960), Folstein, Maiberger, and McHugh (1977) found that the rate and severity of depression were greater in stroke patients than in a control group of patients with severe orthopedic injuries and similar degrees of functional disabilities. Intrigued, this group went on to prospectively study a consecutive series of stroke patients admitted to the University of Maryland Hospital, exploring the interactions between lesion characteristics and subsequent mood disorders. The population consisted of about 100 patients with thromboembolic strokes or intracerebral hemorrhages. African American males from lower socioeconomic groups were somewhat overrepresented. Lesion locations were assessed along left/right, anterior/posterior, and cortical/subcortical dimensions using computed tomography (CT) scans. Several findings are important and appear relevant to mood disorders in MTBI patients.

Major depressive episodes or minor depressive episodes (similar to dysthymia except for the duration criteria) occurred in well over half of the patients in the first 2 years after the event (Lipsey, Spencer, Rabins, & Robinson, 1986; Robinson & Forrester, 1987; Robinson, Starr & Price, 1984; Robinson & Szetela, 1981). The phenomenology of these depressive syndromes is similar to that seen in the absence of neurological precipitants. This is true whether the depressive syndrome occurs acutely or has a delayed onset. Depressive syndromes typically last 6 to 12 months (Robinson, Lipsey, Rao, & Price, 1986; Robinson et al., 1984; Robinson, Starr, Lipsey, Rao, & Price, 1985).

Location of the cerebrovascular event impacts on the risk of developing a depressive syndrome and the severity of depressive symptoms. Left-hemispheric lesions, and particularly left anterior lesions, were found to correlate with increased rate and severity of depressive syndromes (Lipsey, Robinson, Pearlson, Rao, & Price, 1984; Robinson et al., 1987; Robinson, Lipsey, Rao, & Price, 1986; Robinson, Starr, Lipsey, Rao, & Price, 1985; Robinson & Szetela, 1981). Depression in this population was associated with poorer cognitive function (Robinson, Bolla-Wilson, Kaplan, Lipsey, & Price, 1986), recovery, and rehabilitation (Robinson, Lipsey, Rao, & Price, 1986; Robinson et al., 1988; Robinson et al., 1984).

DEPRESSIVE SYNDROMES IN TRAUMATIC BRAIN INJURY

Using similar methodology, this group has also studied a population of patients with traumatic brain injury (Federoff et al., 1992; Jorge et al., 1993b; Jorge, Robinson, Starkstein, & Arndt, 1994). A series of 66 traumatic brain injury patients admitted to a shock-trauma center were the subjects. Patients with spinal cord injuries and significant injuries to other body systems (e.g., multiple fractures, ruptured spleen, etc.) were excluded. There was a spectrum of traumatic brain injury severity, although 20% of the group had Glasgow Coma Scores (GCS; Teasdale & Jennett, 1974) of 12 to 15. Of note is that the GCS administered 24 hr after injury did not correlate with any of the other study findings; this suggests that findings from this and other studies of mixed or more severe traumatic brain injury populations may be generalizable to MTBI patients. Information about past personal and family psychiatric history were obtained. A modified version of the Present State Exam (Wing, Cooper, & Sartorius, 1974), and the Hamilton Rating Scale for Depression (Hamilton, 1960) were used to diagnose and quantify psychiatric symptoms. In addition, CT scans were used to categorize and localize focal lesions. It is important to recall, however, that traumatic brain injury typically results in diffuse injury patterns. When present, focal injury is superimposed on diffuse injury. Thus, the relative contribution of the focal lesion to sequelae of interest can be difficult to sort out from the diffuse injury. In this series of studies, it should be noted that if lesions were present in a given region of interest (e.g., left anterior), scans were considered positive for that location even if lesions were also present in other areas.

Patients were initially assessed approximately one month after their injury (Federoff et al., 1992). At that time, 27% were found to meet *DSM–III* criteria for major depression. There was no difference in the frequency of family history of psychiatric illness between the depressed and nondepressed groups. The depressed group did have a higher rate of personal past psychiatric history, although not when histories of drug and alcohol abuse were excluded. As was found in the population of stroke patients, the strongest correlate of a depressive episode was the presence of left anterior and/or left basal ganglia lesions, although parietal-occipital and right-hemispheric lesions were also associated with depression.

These patients were followed over the year subsequent to their injury (Jorge et al., 1993a, 1993b). The percentage of depressed patients remained about the same (20%–30%). The mean duration of a depressive episode was between 4 and 5 months. Thus, although the percentage of depressed patients did not change significantly at any given assessment interval, the same group of patients may not have been represented. Furthermore, the correlation between left anterior and/or left basal ganglia lesion location and depression was not found 1 year after the injury. Further analysis of the initial 1-month data suggested that the correlation between depression and lesion location was strongest for acute transient depression (resolved within 3 months of the injury). Examination of the effects of depression on outcome (Jorge et al., 1994) suggested that prolonged depression (lasting greater than 6 months) was associated with poorer social and functional outcome. Interestingly, this group was more likely to have a focal right-hemispheric lesion.

Others have also found significant rates of depression in TBI patients. For example, Varney, Martzke, and Roberts (1987) interviewed 120 patients with a history of TBI referred to a Veterans' Administration medical center for neuropsychological evaluation. Duration of unconsciousness in these patients ranged from several minutes to 8 days. Patients were seen an average of 3.4 years after their injury; 77% of these patients met *DSM–III* criteria for major depression. The depression was typically of late onset (6 months or more after the injury). The authors called attention to the fact that although meeting criteria for depression, many of these patients did not appear depressed, and had not sought help for depression.

In general, these findings are supported by a recent survey of traumatic brain injury outpatients (Fann, Katon, Uomoto, & Esselman, 1995), the majority of whom were MTBI patients. When assessed about 2½ years after their injury, 26% were depressed and 24% suffered from a generalized anxiety disorder. Past personal or family history of psychiatric disorder was not associated with current depression or anxiety. Again, injury severity was not correlated with depression or anxiety. Depressed and/or anxious patients were more disabled in general. Of interest, depressed and anxious patients rated their symptoms, including their cognitive deficits, as more severe and disabling than did their nondepressed, nonanxious cohort.

Studies of depression using only patients with MTBI are not common. Although the prevalence rate of depression in MTBI has not been firmly established, reported rates are consistent with the preceding rates of depression in traumatic brain injury of mixed severity (20%–30%). Merskey and Woodforde (1972) found that 20 of their 27 patients had some form of depressive syndrome, although just under 25% had what was termed an "endogenous" depression. Mobayed and Dinan (1990) found that 20% of their 55 MTBI patients met *DSM–III* criteria for depression, and another 10% had evidence of an affective spectrum disorder. In their study of MTBI patients, Schoenhuber and Gentilini (1988) found that patients with MTBI were at increased risk of developing depression, although they did not demonstrate evidence of either state or trait anxiety compared to a group of matched control subjects. There have been several studies of "emotional distress" following MTBI, many of which show that symptoms consistent with depressive spectrum disorders are elevated (Burke, Imhoff, & Kerrigan, 1990; Fordyce, Roueche & Prigatano, 1983; Hinkeldey & Corrigan 1990). Further, there is some evidence to suggest that emotional functioning can deteriorate with time (Fordyce et al., 1983). Although there has been speculation that some emotional distress may be related to increasing awareness of cognitive deficits and social adjustment problems secondary to the injury, other evidence (discussed later) suggests that these mood problems may be primary in nature. However, it is important to note that cognitive and emotional recovery may not coincide.

Thus it is clear that depressive symptoms and depressive spectrum disorders are quite common following MTBI. Major depressive episodes occur in 20%–30% of MTBI patients in the first year after the injury, and probably in similar numbers in the subsequent several years. Although these episodes can be relatively brief (4–5 months), they can also persist and contribute to functional, cognitive, and psychosocial disability.

MANIC SYNDROMES

Mania can also be a complication of MTBI. Once again it is important to put this in an appropriate context. Mania is frequently associated with a wide variety of medical disorders, and is known as secondary mania (Krauthammer & Klerman, 1978). Mania following central nervous system injury is seen much less frequently than depression (Bamrah & Johnson, 1991; Robinson et al., 1988). Although the reasons for this are not clear, some evidence suggests that injury-induced mania requires an interaction between genetic vulnerability, preexisting CNS damage, and lesion location. In a series of papers exploring the correlates of mania after stroke or traumatic brain injury, the Hopkins group (Robinson et al., 1988; Starkstein et al., 1988; Starkstein, Federoff, Berthier, & Robinson, 1991; Starkstein et al., 1990; Starkstein, Pearlson, Boston, & Robinson, 1987) found that manic patients had an increased rate of family history of mood disorders compared to brain-injured patients with depression or no history of mood disorders. The groups also differed in terms of lesion location profiles. Specifically, patients with mania demonstrated a higher rate of right-hemispheric lesions, particularly lesions involving the right orbitofrontal, basotemporal, and basal ganglia areas, as well as indications of subcortical atrophy. These results should be considered preliminary as there appears to be significant overlap in the patient sample described in these papers.

With respect to traumatic brain injury, the collective literature suggests that mania does occur after traumatic brain injury of all degrees of severity. Unfortunately, most of this literature is in the form of single case reports or small case series (e.g., Mas, Prichep, & Alper, 1993). We are aware of no prospective studies exploring the frequency, phenomenology, or neuroanatomical correlates of manic syndromes following traumatic brain injury in general, or MTBI in particular. Nevertheless, the limited existing body of work allows us to make several broad generalizations.

Although manic syndromes have been reported most commonly after moderate and severe traumatic brain injury, they have also been reported after MTBI, even in the absence of clear loss of consciousness (Bracken, 1987; McAllister, 1992a, 1994; Nizamie, Nizamie, Borde, & Sharma, 1988; Pope et al., 1988; Riess, Schwartz, & Klerman, 1987; Zwil, McAllister, Cohen, & Halpern, 1993). Regardless of injury severity, the core symptoms of the manic syndrome appear similar to those in idiopathic mania. Patients with postinjury mania present with alterations in mood, level of activation, sleep, judgment, and reality testing. There is some evidence to suggest that, in these patients, irritable mood, higher rate of relapse, and assaultive behavior may be more common (Hale & Donaldson, 1982; Hoff et al., 1988; McAllister, 1992a, 1994; Shukla, Cook, Mukherjee, Goodwin, & Miller, 1987; Stewart & Hemsath, 1988; Zwil, McAllister, & Raimo, 1990; Zwil et al., 1993). One can see a variety of different longitudinal profiles, including single or recurrent manic episodes, bipolar patterns, rapid cycling, and antidepressant triggering of manic episodes (Cohn, Wright, & DeVaul, 1977; Hale & Donaldson, 1982; McAllister, 1992b; Pope et al., 1988; Shukla et al., 1987; Stewart & Hemsath, 1988).

There is significant overlap between some of the core symptoms of mania or hypomania and what used to be known as Organic Personality Disorder (now Personality Change Secondary to Traumatic Brain Injury) (Zwil et al., 1990, 1993). Irritability, affective lability, increased psychomotor activity, disturbed sleep, silly disinhibited behavior, and poor judgment are commonly reported by patients and their families following brain injury. These symptoms are also common features of a manic episode. It is important to bear this in mind when evaluating patients with these complaints in the context of MTBI, although careful history or observation can usually clarify this. Perhaps the most helpful distinction is that in hypomanic or manic episodes, the core features are more likely to be episodic (usually weeks to months), then remit. There is a driven quality to the person's behavior and level of activity. In contrast, when a person is suffering from a personality change secondary to a traumatic brain injury, these characteristics are present at a lower level of intensity but are more constant in nature.

OTHER MOOD DISORDERS ASSOCIATED
WITH MTBI

Although the most frequently reported mood symptoms following MTBI are depression and mania, other mood symptoms have also been reported in some patients. A wide variety of problems is seen, including anxiety, posttraumatic stress, substance abuse, mood lability, irritability, and decreased frustration tolerance. These may be seen immediately following the injury and may persist for years.

Englander, Hall, Stimpson, and Chaffin (1992) conducted phone interviews with 77 MTBI patients an average of 2 months (range: 26–92 days) postinjury. Twenty-six percent reported complaints, the most frequent of which were fatigue and headaches (18% of total sample), decreased frustration tolerance (17% of total sample), anxiety (16% of total sample), and increased temper (12% of total sample). Yarnell and Rossie (1988) evaluated 27 patients with minor whiplash head injury who were referred for neurological evaluation several months postinjury for worsening symptoms and/or persistent complaints. Affective complaints, in addition to depression, included loss of drive and initiation, increased irritability, and decreased frustration tolerance. Patients also reported features of posttraumatic stress disorder, with obsessive hypochondriacal ruminations, depersonalization, phobias, apathy, and blunted affect. Parker and Rosenblum (1996) report that 31 of 33 patients had a psychiatric disorder (new diagnosis or reemergence of a problem in remission prior to the injury) complicating recovery from their MTBI. The most prevalent *DSM–III—R* diagnosis was posttraumatic stress disorder; anxiety reaction, affective disorder, depression, and conversion reaction were also reported.

Middelboe, Andersen, Birket-Smith, and Friis (1992) evaluated patients 1 year following minor head injury. Twenty-one percent of patients who responded to their mail survey attributed problems with irritability to their head trauma; 18% reported anxiety. Symptoms of depression, including sleep disturbances (18%), fatigue (21%), and memory and concentration problems (25%), were also reported. As noted earlier, a recent survey of predominately MTBI outpatients (Fann et al., 1995) indicated that 24% surveyed suffered from a generalized anxiety disorder approximately 2.5 years postinjury. Current symptoms of anxiety were not associated with either injury severity, past personal history of psychiatric disorder, or family psychiatric history.

MacNiven and Finlayson (1993) have also investigated the nature of the emotional disturbance in patients with traumatic brain injury. They examined 59 patients with traumatic brain injury (severity of injury not reported) 1 year after their injury and were able to assess patients 2 years post-injury. Psychopathology and emotional distress were assessed using the Minnesota Multiphasic Personality Inventory (MMPI). The mean MMPI profile obtained for these patients showed evidence of significant depression and anxiety. On initial assessment (at referral), 73% of the patients had at least one scale elevated above T = 70, with 54% having two or more scale elevations. At 1 year, 66% of patients had at least one elevated scale, and 51% had two or more elevations. Of interest, at 2-year follow-up, a higher prevalence of psychopathology was observed: 93% of participating patients had at least one elevated MMPI scale, and 86% had two or more elevated scales. Similarly, Fenton et al. (1993) evaluated 45 consecutive patients with MTBI (PTA <24 hr). Using the Present State Examination, 39% of the group were diagnosed with "neurotic depression" or anxiety states acutely (6 weeks postinjury), compared with 4% of matched controls. Six months after the injury, 28% of the head injury group endorsed at least three symptoms of chronic social difficulty.

In summary, it appears that the emotional consequences of MTBI are extremely varied and sometimes extreme. This distress can augment the cognitive deficits resulting from the traumatic brain injury and complicate postinjury adaptation. Adjustment may be further complicated by medication side effects as well as mood disturbances. This can set in motion a malignant cycle in which self-esteem is further reduced, leading to increased isolation and worsening emotional distress.

THE POSTCONCUSSION SYNDROME

In addition to the psychological distress commonly encountered as described already, MTBI patients also report cognitive and somatic signs and symptoms (for reviews see Alexander, 1995; Brown, Fann, & Grant,

1994; McAllister, 1994). This clustering of psychological, somatic, and cognitive difficulties is commonly referred to as the postconcussion syndrome. Virtually all patients with MTBI will endorse difficulties in these areas in the first week after their injury (Levin et al., 1987; McAllister, 1994). The great majority of patients recover rapidly. By 3 months, and certainly by 6 or 12 months, most patients are asymptomatic. The literature also suggests that a small percentage of patients will suffer significant and chronic sequelae from their injury (Alves, Macciocchi, & Barth, 1993; Brown & Davidson, 1994; Dikmen, McLean, & Temkin, 1986; Levin et al., 1987; McAllister, 1994; Rutherford, 1989). It is important to point out that not all MTBI patients experience a full complement of these difficulties. For example, some report only a single symptom, such as headache.

In both clinical practice and the medical literature the same signs and symptoms ascribed to the "postconcussion syndrome" following a clear loss of consciousness have also been reported in patients in whom there was no clear loss of consciousness (Brown et al., 1994; Evans, 1994; Hugenholtz et al., 1988; Radanov, Dvorak, & Valach, 1992; Yarnell & Rossie, 1988). There is no universal agreement among clinicians or in the literature about whether loss of consciousness is an absolute prerequisite to having an MTBI or developing a postconcussion syndrome. Some argue that loss of consciousness is necessary and others that any brain trauma sufficient to result in a change in mental state (such as being dazed or confused) is evidence of a concussion (Kelly et al., 1991). This latter position is espoused by the Mild Traumatic Brain Injury Committee of the Head Injury Interdisciplinary Special Interest Group of the American Congress of Rehabilitation Medicine (Kay et al., 1993).

Another source of confusion arises from lack of precision in terminology (concussion, postconcussion syndrome, minor head injury, etc.). Traumatic brain injury occurs along a spectrum of injury severity. Whether the injury is mild, moderate, or severe, it results in a predictable profile of pathophysiological insults to the brain, and a predictable profile of clinical deficits in the domains of sensory-motor function, cognition, and behavior (Adams & Victor, 1985; Auerbach, 1989; Gennarelli, 1987; Graham, Adams & Gennarelli, 1987). These pathophysiological insults and clinical deficits have a generally predictable time course of evolution and recovery (McAllister, 1992a, 1994). In MTBI defined by the most common criteria (e.g., duration of unconsciousness, length of posttraumatic amnesia, Glasgow Coma Score, etc.), the extent of injury is less than that seen in patients with moderate and severe injury. Further, the prognosis for recovery is better. *Mild traumatic brain injury* is not synonymous with terms such as the *postconcussion syndrome*. The former is simply the less severe end of the spectrum of brain injury; the latter is the cluster of signs and symptoms (usually including one or more difficulties from somatic, cognitive, and behavioral domains) that can be seen after traumatic brain injury of any severity. These signs and symptoms are seen in the vast majority of patients shortly after a mild traumatic brain injury, show progressive resolution over the subsequent 1 to 3 months, and in a small percentage of patients will persist 12 months or more after the injury. At this point it may be helpful to refer to the syndrome as a chronic or persistent postconcussion syndrome or disorder.

The etiology of the emotional disturbance following MTBI is unclear. General theories have suggested that the psychological disturbance of patients having MTBI may be reactive in nature, and depend at least partially on their awareness of the severity of their deficits. An alternative theory is that the basis for psychological disturbance after MTBI is related to biochemical or anatomical damage caused at the time of the injury. Animal models and scant human data both suggest that neuronal injury can be seen with even mild trauma, including injuries with brief or unclear periods of unconsciousness (Blumbergs et al., 1994; Jane, Steward, & Gennarelli, 1985; Oppenheimer, 1968; Povlischock & Coburn, 1989). The pattern of injury both microscopically and in terms of anatomical distribution is similar to that seen in more severe injuries. Confusion, disorientation, retrograde amnesia, and anterograde amnesia (even if brief) suggest at least temporary widespread neuronal dysfunction (Gennarelli, 1987).

Thus, it is possible that emotional disturbance following brain trauma may be associated with the pathophysiology of the injury, and that improvement in psychological functioning may be related less to cognitive performance than to biological recovery processes. Further, the mechanisms that lead to the persistence of symptoms have not yet been well delineated. One view is that long-term sequelae are modulated by an individual's personal, psychological, and social adjustment to the injury, its context, and the distressing early symptoms (Lishman, 1988; Russell, 1974). Middelboe et al. (1992) reported considerable morbidity in MTBI patients 1 year postinjury, and they indicated that this can occur with very short or no loss of consciousness. Although they indicated that persistent symptoms such as depression and anxiety are difficult to explain in terms of a "supposedly minimal organic brain lesion" (p. 7), they believed that brain injury is directly related to initial affective symptoms. They proposed that psychological mechanisms are responsible for the sustaining or progression of symptoms in these predisposed individuals. In some patients, however, persistent deficits are clearly related to early dysfunction of the cortex and brainstem (Montgomery, Fenton, McClelland, MacFlynn, & Rutherford, 1991; Watson et al., 1993).

There has been considerable discussion about the interaction between the emotional and cognitive sequelae of MTBI. According to the coping hypothesis, long-term emotional complaints (as well as other symptoms of the postconcussion syndrome) may result from the chronic effort of patients attempting to compensate for their cognitive deficits, which may lead to a chronic stress reaction, depression, or anxiety. That is, symptoms or deficits that appear minor when regarded separately can in aggregate cause a more substantial impact on the recovery and well-being of the MTBI patient. This hypothesis is supported by Bornstein, Miller, and van Schoor (1989), who reported a significant positive correlation between emotional disturbance and cognitive deficits in patients with MTBI. Gasquione (1992) reported that level of dysphoria was correlated with subject awareness of sensory and cognitive changes. Others have reported that cognitive improvements over 1 year may be accompanied by increased psychological distress, which may be related to increasing awareness of cognitive difficulties, increased loneliness and isolation (e.g., Lezak & O'Brien, 1988; Slater, 1989). MacNiven and Finlayson (1993) found that the presence of depression was particularly detrimental to cognitive performance, as assessed by number of errors on the Halstead–Reitan Category Test. Finally, in a recent study of 50 patients with mild and moderate traumatic brain injury, King (1996) reported that measures of emotional factors taken early after injury (rather than neuropsychological or traditional measures) were the best individual predictors of severity of postconcussion syndrome 3 months after traumatic brain injury. Thus, it seems clear that there is an interaction such that awareness of cognitive deficits can exacerbate primary depressive symptoms, and conversely, depression can impair speed of information processing and other cognitive functions.

THE DARTMOUTH DATA

Studies of the frequency and type of complaints following MTBI have generally not excluded depressed patients from their samples. Studies of the rate of depressive disorders following MTBI have not excluded patients with the postconcussion syndrome from their samples. Given that these studies show that 20%–30% of patients suffer from clear-cut depressive disorders, and another 10%–20% from depressive spectrum disorders, it can be argued that what little we actually know about the persistent postconcussion syndrome is confounded by the high rate of depressive illness, and the significant overlap between signs and symptoms that are shared by both depressive disorders and what is commonly called the postconcussion syndrome (dysphoria, fatigue, sleep disturbance, irritability, and trouble with memory, concentration, and attention). This is illustrated by our recent experience at the Darmouth Hitchcock Medical Center.

Sixty consecutive patients with traumatic brain injury were referred to the Neuropsychology Program at Dartmouth Hitchcock Medical Center for neuropsychological evaluation between January 1995 and November 1996. Of these patients, 38 were determined to have a mild traumatic brain injury. This was determined on the basis of either a Glasgow Coma Scale Score of 13 to 15 when available, or a loss of consciousness of less than 30 min. At a minimum, they had a documented alteration of consciousness following a traumatic blow to the head. All patients received a full neuropsychological evaluation, which included assessment of general intellectual functioning, tests of attention and memory, language assessment, evaluation of visuospatial abilities, and assessment of fine motor skills. In addition, patients completed the Beck Depression Inventory (BDI; Beck, Ward, Mendelson, & Erlbaugh, 1961). The BDI is a 21-item self-report questionnaire. Patients rate each item on a 4-point (0–3) scale based on the current severity of that item. Higher scores indicate more severe depression.

Demographic Information

Patients were, on average, 40.4 years of age (SD = 10.8, range: 17–68) at the time of evaluation. They were 2.44 years post-injury (SD = 3.69, range: 14–6,287 days). Of the 38 patients meeting criteria for MTBI, 23 (60%) were male and 15 (40%) were female. Mean Full Scale IQ was 96.9 (SD = 14.1, range 60–128), with no significant differences between VIQ (X = 98.0, SD = 15.4) and PIQ (X = 96.6, SD = 12.4). Twenty-four of the 38 patients were hospitalized immediately following their injury. Consistent with the literature of premorbid risk factors in the MTBI population, 17 (45%) patients reported that they had experienced a prior traumatic brain injury, 9 (24%) patients endorsed a history of prior or current drug abuse, 12 (32%) endorsed a history of prior or current alcohol abuse, and 16 (42%) endorsed prior psychiatric history independent of substance abuse.

Affective Status

Scores on the BDI suggested that this was a very depressed group. Only 7 (18%) of the 38 patients scored in the nondepressed range (total score less than 10). Twelve (32%) were severely depressed (BDI > 25); the rest fell in the mild to moderate range. There was a nonsignificant trend for the depressed patients to perform more poorly on cognitive measures (e.g., correlation between BDI score and FSIQ = –0.33, p < .06). Despite the frequency and severity of depressive symptoms in this group, a surprising number of patients were receiving little or inadequate treatment for their mood disorder. Fourteen (45%) of the 31 depressed patients were not on medication for their mood problems; six of these 14 patients were moderately or severely depressed. Even those that were on mood altering

TABLE 16.1
Level of Depression and Type of Medications

	No Medications	Thymoleptics	Other Medications
Not depressed	2 (5.26%)	1 (2.63%)	4 (10.53%)
Mild depression	4 (10.53%)	3 (7.89%)	4 (10.53%)
Moderate depression	1 (2.63%)	5 (13.16%)	2 (5.26%)
Severe depression	2 (5.26%)	9 (23.68%)	1 (2.63%)
Total [38 (100%)]	9 (23.68)	18 (47.37)	11 (28.95)

Note: Other medications = pain medication, antihypertensives, etc.

medications were very depressed, suggesting that they were inadequately or only partially treated at the time of the assessment (Table 16.1).

Results and Implications

DSM–IV criteria for postconcussion disorder include three or more of the following symptoms: fatigue; sleep disturbance; headache; vertigo or dizziness; irritability; anxiety, depression, or affective lability; changes in personality (social or sexual inappropriateness); and apathy. Of these eight core symptoms, six overlap with items on the BDI (sadness, irritability, avolition, sleep disturbance, fatigue, somatic concerns). In our data, there were 35 patients who would meet criteria for postconcussion disorder on the basis of having endorsed three or more of the relevant six overlapping items on the BDI (with a score of at least 1 point), and 14 patients who would meet criteria by endorsing at least three of the six overlapping items with a score of 2 or 3 (more severe symptomatology). Of the 35 patients identified using the former, less stringent criteria, 89% scored in the mild ($n = 11$), moderate ($n = 8$), or severe ($n = 12$) range of depression. Of the 14 patients with higher scores on the overlapping postconcussion items, 100% scored in the mild ($n = 1$), moderate ($n = 4$), or severe ($n = 9$) range of depression (Fig. 16.1).

These results are not an artifact of these patients scoring very high on just the postconcussion items. When the other 15 nonoverlapping BDI items are examined, 29 of 35 and 13 of 14 subjects endorsed at least five other depressive symptoms.

These data makes the point that it is not enough in this population to simply assess for common postconcussion symptoms alone, but rather one should aggressively assess for the presence of a full-blown depressive syndrome. Failure to explicitly ask about other signs and symptoms that comprise the depressive syndrome could result in labeling a patient as having a postconcussion disorder alone, and missing a patient's depressive illness. We believe that the lack of treatment or relative undertreat-

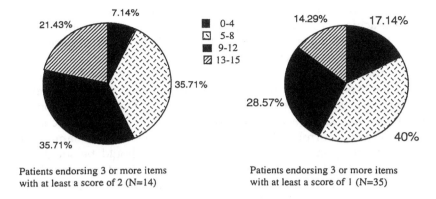

FIG. 16.1. Number of additional (non-postconcussion syndrome) items endorsed on the BDL.

ment of depression in our group suggests that many clinicians are not taking this step and thus are needlessly exposing their patients to excess disability caused by unrecognized and untreated depressive illness.

TREATMENT ISSUES

Assessment Issues

Appropriate treatment always begins with a careful initial evaluation, particularly given the increased rates of comorbid and premorbid conditions in the MTBI population. As previously mentioned, features of those at greatest risk for MTBI include increased rates of previous traumatic brain injury, probable learning disabilities (Dicker, 1992; Silver et al., 1987), and alcohol abuse or dependence syndromes (Sparadeo et al., 1990). It is important to know if current personality traits such as impulsivity, hyperactivity, and risk-taking behavior truly developed after the MTBI or were premorbid characteristics (McAllister, 1992a; Rutter et al., 1983; Silver et al., 1987). Because medical, psychiatric, and psychosocial difficulties occur more frequently in these patients and their families, it is important not to assume that current affective distress is solely attributable to the MTBI and its sequelae (Rutter et al., 1983). Preinjury coping skills should be assessed, as they may have a significant impact on emotional adjustment following injury.

It is important to determine the patient's previous level and type of work. Even subtle declines in speed of information processing, simultaneous information processing, creativity, executive functions, and/or interpersonal sensitivity can be devastating to persons in positions of responsibility (O'Hara, 1988). Seemingly minor declines in "high achievers" or "overachievers" may subsequently lead to a catastrophic response when they are unable to maintain their previous levels of performance or meet their own expectations.

Attention should be paid to the details of the injury. One should inquire about the type of injury, the presence and duration of loss or alteration of consciousness, and the presence or absence of other complications such as contusions, skull fractures, and other systemic or orthopedic injuries. When possible, corroboration from other sources (such as family members, witnesses, emergency room records, etc.) should be sought. This attention to detail serves several purposes. First, it informs the clinician about the circumstances of the injury and to some extent the likely severity of the injury. Second, it indicates that the clinician is informed in this area, that he or she "speaks the language." Time spent on these questions is critical to building a relationship in which the patient feels he or she will be heard. Third, these questions can shed light on the meaning and significance of the accident and injury to that particular individual.

The presentations of mood syndromes in traumatic brain injury including MTBI can be somewhat atypical (McAllister, 1992a, 1994; McAllister & Price, 1990; Saran, 1985; Silver, Yudofsky, & Hales, 1991). It is our observation that depressive syndromes may have fewer neurovegetative signs and symptoms, and more anxiety and somatic complaints. Fatigue and anhedonia remain important key features. The tendency of mania to present with an irritable rather than a euphoric affect has been described earlier (Shukla et al., 1987).

Medication Approaches

Antidepressants. There are few studies comparing the relative efficacy of different antidepressants in brain-injured patients. Saran (1985) reported a poor response to amitriptyline and phenelzine in 10 patients with depression following MTBI, and suggested that depression in this context might be less responsive to antidepressant medications. Dinan and Mobayed (1992) also found a poor response to amitriptyline in 13 patients with depression following MTBI, with only 4 patients improving. Although this might suggest that depressed MTBI patients respond poorly to tricyclic medications, it should be noted that only amitriptyline has been used and in only two studies. Cassidy (1989) reported that 5 of 9 patients had either moderate or marked improvement to fluoxetine, but this was not a blinded study design.

Given the absence of consistent data on large numbers of patients, we feel the usual algorithms for choosing medications in idiopathic mood disorders apply to MTBI patients with mood disorders. Thus serotonin reuptake inhibitors (SSRIs) such as fluoxetine, paroxetine, and sertraline are now commonly used as first-line antidepressant drugs. Their relative lack of side effects makes them attractive, given that MTBI patients seem to have an increased susceptibility to common medication side effects. On the other hand, the SSRIs can have an unpleasant activating effect in some patients, which can present as agitation or anxiety, and they may have a particular propensity to induce manic episodes in traumatic brain injury patients (Jones et al., 1995). It is also possible to see an initial robust antidepressant response followed by apparent relapse several months later despite no change in dose. Increasing the dose in this situation can often be helpful. In the absence of a response to SSRIs, and despite the limited literature just cited, our experience suggests that tricyclic antidepressants remain excellent first-line agents. Desipramine and nortriptyline are good choices because of their relatively low anticholinergic profiles. An additional consideration in patients with prominent complaints of attentional deficits is the cognitive (attentional) enhancing properties of desipramine and bupropion.

Regardless of which agent is used, it is necessary to alter the typical dosing strategy. As noted, patients with MTBI appear to have a heightened sensitivity to medication side effects. In general, one should start at one half to one third the usual starting doses, and increase doses more slowly than one does in the non-brain-injured population.

It is important to distinguish different patterns of medication response. It is common in the MTBI population to see patients with a persistent postconcussion syndrome complicated by a major depressive episode. In these cases, aggressive antidepressant medication trials may alleviate some of the core target symptoms, such as dysphoria, anhedonia, and sleep disturbance. Other symptoms such as various somatic complaints and cognitive disturbances (memory, attention, speed of information processing) may not improve. It can be difficult to distinguish if this represents a good antidepressant response with residual postconcussion symptoms, or rather a partial antidepressant response. If the residual symptoms are severe or disabling, it may be worth a trial of an alternate antidepressant, or augmentation of the current regimen with lithium, thyroid hormone, or stimulants. The latter, perhaps due to dopaminergic agonist properties, can also be helpful in the treatment of attentional deficits, apathy, and impulse dyscontrol often associated with traumatic brain injury (Gualtieri, 1988; Gualtieri et al., 1989; McAllister, 1992b, 1994; Silver et al., 1991).

Mood Stabilizers. There is also little work exploring the use of mood stabilizers in MTBI. The literature suggests that secondary mania is fairly responsive to traditional mood stabilizing regimens (McAllister, 1992b; Pope et al., 1988; Zwil, McAllister, & Raimo, 1992); again, it is reasonable to use the usual treatment algorithms. Lithium is an excellent first-line anti-manic agent. Apart from the general precautions about lower dosing (discussed earlier), it can be used as in the idiopathic psychiatric population. Patients should be warned about potential side effects such as tremor and nausea. Anti-manic effects are usually seen 10 to 14 days after achieving a reasonable serum lithium level. Our practice is to keep serum levels in the 0.6–1.0 mEq/L range, somewhat lower than in the non-brain-injured population. In addition to its anti-manic effects, lithium can be used to reduce the frequency and intensity of impulse dyscontrol syndromes in the brain-injured, and to augment the antidepressant effects of SSRIs and tricyclics (McAllister, 1992b).

Anticonvulsants, particularly valproic acid (Divalproex, Depakote, Depakene) and carbamazepine (Tegretol), are used more and more frequently as first-line agents in mania (McElroy, Keck, Pope, & Hudson, 1989; Post, Uhde, Ballenger, & Squillace, 1983). Although many assume that these agents are preferable to lithium in the management of mania associated with neurological illness, there is little literature to support this contention. Certain clinical features such as a mixed episode (features of both depression and mania) or a rapid cycling pattern may be indicators for valproic acid (American Psychiatric Association, 1994). Varney et al. (1993) reported that carbamazepine may also have a role in the treatment of depressed patients with brain injury who have failed to respond to other antidepressants. Newer anticonvulsants such as gabapentin (Neurontin) and lamotrigine (Lamictal) may also have a place in the management of mood disorders, although little work has been done.

Although sometimes useful in the management of mania, clonazepam (a long-acting benzodiazepine) has not received much attention in the traumatic brain injury literature, and in our experience is not particularly useful in this population. We find that it can sedate without affecting the core symptoms of the manic syndrome, and in some cases leads to further disinhibition.

Psychoeducation and Psychotherapeutic Issues

Despite the prevalence of mood disorders in MTBI, little work has been devoted specifically to identifying the psychotherapeutic techniques that are most efficacious in their treatment. Most of the available literature that might be relevant actually deals with the alleviation of postconcussion symptoms. A number of programs have been developed to assist people after they have suffered a mild traumatic brain injury. These programs consist of several "modules" that provide different information and/or techniques to assist in the recovery process. Even fairly simple standardized information modules appear to reduce the frequency and intensity of common symptoms and the related disability (Gronwall, 1986; Kelly, 1975; Minderhoud, Boelens, Huizenga, & Saan, 1980; Mittenberg, Zielinski, & Fichera, 1993; Wrightson, 1989). Information about the underlying pathophysiology, common symptom profiles, and reassurance about the usual time course of recovery are important to cover. Because the patient may have memory and attentional difficulties, this information should be supplemented with written materials, and shared with family members, significant others, and other relevant caregivers. Mittenberg et al. (1993) developed a treatment manual for MTBI patients that has a cognitive-behavioral framework and has shown preliminary promise in reducing symptom distress. We feel that regardless of the specific structure of the intervention, there appear to be four elements that are important to include in the treatment of postconcussion symptoms and mood disorders: reassurance, education, support (individual and/or group therapy), and regular monitoring of progress (Gronwall, 1986).

Reassurance. By the time many patients are referred for rehabilitation, visible signs of the trauma will probably have disappeared. Patients' expectations, as well as those of family and employers, are that they have recovered from the incident. However, although physical appearances may be unchanged, daily functioning may be affected. Reassurance from health care professionals is important, and the reassurance that comes from other people who have had the same kind of problems after MTBI is equally important.

Education. In our experience, it is impossible to overstate the importance of psychoeducation in addition to reassurance in the management of MTBI patients with or without depression (Gronwall, 1986; Kay et al., 1993; McAllister, 1994; Wrightson, 1989). All patients experience obvious relief when informed that their bewildering array of symptoms is a normal part of the postinjury course. Patients also need to be educated about the interaction between depression and many of the postconcussion symptoms, as described earlier. Those that are depressed find comfort in the knowledge that their emotional distress is at least in part linked to physiological processes set in motion by the brain injury. This often frees them up to describe and elaborate on the nature of their distress and factors that impact on it.

The medical community is in a prime position to alert patients not only to possible residual physical and cognitive deficits, but also to emotional sequelae and the probabilities of recovery. This may be best accomplished through written material, as persons who have undergone such trauma may still be in posttraumatic amnesia, in shock, under stress, and/or highly distractible and therefore may be less likely to store new information presented orally. Review of any available reports with the patient will allow for increased awareness of causality, probable outcome, options for prevention for further injury, and appropriate caution in initial resumption of mental and physical activity immediately following the injury. When possible, this information should be shared with family members in order to engage the support system in setting appropriate expectations. It may be that the specific details of the program are less important than ensuring that either you or someone familiar with the sequelae of MTBI takes the necessary time to educate the patient and their caregivers about the sequelae and time course of recovery associated with MTBI.

Individual Psychotherapy and Cognitive Rehabilitation. Although it is likely that only a small portion of people with MTBI seek or accept referral for counseling immediately postinjury, it is the persistence of symptoms that typically escalates the patient into severe emotional distress and leads to family, physician, or self-referral for an assessment of cognitive and emotional status. Upon documentation of cognitive dysfunction and/or emotional distress, patients with MTBI can be served optimally when rehabilitation efforts address cognition, emotion, and behavior. Emotional skills that can be addressed in psychotherapy include processing and resolving issues related to loss of "self," personality changes, adjustment reactions to trauma and/or losses resulting from the traumatic brain injury, and relationships. In all forms of therapeutic intervention, treating physicians or therapists must take into account the patient's prevailing cognitive difficulties. These difficulties generally include some combination of impairment in attention/concentration, memory, planning and sequencing, increased susceptibility to distraction, and abrupt shifts in emotional state. It is important to remember that cognitive deficits which may result from the MTBI may impact on coping strategies, and new methods of adapting to stress may need to be learned. The goals of psychotherapy must include dealing with loss issues, facilitating psychological adjustment, and helping the person cope with changes resulting from the brain injury.

Group Psychotherapy. Although individual outpatient treatment targets cognitive and emotional/interpersonal problems unique to each person, group treatment allows for peer modeling, risk taking, social and emotional support, interpersonal and self-awareness skills building, and mutual assistance in problem solving.

Vocational Issues. Assisting the patient in the resumption of employment, community activities, and family/social relationships is the final task of psychotherapeutic treatment. One of the more difficult tasks is the setting of realistic time frames and goals for return to work. Some have suggested specific work readiness criteria within the framework of their rehabilitation programs (Gronwall, 1986), and others suggest that gradual transition back to the work place is critical (Kay et al., 1993). Direct discussions and negotiations between the therapist and the patient's employer can sometimes be helpful. The sooner this information is shared with the patient and relevant others, the better. Unfortunately, therapists frequently become involved months or years after the injury when it has become apparent that there are lingering and often disabling symptoms. The apparent discrepancy between the "mild" brain injury, the perception that the patient "should" be better by now, and the persistent severe nature of the symptoms has fostered an adversarial posture between the patient, significant other, insurance carriers, and employers.

At this point, depressive spectrum disorders are often responsible for a significant amount of excess disability. As Kay suggested (Kay et al., 1993; Kay, Newman, Cavallo, Ezrachi, & Resnick, 1992), it is critical to sort out the relative contributions of the affective distress from long-term or permanent neurocognitive deficits. The negativism and sense of hopelessness and helplessness that accompany depression contribute to functional disability and augment the patient's subjective and objective cognitive deficits. Successful treatment can make an enormous difference. It can also set the stage for more willing acceptance of and adaptation to any permanent injury sequelae.

As is the case with idiopathic mood disorders, the combination of pharmacotherapy and talking therapies is most effective. Because of the special nature of the mix of neurological, medical, and psychological factors (Kay et al., 1993) that contribute to the genesis and maintenance of depressive symptoms in this population, cognitive-behavioral approaches coupled with modest adjustments in psychotherapeutic technique are needed (Bennett, 1989; Lewis, Athey, Eyman, & Saeks, 1992; Mittenberg et al., 1993).

SUMMARY

Based on the review in this chapter, several general points can be highlighted:

- Mood disorders, particularly depressive syndromes, are a very common complication of MTBI. Major depressive episodes occur in about 20%–30% of MTBI patients in the first year, and probably in subsequent years. Depressive symptoms occur even more commonly.

- This is similar to rates seen in other disorders affecting the central nervous system, including moderate and severe traumatic brain injury.
- A wide variety of other mood disturbances have also been reported, including mania, anxiety, posttraumatic stress, substance abuse, mood lability, irritability, and decreased frustration tolerance.
- There is considerable overlap between the symptoms of the postconcussion syndrome and depression. It is important to assess MTBI patients for the full range of depressive signs and symptoms and not simply attribute their distress to a persistent postconcussion syndrome.
- The most effective treatment of mood disorders in MTBI patients is a combination of pharmacotherapy and psychoeducational approaches. Although the medication algorithms do not differ from the noninjured population, MTBI patients have an increased susceptibility to common medication side effects, and thus dosing must be altered.

REFERENCES

Adams, R. D., & Victor, M. (1985). Craniocerebral trauma. In R. D. Adams & M. Victor (Eds.), *Principles of neurology* (3rd ed., pp. 641–644). New York: McGraw-Hill.

Alexander, M. P. (1995). Mild traumatic brain injury: Pathophysiology, natural history, and clinical management. *Neurology, 45*, 1253–1260.

Alves, W., Macciocchi, S. N., & Barth, J T. (1993). Postconcussive symptoms after uncomplicated mild brain injury. *Journal of Head Trauma Rehabilitation. 8*, 48–59.

American Psychiatric Association. (1994). Practice guideline for the treatment of patients with bipolar disorder. *American Journal of Psychiatry, 151*(12), 1–36.

Auerbach, S. H. (1989). The pathophysiology of traumatic brain injury. In L. J. Horn & D. N. Cope (Eds.), *Physical medicine and rehabilitation state of the art reviews: Traumatic brain injury* (Vol. 3, pp. 1–11). Philadelphia: Hanley and Belfus.

Bamrah, J. S., & Johnson, J. (1991). Bipolar affective disorder following head injury. *British Journal of Psychiatry, 158*, 117–119.

Beck, A. T., Ward, C. H., Mendelson, M., & Erlbaugh, J. (1961). An inventory for measuring depression. *Archives of General Psychiatry. 4*, 561–571.

Bennett, T. L. (1989). Individual psychotherapy and minor head injury. *Cognitive Rehabilitation* (September/October), 20–25.

Blumbergs, P. C., Scott, G., Manavis, J., Wainwright, H., Simpson, D. A., & McLean, A. J. (1994). Staining of amyloid precursor protein to study axonal damage in mild head injury. *Lancet, 344*, 1055–1056.

Bornstein, R. A., Miller, H. B., & van Schoor, J. T. (1989). Neuropsychological deficit and emotional disturbance in head-injured patients. *Journal of Neurosurgery, 70*, 509–513.

Bracken, P. (1987). Mania following head injury. *British Journal of Psychiatry, 150*, 690–692.

Brown, G. W., & Davidson, S. (1978). Social class, psychiatric disorder, and accidents to children. *Lancet, i*, 378–381.

Brown, S. J., Fann, J. R., & Grant, I. (1994). Postconcussional disorder: Time to acknowledge a common source of neurobehavioral morbidity. *Journal of Neuropsychiatry and Clinical Neurosciences, 6*, 15–22.

Burke, J. M., Imhoff, C. L., & Kerrigan, J. M. (1990). MMPI correlates among post-acute TBI patients. *Brain Injury, 4*, 223–231.

Cassidy, J. W. (1989). Fluoxetine: A new serotonergically active antidepressant. *Journal of Head Trauma Rehabilitation, 4*, 67–69.

Cohn, C. K., Wright, J. R., & DeVaul, R. A. (1977). Post head trauma syndrome in an adolescent treated with lithium carbonate: Case report. *Diseases of the Nervous System, 38*, 630–631.

Department of Health and Human Services. (1989, February). *Interagency Head Injury Task Force report.* Washington, DC: US Dept of Health & Human Services.

Dicker, B. G. (1992). Profile of those at risk for minor head injury. *Journal of Head Trauma Rehabilitation, 7*, 83–91.

Dikmen, S., McLean, A., & Temkin, N. (1986). Neuropsychological and psychosocial consequences of minor head injury. *Journal of Neurology, Neurosurgery and Psychiatry, 49*, 1227–1232.

Dinan, T. G., & Mobayed, M. (1992). Treatment resistance of depression after head injury: A preliminary study of amitriptyline response. *Acta Psychiatrica Scandinavica, 85*, 292–294.

Englander, J., Hall, K., Stimpson, T., & Chaffin, S. (1992). Mild traumatic brain injury in an insured population: Subjective complaints and return to employment. *Brain Injury, 6*(2), 161–166.

Evans, R. W. (1994). The postconcussion syndrome: 130 Years of controversy. *Seminars in Neurology, 14*, 32–39.

Fann, J. R., Katon, W. J., Uomoto, J. M., & Esselman, P. C. (1995). Psychiatric disorders and functional disability in outpatients with traumatic brain injuries. *American Journal of Psychiatry, 152*, 1493–1499.

Federoff, J. P., Starkstein, S. E., Forrester, A. W., Geisler, F. H., Jorge, R. E., Arndt, S. V., & Robinson, R. G. (1992). Depression in patients with acute traumatic brain injury. *American Journal of Psychiatry, 149*, 918–923.

Fenton, G., McClelland, R., Montgomery, A., MacFlynn, G., & Rutherford, W. (1993). The postconcussional syndrome: Social antecedents and psychological sequelae. *British Journal of Psychiatry, 162*, 493–497.

Fisher, S. H. (1961). Psychiatric considerations of cerebral vascular disease. *American Journal of Cardiology, 7*, 379–385.

Folstein, M. F., Maiberger, R., & McHugh, P. R. (1977). Mood disorder as a specific complication of stroke. *Journal of Neurology, Neurosurgery, and Psychiatry, 40*, 1018–1020.

Fordyce, D. J., Roueche, J. R., & Prigatano, G. P. (1983). Enhanced emotional reactions in chronic head trauma patients. *Journal of Neurology, Neurosurgery, Psychiatry, 46*, 620–624.

Gasquione, P. G. (1992). Affective state and awareness of sensory and cognitive effects after closed head injury. *Neuropsychology, 6*, 187–196.

Gennarelli, T. A. (1987). Cerebral concussions and diffuse brain injuries. In P. R. Cooper (Ed.), *Head injury* (2nd ed., pp. 108–124). Baltimore, MD: Williams & Wilkins.

Graham, D. I., Adams, J. H., & Gennarelli, T. A. (1987). Pathology of brain damage in head injury. In P. R. Cooper (Ed.), *Head injury* (2nd ed., pp. 72–88). Baltimore, MD: Williams & Wilkins.

Gronwall, D. (1986). Rehabilitation programs for patients with mild head injury: Components, problems, and evaluation. *Journal of Head Trauma Rehabilitation, 1*, 53–62.

Gualtieri, C. T. (1988). Pharmacotherapy and the neurobehavioral sequelae of traumatic brain injury. *Brain Injury, 2*, 101–129.

Gualtieri, C. T., Chandler, M., Coons, T. B., & Brown, L. T. (1989). Amantadine: A new clinical profile for traumatic brain injury. *Clinical Neuropharmacology, 12*, 258–270.

Hale, M. S., & Donaldson, J. O. (1982). Lithium carbonate in the treatment of organic brain syndrome. *Journal of Nervous Mental Disease, 170,* 362–365.

Hamilton, M. (1960). A rating scale for depression. *Journal of Neurology, Neurosurgery, and Psychiatry, 23,* 56–62.

Hinkeldey, N. S., & Corrigan, J. D. (1990). The structure of head injured patients' neurobehavioral complaints: A preliminary study. *Brain Injury, 4,* 115–133.

Hoff, A. L., Shukla, S., Cook, B. L., & Aronson, T. A., Ollo, C. L., & Pass, H. L. (1988). Cognitive function in manics with associated neurologic factors. *Journal of Affective Disorders, 14,* 251–255.

Hugenholtz, H., Stuss, D. T., Stethem, L. L., & Richard, M. T. (1988). How long does it take to recover from a mild concussion? *Neurosurgery, 22,* 853–858.

Jane, J. A., Steward, O., & Gennarelli, T. A. (1985). Axonal degeneration induced by experimental noninvasive minor head injury. *Journal of Neurosurgery, 62,* 96–100.

Jones, K. T., Zwil, A. S., McAllister, T., Rogers, C., & Brennan, S. (1995). Mania secondary to antidepressant medications in brain-injured patients. *Journal of Neuropsychiatry and Clinical Neuroscience, 7,* 417.

Jorge, R. E., Robinson, R. G., Arndt, S. V., Forrester, A. W., Geisler, F., & Starkstein, S. E. (1993a). Comparison between acute- and delayed-onset depression following traumatic brain injury. *Journal of Neuropsychiatry and Clinical Neurosciences, 5,* 43–49.

Jorge, R. E., Robinson, R. G., Arndt, S. V., Forrester, A. W., Geisler, F., & Starkstein, S. E. (1993b). Depression following traumatic brain injury: A 1 year longitudinal study. *Journal of Affective Disorders, 27,* 233–243.

Jorge, R. E., Robinson, R. G., Starkstein, S. E., & Arndt, S. V. (1994). Influence of major depression on 1-year outcome in patients with traumatic brain injury. *Journal of Neurosurgery, 81,* 726–733.

Kay, T., Harrington, D. E., Adams, R., Anderson, T., Berrol, S., Cicerone, K., Dahlberg, C., Gerber, D., Goka, R., Harley, P., Hilt, J., Horn, L., Lehmkuhl, D., & Malec, J. (1993). Definition of mild traumatic brain injury. *Journal of Head Trauma Rehabilitation, 8*(3), 86–87.

Kay, T., Newman, B., Cavallo, M., Ezrachi, O., & Resnick, M. (1992). Toward a neuropsychological model of functional disability after mild traumatic brain injury. *Neuropsychology, 6,* 371–384.

Kelly, J. P., Nichols, J. S., Filley, C. M., Lillehei, K. O., Rubinstein, D., & Kleinschmidt-DeMasters, B. K. (1991). Concussion in sports: Guidelines for the prevention of catastrophic outcome. *JAMA, 266*(20), 2867–2869.

Kelly, R. (1975). The post-traumatic syndrome: An iatrogenic disease. *Forensic Science, 6,* 17–24.

King, N. S. (1996). Emotional, neuropsychological, and organic factors: Their use in the prediction of persisting postconcussion symptoms after moderate and mild head injuries. *Journal of Neurology, Neurosurgery, and Psychiatry, 61,* 75–81.

Kraus, J. F., & Nourjah, P. (1988). The epidemiology of mild, uncomplicated brain injury. *Journal of Trauma, 28,* 1637–1643.

Kraus, J. F., & Nourjah, P. (1989). The epidemiology of mild head injury. In H. S. Levin, H. M. Eisenberg, & A. L. Benton (Eds.), *Mild head injury* (pp. 8–22). New York: Oxford University Press.

Krauthammer, C., & Klerman, G. L. (1978). Secondary mania. *Archives of General Psychiatry, 35,* 1333–1339.

Levin, H. S., Mattis, S., Ruff, R. M., Eisenberg, H. M., Marshall, L. F., Tabaddor, K., High, Jr., W. M., & Frankowski, R. F. (1987). Neurobehavioral outcome following minor head injury: A three center study. *Journal of Neurosurgery, 66,* 234–243.

Lewis, L., Athey Jr., G. I., Eyman, J., & Saeks, S. (1992). Psychological treatment of adult psychiatric patients with traumatic frontal lobe injury. *Journal of Neuropsychiatry, 4*(3), 323–325.

Lezak, M. D., & O'Brien, K. P. (1988). Longitudinal study of emotional, social, and physical changes after traumatic brain injury. *Journal of Learning Disabilities, 21,* 456–463.

Lipsey, J. R., Robinson, R. G., Pearlson, G. D., Rao, K., & Price, T. R. (1984). Nortriptyline treatment of post-stroke depression: A double-blind treatment trial. *Lancet, 1,* 297–300.

Lipsey, J. R., Spencer, W. C., Rabins, P. V., & Robinson, R. G. (1986). Phenomenological comparison of poststroke depression and functional depression. *American Journal of Psychiatry, 143,* 527–529.

Lishman, W. A. (1988). Physiogenesis and psychogenesis in the "post-concussive syndrome." *British Journal of Psychiatry, 153,* 460–469.

MacNiven, E., & Finlayson, M. A. J. (1993). The interplay between emotional and cognitive recovery after closed head injury. *Brain Injury, 7*(3), 241–246.

Mas, F., Prichep, L. S., & Alper, K. (1993). Treatment resistant depression in a case of minor head injury: An electrophysiological hypothesis. *Clinical Electroencephalography, 24*(3), 118–122.

McAllister, T. W. (1992a). Neuropsychiatric sequelae of head injuries. *Psychiatric Clinics of North America, 15*(2), 395–413.

McAllister, T. W. (1992b). Mixed neurologic and psychiatric disorders: Pharmacological issues. *Comprehensive Psychiatry, 33*(5), 296–304.

McAllister, T. W. (1994). Mild traumatic brain injury and the post-concussive syndrome. In J. Silver, S. C. Yudofsky, & R. E. Hales (Eds.), *Neuropsychiatry of traumatic brain injury* (pp. 357–392). Washington, DC: American Psychiatric Press.

McAllister, T. W., & Price, T. R. P. (1990). Depression in the brain-injured: Phenomenology and treatment. In N. S. Endler & C. D. McCann (Eds.), *Depression: New directions in theory, research and practice* (pp. 361–387). Toronto: Wall and Emerson.

McElroy, S. L., Keck, P. E., Pope, H. G., & Hudson, J. I. (1989). Valproate in psychiatric disorders: Literature review and clinical guidelines. *Journal of Clinical Psychiatry, 50(Suppl.),* 23–29.

Merskey, H., & Woodforde, J. M. (1972). Psychiatric sequelae of minor head injury. *Brain, 95,* 521–528.

Middelboe, T., Andersen, H. S., Birket-Smith, M., & Friis, M. L. (1992). Minor head injury: Impact on general health after 1 year. A prospective follow-up study. *Acta Neurologica Scandinavica, 85,* 5–9.

Minderhoud, J. M., Boelens, M. E. M., Huizenga, J., & Saan, R. J. (1980). Treatment of minor head injuries. *Clinical Neurology and Neurosurgery, 82,* 127–140.

Mittenberg, W., Zielinski, R., & Fichera, S. (1993). Recovery from mild head injury: A treatment manual for patients. *Psychotherapy in Private Practice, 12*(2), 37–52.

Mobayed, M., & Dinan, T. G. (1990). Buspirone/prolactin response in post head injury depression. *Journal of Affective Disorders, 19,* 237–241.

Montgomery, A., Fenton, G. W., McClelland, R. J., MacFlynn, G., & Rutherford, W. H. (1991). The psychobiology of minor head injury. *Psychological Medicine, 21*(2), 375–384.

Nizamie, S. H., Nizamie, A., Borde, M., & Sharma, S. (1988). Mania following head injury: Case reports and neuropsychological findings. *Acta Psychiatrica Scandinavica, 77,* 637–639.

O'Hara, C. (1988). Emotional adjustment following minor head injury. *Cognitive Rehabilitation* (March/April), 26–33.

Oppenheimer, D. R. (1968). Microscopic lesions in the brain following head injury. *Journal of Neurology, 31,* 299–306.

Parker, R. S., & Rosenblum, A. (1996). IQ loss and emotional dysfunctions after mild head injury incurred in a motor vehicle accident. *Journal of Clinical Psychology, 52*(1), 32–43.

Pope, H. G., McElroy, S. L., Satlin, A., Hudson, J. I., Keck, Jr., P. E., & Kalish, R. (1988). Head injury, bipolar disorder, and response to valproate. *Comprehensive Psychiatry, 29,* 34–38.

Post, R. M., Uhde, T. W., Ballenger, J. C., & Squillace, K. M. (1983). Prophylactic efficacy of carbamazepine in manic-depressive illness. *American Journal of Psychiatry, 140,* 1602–1604.

Povlishock, J. T., & Coburn, T. H. (1989). Morphopathological change associated with mild head injury. In H. S. Levin, H. M. Eisenberg, & A. L. Benton (Eds.), *Mild head injury* (pp. 37–53). New York: Oxford University Press.

Radanov, B. P., Dvorak, J., & Valach, L. (1992). Cognitive deficits in patients after soft tissue injury of the cervical spine. *Spine, 17,* 127–131.

Riess, H., Schwartz, C. E., & Klerman, G. L. (1987). Manic syndrome following head injury: Another form of secondary mania. *Journal of Clinical Psychiatry, 48,* 29–30.

Robinson, R. G., Bolla-Wilson, K., Kaplan, E., Lipsey, J. R., & Price, T. R. (1986). Depression influences intellectual impairment in stroke patients. *British Journal of Psychiatry, 148,* 541–547.

Robinson, R. G., Boston, J. D., Starkstein, S. E., & Price, T. R. (1988). Comparison of mania and depression after brain injury: Causal factors. *American Journal of Psychiatry, 145,* 172–178.

Robinson, R. G., & Forrester, A. W. (1987). Neuropsychiatric aspects of cerebrovascular disease. In R. E. Hales & S. C. Yudofsky (Eds.), *Textbook of neuropsychiatry* (pp. 191–208). Washington, DC: American Psychiatric Press.

Robinson, R. G., Lipsey, J. R., Rao, K., & Price, T. R. (1986). Two-year longitudinal study of poststroke mood disorders: Comparison of acute-onset with delayed-onset depression. *American Journal of Psychiatry, 143,* 1238–1244.

Robinson, R. G., Starr, L. B., Lipsey, J. R., Rao, K., & Price, T. R. (1985). A two-year longitudinal study of poststroke mood disorders: In-hospital prognostic factors associated with six-month outcome. *Journal of Nervous and Mental Disease, 173,* 221–226.

Robinson, R. G., Starr, L. B., & Price, T. R. (1984). A two-year longitudinal study of mood disorders following stroke: Prevalence and duration at six months follow-up. *British Journal of Psychiatry, 144,* 256–262.

Robinson, R. G., & Szetela, B. (1981). Mood change following left hemispheric brain injury. *Annals of Neurology, 9,* 447–453.

Russell, W. R. (1974). Recovery after minor head injury. *Lancet, ii,* 13–15.

Rutherford, W. H. (1989). Postconcussive symptoms: Relationship to acute neurological indices, individual differences, and circumstances of injury. In H. S. Levin, H. M. Eisenberg, & A. L. Benton (Eds.), *Mild head injury* (pp. 217–228). New York: Oxford University Press.

Rutter, M., Chadwick, O., & Shaffer, D. (1983). Head injury. In M. Rutter (Ed.), *Developmental neuropsychiatry* (pp. 83–111). New York: Guilford Press.

Saran, A. S. (1985). Depression after minor closed head injury: Role of dexamethasone suppression test and antidepressants. *Journal of Clinical Psychiatry, 46,* 335–338.

Schoenhuber, R., & Gentilini, M. (1988). Anxiety and depression after mild head injury: A case control study. *Journal of Neurology, Neurosurgery, and Psychiatry, 51,* 722–724.

Shukla, S., Cook, B. L., Mukherjee, S., Godwin, C., & Miller, M. G. (1987). Mania following head trauma. *American Journal of Psychiatry, 144,* 93–96.

Silver, J. M., & McAllister, T. W. (1997). Forensic issues in the neuropsychiatric evaluation of the patient with mild traumatic brain injury. *Journal of Neuropsychiatry and Clinical Neurosciences, 9,* 102–113.

Silver, J. M., Yudofsky, S. C., & Hales, R. E. (1987). Neuropsychiatric aspects of traumatic brain injury. In R. E. Hales & S. C. Yudofsky (Eds.), *The American Psychiatric Press textbook of neuropsychiatry* (pp. 179–190). Washington, DC: American Psychiatric Press.

Silver, J. M., Yudofsky, S. C., & Hales, R. E. (1991). Depression in traumatic brain injury. *Neurology, Neuropsychology and Behavioral Neurology, 4,* 12–23.

Slater, E. J. (1989). Does mild mean minor? Recovery after closed head injury. *Journal of Adolescent Health Care, 10,* 237–240.

Sparadeo, F. R., Strauss, D., & Barth, J. T. (1990). The incidence, impact, and treatment of substance abuse in head trauma rehabilitation. *Journal of Head Trauma Rehabilitation, 5,* 1–8.

Starkstein, S. E., Boston, J. D., & Robinson, R. G. (1988). Mechanisms of mania after brain injury: 12 Case reports and review of the literature. *Journal of Nervous and Mental Disease, 176,* 87–100.

Starkstein, S. E., Federoff, P., Berthier, M. L., & Robinson, R. G. (1991). Manic-depressive and pure manic states after brain lesions. *Biological Psychiatry, 29,* 149–158.

Starkstein, S. E., Mayberg, H. S., Berthier, M. L., Fedoroff, P., Price, T. R., Dannals, R. F., Wagner, H. N., Leiguarda, R., & Robinson, R. G. (1990). Mania after brain injury: Neuroradiological and metabolic findings. *Annals of Neurology, 27*(6), 652–659.

Starkstein, S. E., Pearlson, G. D., Boston, J. D., & Robinson, R. G. (1987). Mania after brain injury: A controlled study of causative factors. *Archives of Neurology, 44,* 1069–1073.

Starkstein, S. E., & Robinson, R. G. (1992). Neuropsychiatric aspects of cerebral vascular disorders. In S. C. Yudofsky & R. E. Hales (Eds.), *Textbook of neuropsychiatry* (pp. 449–472). Washington, DC: American Psychiatric Press.

Stewart, J. T., & Hemsath, R. N. (1988). Bipolar illness following traumatic brain injury: Treatment with lithium and carbamazepine. *Journal of Clinical Psychiatry, 49,* 74–75.

Teasdale, G., & Jennett, B. (1974). Assessment of coma and impaired consciousness: A practical scale. *Lancet, 2,* 81–84.

Ullman, M., & Gruen, A. (1960). Behavioral changes in patients with strokes. *American Journal of Psychiatry, 117,* 1004–1009.

Varney, N. R., Martzke, J. S., & Roberts, R. J. (1987). Major depression in patients with closed head injury. *Neuropsychology, 1*(1), 7–9.

Varney, N. R., Garvey, M. J., Cook, B. L., Campbell, D. A., & Roberts, R. J. (1993). Identification of treatment-resistant depressives who respond favorably to carbamazepine. *Annals of Clinical Psychiatry, 5,* 117–122.

Watson, M. R., Fenton, G. W., McLelland, R. J., Lumsden, J., Headley, M., & Rutherford, W. H. (1995). The post-concussional state: Neurophysiological aspects. *British Journal of Psychiatry, 167,* 514–521.

Wing, J. K., Cooper, E., & Sartorius, N. (1974). *Measurement and classification of psychiatric symptoms.* Cambridge: Cambridge University Press.

Wrightson, P. (1989). Management of disability and rehabilitation services after mild head injury. In H. S. Levin, H. M. Eisenberg, & A. L. Benton (Eds.), *Mild head injury* (pp. 245–256). New York: Oxford University Press.

Yarnell, P. R., & Rossie, G. V. (1988). Minor whiplash head injury with major debilitation. *Brain Injury, 2,* 255–258.

Zwil, A. S., McAllister, T. W., Cohen, I., & Halpern, L. (1993). Ultra-rapid cycling bipolar affective disorder following a closed head injury. *Brain Injury, 7*(2), 147–152.

Zwil, A. S., McAllister, T. W., & Raimo, E. (1990). Expression of bipolar spectrum disorders in brain-injured patients. *Biological Psychiatry, 27*(9A), 55A–56A.

Zwil, A. S., McAllister, T. W., & Raimo, E. (1992). The expression of bipolar affective disorders in brain injured patients. *International Journal of Psychiatry in Medicine, 22*(4), 377–395.

Posttraumatic Headaches

Marc E. Hines
*Southeast Iowa Neurological Associates, P.C.,
and Kirksville College of Osteopathic Medicine*

Headache is the most common of the many symptoms seen after concussion or even seemingly trivial head injury, and, as such, is an important component of the controversial and often difficult-to-treat postconcussion syndrome (PCS). Because PCS, or its equivalent is seen in occasional patients with whiplash, it has also been referred to as posttraumatic syndrome. Unfortunately, this terminology is too easily confused with posttraumatic stress disorder. PCS has therefore remained the prevalent terminology in describing the bulk of posttraumatic symptoms. An extensive literature is available regarding posttraumatic headache (PTH). Among the resources is the International Headache Society (IHS) Classification System. The IHS criteria, which were developed in 1988, have never taken hold in primary care as a practical clinical classification system. This is largely due to their unwieldy length and thoroughness and partly due to a tendency for physicians to utilize preceding classifications already well understood.

The IHS criteria for a diagnosis of PTH require a loss of consciousness, posttraumatic amnesia lasting more than 10 min, and at least two abnormalities in the following evaluations: neurologic exam, skull films, central nervous system (CNS) imaging, evoked potentials, cerebrospinal fluid (CSF), vestibular function tests, or neuropsychological tests. These criteria, although serving an important purpose of ensuring a standard degree of trauma, unfortunately exclude the patients who comprise the greater number of cases with PTH. It has been repeatedly demonstrated that PTH is most common and indeed often most severe in patients with the least injury. Because we know that many patients develop a headache after trauma insufficient to meet these criteria, it begs the as yet unsettled question of etiology to exclude them a priori. I have therefore chosen to continue the common practice of calling a headache posttraumatic when the headache seems to be reasonably temporally related to trauma to the head or neck and no other etiology seems to readily explain the patient's current symptoms.

INTRODUCTION

Posttraumatic headaches and the postconcussion or posttraumatic syndrome (do not confuse with posttraumatic stress disorder) are inextricably tied together. Although one can occur without the other, headache is the most common manifestation of the posttraumatic syndrome, and the majority of patients with posttraumatic headaches have other symptoms typical of the posttraumatic syndrome. It is therefore necessary in discussing posttraumatic headaches to frequently refer to the posttraumatic syndrome. A second reason that the two are linked is for the sake of therapy. Many times it is necessary to deal with neck pain, vertigo, cognitive difficulties, and depression before the trigger to the patient's headaches can be adequately controlled.

Taken as a group, patients with posttraumatic headaches generally do well. According to Speed (1986), although most individuals who injure their heads have pain and tenderness at the site of impact for hours to days and then become symptom free, one third to one half will have symptoms persisting more than 2 months. Interventions for headache when informed by careful diagnosis are most often helpful. However, Packard (1994) pointed out that patients with posttraumatic headaches frequently have a variety of other complaints.

The study by Sturzenegger (1994) clarified that the typical individual who has experienced whiplash may have difficulties similar to those seen in some patients with postconcussion syndrome. Radanov et al. (1992), in a study of patients with acceleration and deceleration injury to the neck, demonstrated that such neck injuries may be coincident with head trauma, and Winston (1987) and Sturzenegger et al. (1994), in discussing the relationship of migraine to whiplash, concluded that soft tissue injury to the neck may induce headache via musculoskeletal mechanisms stemming from the neck and shoulders. It is also notable that the synaptic field of the upper cervical first-order pain neurons intersects with the terminal portion of the descending nucleus of cranial nerve V (a nociceptive receptor field with the upper portions of the head being in the most inferior position anatomically). Because of this odd anatomical fact, pain in the upper cervical segments can easily cause generalization of pain into the head.

The frequent early complaints in either head trauma or whiplash include pain in the head and/or neck, often with nausea, dizziness, and disorientation (at least initially), as well as complaints from other somatic injuries. As recovery ensues, if symptoms persist, as Ham et al. (1994) explained, there is virtually always a compensatory emotional reaction to the symptoms and any perceived disability. The symptoms of these posttrauma patients have been summarized elsewhere and so are only briefly reviewed in Table 17.1.

A SIMPLIFIED DISCUSSION OF PAIN

Important, perhaps even critical, to any discussion of pain is the concept that hurt does not equal harm. In chronic pain, the hurt the patient experiences does not necessarily reflect any tissue damage, and the insistence of the pain may convince the patient to be inactive and dependent. The resulting spiral of muscle atrophy, poor tolerance for exercise, and lowered self-esteem drops the patient into a progressive decline in function. The vicious cycle, known all too well to those of us who see pain patients regularly, becomes a self-reinforcing process.

Pain is often defined as an unpleasant sensory and emotional experience associated with actual or potential tissue damage, or described in terms of such damage. However, many individuals learn the application of the word for instances in which there is no tissue damage, nor is there likely to be any damage. The clinician might at first be inclined to disagree

TABLE 17.1
Symptoms: Posttraumatic Syndrome and
Sequelae of Mild Head Injury (Evans, 1994)

Headaches
  Muscle contraction type
  Migraine
  Cluster
  Occipital neuralgia
  Supraorbital and infraorbital neuralgia
  Secondary to neck injury
  Secondary to temporomandibular joint syndrome
  Owing to scalp laceration or local trauma
  Dysautonomic
  Mixed

(Continued)

TABLE 17 1
(Continued)

Cranial nerve symptoms and signs
  Dizziness and lightheadedness
  Vertigo
  Tinnitus
  Hearing loss
  Hyperacusis
  Blurred vision
  Diplopia
  Convergence insufficiency
  Light and noise sensitivity
  Diminished taste and smell
Psychologic and somatic complaints
  Irritability
  Anxiety
  Frustration
  Depression
  Personality change
  Easy fatigability
  Sleep disturbances
  Decreased libido
  Increased or decreased appetite
  Anger outbursts
  Emotional callousness
  Blunting or lability of emotional response
  Mood swings
Cognitive impairments
  Impaired memory
  Reduced attention span
  Decreased ability to concentrate
  Slowing of reaction time
  Slowing of information processing speed
  Heightened distractibility
  Difficulty in turning from one subject to another
  Deterioration of synthetic thinking
  Inability to grasp new or abstract concepts
  Lack of spontaneity accompanied by apathy and loss of initiative
  Reduced motivation
Other
  Alcohol intolerance
  Increased sensitivity to weather or temperature change
  Syncope
Less common sequelae
  Subdural and epidural hematomas
  Seizures
  Transient global amnesia
  Tremor
  Dystonia

with this use of the word, but on more careful reflection realizes that many situations occur in which pain seems to be present, either through observation of patient behavior, or because of the overall clinical presentation, and yet no tissue damage is apparent. Degree of tissue damage does not always correlate with the quality, duration, or severity of pain. Headache is a typical example of just such a condition.

Severe pain can occur in many conditions long after injury has healed. Examples include phantom limb pain, thalamic infarction, postherpetic neuralgia, trigeminal neuralgia, and others. The discovery that many factors, other than simple peripheral pain receptor mechanisms, have an impact on pain experience should be no surprise to the experienced clinician. Most of our models for pain transmission come from lower animal species and cannot involve understanding of the mental processes subserving pain control or lack of it. A key concept in understanding pain is that neither an entirely peripheral or an entirely central model suffices to explain all phenomena.

For instance, the following case is presented by McDonald Critchley and referred to by Adler, Adler, and Packard (1987).

> A male, age 57, at the age of 35 had sustained a crushing injury to the right foot. Though no bones were broken, the resulting pain was severe. Twelve months later, after months in the hospital, the foot was amputated just above the ankle joint on account of the persisting pain. The pain, however, continued not only in the stump but in the phantom. Two months later a second amputation was carried out in the upper third of the thigh, but with no effect on the pain. A year after that, the stump was explored and the ends of the severed nerves freed and sectioned at a higher level. Because this measure was ineffectual, the sciatic nerve was exposed and divided in two places. No benefit followed. Nine years after the original trauma, a posterior rhizotomy of the lumbosacral plexus was performed, and because this operation did not help, a chordotomy was conducted in the upper dorsal region. Even this measure failed to assuage pain. . . . When seen 22 years after the original accident, the patient was still complaining of severe and immutable pain in the stump. (p. 25)

I do not have time in this discussion to cover all of the intricacies of the pain transmission pathways. But to be succinct, according to the original model of pain transmission of Melzack and Wall, the modalities of touch, vibration, and position sense form an inhibitory network that serves to "gait" "pain" transmission. Even though the particulars of the Melzack and Wall hypothesis have changed, the overall principle stands. We can rub the area we have bruised and reduce "pain" transmission; we can apply a TENS unit and reduce "pain" transmission. Despite this seeming dedicated "pain" transmission and control system, we cannot assign "pain" to the system, because pain is a perception not solely dependent on the peripheral pathways alone. By hypnosis, rage reaction, stress, euphoria, dissociative states, and even placebo, the individual can be essentially divorced from the experience of pain.

Signal interpretation centrally has generally been explained on the basis of two theories, both of which probably are partially active. The labeled line theory postulates that pain is processed by a specific system from the receptor to the cortical receiving areas. The pattern theory proposes that pain is due to excessive stimulation in any modality that produces a pattern of nerve impulses interpreted centrally as pain. The labeled line system works well for explanations of peripheral pain but is less readily capable of explaining events at the central level. Descending influences on the spinal "pain" system output have been demonstrated to descend from the periaquaductal gray in the midbrain (PGA) and from the nucleus raphé magnus (NRM). These systems are controlled by opiate receptors and give rise to descending seritonergic pathways that presynaptically inhibit release of substance P (pain neurotransmitter) from the nociceptive efferents as they attempt to synapse in the spinal cord. Other mechanisms of direct spinal opiate-induced inhibition of pain and even histamine-related inhibition of pain have all been described.

How does all this relate to headache and how much pain the patient is suffering? The mechanisms whereby pain is created anywhere in the body are largely mimicked by one form of headache or another. It is useful in evaluating headache to try to keep in mind the chronicity versus the acuteness of the headache problem. Is the pain a needless pain, versus a purposeful pain? Is the pain of peripheral or central origin? Not all headaches can be easily classified in this way. But treatment decisions frequently are specifically clarified by an unclouded attempt to categorize the pain. Each pain situation, even in the most "organic" circumstances, becomes manifest as a group of coping behaviors that have been the result of the patient's perception of pain and its significance. Likewise, even in the least "organic" circumstance, pain often creates physiologic change that may become dysfunctional (minor injury with anxiety/depression leading to chronic increased muscle tone and sleep loss leading to some patients developing fibromyalgia).

If a patient has meningitis, a relatively acute and purposeful pain, with a presumptively peripheral mechanism of irritation of the meninges, our treatment regimen is oriented toward the cause and ameliorating the pain with necessary narcotic analgesia, if clinical status is stable enough that critical information regarding the patients course will not be lost. On the other hand, a patient presenting with 20 years of continuous headache, a normal neurological exam, and a depressed affect with markedly accentuated descriptions of their pain perception may receive therapy more oriented to the central process of pain control. A seritonergic antidepressant and counseling for realistic goals of therapy and gradually increasing activity through coached exercises all come to mind.

Whatever the etiology, physiology impacts psychology, which impacts physiology. The two faces of pain can sometimes be unfolded for our intellectual review, but we must not confuse this theoretical activity with reality.

PHYSIOLOGIC VERSUS PSYCHOGENIC CONCEPTS, NOT OPPOSITES

In an attempt to describe the PCS symptom complex, including headache, investigators and academicians (depending on their point of view on the subject) attribute PCS and head pain to a seeming "wastebasket" of psychosocial stressors, preexisting personality traits, and litigation-related motivations on the one hand, or they attribute PCS to somewhat less than perfectly defined physiologic mechanisms. It has also been maintained that PCS patients improve with the completion of litigation. In one survey (Evans, Evans, & Sharp, 1994), 24% of neurologists believed that once litigation is settled, symptoms quickly resolve. Guthkelch (1980) in an earlier review demonstrated what more recent studies (see Mendelson, 1982; also Fee & Rutherford, 1988) have shown: that the majority of patients with PCS do not have full improvement following the completion of litigation.

It is pleasing to note that the early literature, including Denny-Brown cited in Brenner (1944), supported the proposition set out in their introduction that "psychogenic and physiologic factors are so closely interwoven when there is organic cerebral damage that a separation between them is unnatural and the practice of dividing cases of postconcussion syndrome into two groups, labeling the syndrome organic in one and functional in the other, is unprofitable and misleading" (p. 382). I spend a moment on this study because it closely reflects the final outcome of over 50 years of additional research. This 1944 article consisted of 200 consecutive cases of head injuries admitted to Boston City Hospital. Any cases in which other factors contributed to duration of loss of conciousness, or exact information could not be confirmed, were excluded from the study.

The high degree of correlation between the incidence of prolonged headache and the incidence of post-traumatic nervous reactions (fears, anxieties, nervousness, fatigue, and an inability to concentrate) as well as prolonged dizziness is, of course, merely a statistical validation of the concept of posttraumatic syndrome. . . . On the other hand . . . a high incidence [of headache post-traumatically] among patients with scalp lacerations . . . indicate[s] that the severity of the physical injury plays some part as well as the degree of emotional and environmental stress. (p. 383)

These situations might seem cripplingly overburdened with difficulties but for the fact that most of the problems once identified are manageable. The seemingly ever-present disadvantage of struggling with the distinction between "organic" and "psychologic" mechanisms of symptom production is lessened by realization that the tension between these two distinctions is generally less necessary for medical purposes than for legal. For purely medical purposes their is no conflict created by simultaneously understanding an individual's posttraumatic problems as consisting of both "organic" and "psychological" components. Perhaps some of the problems develop from far too static a view of brain injury, combined with a tendency to believe that psychological difficulties are by their nature not organic.

The computer analogy of brain function is prevalent in popular and even in scientific literature. I notice that although it is often pointed out that the human brain is self-programming, it is frequently overlooked that, to a degree, it is self-creating. Self-creation occurs at the level of axonal branching, synaptic density, and certainly biochemically. At this level, significant psychologic change can become structural. The distinction between "psychological" and "organic" factors, although convenient, is not always genuinely intrinsic to the system being studied but rather to the convenience of evaluation.

A practical guide to the evaluation and treatment of posttraumatic head pain can be traced back to three concepts: first, psychodynamics and physical attributes of the problem are interactive at all moments and often in a multiplicity of fashions; second, headache is but one of the patient's symptoms; and third, all headache types can be seen with PTH, and many respond as they would if of any other etiology.

It is widely agreed that in patients with posttraumatic headache with or without postconcussion syndrome, attitudes conveyed by medical personnel can influence outcome. Kelly (1973, 1983) was especially forceful in espousing this viewpoint and related the following information concerning a follow-up study of patient outcomes as related to physician attitudes:

One hundred and twenty-nine patients were studied with specific inquiry as to what treatment was offered.

Seventy-six patients with posttraumatic syndrome were given little treatment. Of these:

19—The physician refused any treatment whatever.

34—Physician failure to inform that any further treatment was available.

10—Received only 10 days of treatment on the physician's grounds that "everybody knows it is a waste of time treating patients who have made a claim."

13—Patients had refused treatment on the basis that previous doctors declared them to be untreatable so they supposed themselves dreadfully ill.

Only 11 of these 76 patients returned to work within a period halfway between the accident and settlement of their claim.

Thirty additional patients had been vigorously treated soon after the accident; 25 had returned to work within 12 months of the onset of their symptoms and long before the settlement of their claim.

It is therefore important to emphasize our duty to assist the patients in understanding their symptoms and experience. Given the very wide array of seemingly inexplicable symptoms, it is valuable for patients to hear that their experience is valid. Failure to clarify that a patient's experience is not bizarre (unless of course it is) leads to cognitive dissonance. The patients are stressed by symptoms they feel cannot be explained. Unfortunately, many physicians have not taken the opportunity of becoming familiar with all the myriad symptoms of the posttraumatic syndrome. It is easy to pass off symptoms as bizarre whenever those symptoms seem inappropriate because the physician is less than fully informed.

A patient can be reassured as to the meaning of symptoms even as the physician is emphasizing the high likelihood of recovery. What seems to most engender an attitude of disbelief or anger from patients is the flippant answer or the minimal exam. A thorough history gathering that allows the patient to voice complaints followed by an exam that at least includes all areas of complaint often does more toward reassurance than a mountain of polysyllabic rhetoric or a frenzy of white coats.

The genuinely tough problems usually begin as the patient runs out of patience with persisting symptoms and shows signs of clinical depression. As the patient continues to be symptomatic for a period of months, the clinical course has certain increasingly stereotypical features. Typically, chronic pain creates an environment of frustration, distraction, discouragement, and loss of sleep. Depression, anger, and incomplete recovery from muscle fatigue during sleep often result. Many patients develop or have prolongation of cognitive symptoms, enhanced by the distractibility of pain, depression, and sleep deprivation.

Posttraumatic headaches that persist late (more than 6 months) are virtually self-selected to be considerably more complex. Frequently, patients have more symptoms and may have suffered more injury than was at first expected. Alternately, the headaches may have evolved to new or more complex mechanisms (neuralgias, migraine, trigger points with chronic cervical inflammation, cervical facet arthropathies, or combinations of headache type). Finally, and importantly, emotional factors including depression, anxiety, posttraumatic stress disorder, personality disorders, or merely personality style may play a substantial role in keeping headaches triggered. Many patients acquire a combination of these factors, added to which they may develop some cynicism about treatment and care providers. This complexity does not lend itself well to the sorting functions of insurance and litigatory processes.

THE LEGAL CLIMATE AND PREEXISTING CONDITIONS

Many preexisting conditions, like headache, are common so that members of the general public, including lawyers, judges, and jurors, often have preconceived notions regarding which preexisting conditions may cause symptomatology. It is sometimes necessary, in order to assist everyone in understanding these preexisting conditions and their impact on a compensable situation, that we educate both ourselves and others regarding the extent to which injury is more marked, may have no impact on the current situation, or may completely explain the patient's present complaints.

Preexisting conditions represent a wide array of difficulties, which may complicate the evaluation of a variety of compensable situations. Headache is assuredly a common preexisting condition. Whether serious or trivial, the prior headache history of the patient is potentially relevant diagnostically, prognostically, and medical-legally. Many preexisting conditions are less than trivial. The application of concern about a preexisting condition can, in certain situations, be trite and inane. (I have witnessed the contention that webbed toe deformity caused a patient's chronic low back pain, rather than the accident after which it had immediately developed.) However, other preexisting conditions represent serious disease, and some of the properties of the preexisting conditions present the examiner and the judicial system with significant questions of fact and principle. (How does preexisting headache interact with head trauma?—see later discussion). The application of fact varies as widely as the access to specific relevant information. We can only begin to touch on some of that information in this review.

For example, a recent study by Russell and Olesen (1996) suggested that migraine without aura is caused by a different mechanism than migraine with aura. Even further, their study, which specifically looked at posttraumatic migraine, demonstrated that posttraumatic migraine without aura was 7 times more likely after trauma than migraine with aura, whereas spontaneous migraine without aura is only 2 times more likely than migraine with aura. This information suggested to the investigators that head trauma produces (causes) migraine without aura as opposed to merely triggering migraine. Therefore, contrary to the opinion that head trauma triggers migraine primarily in susceptible individuals, this evidence seems to demonstrate that head trauma may in fact cause the headache process de novo.

The impact on our better comprehension of preexisting conditions by recent research is well illustrated in the following example. Wallis, Lord, and Bogduk (1997) investigated the remediability of psychological symptoms in patients who have chronic whiplash symptomatology. The finding of increased incidence of psychological distress, anxiety, and depressive symptoms in patients with chronic whiplash has often been equated with a reverse causality; that is, the increased incidence in such patients is equated with the psychological problems being part or all of the cause of the patients' prolonged symptomatology. Furthermore, the psychological condition is assumed to be preexisting as a fundamental part of the patient's personality, which is in turn supposed to be stable and well delineated by our testing procedures. In this study, the issue of psychological factors as an etiology in the chronic whiplash pain syndrome is markedly simplified by studying a group of patients in whom good or excellent pain relief can be obtained. When this was done, it became immediately obvious that the pain was the principal cause of the psychological distress of these patients and not the other way around. This study demonstrated that when chronic pain was alleviated, patients who had experienced an equal incidence of "psychological" symptomatology with others who did not improve had a dramatic reduction in their psychological symptoms. This reduction in "psychological" symptoms was so complete that testing and interviews reverted to normal. This information was correlated with the data demonstrating that patients with chronic posttraumatic headache and whiplash symptoms do not have an elevation in measures of preexisting psychological conditions when compared to the general populace. Many physicians are unaware of these data and have long used (or is it abused?) the information that chronic pain in many settings is associated with increased psychological distress, to conclude that such patients have preexisting personality types which lead to the chronicity of the problem. These assertions are typical of many overgeneralizations: undoubtedly excessive and at least partially incorrect. The difficulty has been deeper still. A physician's responsibility to assist a patient is significantly proscribed and reduced if one can ascribe the problem to a fundamental unchanging aspect of the patient's personality. Patients with chronic pain are typically time-consuming and demanding; therefore, the ability to reduce responsibility to them and distance ourselves from their needs is beneficial to the busy physician who is often under pressure to quickly either find improvement or move the patient to a category of maximum benefit in therapies and reduce treatment and visits.

Unfortunately, not all patients with chronic whiplash pain respond to aggressive management. This leaves even this study open to a criticism that those not responding may be at risk due to latent psychological pathology. Because the preexisting state of the psychological health had been formerly assumed to be in question for anyone not responding to conventional therapy—and in fact, by extension, to anyone not sponta-neously recovering—we can at least relate that the logic of such assump-tions was not only flawed but that the conclusions were clearly incorrect. Plainly speaking in this study: Patients' chronic pain was the cause of psychological distress, and as our patients generally relate to us, "when the pain goes away, I will no longer be depressed or upset."

TYPES OF POSTTRAUMATIC HEADACHES

Posttraumatic headaches present in a number of different manners and with a variety of patterns. Just as it has become potentially valuable to separate the types of posttraumatic syndrome (see Cicerone, 1996), it is useful to separate types of posttraumatic headaches in order to better describe treatment options and prognosis. There are often substantial etiologic differences between early and late presentation headaches, scar pain, purely facial pain, occipital neuralgia, cervicogenic tension-type headaches, and migraines. Among the important etiologic considerations we must also include headaches with contributions from anxiety and posttraumatic stress disorder and depression.

After completing a listing of the various types of headaches by location, duration, severity, and type of pain, it is still necessary to divide these headaches into acute, subacute, and chronic. The etiology, prognosis and behavior of headaches are likely to be quite different depending on the duration. In patients with severe or moderate head injury it is critical to develop an understanding of the phase of recovery that a patient is currently experiencing. This knowledge assists in understanding various aspects of the return of abilities and response to rehabilitation and to medications. The same sophistication should at least be looked for in rehabilitation of patients with mild head injury.

Simons and Wolff (1946) were probably the first to divide posttraumatic headaches into subtypes. The first headache subtype was described as steady pressure or aching in a caplike distribution or in a circumscribed area (not at the site of injury) and deep tenderness on manual palpation. The second was a circumscribed area of relatively superficial tenderness at the site of impact or in a scar with aching pain of moderate intensity. The third type was described as an aching pain, often throbbing, occurring in attacks, usually unilateral in onset, and chiefly in the temporal, frontal, postauricular or occipital region, occasionally combined with headache type 1.

Speed (1983) concluded that posttraumatic headaches may mimic virtually any other type of headache. There are, however, certain patterns that reflect the descriptions originally utilized by Simons and Wolff. Type 1 would now be called tension-type PTH, type 2 scalp injury or scar pain, and type 3 probably corresponds to posttraumatic migraine.

Scherokman and Massey (1983) added a type 4 to the original three. This fourth type is characterized by injury that includes the anterior compartment of the neck and probably represents a dysautonomic cephalgia. This variety was first described by Vijayan (1977) and was a recurrent headache that occurred episodically, unilaterally, as a frontotemporal pain associated with mydriasis and facial hyperhydrosis. Vijayan postulated that the injury involved third-order sympathetic neurons in the neck. The patients are known to improve with propranolol but not ergotamine. Another type of PTH that can be included in this dysautonomic group is cluster. Cluster is characterized by unilateral lancinating pain in the periorbital area associated with rhinorrhea, lacrimation, and local erythema.

In addition to these types it seems necessary to add a fifth type. Treleaven et al. (1994) described cervicogenic headache, which should be given a separate major subtype designation (type 5), particularly because it may not simply correspond to the pattern of tension-type PTH. This headache may be a consequence of head injury or of whiplash with or without head injury per se. It usually begins in the neck or low occipital area and extends forward, with aching pain associated with significant complaints of tenderness and tightness of muscles. Some patients develop trigger points in the cervical area, shoulders, or posteriorly between the shoulder blades.

Katayama (1970), Unterharnscheidt (1986), and Wickstrom et al. (1967) described studies of experimentally induced whiplash in animals. Hyperflexion injuries have demonstrated hemorrhages due to tears and ruptures of muscle near their origins. Tectorial membranes and posterior longitudinal ligaments were frequently disrupted, as were transverse and cruciate ligaments. Hyperextension causes multiple hematomas and hemorrhages in the neck musculature, particularly the sternocleidomastoids. Wickstrom (1965) also noted that more severe g forces (peak sled accelerations induced by pendulum strikes or air cylinders) of 64 gs or more are associated with much more severe cervical injuries such as fractures, dislocations, intervertebral disc herniations, and in some cases even brain injuries.

Neuropathic pain is seen in two types of headache that often respond dramatically to local injections of steroids and anesthetic. Occipital neuralgia is a distinct although slightly related entity in which a blow to the back of the head results in exquisite tenderness over the area of penetration of the occipital nerve into the far posterior aspect of the musculature over the occipital area. Presumptively, injury leads to swelling and then entrapment, which in turn perpetuates inflammatory responses and further swelling. Early identification and injection locally with steroids can be beneficial.

Possibly related to similar mechanisms is a scar or scalp contusion, which in some patients develops into sharp stabbing pains, some with electric-like sensations when pressure is applied in the area of a scar or scalp injury. This is distinct from other types of scalp pain in its clear neuralgic nature (sharp, lancinating, or burning, with symptoms usually demonstrated on tapping or pressure to a discreet area—presumptively the neuroma). Again, some patients respond to injection of the area with steroids. These neuralgic pains probably deserve a separate type 6 categorization because of their distinct qualities including response to local therapy.

In summary, the "classic" PTH headache subtypes include:

Type 1: Tension type.
Type 2: Local injury or scar pain without neuralgia.
Type 3: Migraine.
Type 4: Dysautonomic cephalgia.
Type 5: Cervicogenic.
Type 6: Neuralgic.

In fact, headache subtypes often coexist and may mix with other headaches due to additional mechanisms (Table 17.2).

MANAGEMENT

"Treat whatever you see," by which I mean, "don't nihilistically simply sit back and observe," was a simple principle that I felt could guide therapy for many patients with headache. Unfortunately, what any individual "sees" in a given case is highly dependent on background, experience, attitudes, training, and specialty. Considerable disagreement can therefore occur depending on the vantage point of the practitioner. Per-

TABLE 17.2
Potential Mechanisms of Posttraumatic Cephalgia
(Levin & Turkewitz, 1993)

Immediate extracranial
  Lacerations
  Abrasions
  Skull or cervical spine fractures
  Whiplash (apophyseal joint injury, musculoskeletal injury, C2 root injury)
Immediate intracranial
  Arterial dilatation (nonmigrainous vascular headache)
  Traumatic subarachnoid hemorrhage
  Arterial occlusion
Delayed extracranial
  Muscle contraction headache
  Entrapment or neuroma of sensory nerves (neuralgia)
  Carotid dissection
  Dysautonomia
Delayed intracranial
  Subdural hematoma
  Epidural hematoma
  Cerebral contusion with edema
  Cerebral spinal fluid leak (low pressure headache)
  Hydrocephalus
Other
  Sinus pathology
  Orbital pathology
  Temporomandibular joint dysfunction
  Posttraumatic migraine
  Posttraumatic cluster headache
  Psychiatric factors
    Psychosocial stress
    Anxiety
    Depression
    Delusional disorder, somatic type or somatiform disorder
  Drug overuse
Combination

haps a more dependable approach to the development of some still simple guides to therapy could include the following.

The symptoms in PTH go through an evolution in variety, severity, and in specificity for underlying mechanisms of headache production. Therefore, evaluation of the patient should be looked on with reference to the time following injury. Many disagreements of practitioners observing the same patient can occur over nothing more than a misunderstanding about the evolution of PTH symptomatology and indeed evolution of the attitudes and reactions of the PTH patient. Six concerns I always look carefully for are:

1. Undiagnosed migraine.
2. Undiagnosed depression.
3. Undertreatment of trigger points.
4. Missed cases of neuralgia.
5. Mixed headache.
6. Sleep disturbances.

The following are "tips" sometimes not seen in reviews on the subject.

Early PTH (<2 Months)

General Recommendations.

1. Most patients improve. Therefore, after an exam and history to exclude the possibility of more serious problems, simple analgesics and reassurance are the most useful approach.

2. Steroid use during the first few days after the concussion can assist with control of pain and headache but must be balanced against the risk of side effects.

Specific Recommendations.

3. Patients with a prior history of migraine should be treated early. Patients with a strong family history of migraine often develop migrainous headaches posttraumatically. Specific therapy for migraine may be necessary for these patients early in their course, and a high index of suspicion for the development of migraine should be maintained.

4. Prior psychiatric concerns should be reevaluated. Patients with a prior history of depression, anxiety, or psychiatric disturbance should consider early counseling for the posttraumatic experience and should be closely monitored for redevelopment of psychological or psychiatric symptoms.

5. Anger should be addressed. Patients who are very angry should have early psychological intervention, should be taught relaxation techniques, and should be encouraged to exercise.

6. Neck injury must be addressed. Patients with neck injury should be placed in a coached exercise program for the neck after initial "cooling down" and after evaluation has reasonably excluded serious structural disease. Chiropractic therapy, which is used by many patients in this setting, has been demonstrated to have an equal or superior effectiveness

to PT. Either approach can be utilized for the several weeks required to calm the acute muscle spasm in the neck. Evaluation for trigger points should then occur if the patient has not had further improvement.

7. Age, prior head injury, alcoholism, or multiple trauma worsens prognosis. Elderly patients, patients with prior head injury, patients with a history of alcohol abuse, or patients with multiple trauma (other orthopedic and soft tissue injuries) with early cognitive complaints should definitely be evaluated by neuropsychology (Evans, 1992).

8. Extensive or severe postconcussion symptoms worsen prognosis. According to Walker and Erculei (1969), the longer patients continue to experience multiple postconcussion symptoms, the worse the prognosis becomes for headache resolution.

Intermediate PTH (2–6 Months)

1. Headache patterns emerge. The headache early on in PTH is often nondescript and difficult to manage other than with simple supportive measures. It is important to note that there is a transformation in many patients during the months following initial injury with the development of clearly recognizable syndromes. These often emerge in this time frame.

2. Migraine, neuralgias, and cervicogenic headache are quite treatable. Look for specific headache patterns because these are often identified in this period if not before. Treatment aimed at each headache type can be effective in significantly reducing symptoms and encouraging confidence in the care being given.

3. Common migraine is often overlooked. Migraine, particularly common migraine, which is often not associated with unilateral headache or visual phenomena, is frequently overlooked as a potentially treatable component of PTH. It is very important to recall that the patient often will be experiencing more than one headache type (mixed headache).

4. Depression is often overlooked. Depression is seen with strikingly high frequency in patients during this period. The classic vegetative symptoms may be missing or only just beginning so that the diagnosis is often overlooked. Newer treatment regimens of chronic daily headache that include seritonergic antidepressants probably will assist in preventing some of the development of these problems.

5. Persistent specific neuropsychological complaints emerge. Neuropsychological evaluation is frequently necessary for patients with persistent complaints of cognitive dysfunction, mood swings, or family complaints of personality change and/or problems managing motivation and decision making. Positron emission tomography (PET) scans have demonstrated frontal deficits in many patients even when neuropsychological testing is

only suggestive. In others the PET studies have demonstrated temporal-lobe deficits.

6. Strikingly episodic symptoms are sometimes seen. Some patients emerge with very episodic symptomatology that often leads to electro-encephalographs (EEGs) being performed to exclude seizures. More often than not, the EEG is negative, yet many of these patients experience improvement in symptoms from the use of anticonvulsants. Depakote also treats headache, anxiety, and mood swings. Tegretol is valuable for mood swings as well as other episodic symptoms. These two anticonvulsants are often preferable because of their additional benefits.

7. Stressors and patient nihilism contribute to triggering headaches. Legal problems, bills for health care, time lost from work, and stress-related marriage and family problems all lead to considerable increase in emotional turmoil, particularly when added to the patient's perception that the problem appears unlikely to improve at an early date. Counseling for all these problems can be helpful, except the legal aspects. Patients with legal activities should be encouraged to spend as little time concerned about these problems as feasible. I encourage the patient to leave the endeavor to the lawyers.

Late (>6 Months)

General Recommendations.

1. Improvement is still possible (National Headache Foundation [NHF], 1996).

2. Complexity combined with mixed presentation is typical. These patients are often very complex with multiple, and sometimes unusual, posttraumatic symptoms. Bipolar illness, anxiety, and depression have all been reported after head trauma. Family psychodynamics are frequently very strained. In this group a very high percentage will have both previously unrecognized "organic" pathology and a very high percentage will also have previously unrecognized "psychological" pathology.

3. Pain is a common thread in failed improvement. The NHF (1996) guidlines specifiy that pain syndromes in addition to headache often play a substantial role in the continuing disability of these patients.

4. Legal concerns must be handled without emotional overinvestment. Legal matters often take a prominent role in undertaking care of such individuals. This is only temporary, but such considerations may be present for several years if litigation is deemed necessary.

Once diagnoses have been evolved, therapeutic decisions may begin.

Data Necessary to Individualize Therapy Selections (NHF, 1996)

1. What are the patient's age, weight, and gender?
2. Does the patient have other physical/medical and/or psychiatric comorbidities? What medications (prescribed and over-the-counter) is the patient taking?
3. What is the patient's reproductive status? Is the patient concerned about compromising libido or fertility? Is the patient pregnant?
4. Does the patient have known drug sensitivities?
5. What time of day do headache attacks occur?
6. Does the headache develop slowly, begin abruptly, or awaken the patient from sleep?
7. Are headache attacks associated with menses or ovulation?
8. Where is patient during attacks?
9. Does each attack create the same level of disability?
10. Does the patient work? If so, does the work involve the operation of dangerous machinery?
11. Does the patient have childcare responsibilities?
12. Is the patient an athlete or does he or she participate in recreational activities that involve strenuous physical excercise or the use of dangerous equipment?

Treatment Regimens of Non-Headache-Related Posttraumatic Complaints

1. Ligamentous and muscle injury, cervical and lumbosacral strains: Rest and acute pain relief only transiently, then physical therapy, followed by *progressive exercise*. Muscle relaxants and nonsteroidals are frequently of moderate benefit.
2. Disc herniations, radiculopathy: Traction, muscle relaxants, steroids acutely, physical therapy (PT), TENS, epidural steroids with surgery as last resort.
3. Fractures: Referral to orthopedics or neurosurgery is usually necessary.
4. Dislocations: Referral to orthopedics or neurosurgery is usually necessary.
5. Root and plexus stretch injuries: Treat as a neuropathic pain syndrome, often even as a sympathetically maintained pain. Utilize a generous amount of PT to strengthen and maintain range of motion. Elavil, 10–50 mg/day; Dilantin, 200–600 mg; Tegretol, 200–2000 mg;

Baclofen, 10–60 mg; Mexitil or Tonocard: Mexitil, 150–600 mg/day; Tonocard, 400 mg tid; Prozac, Paxil, or Zoloft: Prozac, 20–60 mg; Paxil, 20–60 mg; Zoloft, 50–200 mg.

6. Reflex sympathetic dystrophies: Early trial sympathetic block, possible sympathectomy, TENS, ultrasound, progressive exercise. Mexitil, 150–600 mg/day. Pharmacologic sympathectomy: phenoxybenzamine 10–40 mg/day or propranolol or reserpine or one of the newer "alpha and beta" antagonists.

7. Canal hematomas and contusions: Can be an acute neurologic emergency due to mass effect and compression of neural structures. These also may develop a neuralgic component late in their course.

8. Trigger-point dysfunction: Injections to the specific trigger points with lidocaine or marcaine and a local steroid such as Depomedrol.

9. Osteoarthritic aggravation: Gentle ultrasound, ice initially, heat later, along with nonsteroidal anti-inflammatory drugs (NSAIDs) and muscle relaxants, may need to be followed by a short course of steroids. Exercise to maintain strength and mobility can be done carefully. Soft collars used in the car or with prolonged sitting can be useful. Cervical pillows are not usually tolerated initially, but later in course may be beneficial.

The most critical information determining treatment of headache is headache type. In the following sections, detailed attributes of headache types are reviewed and then recommendations for abortive and prophylactic therapy are reviewed.

Type 1: Tension Type (So-Called Muscle-Contraction Type) Characteristics

1. Gradual onset and offset.
2. Usually bilateral, diffuse nonthrobbing pain.
3. Pain is often continuous, aching, or dull.
4. Pain is often frontal, temporal, occipital, diffuse, or bandlike.
5. Muscular aching common.
6. Tightness of the neck common.
7. Tenderness of the neck and scalp.
8. Steady pain of extended duration (in a study of 1,000 tension headaches.
9. Often precipitated by stress, anxiety, overwork, eyestrain, fatigue, and so on.

10. Often relieved by ordinary analgesics and rest or removal of inciting factors.
11. Often associated with underlying psychiatric conditions such as anxiety, depression, or personality disorders.
12. Insomnia from headache is frequent.
13. More than one headache type is common.

Cervical Osteoarthritis With Tension Type Headache.

1. As in tension type but with prominent neck complaints
2. Often responds to a cervical pillow at night, NSAID, PT; if foramina are stenosed, then cervical traction may be useful.
3. Occasionally simply supporting the neck during the examination is beneficial in relieving the pain.

Conversion Disorders.

1. The headache is often tension type but with bizarre or exaggerated descriptions and may not respond at all to significant doses of analgesics or appropriate agents; or responds transiently to virtually anything including placebo but always eventually escapes control.
2. A history of similar or other symptoms not following typical physiologic patterns.

Temporomandibular Joint Syndrome (Can Mimic Tension Type). Recurrent facial pain associated with tenderness over the temporomandibular joint is most probably temporomandibular cephalgia. Usually unilateral, constant, aching pain around the temporomandibular joint sometimes radiating to the jaws, exacerbated by movement of the lower jaw (chewing, yawning). The patient may report an associated clicking or grating sound. The pain may be associated with bruxism during sleep; depression or insomnia may also be present.

Palpation of the temporalis muscle or direct pressure on the temporomandibular joint may result in pain. Special x-ray techniques often reveal asymmetric temporomandibular joints with degenerative changes in the cartilage. Palpation over the joint often reveals subluxation.

Treatment is often unsatisfactory. Correction of dental malocclusion may or may not relieve the pain. Conservative therapy includes heat applied to the affected area, a diet of soft foods, limitation of mouth opening, dental prostheses, mild analgesics, NSAIDs, muscle relaxants, or antidepressants.

Treatment. See Tables 17.3 and 17.4.

Type 2: Local Injury or Scar Pain

Scar Pain. Neuroma formation may play a prominent role in the development of these problem areas. Scar pain may require injection of local anesthetics and locally deposited steroids, but sometimes requires local surgical recision of the scar.

Trigger-Point Dysfunction. Local areas of extreme point tenderness in stereotypic distribution can be treated with NSAIDs, muscle relaxants, and local physical therapy but often does not respond to anything short of injection utilizing local anesthetics and locally deposited steroids.

Type 3: Migraine

The somewhat less precise but better understood phenomenological nomenclature is used to promote clinical utility for the nonheadache specialist reader.

Classical Migraine. This may display the following:

1. Visual prodrome or accompaniment, scintillating, fortification, blurring, dark spots, and so on. Less commonly, visual illusions, distortions, binocular blindness, and so on.
2. Unilateral pain.
3. Throbbing.
4. Prodrome euphoria or neurologic symptoms.
5. Nausea and vomiting.
6. Photophobia and audiophobia.
7. Family history.
8. Response to ergotamines.
9. Relation to menstrual periods, pregnancy, or birth control pills.
10. Polyuria, chills, blushing, edema.
11. Malaise.
12. Incapacitation.

Common Migraine.

1. Bilateral or unilateral pain.
2. Visual disorders less common.
3. Nausea.

TABLE 17.3
Recommendations for Selected Abortive Therapies in the
Treatment of Tension-Type Headache (NHF, 1996)

Medication	Route	Dose	Comments
NSAIDs			
Ibuprofen	po	1200 mg stat, then 600 mg q4h × 2	Side effects of NSAID therapy may include dyspepsia,
Diclofenac	po	50–100 mg	heartburn, upper GI bleeding, diarrhea, constipation,
Ketorolac	im	60 mg	nausea, and vomiting.
Flurbiprofen	po	100 mg, repeat × 1 after 1 hr	
Meclofenac	po	200 mg, repeat × 1 after 1 hr	
Muscle relaxants/analgesics			
Carisprodol	po	350 mg tid	Side effects may include
Carisprodol/aspirin	po	200 mg/325 mg, 1 tab tid	fatigue, sedation, stomach upset, and dizziness. Some
Orphenadrine citrate	po	100 mg bid	of these drugs are potentially habit-forming but
Orphenadrine citrate, aspirin, caffeine	po	50 mg/ 770 mg/ 60 mg, 1 tab bid-tid	may be used continuously as needed over the course of several days. Some of
Chlorzoxazone	po	500 mg qid	these drugs have been abused by users of illicit
Methocarbamol	po	750 mg, 1–2 tabs qid	drugs.
Cyclobenzaprine HCl	po	10 mg bid	
Metaxalone	po	400 mg, 2 tabs tid– qid	
Baclofen	po	5–20 mg tid–qid	Do not abruptly discontinue drug. Contraindicated in pregnancy.
Other			
Isometheptene mucate	po	65 mg/	Use 2 caps stat, then 1qh to a
Dichloralphenazone		100 mg/	max of 5 caps/24 h or 2 stat,
Acetaminophen		325 mg	then repeat 2 caps in 1 hr, then stop. Contraindicated in presence of uncontrolled HTN, history of MI, ischemic or structural heart disease, cerebrovascular disease, peripheral vascular disease, hepatic or renal dysfunction.

TABLE 17.4
Recommendations for Selected Prophylactic Therapies
in the Treatment of Tension-Type Headache (NHF, 1996)

Medication	Route	Dose	Comments
NSAIDs			Common side effects may
Fenoprofen	po	600 mg tid	include dyspepsia, heartburn,
Flurbiprofen	po	100 mg bid	upper GI bleeding, diarrhea,
Ketoprofen	po	75 mg tid	constipation, nausea and
Naproxen	po	250–500 mg bid	vomiting.
Nabumetone	po	1000 mg qd	
Antidepressants, tricyclics			Side effects may include
Nonsedating			constipation, dry mouth,
Protryptyline	po	5–30 mg/day	weight gain, blurred vision,
Desipramine	po	25–150 mg/day	sedation, tachycardia,
Sedating			orthostatic hypotension, and
Amitriptyline	po	10–150 mg/day	urinary retention. Avoid in
Doxepin	po	10–150 mg/day	patients with narrow-angle
Nortripyiline	po	10–150 mg/day	glaucoma, prostatic
Imipramine	po	10–150 mg/day	hypertrophy, or cardiac
Antidepressants, serotonin reuptake inhibitors			conduction disturbances. Side
Fluoxetine[a]	po	10–80 mg/day	effects may include nausea,
Sertraline	po	50–200 mg/day	diarrhea, insomnia, agitation,
Paroxetine	po	20–60 mg/day	sexual dysfunction.
Others			
Trazedone	po	50–300 mg/day	Use in males may result in priapism.
Bupropion[b]	po	200–300 mg/day	Side effects may include CNS agitation and seizures.
Nefazodone	po	200–600 mg/day	Side effects may include nausea, constipation, dizziness, dry mouth, fatigue insomnia, asthenia, and agitation.
Venlafaxine	po	75–225 mg/day	Side effects may include nausea, constipation, dizziness, dry mouth, fatigue insomnia, asthenia, agitation, and sweating.
Phenelizine (monoamine oxidase inhibitors, MAOI)	po	15–60 mg/day	Significant food and drug interactions severely restrict use of this drug. Ingestion of tyramine may result in hypertensive crisis, myocardial infarction, or cerebrovascular accident.

[a]Fluoxetine must be discontinued for at least 5 weeks before initiating MAOIs.
[b]Must allow 14 days after discontinuation to begin use of MAOIs.

4. Throbbing or pressure.
5. Photophobia or audiophobia.
6. Family history less common.
7. Often associated with and mistaken for tension headache.
8. Often associated with menstrual periods, pregnancy, or birth control pills.

Complicated Migraine. The hemiplegic form may demonstrate any combination of the following:

1. Hemiplegia.
2. Hemianesthesia.
3. Confusion.
4. EEG abnormalities.
5. Visual disturbances.
6. Unilateral pain more common.
7. Throbbing pain.
8. Usually discrete self-limited episodes but can lead to stroke.
9. Ten times more common in women who smoke and 10 times more common in women who are on birth control pills.
10. Vertigo, dysarthria.
11. Nausea, malaise.
12. Photophobia, audiophobia.
13. Easily mistaken for catastrophic illness, but patient must have appropriate studies to exclude stroke, hemorrhage, aneurysm, seizures, and so forth.

Ophthalmic Migraine.

1. Duration 10–30 min.
2. Hemianopic.
3. Variable visual loss.
4. Scotoma: scintillating, fortification, spectra.
5. Family history of migraine is frequent.
6. Risk factors for stroke absent or minimal.

Ophthalmoplegic Migraine.

1. Diplopia, third cranial nerve involvement most frequent, fourth and sixth cranial nerves next in frequency, ptosis may be present.

2. Pain most often in the ipsilateral eye.
3. More common in children.
4. Deficits are generally not an aura occurring during the headache phase.
5. Brain tumor and aneurysm must be excluded.

Basilar Migraine.

1. Adolescent females.
2. Equal male and female prevalence in children.
3. Posterior circulatory symptoms.
4. Symptoms precede headache as with aura.
5. Syncope.
6. Vertigo, ataxia.
7. Dysphagia, dysarthria.
8. Tinnitus, hearing loss.
9. Hemianopsia.
10. Nausea and vomiting.
11. Occipital pain, throbbing pain.
12. Prostration.

Dysphrenic Migraine.

1. Mental disturbance with migraine.
2. Mental disturbance without headache but with a history of migraine.
3. Transient global amnesia.
4. Disorientation.
5. Loss of consciousness (may be basilar migraine).
6. Family history of migraine is usually present.

Mixed Headache.

1. Mixed features of both migraine and tension.
2. Tension headache triggers migraine or the reverse.
3. Common after trauma and accompanied by cervicogenic headache, whiplash, shoulder injuries, and scar pain.

Treatment. See Tables 17.5 and 17.6.

TABLE 17.5
Recommendations for Selected Abortive Therapies
in the Treatment of Migraine (NHF, 1996)

Medication	Route	Dose	Comments
NSAIDs			Side effects of NSAID therapy
Ibuprofen	po	1200 mg stat, then 600 mg qh4 × 2,	may include dyspepsia, heartburn, upper GI bleeding,
Diclofenac	po	50–100 mg	diarrhea, constipation, nausea,
Ketorolac	im	60 mg	and vomiting.
Flurbiprofen	po	100 mg, repeat × 1 after 1 hr	
Meclofenamate	po	200 mg, repeat × 1 after 1 hr	
Glucocorticoids			
Dexamethasone	im	16 mg	Use should be limited to less than
Dexamethasone	po	1.5 mg bid for 2 days	one treatment/month. Observe
Prednisone	po	20 mg qid for 2 days	general precautions for
Methylprednisolone	po	4 mg × 21 tabs over 6 days (dose pack)	glucocorticoids.
Acute abortives			
Sumatriptan	sc	6 mg	May repeat × 1, after 1 hr. Up to 12 mg. Do not use concomitantly with ergot alkaloids. Contraindicated in presence of uncontrolled hypertension, history of MI, ischemic or structural heart disease, peripheral vascular disease, hepatic or renal dysfunction, or pregnancy.
Sumatriptan (other "triptans" are essentially similar)	po	25, 50, 100 mg	As above. Start with 25–50 mg. If ineffective, dose can be repeated in 2 hr. Oral response rates lower than parenteral route.
Dihydroergotamine	iv, im, sc, ns		Often coadministered with metaclopramide or other antiemetic when used parenterally. Individualize dose to patient, usually in range of 0.5 to 1.5 mg; iv, im usually administered in hospital or office; sc useful in home. Contraindicated in presence of uncontrolled hypertension, history of MI, ischemic or structural heart disease, peripheral vascular disease, hepatic or renal dysfunction, or pregnancy.

(Continued)

TABLE 17.5
(Continued)

Medication	Route	Dose	Comments
Ergotamine tartrate	sl	2 mg	One tab sl at earliest sign of headache. May repeat every 30 min. up to 3 tabs/d, 5 tabs/week.[a]
Ergotamine tartrate	po	1 mg/	Two tabs at earliest sign of headache.
Caffeine		100 mg	May repeat 1 tab every 30 min up to 6 tabs/day, 10 weeks.[a]
Ergotamine tartrate Caffeine	pr	2 mg/100 mg	May begin with ¼ to ½ suppository. May repeat dose at 60 min up to 2/day, 5/week.
Isometheptene mucate	po	65 mg/100 mg/ 325 mg	Use 2 caps stat, then 1qh to a max of 5 caps/24 hr or 2 stat, then repeat 2 caps in 1 hr, then stop.
Dichloral phenazone			Contraindicated in presence of uncontrolled hypertension, history of MI, ischemic or structural heart disease, cerebrovascular disease, peripheral vascular disease, hepatic or renal dysfunction.
Acetaminophen			

[a]Must maintain strict hiatus of 4 days between treatment days to avoid rebound headache. Contraindicated in presence of uncontrolled hypertension, history of MI, ischemic or structural heart disease, cerebrovascular disease, peripheral vascular disease, hepatic or renal dysfunction, or pregnancy.

TABLE 17.6
Recommendations for Selected Prophylactic Therapies
in the Treatment of Migraine (NHF, 1996)

Medication	Route	Dose	Comments
Beta blockers			
Propranolol	po	60–160 mg/day	Side effects may include fatigue,
Timolol	po	10–20 mg/day	GI upset, sleep disturbances,
Nadolol	po	20–120 mg/day	hypotension, cold extremities,
Metoprolol	po	100–200 mg/day	bradycardia, and sexual
Atenolol	po	25–100 mg/day	dysfunction. Avoid use in patients with asthma, COPD, CHF, A-V heart block, bradycardia, insulin-dependent diabetes, and peripheral vascular disease.
Calcium channel blockers			
Verapamil	po	120–480 mg/day	May cause hypotension,
Diltiazem	po	90–360 mg/day	constipation, nausea, flushing,
Nicardipine	po	20–30 mg bid–tid	light-headedness, edema.

(Continued)

TABLE 17.6
(Continued)

Medication	Route	Dose	Comments
NSAIDs			Common side effects may include
Fenprofen	po	600 mg tid	dyspepsia, heartburn, upper GI
Flurbiprofen	po	100 mg bid	bleeding, diarrhea, constipation,
Ketoprophen	po	75 mg tid	nausea and vomiting.
Naproxen	po	250–500 mg bid	
Nabumetone	po	1,000 mg qd	
Antidepressants			
Tricyclics			Most drugs in this category have not been studied in controlled clinical trials for headache. Side-effect profile and cost should be major considerations when making selections within this group.
Non-sedating			Side effects may include
Protriptyline	po	5–30 mg/day	constipation, dry mouth,
Desipramine	po	25–150 mg/day	weight gain, blurred vision,
Sedating			sedation, tachycardia,
Amitriptyline	po	10–150 mg/day	orthostatic hypotension, and
Doxepin	po	10–150 mg/day	urinary retention. Avoid in
Nortriptyline	po	10–150 mg/day	patients with narrow-angle
Imipramine	po	10–150 mg/day	glaucoma, prostatic hypertrophy, or cardiac conduction disturbances.[a]
Serotonin reuptake inhibitors			Side effects may include nausea, diarrhea, insomnia, agitation,
Fluoxetine	po	10–80 mg/day	sexual dysfunction.[a] Fluoxetine
Sertraline	po	50–200 mg/day	must be discontinued for at
Paroxetine	po	20–60 mg/day	least 5 weeks before initiating
Fluvoxamine	po	50–300 mg/day	MAOI therapy. Fluoxetine has not been shown to be effective in migraine prophylaxis in a published clinical study.
Other antidepressants			
Trazedone	po	50–300 mg/day	Use in males may result in priapism.
Bupropion	po	200–300 mg/day	Side effects may include CNS agitation and seizures.[a]
Nefazodone	po	200–600 mg/day	Side effects may include nausea, constipation, dizziness, dry mouth, fatigue insomnia, asthenia, and agitation.
Venlafaxine	po	75–225 mg/day	Side effects may include nausea, constipation, dizziness, dry mouth, fatigue insomnia, asthenia, agitation, and sweating.

(Continued)

TABLE 17.6
(Continued)

Medication	Route	Dose	Comments
Other Therapies			
Methylergonovine	po	0.2 mg bid–qid	4–6 months max. with 1 month drug holiday may be appropriate.
Phenobarbitol	po	40 mg	May cause rash, dry mouth, fatigue.
Ergotamine tartrate		0.6 mg	
Bellafoline		0.2 mg	
		1 tab bid	
Cyproheptadine	po	Up to 4–8 mg qid; begin with 4–8 mg qpm, increase to max. if needed.	Commonly used in children. Commonly causes weight gain and sedation. Other anticholinergic effects may also occur.
Methysergide	po	2 mg bid–qid	One month drug holiday should follow 6 months consecutive use due to possible fibrotic complications. Peripheral ischemia, hallucinations, and peptic ulcer disease may occur.
Phenelzine	po	Same as with tension type.	Same as tension type.
Divalproex sodium	po	250–2000 mg/d	Side effects may include hepatic dysfunction (especially in children), GI upset, tremor, sedation, nausea, weight gain, alopecia, pancreatitis, and bone marrow suppression; polypharmacy (especially barbiturates and anticonvulsants) increases incidence of hepatic complications. Avoid in patients with hepatic disease. Liver function tests should be performed prior to therapy.

[a]Must allow 14 days after discontinuing use of MAOIs to begin use.

Type 4: Dysautonomic Cephalgia

Cluster

Episodic Form (Most Frequent Pattern).

1. Attacks in stereotypic series.
2. Unilateral, sharp, boring, severe, periorbital facial pain.

3. Conjunctival injection.
4. Nasal congestion.
5. Watery rhinorrhea.
6. Lacrimation.
7. Ptosis, miosis.
8. Photophobia.
9. Patient is restless, pacing.
10. Family history.
11. More frequent in men.

Chronic Form. Similar to episodic, but attacks either continue for very prolonged periods or never fully remit. This chronicity may be primary or may develop after the disease process has proceeded for a time.

Treatment of Cluster Headache. See Tables 17.7 and 17.8.

"Red Flags" in the Diagnosis of Headache (NHF, 1996)

1. Onset of headache after age 50.
2. Onset of new or different headache.
3. "Worst" headache ever experienced.
4. Onset of subacute headache that progressively worsens.
5. Onset of headache with exertion, sexual activity, coughing, or sneezing.
6. Headache associated with any of the following changes in neurological evaluation:
    a. Drowsiness, confusion, memory impairment.
    b. Weakness, ataxia, loss of coordination.
    c. Numbness and/or tingling.
    d. Paralysis.
    e. Sensory loss associated with headache.
    f. Asymmetry of pupillary response, deep tendon reflexes, or Babinski response.
    g. Signs of meningeal irritation.
    h. Progressive visual or neurological changes.
    i. Other evidence to suggest an underlying neurological disorder, such as persistent tinnitus, loss of sense of smell, loss of sensation over the face, dysphagia.
7. Abnormal medical evaluation:
    a. Fever.
    b. Stiff neck.
    c. Hypertension.

TABLE 17.7
Recommendations for Selected Abortive Therapies
in the Treatment of Cluster Headache (NHF, 1996)

Medication	Route	Dose	Comments
Oxygen	Inhalation	7–10 L/min for 10 min	Patient should be seated, leaning forward, sinuses draining.
Dihydroergotamine	im, sc, iv		Often coadministered with metaclopramide or other antiemetic. Individualize dose to patient, usually in range of 0.5 to 1 mg; iv, im usually administered in hospital or office; sc in home. Contraindicated in presence of uncontrolled hypertension, history of MI, ischemic or structural heart disease, cerebrovascular disease, peripheral vascular disease, hepatic or renal dysfunction, or pregnancy.
Sumatriptin	sc	6 mg	May repeat ×1, after 1 hr. Up to 12 mg/24hr. Do not use concomitantly with ergot alkaloids. Contraindicated in presence of uncontrolled hypertension, history of MI, ischemic or structural heart disease, cerebrovascular disease, peripheral vascular disease, hepatic or renal dysfunction, or pregnancy.
Lidocaine	Nose drops	4%	Apply 15 drops into the nostril of the affected side with head turned in that direction and tilted backward. Dose may be repeated in 15 min if necessary up to 2 times per headache and up to 4 times/day. May cause dizziness and nervousness. Some patients may experience hypersensitivity reaction. Prior to application patient may use phenylephrine HCl nasal drops to clear congestion.

    d. Weight loss.

    e. Tender, poorly pulsatile temporal arteries.

    f. Papilledema.

    g. Chronic cough, lymphadenopathy, recurrent nasal drainage/ discharge, or other evidence to suggest a systemic illness.

TABLE 17.8
Recommendations for Selected Prophylactic Therapies
in the Treatment of Cluster Headache (NHF, 1996)

Medication	Route	Dose	Comments
Verapamil	po	240–480 mg/day	As in migraine tables.
Prednisone	po	10–60 mg/day	Avoid long-term use. Observe general precautions for gluco-corticoids.
Ergotamine tartrate	po	1–2 mg qPM or 1 mg bid	As in migraine tables.
Methysergide	po	2–8 mg/day	One month drug holiday should follow 6 months of consecutive use due to possible fibrotic complications. Peripheral ischemia, hallucinations, and peptic ulcer disease may occur.
Lithium carbonate	po	300–1200 mg/day	In divided doses, bid–qid. Patient's serum lithum should stay below 1.5 mEq/L to prevent toxicity. Verapamil may be added in resistant cases, but with possible drug interaction.
Divalproex sodium	po	250–2000 mg/day	Side effects may include hepatic dysfunction (especially in children), GI upset, tremor, sedation, nausea, weight gain, alopecia, pancreatitis, and bone marrow suppression; polypharmacy (especially barbiturates and anti-convulsants) increases incidence of hepatic complications. Avoid in patients with hepatic disease. Liver function tests should be performed prior to therapy.
Histamine acid phosphate	iv	2.75 mg in 250 ml normal saline	Use 6 to 10 drops/min on first administration for 30 min with patient sitting in chair. If given too rapidly or if dose is too strong, can precipitate headache.

Imaging Decisions

Acute Headache. Use computed tomography (CT) if:

1. Recent trauma with neurological abnormality.
2. Subarachnoid hemorrhage is suspected.

3. Cause of headache is unclear and patient does not respond to usual maneuvers to control head pain.
4. Decreased alertness or cognition.
5. Onset of pain with exertion, coitus, coughing, or sneezing.
6. Worsening under observation.
7. Nuchal rigidity.
8. Focal neurological signs.
9. First headache in a patient over 50.
10. Worst headache ever experienced.
11. Headache not fitting a defined pattern.

Use magnetic resonance imaging (MRI) in the preceding circumstances if it is available, and the patient is not agitated or can tolerate the longer procedure. Bony injuries are often difficult to identify by MRI, and acute blood may be easier to identify with CT, although MRI demonstrates petichial hemorrhages more easily than CT. MRI is quite superior in identification of diffuse axonal injury.

Chronic Headache. Use MRI if:

1. A neurologic abnormality is present.
2. Persistent or exertional headache is present.
3. There is a substantial change in the character of the headache.
4. Seizures are associated.
5. Syncope has occurred.
6. Personality change has occurred.
7. There is a history of additional trauma.
Neuroimaging is generally *not necessary* if all of the following are present:

1. History of similar headaches.
2. Normal vital signs.
3. Alertness and cognition intact.
4. Supple neck.
5. No neurological signs.
6. Improvement in headache without analgesics or abortive medications.

EPILOGUE

Epilogues are often most useful to emphasize some critical issue already examined in the text of an essay, speech or book. Here I feel it is sufficient to state that the guidelines presented are merely suggestions derived from extensive exposure to many patients relief or lack of it. The most succinct message I could relate is to listen to these patients. If physicians listen and if they see enough of these patients with an open frame of mind, the similarity of concerns from one patient to the next can be striking. Such uniformity from patient to patient is also reflected over time (in the literature), culture, sex, and age group. Even in settings where litigation is less necessary or less accepted, these patients, if questioned, relate similar difficulties.

Prolonged symptomatology is a complex montage of interacting factors, but treating whatever is treatable can provide a convenient point of reference for any practitioner. Everyone stands to benefit from reduced symptoms, whatever their etiology. It is my sincere hope that this chapter adds to ideas already tried in your next difficult and challenging posttraumatic head injury case.

REFERENCES

Adler, C. S., Adler, S. M., & Packard, R. C. (1977). The inscrutability of pain, with particular reference to migraine and to headache. In Adler, Adler, & Packard (Eds.), *Psychiatric aspects of headache* (p. 25).

Brenner, C. (1944). Post-traumatic headache. *Journal of Neurosurgery, 1*, 379–391.

Cicerone, K. D. (1996, November). *Post-concussive syndrome: Is this a disorder which neuropsycholgists can diagnose and treat?* Presentation to the National Academy of Neuropsychology.

Evans, R. W. (1992). The postconcussion syndrome and the sequelae of mild head injury. *Neurology Clinics, 10*(4), 815–847.

Evans, R. W. (1994). The postconcussion syndrome: 130 Years of controversy. *Seminars in Neurology*, 32–39.

Evans, R. W., Evans, R. I., & Sharp, M. J. (1994). The physician survey on the post-concussion and whiplash syndromes. *Headache.*

Fee, C. R. A., & Rutherford, W. H. (1988). A study of the effect of legal settlement on post-concussion symptoms. *Archives of Emergency Medicine, 5*, 12–17.

Guthkelch, A. N. (1980). Post-traumatic amnesia, post-concussional symptoms and accident neurosis. *European Neurology, 19*, 91–102.

Ham, L. P., et al. (1994). Psychopathology in individuals with post-traumatic headaches and other pain types. *Cephalgia, 14*(2), 118–126.

Katayama, K. (1970). Histopathological study of the whiplash injury. *Journal of the Japanese Orthopedics Association, 44*, 439–453.

Kelly, R. E. (1973). *The post-traumatic syndrome—An iatrogenic disease.* Amsterdam: Excerpta Medica.

Kelly, R. E. (1983). Post-traumatic headache. In P. J. Vinken, G. W. Bruyn, & H. L. Klawans (Eds.), *Handbook of clinical neurology* (Vol. 48, pp. 383–390). Amsterdam: Elsevier.

Levin, M., & Turkewitz, J. (1993). Post-traumatic cephalgia. In A. M. Rapoport & F. D. Sheftell (Eds.), *Headache: A clinician's guide to diagnosis, pathophysiology, and treatment strategies* (pp. 197–205). Costa Mesa, CA: PMA Publishing.

Mendelson, G. (1982). Not "cured by a verdict": Effect of legal settlement on compensation claimants. *Medical Journal of Australia, 2*, 132–134.

National Headache Foundation. (1996). *Standards of care for headache diagnosis and treatment as established by the National Headache Foundation* (pp. 5, 9, 14, 15, 16, 18–19, 20, 21). Chicago, IL: Author.

Packard, R. C. (1994). Posttraumatic headache. *Seminars in Neurology, March,* 40–45.

Radanov, B. P., Dvorak, J., & Valach, L. (1992). Cognitive deficits in patients after soft tissue injury of the cervical spine. *Spine, 17*(2), 127–131.

Russell, M. B., & Olesen, J. (1996). Migraine associated with head trauma. *European Journal of Neurology,* 424–428.

Sherkoman, B., & Massey, W. (1983). Post-traumatic headaches. *Neurologic Clinics, 1*(2), 457–463.

Simons, D. J., & Wolff, W. G. (1946). Studies on headache: Mechanisms of chronic post-traumatic headache. *Psychosomatic Medicine,* 227–242.

Speed, W. G. III. (1986). Posttraumatic headache. In S. Diamond & D. J. Dalessio (Eds.), *The practicing physician's approach to headache* (4th ed., pp. 113–119). Baltimore, MD: Williams & Wilkins.

Sturzenegger, M., et al. (1994). Presenting symptoms and signs after whiplash injury: The influence of accident mechanisms. *Neurology, 44*(4), 688–693.

Treleaven, J., et al. (1994). Cervical musculoskeletal dysfunction in post-concussional headache. *Cephalgia, 14*(4), 273–279; discussion 257.

Unterharnscheidt, F. (1986). Pathological and neuropathological findings in rhesus monkeys subjected to −Gx and +Gx indirect impact acceleration. In D. J. Thomas et al. (Eds.), *Mechanisms of head and spine trauma* (pp. 565–663). Goshen, NY: Aloray.

Vijayan, N. (1977). A new post-traumatic headache syndrome: Clinical and therapeutic observations. *Headache, 17,* 19–22.

Walker, A. E., & Erculei, F. (1969). *Head injured men* (pp. 44–55). Springfield, IL: Charles C. Thomas.

Wallis, B. J., Lord, S. M., & Bogduk, N. (1997). Resolution of psychological distress of whiplash patients following treatment of radiofrequency neurotomy: A randomized, double-blind, placebo-controlled trial. *Pain,* 15–22.

Wickstrom, J. (1965). Effects of whiplash injury. *JAMA, 194,* 40.

Wickstrom, J., et al. (1967). Cervical sprain syndrome: Experimental acceleration injuries of the head and neck. *Proceedings, Prevention of Highway Injury, Highway Safety Research Institute* (pp. 182–187). Ann Arbor: University of Michigan.

Winston, K. R. (1987). Whiplash and its relationship to migraine. *Headache, 27,* 452–457.

18

The Pharmacologic Treatment of Mild Brain Injury

C. Thomas Gualtieri
North Carolina Neuropsychiatry,
Chapel Hill, North Carolina

> *The symptoms of mild brain injury (MBI) are sometimes severe, but severe symptoms are almost always transient. The symptoms may be persistent, but persistent symptoms are almost always mild, and hardly ever debilitating. In young, healthy individuals, the prognosis of a single concussion is almost always very good. When complications arise, or when severe symptoms are persistent, it is likely that the patient had more than a mild brain injury, or that the effects of concussion interacted, in an untoward way, with some other pathological condition.*
>
> —Gualtieri (1995)

The treatment of a medical condition that is benign and self-limiting is always a challenge to the first principle of medical practise: *primum non nocere* (first, do no harm). MBI, or concussion, is a benign condition, in the scheme of things, and for the vast majority of patients, the symptoms are short-lived. Therefore, drug treatment for MBI is seldom necessary. Treatment, in general, should always be conservative, and no treatment should ever be undertaken that is likely to make the condition worse.

What treatments can make the postconcussion syndrome (PCS) worse? Two examples stand out. One is the prescription of heroic headache treatments, which can sometimes lead to rebound headache and drug dependence. This is as true of drugs like the nonsteroidal anti-inflammatory drugs (NSAIDs) and sumatriptan as it is of the opiates. Posttraumatic headache can be the devil to treat; one of the ironies of traumatic brain injury is that the most severe problems with cephalgia often attend the least severe head injuries.

411

Elaborate recourse to neurodiagnostic tests, psychodiagnostics, and "rehabilitation" is another form of intervention that can do more harm than good. The power of suggestion is very strong, especially among simple people, and especially in the context of the compensation system. To place undue emphasis on the severity of the symptoms of the post-concussion syndrome, and to understate their transient nature, is to do the patient a great disservice. It is possible to create an iatrogenic cripple.

We are indeed fortunate that among the 2 million people who fall victim to MBI every year in the United States, only a very small number are prey to practitioners who promote such artless methods. We are also fortunate that the vast majority of concussives are well treated pharmacologically, even if they are somewhat undertreated.

It is possible, however, to improve the condition of *some* postconcussive patients with a well-timed pharmacologic intervention. The recommendations that follow are an outline for such practice. They comprise a method that is well proven in the clinical arena, even though it has never been the subject of controlled studies or clinical trials.

(The author is not one to propose that "more research is clearly needed" about the drug treatment of the postconcussion syndrome. It is sufficient to be guided by what we know about the pathophysiology of the condition, its usual course and its occasional complications, and how its symptoms respond to drugs whose pharmacology is well understood. There are few questions that cannot be answered on the basis of wide experience. What is required is not a new body of data, but to present systematically information that is already at hand.)

The diagnosis of MBI, its pathophysiology, and its wide range of symptoms have been amply reviewed on several occasions. Concussion represents a transient encephalopathy that is extremely short-lived, characterized by the acute symptoms of nausea, blurred vision, amnesia, and somnolence. In a substantial proportion of patients—how many, we do not really know—a more persistent symptom complex develops, referred to as the postconcussion syndrome (PCS). The PCS may last for days, weeks, or months, but it invariably subsides, and it usually remits entirely in a year or two, at most. Nevertheless, in some patients, even young, healthy patients, isolated symptoms of the PCS, like headache, inattention, and memory deficits, can persist indefinitely. Some problems, like depression, somatization, and migraine, can actually grow in severity, even as other PCS symptoms disappear.

The transient encephalopathy that attends concussion rarely requires pharmacological intervention; indeed, it is unwise to prescribe a psychotropic drug to any patient whose level of arousal may be the first indicator of a catastrophic intracranial event. Drug treatment is, however, appropriate for patients with severe or persistent postconcussive symptoms, and it is always necessary for patients who develop major depression or debilitating migraine over the long term.

DRUG TREATMENT FOR THE POSTCONCUSSION SYNDROME

Somatic Symptoms

The most common postconcussive symptoms are somatic (headache, dizziness, alcohol intolerance), cognitive (inattention, poor memory, slowness), psychosomatic (fatigue, anergia, insomnia, hyposexuality), and psychiatric (anxiety, depression, irritability). Headache is the most frequent symptom, and because the patient may also have pain from associated injuries, like neck sprain, analgesics are often prescribed in the emergency department. These are usually the nonsteroidal anti-inflammatory drugs (NSAIDs). There are rarely complications to their use, at least from the neuropsychiatric perspective, and they are effective. Sometimes opiates and muscle relaxants are prescribed. These are potentially problematic, but short-term use is harmless.

Posttraumatic dizziness or vertigo (so-called "labyrinthine concussion") is the second most common somatic symptom of the PCS, and it may be debilitating, at least for a while. The specialists who treat this condition do not resort to medications, but they do recommend postural exercises that may (but all too often don't) fatigue the response. They also suggest that neuroactive drugs, especially sedating drugs, may aggravate the condition. Thus, they will advise the patients against using benzodiazepines, muscle relaxants, opiates, tricyclic antidepressants, antihistamines, and so on. They rarely prescribe meclizine, although almost everyone else does.

Whatever you may think of this nihilistic regime, it seems to work, because posttraumatic dizziness rarely persists beyond 12 months.

Photosensitivity and sonosensitivity are transient symptoms that are usually amenable to temporary environmental modifications. Drug treatment is not indicated.

Neurocognitive and Psychosomatic Symptoms

The classic neuropsychological symptoms include inattention, memory deficits, cognitive slowing, and loss of perseverance. Related symptoms include fatigue, anergia, lack of initiative or motivation, disorganization, stuttering, word-retrieval problems, and dyslexia. They are among the most debilitating of all the postconcussive symptoms, especially after the patient has returned to work or to school.

The basic treatment is reassurance. If patients understand that the problems are time-limited, they can usually make the necessary accommodations.

The second treatment is to avoid fatigue or overwork. The patient will do much better by pacing himself or herself, dealing with work in smaller bites, and taking frequent rests. Routine work is preferred to activities that demand a high level of concentration or activity.

The third treatment is to sleep well. Daytime fatigue will remain a problem, and will aggravate all of the other postconcussive symptoms, as long as the patient sleeps poorly at night. That means that dealing with insomnia is often the first opportunity for intelligent psychopharmacology. On the other hand, one would prefer to avoid sedating drugs; sedation, as we have seen, can exacerbate the problem of posttraumatic vertigo. Sedating drugs taken at night may lead to daytime hangovers, morning irritability, memory impairment, and depression.

Amytryptaline in low to moderate doses (10–50 mg qhs) is a venerable treatment for postconcussive insomnia and may also improve headache, other painful conditions, and daytime irritability. It is used less frequently, these days, than trazodone, a heterocyclic antidepressant, with no anticholinergic properties and no danger whatever of fatal overdose. Doses of trazodone ranging from 50 to 150 mg are highly effective for posttraumatic insomnia, with only occasional hangover. Effects on depression and anxiety are often sanguine, even if unsought. Benzodiazepines and related compounds are second-choice agents; their problems have probably been overstated in the literature.

Melatonin is a nonsedating hypnotic that is available without a prescription. Valerian root is an herbal remedy that is also a mild but effective hypnotic. Neither can be recommended on the basis of medical research or clinical experience. We know of a number of people who have taken melatonin or valerian root for posttraumatic insomnia, without ill effects. One is not surprised.

The neurocognitive problems that follow concussion usually abate with the passage of time, with proper rest and the avoidance of fatigue, and with the appropriate control of posttraumatic insomnia. Their occasional persistence, however, may be the occasion of more aggressive pharmacotherapy.

The psychostimulants (methylphenidate, amphetamine, methamphetamine) are extremely effective for neurovegetative symptoms like fatigue and anergia, as well as for cognitive deficits in attention, memory, or organization. They are perhaps the best studied class of drugs among brain injury patients, and there is even a body of literature to suggest that they actually may augment the recovery process (Feeney, Gonzalez, & Law, 1982). The effective dose is low (e.g., methylphenidate 10–20 mg bid or tid), and the positive effects are felt almost immediately. A single test dose of a stimulant may improve the performance of a patient on a laboratory measure like the Paced Auditory Serial Addition Test (PASAT) or the Continuous Performance Test within 60–90 min of administration; thus, the utility of treatment can be measured in the office. Most patients experience positive subjective effects that correlate with improvement on neuropsychological measures. The side effects of stimulants are easy to predict and easy to control, and treatment is rarely necessary for more than a few weeks.

The stimulants are not recommended as "tonics" to be routinely administered to postconcussive patients. In our practice, they are seldom administered to patients whose symptoms have not persisted for at least 6 months; students and high-powered professionals may be treated as early as 3 months. It is not clear that early treatment is associated with any particular dangers, but it is usually unnecessary.

The new acetylcholinesterase inhibitor donepizil is a likely alternative to the psychostimulants for persistent neurocognitive problems associated with the PCS. It is the first cholinergic stimulant that is effective, safe, and easy to administer. Although cholinergics sometimes cause depression, that does not seem to be a problem with donepizil, which is, indeed, a mildly activating drug. It has virtually supplanted tacrine as the treatment of choice for Alzheimer's disease, and as one expects from a drug that stimulates cholinergic neurotransmission, it has a positive effect on memory, concentration, and lucidity of thought.

Psychiatric Symptoms

Anxiety, depression, irritability, temper outbursts, stress intolerance, and nightmares are all psychiatric symptoms that typify the postconcussive state. As we have already mentioned, they improve with time, and they may be improved by most of the treatments we have already suggested. It is rare to propose additional psychotropic treatment for these problems, mild and self-limiting as they usually are, especially in the first 6 months following concussion.

Persistent problems in this vein, or severe problems even before the 6-month benchmark, may be treated, usually with one of the modern antidepressants. Never be surprised, though, when antidepressants fail but the patient responds to a psychostimulant.

DRUG TREATMENT FOR POSTCONCUSSIVE
DEPRESSION

The PCS may develop over the months into a more malignant state. Major depression is perhaps the single most serious consequence of mild brain injury. It is not an early problem, as a rule, although depressive symptoms are not uncommon in the first few months. Rather, it appears to evolve. Whether this is the result of chronic frustration and dismay, financial or interpersonal problems, or a biological event like diaschisis or receptor downregulation or some combination of factors, the author cannot say.

Toward the end of the first year following MBI, a patient with persistent postconcussive symptoms may experience a change in his or her emotional state. Moodiness and irritability give way to a deeper and more pervasive feeling of sadness, discouragement, and despair. The frustration that comes of trying to cope leads to demoralization, apathy, and withdrawal. The neurocognitive and neurovegetative symptoms incorporate themselves neatly into the total picture of a major depressive episode. Low doses of antidepressants like amitryptiline or trazodone may not avert this transformation. Continued treatment with stimulants may actually aggravate the depression. The patient is caught in a vicious circle. His or her depressed state begins to work against the process of natural recovery; the prolonged disability compounds the depression.

It is at this point that a treating physician considers an aggressive course of antidepressant treatment. One selects a potent first-line antidepressant, preferably one whose side-effect profile may be agreeable to the patient's ancillary symptoms. To begin, the modern antidepressants (the serotonin reuptake inhibitors [SSRIs], buproprion, venlafaxine, mirtazapine) are preferred to the tricyclics, although two failed trials should lead to a tricyclic and/or an augmentation strategy. The best antidepressant augmenter is probably lithium, but one usually tries a less complicated approach first: amantadine, a stimulant, a second antidepressant, buspirone or pindalol.

The treatment of posttraumatic depression usually requires 3–6 months of maintenance therapy, while the patient is perfectly euthymic, before the antidepressant is gradually withdrawn. Patients with more profound depressions, or with a significant premorbid history of affective disorder, may require long-term therapy.

From time to time, aggressive antidepressant therapy may aggravate one of the concomitant symptoms of the PCS, like vertigo, dysnomia, or memory impairment. That is why lithium and the tricyclic antidepressants tend to be second-choice drugs. One certainly prefers to treat depression with drugs that are free of side effects. But major depression is a disease that carries significant morbidity and mortality, and its proper treatment usually takes primacy.

There are no longitudinal studies of posttraumatic depression following MBI. It does not seem to be one of the more difficult depressions to treat, and is rarely, if ever, refractory to aggressive pharmacotherapy. Depression, however, is frequently undertreated, even by psychiatrists.

DRUG TREATMENT FOR POSTTRAUMATIC MIGRAINE

Posttraumatic headache begins as a generalized dull or pounding headache, which is continuous and unaccompanied by migranoid features. If the patient also sustained a neck or back injury, it may present as a typical "tension" headache. The treatment is entirely symptomatic: rest, mild analgesics, and sometimes muscle relaxants.

As time passes, posttraumatic headache gradually remits. In some cases, however, it may evolve, as the patient grows increasingly sensitive to the continuing ill effects of muscle tension or fibrositis, or as the typical features of vascular headache begin to emerge. The classical posttraumatic headache, several months following concussion, has mixed features: the dull, generalized background headache, the intense occipital headache that radiates anteriorly in response to muscular tension, and migranoid symptoms like nausea, photosensitivity, exercise intolerance, and so forth. By this time, the effects of conservative measures have weakened, and the patient may even develop rebound headache as the result of excessive drug intake.

Chronic posttraumatic headaches may be formidable, even refractory to treatment. They may be complicated by the problems of drug dependence, drug rebound, and compensation. And when headaches are difficult, an enterprising physician will unleash a veritable parade of medications, many of which have psychotropic effects or the potential for neurotoxicity. Chronic pain is accompanied by frustration, dismay, or outright depression, a state of mind that is hardly ever relieved by amitryptiline, doxepin, fluoxetine, sertraline, valproate, diazepam, carbamazepine, chlorpromazine, lithium, or any of the other psychotropics that are prescribed by headache doctors. (It is always remarkable when drugs that have a record of success for the most severe major affective disorders fail to alleviate the psychological distress that accompanies posttraumatic cephalgia.)

The kind of accident that often causes MBI is often associated with cervical strain or back injury. The latter may also evolve, as headache does, to a more complex state, variously described as "myofascial pain syndrome," "fibrositis," "fibromyalgia," or "chronic fatigue syndrome." Without venturing into a controversial literature that never seems to find sucessful resolution, it is appropriate to inidicate that the symptoms of persistent PCS are quite similar to those of chronic fatigue syndrome/fibromyalgia. The pharmacologic treatment of the latter can be as frustrating as posttraumatic headache. Virtually everything has been tried, and hardly anything works, with any degree of regularity or predictability.

SPECIAL PHARMACOLOGICAL INTERVENTIONS

Mild brain injury almost always has a good prognosis, and the symptoms of PCS usually recede with time, and the prescription of mild, conservative treatments. But "almost always" and "usually" are not "always" or "invariably," and in the large set of MBI patients there are very small subsets with unremitting symptoms and a poor prognosis. Because there are 2 million MBI patients in the United States every year, even a small proportion of bad-prognosis patients constitutes a formidable medical problem.

In a recent paper, we addressed the problem of MBI patients who do, indeed, have severe and persistent symptoms (Gualtieri, 1995). We concluded that they fall into four broad categories:

1. Patients whose original injury was, in fact, more severe than it was originally thought to be.
2. Patients with significant premorbid pathology.
3. Patients who develop posttraumatic depression, or posttraumatic headache, but who are undertreated, or mistreated.
4. Patients with somatoform disorders (i.e., hysteria), compensation neurosis, or malingering.

Within the limits of this contribution, categories 1 and 4 are beyond the scope of a targeted discussion of MBI, and category 3 has been addressed already.

The most troublesome cases of MBI patients have premorbid pathology. These are either neurological or psychiatric.

Patients with premorbid conditions that effect the central nervous system are necessarily more vulnerable to the effects of concussion. The most common such conditions are the nonspecific changes that occur to brain in association with aging, and the specific white matter changes that occur, even in young brain, as a result of hypertension, diabetes, hyperlipidemia, alcoholism, and cigarette smoking. A mild brain injury may effect such a person just as a severe brain injury would effect someone else. Postconcussive symptoms tend to be more persistent. The cognitive and emotional sequelae of concussion are particularly troublesome. The same pharmacological treatments are brought to bear, but sooner, and more aggressively.

The epileptic patient who has tolerated a drug like phenytoin without overt neurotoxic effects may develop a relative intolerance following concussion. The same principle of "cerebral" reserve is operative here. The healthy brain (albeit epileptic) was able to accommodate the mildly sedating effects of the drug; when the brain was concussed, it decompensated.

Developmental problems—mild ones like attention deficit disorder (ADD) and the learning disabilities, and severe ones, like mental retardation and cerebral palsy—may similarly complicate the recovery from concussion.

Concussions do not cause dementia, but in an elderly patient with subclinical dementia, an MBI may unmask the disorder, and the patient may not necessarily attain his or her premorbid state of adjustment. The new cholinesterase inhibitor donepizil is as well tolerated by traumatic brain injury (TBI) patients as it is by demented patients, so there is no contraindication to its use in such cases.

Psychiatric disorders are very common in the population at large and even more common in the broad group of TBI patients. Even MBI may be expected to complicate the course and treatment of a psychiatric disorder. And there is an inverse rule, just as there is for headache. It seems that the comparatively mild psychiatric conditions, like the anxiety disorders and chronic depressions, are more likely to be aggravated by MBI than the major psychiatric disorders like schizophrenia or manic depression. Psychiatric disorders that are characterized by self-absorption, narcissism, or somatization are particularly prone to interact with the symptoms of concussion, as well as with the compensation issues that inevitably arise.

REFERENCES

Feeney, D. M., Gonzalez, A., & Law, W. A. (1982). Amphetamine, haloperidol and experience interact to affect rate of recovery after motor cortex surgery. *Science, 217,* 855–857.

Gualtieri, C. T. (1995). The problem of mild brain injury. *Neuropsychiatry, Neuropsychology, and Behavioral Neurology, 8,* 127–136.

19

Integration of the Evaluation and Management of the Transient Closed Head Injury Patient: Some Directions

Vernon M. Neppe
Pacific Neuropsychiatric Institute, Seattle, Washington,
St. Louis University, St. Louis, Missouri,
and University of Washington, Seattle, Washington

BACKGROUND TO ASSESSMENT OF THE CHIT

We have defined the *closed head injury syndrome of transient kind* (CHIT) as having several subtypes: a physiological brain injury of the postconcussional dimension (PCCHITS), a psychological dysfunction of posttraumatic kind (PTCHITS), a focal residual kind (FRCHITS), or combinations mixed with these (MCHITS). Further, there is a synergistic physical, cognitive, and psychological synergism across the posttraumatic functional syndrome, and legitimate brain injury and predisposing factors and degrees of physiological brain reserve may determine exact manifestations of a CHIT (Neppe & Goodwin, chap. 10., this volume).

We have seen how "minor" CHI is often not minor. The misnomer of *mild* often is linked with significant and brief, or no impairments of consciousness may be associated with significant residua of the CHIT. Some patients may manifest pathoplastic compensations less with preexisting conditions such that the symptoms of the CHIT may relate to the straw that broke the camel's back. Additionally, the actual pathogenetic changes in CHITs may manifest in both focal and generalized forms (Neppe & Goodwin, chap. 10, this volume).

We have demonstrated how time-based evaluations of comprehensive kind may be the most valuable way of monitoring of the headache, dizziness, concentration, myalgic pains, memory disturbance and sleep disturbance, and specific complications including seizure disorders, atypi-

421

cal spells, and fibromyalgia that may follow CHITs. The neuropsychiatric evaluation is not a single interview over 40 min or an hour. It cannot be done in one interview; it is too complex and, moreover, the time-based evaluation allows a filmstrip view in which the whole system, all the biopsychofamiliosociocultural elements, must be taken into account (Neppe & Goodwin, chap. 10, this volume).

The sequence of such a basic exam involves outside sources of history and information, demographics analysis, a detailed main complaint with injury information, relevant past psychiatric and neurologic history including any other injuries and any links with lawsuits, a detailed pharmacologic history including doses, duration, combinations, responsiveness, and side effects, a history of abuse of recreational drugs, basic habits, a detailed computerized history of social and medical facets, psychological and personality evaluations, obtaining of collateral information, and detailed neurologic, psychiatric, mental status, and neuropsychiatric cerebral cortical evaluations. Furthermore, specialized testing is then done. All this information is then elaborated and examined, producing diagnoses using a multiaxial framework of both neurologic and psychiatric kind. Consequently, management of the patient with a CHIT requires comprehensive time-based evaluations and significant planning. Such handling is both pharmacological and nonpharmacological (Neppe & Goodwin, chap. 10, this volume).

Although we have always had pharmacologic agents that had behavioral effects on brain-injured patients, it was only with the investigations associated with modern pharmacology that we began to understand the neurotransmitter systems affected by these agents and particularly began to notice that some of these neurotransmitter systems appeared to be disturbed in various mental illnesses. These studies into the pathophysiology of head injury have extended, inter alia, to electrophysiologic measures of sleep, evoked potentials, reaction times, and ambulatory electroencephalography. They have further continued with sophisticated imaging techniques such as magnetic resonance imaging (MRI), including functional MRI (fMRI), computerized axial tomography (CT or CAT) scanning, positron emission tomography (PET), and single-photon emission tomography (SPECT). The findings of molecular biology, including genetics, endocrine tests, and psychopharmacologic probes, all have greatly complicated an area once regarded as psychological. The biological perception of "behind every twisted thought is a twisted molecule" has shifted currently to a balance between the exploration for psychologic factors and biologic factors—the *biopsychofamiliosociocultural* approach (Neppe, 1999).

This chapter is not intended to be complete. It simply highlights several areas of management in the CHIT patient with the awareness that management involves two components: further investigations as necessary, and pharmacologic and other therapeutic interventions.

MANAGEMENT OF THE CHIT PATIENT

Four levels of management exist in the CHIT patient, namely, further investigations, cognitive rehabilitation, nonpharmacologic approaches, and pharmacologic interventions. This chapter focuses on the last—the pharmacologic—but all four areas are critical.

Further Investigations

After the longitudinal time-based initial evaluation, additional tests are based on the specific evaluation. Early on such tests as MRI, CT, and routine sleep and wake electroencephalography plus supporting blood tests should be performed as indicated in the previous section (Neppe & Goodwin, in press).

Changes in behavior should be carefully monitored, as accurate diagnosis and evaluation are key to appropriate management, and further tests should be done as indicated.

Cognitive Rehabilitation of the CHIT Patient

Cognitive rehabilitation is exceedingly important. The potential use of computers in this regard is an area in its infancy that will rapidly grow over the next decade. This is also not specifically focused on in this chapter.

Nonpharmacologic Approaches: Basic Guidelines and Habits

The following guidelines have been prepared for the CHIT patient.

Dietary Recommendations

Three regular meals per day are essential. Vegetables and fruit are particularly useful. Avoid highly refined sugars such as candies. Consideration of supplementation with vitamins such as E, D, B_6, and C or a complex of multivitamins is warranted. Even vitamins can be toxic in high doses, so appropriate dosing is important. Additionally, drug interactions can occur, given the fat solubility of such vitamins as A, E, and D. Avoid saccharins and Nutrasweet until it is established that no specific behavioral effects occur correlating with these.

Significant water intake is useful (hence the value of water filters).

Plenty of exercise, regulated appropriately by the primary care physician, is valuable—use graded aerobic elements.

Habitual Consumption Change

Cut Down on Any Caffeinated Beverage Consumption. Because of the presence of symptomatology that may in part be attributed to caffeine intake, we recommend the patient to taper totally off such beverages—coffee, tea, cola drinks—at the rate of 1 cup per day. Decaffeinated beverages can be taken as needed instead. Withdrawal effects such as caffeine withdrawal headache can be managed with acetaminophen and a slower taper of the caffeine.

Cut Down on Any Alcohol. Besides direct effects, this will commonly interact with medications at one or more of four levels: absorption, altered metabolism, modified responsiveness at receptor levels, and behavioral effects. Unless there are specific reasons, such as seizures triggered by a tot of wine, previous or current alcohol or drug difficulties, or such predisposition, aggression, or bizarre previous reactions to alcohol, or driving, the occasional small amount of low-potency alcohol (e.g., beer) or medium-potency alcohol (e.g., wine) is acceptable.

Clearly the Use of Any Pleasure Drugs of Abuse Should Be Avoided.

Cut Down on Smoking. This can also be done using a slow taper. The availability of either Nicorette gum or Habitrol is a useful usable adjunct in this regard. Smoking withdrawal is commonly associated with weight gain, and I have recommended that noncalorific fluids such as water be used instead; appropriate solids would be lentils, carrots, and tomatoes, which can be eaten instead. Moreover, changes in cigarette habit may result in different prescription needs, because drug interactions or hepatic metabolism may change.

Proper Hygiene

Allergy. An air filter in the home may be useful, particularly in the context of any allergy history.

Bed and Sleep. The mattress should be good and firm; it should be turned regularly. The pillow should be comfortable; a neck pillow should be used in the event of neck pain. Any snoring should be taken seriously and its association with any other features of possible sleep apnea, such as daytime fatigue or periods of not breathing, noted by others and handled. The value of adequate temperature in the room—neither hot nor cold—cannot be overestimated. During winter, if greater fatigue or seasonal variations of mood arise, the use of a simple timer switch to create artificial light may be valuable; failing this, more appropriate light therapy may be used, if necessary and severe enough.

Neck. A nodule vibrator or equivalent for the neck in the event of any neck pain may be useful.

Special Issues

Memory. Most so-called memory deficits have a significant functional component, frequently relating to the nonspecific symptoms of poor concentration. Valuable is the habit of recording information in a notebook to be carried around everywhere. This should include a list of "To Do" items and an address book. A cheap watch with multiple alarms is useful to ensure compliance with medications and relevant arrangements.

Speech. The use of computerized software (such as the program Word Foundry by Nordic software) may be useful for receptive or executive-level mild aphasia. If the initial evaluation is suggestive of speech pathology, subtle elements could have been missed such as specific reading disability, and an educational evaluation should be performed.

Psychological. Express *anger* by using a punching bag. *Exercise* may be useful. *Loneliness* may be alleviated by joining a social club. Write *notes to self* to express distress.

Driving. The operation of any motor or any other vehicle is always controversial. Most medications sedate somewhat, and even those that do not may cause paradoxic reactions. On the other hand, certain conditions such as anxiety, daytime sleepiness, seizures, poor concentration, or memory disturbance aggravate driving risk, and the treatment may be assisting these problems. Extreme care should be used when driving, and even when it is deemed safe to drive short distances in familiar areas, it may be unsafe on longer or unfamiliar drives. Driving should be avoided in the event of doubt as to safety to drive, not only on behalf of the patient but for the family. Driving a car is always the ultimate responsibility of the individual driving it. The physician can advise in cases of uncertainty—frequently, medication control is safer than the untreated underlying condition, but any sedation or slowed reaction times or impaired consciousness, or sleep, visual, or memory impairment, is a good reason not to drive.

Psychotherapeutic Support. Supportive psychotherapy with an appropriately trained therapist is useful. This should be directed at support with regard to current problems as well as allowing the patient a smoother transition as readjustments back to a healthy core occurs.

Depth therapeutic probing, uncovering many layers of the patient's psyche, should be approached only with extreme caution as this may lead to further decompensation.

Behavioral Elements. Access to a firearm, in the context of significant psychopathology linked with the CHIT, is dangerous. This should be avoided if at all possible.

Follow-Up. The patient should always have a regular follow-up primary care physician to handle any acute problems.

Pharmacologic Interventions

Pharmacologic interventions are dependent on diagnostic evaluation. The four major intervention groups are:

1. The azapirone, buspirone, technically an anxioselective agent, is the most versatile and possibly the safest of all medications in the CHIT. However, because of the organicity, even buspirone is sometimes associated with paradoxic reactions, such as irritability instead of antiaggressive effects.
2. The use of anticonvulsant medication for focal residual CHITs is critical at times.
3. Assistance with disruption of the biological cycle of sleep.
4. Antidepressant medication is commonly used to manage the depression and also the pain syndromes.

More uncommon interventions are linked with:

1. Beta-adrenergic blocking agents like nadolol and propranolol, which are sometimes useful in situations of autonomic instability with significant somatization.
2. Occasional psychostimulant medication is used for the apathy or for an attention deficit disorder-like condition or for profound sleepiness.
3. Use of antipsychotic medication such as perphenazine.
4. Supplements such as minerals, vitamins, and the various fatty acids are all speculative approaches generally characterized by the absence of specific medical prescription.

Finally, analgesics and muscle relaxants may be necessary to treat pain syndromes. This is not specifically dealt with later.

Highlights of use of these various medications and the conditions in which they should be considered are outlined next, with emphasis on specific practical clinical approaches and needs.

Pharmacological Preliminaries

One should take only the medication that is needed, the patient should be informed about the prescription medications, and compliance with treatment is essential.

Tapering of Unnecessary Medications. Prior to medicating with extras, one approach is often to establish that a drug is indeed doing more good than harm. Tapering or cessation of any medication prescribed in a CHIT is a reasonable approach when side effects are significant or there is a lack of therapeutic effects

Specific Schedules on Medications. Whenever prescribed, the patient should ensure that the pharmacist dispensing the prescription give a package insert, which can be read to ensure familiarity with side effects. However, this should be in the context of appropriate medical education by the prescribing physician and the pharmacist, lest the patient distort side effects and therapeutic indication, which in the CHIT context is frequently outside labeling. It is good practice for physicians to develop specific schedules in this regard, prioritizing relevant side effects and dosing difficulties. Frequently, side effects pertaining to weight gain on such medications as valproate, tricyclic antidepressants, and neuroleptics are not listed in such inserts. Some effects listed are very uncommon or may not necessarily be associated with the medication specifically but may have been coincidental. The patient should feel free to further discuss these with the physician.

Compliance. Compliance with medication and cognitive rehabilitation is critical. Because of memory impairments and amotivation, it is often necessary to assist with compliance in the CHIT patient. Medication compliance may be increased by:

1. Buying a cheap alarm watch with, if necessary, multiple alarms.
2. Mediset or tablet dispensers and medication being prepared once per week in these dispenser medisets.
3. One regular pattern is to take medication at specific times linked with actions. Patterns of regularity that are individually determined, such as breakfast, lunch, and dinner, are useful.

4. Take medication with water, and avoid chocolate milk or cola drinks or beverages for about half and hour before and after. Alterations in absorption pattern may otherwise result.

5. If taking nonprescribed tablets such as minerals or vitamins or health-store medications, then preferably take them at a different time so that absorption interactions will be diminished.

6. Consistency is important.

7. If a dose is missed, in general, take that dose as soon as the error is discovered—this may mean taking one double dose. If several doses have been missed, take one double dose with the next dose, then with the following dose a dose and a half, then regular prescription.

Medication Prescription

Unless specifically indicated, medications are generally not necessary in a CHIT. However, even if they may not be necessary at one point, these ideas may serve as a guide for future management of individual patients. Treatment is commonly based on symptom alleviation, although chemical regulation with buspirone or putting out fires with anticonvulsants is sometimes based on treating the underlying cause.

The four major groups of treatment (neuromodulation, anticonvulsants, sleep disruption, antidepressants) and the specific conditions linked with these medications are given next.

Neuromodulation Options

Posttraumatic Head Injury Characterologic Changes and Personality Disorders and Anxiety Disorders. Following transient traumatic head injury, a range of central nervous system dysfunctions may ultimately influence the behavior we site as characterological disturbances. Organic links (from diverse etiologies) have been noted particularly in antisocial personality by Robins (1966), Thomas and Chess (1977), and Tucker and Pincus (1980). Usually these correlate with antisocial behavior and delinquency that relates to electroencepholograph (EEG) abnormalities, delayed reaction times, and seizure disorders (Tucker & Neppe, 1988).

The heterogeneous and poorly validated condition of borderline personality disorder with fluctuations in affect, intensity of experience, irritability, frequent suicidal behaviors, aberrant behavior spells, and brief psychotic features with total recovery all suggest some temporolimbic instability (Tucker & Neppe, 1988, 1994; Tucker et al., 1986).

Anxiety is a ubiquitous psychiatric symptom. Episodes of anxiety, particularly so-called "panic attacks," may correlate in our experience with complex partial seizures. Such events were recognized by Hughlings Jackson in the last century (Neppe, 1984a). Most anxieties with head injuries are likely to be on the psychological side, not due to brain injury.

Buspirone (Buspar) medication is a prime drug for the patient with a CHIT because of its versatility and safety. Buspirone can be used for the approved usage of relieving anxiety/mixed anxiety depression in the posttraumatic CHIT. In this instance, the postsynaptic serotonin 1A partial agonist effect comes into play. The usual dose for anxiety is 10 mg t.i.d., and for mixed-anxiety depression is 15 mg t.i.d. (Neppe, 1989a, 1990a, 1993a). However, it should alleviate the following symptoms, which are not FDA approved and which frequently relate to postconcussional phenomena of the CHIT: concentration disturbance and also the spectrum of agitation, irritability, frustration, anger, and aggression (where no FDA-approved drugs exist): Two dose levels of dosage are useful: low (e.g., 5 mg t.i.d.), which probably reflects autoreceptor raphé serotonergic nuclei effects, and high for considerable agitation and coexisting other symptoms (e.g., 20 mg t.i.d.), probably reflecting a predominantly serotonin 1A weak agonist effect. The low dose is based on uncontrolled work of Neppe on nonorganic patients and by Ratey on mental retardates, and on the higher dose on Neppe's research.

In many patients, we suggest initiating dosage at 5 mg t.i.d. built up gradually by increasing by 5 mg every 3 days to a initial aim level of 60 mg/day; if the patient develops nonvertiginous dizziness, then drop the dose by 5 mg/day and continue the taper of dose until no dizziness occurs.

Additionally, many CHIT patients reveal a predisposition towards obsessionality. Doses of, for example, 20 mg t.i.d. probably reflect a predominantly serotonin 1A weak agonist effect and could be useful here. The only approved drugs for obsessive compulsive disorder—clomipramine (Anafranil)—and serotonin reuptake inhibitor (SSRI) drugs like fluoxetine (Prozac) often have significant side effects in this population. Important relevant side effects are:

1. Nonvertiginous dizziness. If this occurs the patient could cut down the dose by 5 mg/day. The patient should contact the treating physician and continue the dose at this lower level without continuing to build up the dose at that time.
2. Nausea. This suggests that the medication should be taken at mealtimes—breakfast, lunch, and dinner.
3. Headache and restlessness.
4. The occasional paradoxic accentuation of anger or confusion in the organic CHIT patient—usually an indication that anticonvulsant is necessary.

Anticonvulsant Options

Seizure Disorders. A person is only epileptic when he or she has seizures recurrently. An epileptic seizure involves paroxysmal cerebral neuronal firing, which may or may not produce disturbed consciousness and/or other perceptual or motor alterations (Neppe & Tucker, 1988a, 1988b). The most classical and common epileptic seizures are of the "grand mal" or generalized "tonic–clonic" kind. These usually involve relatively short (10–30 sec) tonic movements with marked extension/flexion of muscles but no shaking and then a longer (15–60 sec) clonic-tonic manifesting as rhythmic muscle group shaking. These movements may be associated with a phase of laryngeal stridor due to tonic muscles, manifesting as a high-pitched scream sound. Urinary and occasionally fecal incontinence may occur due to sphincteric change, and the seizures are almost invariably followed by headache, sleepiness, and/or confusion. When preceded by perceptual, autonomic, affective, or cognitive alterations, such seizures are secondarily generalized, as opposed to no original locus of firing producing focal features prior to the tonic-clonic movements (generalized from the start) (Neppe, 1982a). The different epileptic seizures are classified in Table 19.1.

Seizures or other paroxysmal neurobehavioral disturbances that may not qualify as seizures because the actual phenomena are not proven to be

TABLE 19.1
International League Against Epilepsy
Revised Classification of Epileptic Seizures
(See International League Against Epilepsy Commission, 1981)

1. Partial (focal, local) seizures:
   A. Simple—motor, somatosensory, autonomic, psychic
   B. Complex
      1. Impaired consciousness at outset
      2. Simple partial followed by impaired consciousness
   C. Partial seizures evolving to generalized tonic-clonic (GTC)
      1. Simple to GTC
      2. Complex to GTC
2. Generalized seizures (convulsive or nonconvulsive)
   A. Absences
      1. Absence seizures
      2. Atypical absences
   B. Myoclonic
   C. Clonic
   D. Tonic
   E. Tonic-clonic
   F. Atonic
   G. Combinations
3. Unclassified epileptic seizures

seizures are not insignificant posttraumatically. Until all variants are measured, it would be difficult to estimate exact incidence. This is particularly so in the context of transient closed head injury (CHIT). There is a dichotomy of the possibly 90% of epileptics who constitute the epilepsy standard patient, who have no more psychopathology than the average patient, and the epilepsy plus patient, a minority of epilepsy patients having behavioral or psychiatric abnormalities (Neppe & Tucker, 1992).

Seizure disorders present with a high incidence of behavioral disturbance, which may initially be interpreted as psychiatric in origin (Neppe & Tucker, 1989, 1994). Many of these relate to the temporal-lobe of the brain. The features of temporal-lobe epilepsy are so varied and so protean that it is necessary to classify them. I have suggested the term *possible temporal lobe symptoms* (PTLSs) for this (Neppe, 1983a). These are features that can be induced by stimulating areas of the temporal lobe during neurosurgery. These symptoms only become specific symptoms of temporal-lobe dysfunction if their occurrence is validated empirically during a seizure—either through observation or by the electroencephalogram (hence the word *possible* in possible temporal lobe seizures) (Table 19.2) (Neppe, 1983b). Using a phenomenological analysis, I was able to demonstrate that the symptom of déjà vu commonly regarded as symptomatic of temporal-lobe epilepsy indeed had a very special phenomenologic quality in patients with temporal lobe epilepsy (Neppe, 1983a, 1983c). This involves its association with postictal features such as sleepiness, headache, and clouded consciousness and its link in time with these features. This association provides an excellent clue to the existence of temporal lobe epilepsy. Déjà vu is a normal phenomenon occurring in 70% of the population, and unless such phenomenological detail is obtained, patients' symptomatology may be misinterpreted. Neppe has similarly done such a study with olfactory hallucinations (Neppe, 1982b, 1983b, 1983d). A specific type of temporal-lobe epilepsy olfactory hallucination could not be demonstrated, although there were suggestive features (Neppe, 1984b).

A major message, therefore, may be the relevance of adequately assessing the symptomatology of patients presenting with epilepsy. It may be that this is a direction as relevant as electroencephalographic monitoring (Neppe, 1999b).

There are also theoretical biases described as kindling and chindling. Kindling may be relevant in head injury. Generally several events would be required to trigger such a phenomenon, but CHIT theoretically may be the straw that broke the camel's back. We discuss kindling briefly here.

Kindling involves the progression of increasingly severe seizure manifestations in response to electrical stimuli of various areas of the brain such as the hippocampus, amygdala, pyriform cortex, or basal ganglia.

TABLE 19.2
Possible Temporal Lobe Symptoms (PTLSs)

Controversial PTLSs (CPTLSs)
 1. Severe hypergraphia.
 2. Severe hyperreligiosity.
 3. Polymodal hallucinatory experience.
Paroxysmal (recurrent) episodes of:
 3. Profound mood changes within hours.
 4. Frequent subjective paranormal experiences, e.g., telepathy, mediumistic trance, writing automatisms, visualization of presences or of lights/colors round people, dream ESP, out-of-body experiences, alleged healing abilities.
 5. Intense libidinal change.
 6. Uncontrolled, lowly precipitated, directed, nonamnesic aggressive episodes.
 7. Recurrent nightmares of stereotyped kind.
 8. Episodes of blurred vision or diplopia.
Not necessarily disintegrative PTLSs (NPTLSs)
Symptoms not necessarily requiring treatment:
 1. Paroxysmal (recurrent) episodes of complex visual hallucinations linked to other qualities of perception such as voices, emotions, or time.
Any form of:
 2. Auditory perceptual abnormality.
 3. Olfactory hallucinations.
 4. Gustatory hallucinations.
 5. Rotation or disequilibrium feelings linked to other perceptual qualities.
 6. Unexplained "sinking," "rising," or "gripping" epigastric sensations.
 7. Flashbacks.
 8. Illusions of distance, size (micropsia, macroscopy), loudness, tempo, strangeness, unreality, fear, sorrow.
 9. Hallucinations of indescribable modality.
10. Temporal-lobe epileptic déjà vu (has associated ictal or postictal features [headache, sleepiness, confusion] linked to the experience in clear or altered consciousness).
11. Any CPTLSs that appear to improve after administration of an anticonvulsant agent such as carbamazepine.
Disintegrative PTLSs (DPTLSs)
Symptoms requiring treatment: Paroxysmal (recurrent) episodes of:
 1. Epileptic amnesia.
 2. Lapses in consciousness.
 3. Conscious "confusion" ("clear" consciousness but abnormal orientation, attention, and behavior).
 4. Epileptic automatisms.
 5. Masticatory-salivatory episodes.
 6. Speech automatisms.
 7. "Fear which comes of itself" linked to other disorders (hallucinatory or unusual autonomic).
 8. Uncontrolled, unprecipitated, undirected, amnesic aggressive episodes.
 9. Superior quadrantic homonymous hemianopia.
10. Receptive (Wernicke's) aphasia.
11. Any CPTLSs or NPTLSs with ictal EEG correlates.
Seizure-related features (SZs)
 Any typical absence, tonic or clonic or tonic-clonic or bilateral myoclonic seizures in the absence of metabolic, intoxication, or withdrawal-related phenomena.

Such stimulation is initially subthreshold, but becomes threshold when administered repetitively. These subthreshold changes, which have been demonstrated in numerous animal species, at times manifest with behavioral changes sometimes preceding the motor seizures (Neppe, 1985a, 1985b, 1985c). There are distinct biochemical and other differences between so-called electrical kindling and the chemical induction of the process, so I developed the term *chindling* for the chemical induction of increasingly severe seizure manifestations in response to general chemical stimuli (Neppe, 1989b).

Kindling is increasingly difficult to induce with the added degrees of encephalization in primates (Neppe, in press). If, indeed, the kindling phenomenon occurs in humans, it would probably take many years. There is indirect evidence for its occurrence in the development of mirror foci, generalization of seizures, the alcohol withdrawal paradigm, and possibly paradigms of response pertaining to nonresponsive psychosis (Tucker & Neppe, 1988, 1991). However, kindling has become a very useful theoretical concept to rationalize interventions pertaining to adjunctive drugs, particularly anticonvulsants. Whether or not kindling is shown to be an artifact is probably not of vital importance, for its role may be as a stimulant to further research.

Anticonvulsant Prescription

The preferential anticonvulsants in this instance are not necessarily for a seizure indication per se. The subpopulation of CHIT being treated is the focal residual group. They may manifest with frank posttraumatic seizures; however, they may have atypical spells manifesting as the various kinds of episodic events that we have called *paroxysmal neurobehavioral disorder (PND)*. Diagnosis is based clinically, on EEG and on anticonvulsant responsiveness.

The management of epileptics presenting with behavior disturbance is closely linked to the discussion of epilepsy in relation to psychopathology. The heterogeneity of such conditions implies a heterogeneity of management, which is patient based and individually tailored (Neppe, 1988).

The most important single principle is anticonvulsant monotherapy. It has been well demonstrated that the degree of seizure control is not increased by increasing the number of anticonvulsant medications (Neppe & Tucker, 1988a, 1988b). It is more important to achieve adequate anticonvulsant dosage, and therapeutic ranges on blood levels are often helpful indicators. However, the object should be to adequately control all the patient's seizures and the choice of anticonvulsant is equally important. Management of patients with seizure disorders involves primarily appropriate use of anticonvulsants (Neppe & Tucker, 1988b). In addition, counseling and the various aspects of psychosocial support, allowing the patient to live as normal a life as possible, and to be supported within the framework of the environment, are also important.

Carbamazepine (Tegretol) is the primary drug in this group for the CHIT indication as it seems to have a specific psychotropic effect. We use it predominantly in the context of temporal lobe phenomena. It should not to be generically substituted (Neppe, Tucker, & Wilensky, 1988c).

The carbamazepine in this instance can be used for the approved usage of relieving seizure disorders or any incidental neuralgia and sometimes fibromyalgia (unapproved and unproven). In seizures, the anticonvulsant effect comes into play. The usual dose for seizures is 200–400 mg t.i.d. or q.i.d. based on monitoring serum levels to 8–12 μ/100 ml and clinical responsiveness, and we have found usually slightly lower doses to be adequate in atypical spells, PND, and temporal-lobe dysfunction (e.g., 200 mg tid) (Neppe, 1999).

Carbamazepine should alleviate the following symptoms that are not FDA approved (and no FDA-approved drugs exist): agitation, irritability, frustration, anger, aggression, mood lability, temporal-lobe symptomatology: The dose levels are probably in the low therapeutic anticonvulsant range (e.g., 6–9 μg/100 ml) and frequently correspond with an initial target dose of 200 mg t.i.d. The low dose is based on our double-blind controlled work on patients with EEG temporal lobe abnormalities and refractory psychosis with hostility and a follow-up retrospective chart review on hostile atypical psychotics (Neppe, Bowman, & Sawchuck, 1991) in which the EEG was normal. The mechanism may be via kindling or chindling, and episodic phenomena respond best (Neppe, 1990b).

Generally, a starting dose of 100 mg b.i.d. is built up by 100 mg every 3 days to an initial target dose of 200 mg t.i.d. Important side effects relevant for the patient include:

1. Signs of neurotoxicity: dizziness, sedation, diplopia, and nausea. Each of these symptoms may reflect toxicity, so that consideration can be given to one dose being held and the dose dropped by 100 mg/day pending a blood level if necessary.

2. Allergy: Usually a rash—possibly in as many as one in eight patients—occurs; far less commonly and more seriously, a sore throat, fever, or mouth ulceration may happen: The patient should stop the medication pending discussion with the treating physician to establish if the reaction is drug related.

3. Extremely rare is the occurrence of bone-marrow depression, which is an idiosyncratic reaction. There appears to be no correlation of the frequent and expected drop in white cell count with this or other immunologic infection predisposition.

4. Tegretol induces enzymes and may impair control of conception by oral contraceptives. The usual practice has been to increase the oral contraceptive dose slightly if not contraindicated for any reason, but it is safer to add a second contraceptive method as well.

Prior to beginning the carbamazepine treatment, the following baseline blood tests should be performed:

Complete blood count (CBC) including differential cell count with optional platelet and reticulocyte count. Hepatic enzymes including gamma-glutamyltransferase (GGT).
Electrolytes.

At subsequent visits, the carbamazepine levels can be measured and after establishing a new baseline the CBC and GGT can be monitored as necessary.

Folate (a B vitamin) supplementation is often necessary based on possible subclinical deficiency induced by carbamazepine, which induces hepatic enzymes; folate is a coenzyme in this cycle. Doses of 5 mg daily are recommended.

Calcium supplementation (e.g., as gluconate) is also relevant sometimes. One mechanism may be carbamazepine enzyme induction, producing subclinical vitamin D deficiency, particularly in a cloudy climate (Neppe, 1999).

Other anticonvulsant options are briefly outlined next:

Phenytoin (Dilantin). Adequate control of seizures with only occasional episodes suggests maintaining this drug. However, high therapeutic levels (e.g., 20 µg/ml) are associated with significantly more cognitive side effects than lower levels. Rigidity, slowed thinking, irritability, sedation, poor psychomotor control, and responsiveness are examples. Consequently, lower doses may be more logical even with adjunctive second anticonvulsant, if necessary. Folate, vitamin D, and calcium supplementation should be considered. The initial aim dosage is 300 mg daily, as a t.i.d. or q.d. dosing. Phenytoin can be given intravenously if necessary.

Important side effects relevant for the patient include:

1. The change to zero-order pharmacokinetics with potential toxicity with slight dose alterations or other drugs added.
2. The gum hyperplasia is a somewhat disabling long-term effect that is extremely common.
3. Allergic reactions include rash commonly, neurotoxicity frequently, and very rarely bone-marrow phenomena.

4. Potent enzyme induction with raised hepatic enzymes produces common drug interactions.

Divalproex Sodium (Depakote). Initiation of divalproex sodium (also called Valproate) (Depakote—not a generic) may be useful particularly with residual focal frontal-lobe phenomena. Valproate has an approved usage of relieving seizure disorders and for prophylaxis of bipolar illness and for headache prophylaxis. However, it could alleviate the following symptoms, which are not FDA approved: agitation, irritability, frustration, anger, aggression, mood lability, and temporal-lobe symptomatology (no FDA-approved drugs exist), but there is limited clinical use in these areas because frequently there is limited effectiveness.

A starting dose of 250 mg t.i.d. is suggested. The usual dose for seizures are 250–1,000 mg t.i.d. or q.i.d. based on clinical responsiveness mainly but also—far less reliable with valproate—monitoring of serum levels to 70–100 μg/100 ml. For nonapproved uses, slightly lower doses (e.g., 250 mg–500 mg t.i.d. or q.i.d.) with similar blood levels to seizures may be appropriate. Whether the mechanism then is anticonvulsant or psychotropic is unknown.

A major advantage of valproate is that it is generally well tolerated with few side effects and is less sedative than carbamazepine. Important side effects relevant for the patient include:

1. Nausea is common; give with meals.
2. Dizziness, sedation, and diplopia, but these are uncommon. Each of these symptoms may reflect toxicity, so that consideration can be given to one dose being held and the dose dropped by 250 mg/day pending a blood level if necessary. Supplemental carnitine has been suggested to both prevent hepatotoxicity and diminish any cognitive side effects. Dosing is disputed, but 500 mg q.d. may be reasonable.
3. Allergy is rare.
4. Extremely rare is the occurrence of hepatotoxicity. There appears to be a correlation with anticonvulsant polytherapy in infants, and in adults the drug should be safe.
5. Most psychotropics will push up the valproate level, and it will do likewise. Carbamazepine may lower it. Valproate does not induce enzymes.
6. Many patients complain of weight gain, which may be the most significant common side effect and reason for discontinuation.

Prior to beginning valproate treatment, the following baseline blood tests should be performed:

Complete blood count including differential cell count with optional platelet and reticulocyte count.

Hepatic enzymes including gamma-glutamyltransferase, bilirubin, prothrombin.

Electrolytes.

At subsequent visits, the valproate levels can be measured and after establishing a new baseline the CBC and GGT can be monitored as necessary.

Gabapentin (Neurontin). This new anticonvulsant has the advantage of low toxicity, low range of side effects, and no known drug interactions. Serum levels are not helpful for clinical practice, as they are noncorrelative with therapeutic range or toxicity and they are, in general, unavailable. Technically, gabapentin is an adjunctive anticonvulsant, but it may be tried in monotherapy for specific symptoms. Doses of 100 mg t.i.d. are low average, although 20% get sedated, so start low (100 mg daily, building by 100 mg q.o.d. till better control, e.g., 300 mg t.i.d.).

Lamotrigine (Lamictal). This new anticonvulsant in the United States has been marketed in numerous countries. It has remarkable effects on some, although in our experience patients may initially become paradoxically worse with each increase in dose. Like gabapentin, serum levels are unnecessary and unavailable. Technically, it too is an adjunctive anticonvulsant, but it may be tried in monotherapy for specific symptoms. Doses of 25 mg daily built up to 100–200 mg b.i.d. over several weeks are average.

Topiramate (Topimax) and Tiagabine. These are new anticonvulsants in the United States. (Tiagabine marketed late in 1997.) Topiramate comes in 25 mg, 100 mg, and 200 mg sizes. Begin with 25 mg b.i.d. and build if necessary to up to 400 mg daily.

Tiagabine has small milligram sizes, with the starting dosage of about 4 mg daily and the usual dosage of 12 through 40 mg/day. Both drugs are useful as adjunctive therapy in patients whose seizures are uncontrolled on monotherapy, particularly in partial seizures. Side effects for both are rather typical for anticonvulsants, namely, fatigue and psychomotor impairments.

Biological Sleep Cycle Disruption

One of the most common complaints after CHIT is sleep disturbance, which may take months or years to fully improve. Many such complaints may be psychiatrically linked; however, some may have biological bases, linked with the conditions given earlier.

Sleep disorders are among the most fundamental of all psychiatric disorders, and certain psychiatric illnesses may well have a very profound base with regard to sleep disturbance. For example, a diagnosis of mania may be nearly impossible without a profound decrease in total sleep time, and, in fact, most manics have a period of at least 36 hr where they do not sleep at all and during which they do not feel fatigued (Tucker & Neppe, 1988) Similarly, a shift with phase advance and a decreased latency to rapid eye movement sleep is characteristic of a biological depression. Another common symptom in this condition is terminal insomnia—early morning waking. This may or may not be correlated with this phase advancement, as the two have not been investigated (Tucker & Neppe, 1988).

Sleep disturbance is of profound importance in the CHIT but may reflect underlying affective disorder or personality. Many patients with profound degrees of antisocial personality give a history of sleep disturbance involving paroxysmal wakenings since childhood. Many brain-impaired individuals may have periods during which they nap during the day.

When sleep is impaired significantly, hypnotics may be considered. Options include zolpidem (FDA approved), trazodone (approved as antidepressant but commonly used), and melatonin (nonprescription hormone).

Zolpidem Tartrate (Ambien). This is an imidazopyridine nonbenzodiazepine hypnotic with no apparent dependence, and normalization of sleep cycles with extensive European experience (5 mg pink or 10 mg white tabs, breakable). It acts at the omega 1 sites of gamma-aminobutyric acid (GABA)-a receptor preferentially. It is FDA indicated for short-term management of insomnia. It has rapid onset, and short half-life (2–3 hr).

Trazodone (Desyrel). Trazodone is marketed as an antidepressant. It does not have anticholinergic side effects and has little cardiotoxicity. In sub-antidepressant doses such as 50–100 mg, it is frequently used as a hypnotic because it is sedative with little carryover to the next day and has excellent physiological effects on slow-wave sleep.

Patients should be warned that it may drop blood pressure and induce tachycardia; hence they should go to bed after taking it until they know what effects it has on them.

In males there is a rare side effect of priapism (1 in 8,000 males), which can usually effectively be treated with pseudoephedrine hydrochloride and immediately packing the penis with ice.

Melatonin. Given the biological sleep disturbance component and disturbances in diurnal rhythms, Melatonin is a nonprescribed option left to the patient's choice. The following key information should be communicated:

1. The lack of research on the drug.
2. Questions on purity of the preparations, which could lead to unusual reactions (other health-food store preparations could have the same problem).
3. Interactions with other drugs.
4. Possible long-term suppression of the pineal (speculative only) based on other neuroendocrine responses to, for example, thyroxin and steroid in thyroid and adrenal suppression, which implies tapering of the melatonin in the event of stopping.
5. Other unknown effects, pharmacokinetic and pharmacodynamic.

On the other hand, melatonin remodulation appears physiological. This has not been prescribed per se but is available in certain health food stores in a 3 mg and 5 mg size. Preferable is the smallest possible dose, as physiologically it is thought only 0.5 mg–1 mg is necessary in the normal person. Preparations of animal extraction should be avoided at this point: Vegetable or synthetic melatonin may prove less risky. The drug is best taken an hour before dusk and should take several weeks to work fully.

Benzodiazepines. Benzodiazepines should be avoided, if possible, because of their addictive qualities and impairments at the psychomotor, cognitive, amnesic, and drug interactional levels. Benzodiazepine may relieve symptoms nonspecifically and incompletely, but it has all the cognitive, psychomotor, and dependence/addictive problems of this drug group. This may be aggravated by previous abuse history and symptomatic status.

Management. Sleep disturbance usually appears secondary in the CHIT and should be managed with no napping during the day.

Management of Depression and Mood Disorder

Affective Disorders and Head Injury. The area of mood disorders allows possible practical and theoretical understanding of the role of the central nervous system in behavior disorders. Affective disturbances may be triggered or induced by head injury with or without traumatic temporal-lobe epilepsy (Neppe & Tucker, 1994) and head trauma (Neppe & Tucker, 1994; Tucker & Neppe 1991).

We believe that CHIT may trigger "depressive pseudodementia" in patients with limited cerebral reserve (McAllister, 1983, 1992). This refers to the organic symptomatology, particularly dementing symptoms in affectively disturbed patients. Cognitive and neuropsychologic disturbances are associated with affective disturbances generally reversible with treatment. Consequently, in dealing with the demented patient, one must rule out affective disturbance in the older patient (Neppe & Tucker, 1994).

Lithium Carbonate (Eskalith and Others—Choice Is Optional). Occasionally lithium is useful when patients manifest cyclical phenomena of their residual focal CHIT. Medication problems with lithium are linked commonly to tremor, which is a rather coarse static one that patients find impairing in functionality and embarrassing. Some patients become nauseous and/ or confused. Our preference is to lower dosage in the event of any of these symptoms.

Baseline blood tests of electrolytes and renal functions are important, as is frequent monitoring for a major but neglected long-term complication nephrogenic diabetes insipidus commonly presenting as polyuria or nocturia.

One way to initiate lithium is by giving 600 mg on the first day and check a level after 24 hr. This will also screen for those who become lithium toxic rather quickly. Lithium is an extremely lethal compound and should be used under supervision of a psychiatrist.

Two different blood levels can be considered: low dose with less side-effect potential but possibly less control—aim at a blood level of 0.4–0.6 mEq/L, or high dose with more side-effect potential but possibly more control—aim at a blood level of 0.7–0.9 mEq/L. Many colleagues use higher doses, but this would not be my preference in this instance.

Antidepressant. These options can be applied in the context of mobilization of significant or major depression either posttraumatically or postconcussionally in the CHIT or in alleviation of pain (not approved). Our preference is to avoid the SSRIs group as well as the tricyclics and to use nefazodone or venlafaxine as selective drugs acting reasonably physiologically at the norepinephrine and serotonin receptor levels. Bupropion may also be of value.

Nefazodone (Serzone). This antidepressant of triazolopyridine structure has ideal theoretical elements both for agitated and retarded depression. The reason relates to its modulating SSRI properties, which implies less side effects such as agitation, anxiety, sexual-related pathology, nausea, akathisia, and suicidality. It has additionally serotonin 2 blocking effects, which should enhance both antidepressant and antiaggressive properties and further diminish SSRI side effects. It is more sedative than the other SSRIs but far less so than the triazolopyridine, trazodone. My preference is to start with doses of 50 mg b.i.d. and increase every 3 days by 50 mg daily, always giving b.i.d. dosing until an initial dose of 150 mg b.i.d. is achieved. Doses should best be given in the morning and afternoon because of its short half-life and uneven kinetics. Costs of all sizes are equal: 100 mg, 150 mg, 200 mg, 250 mg.

Serzone inhibits the 3A4 part of the cytochrome P-450 enzyme system in the liver. This increases levels of certain chemicals such as ketoconazole, alprazolam, triazolam, and probably SSRIs like fluoxetine, as well as some calcium channel blockers. These substances should increase nefazodone levels as well, and a 50% dose adjustment is general rule. Particularly, do not give with Seldane (terfenadine) and Hismanal (astemizole); if necessary change to claritin (Loratadine) (10 mg claritin usually equal to 10 mg Hismanal, 60 mg b.i.d. of Seldane).

Venlafaxine (Effexor). This has the advantage of acting at both serotonin ("sledgehammer" pharmacologic) and norepinephrine ("chisel" and more physiologic) and should not produce the sexual dysfunction of the SSRIs. Its limitations relate to possible nausea, escalated blood pressure, and agitation. It is logical in the retarded depressive patient.

Bupropion (Wellbutrin). This antidepressant likely acts clinically through a somewhat irreversible norepinephric reuptake inhibitor effect of an active metabolite hydroxy bupropion and not the dopaminergic effect previously thought.

Bupropion differs from most antidepressants in its absence of effect on serotonin.

Given the availability of a long-acting form, twice daily dosing is logical, with a starting dose of 75 mg twice per day, building if necessary to 300 mg daily.

Likely choice is based on amotivation, with the norepinephric effect supplementing serotonergic drugs if necessary, lack of sexual dysfunction, overweight status, and need for some activating action.

Others. In our opinion, the following antidepressants are not usually recommended in the CHIT patient with depression, but are commonly prescribed by some—the tricyclic antidepressant and the selective serotonin reuptake inhibitor groups.

1. Tricyclic antidepressants like nortriptyline, imipramine, and desipramine. The tricyclic group has problematic side effects, namely, potential epileptogenicity, memory impairments, cardiotoxicity due to arrhythmias, anticholinergic effects such as urinary retention, dry mouth, blurred vision and constipation, interaction with alcohol, and sedation. In the CHIT patient, the dysmnesic and seizure elements are particularly troublesome.

Nortriptyline (Aventyl, Pamelor) medication is potent and can be used frequently in doses of 75 mg/day in instances requiring 150 mg of similar other tricyclic agents. Moreover the monitoring of blood levels to an antidepressant therapeutic window allows easy evaluation, particularly in the complex patient on carbamazepine. Its effects are predominantly serotonergic.

Imipramine (Tofranil) medication for biological depression is linked with seizures This is two-edged as it may exacerbate seizure phenomena. This tricyclic antidepressant is potent and can be used frequently in doses of 75–150 mg/day in this case. Its effects are predominantly adrenergic.

Desipramine (Norpramin) medication is not very potent milligram for milligram and is used frequently in doses of 150–225 mg/day. It is a breakdown product of imipramine. In practice, it is more activating, less sedating, and causes more sweating than the more sedative tricyclics. Its effects are predominantly noradrenergic.

2. Selective serotonin reuptake inhibitors (SSRIs) like fluoxetine, paroxetine, and sertraline do not have the anticholinergic nor cardiotoxic side effects of the tricyclic antidepressants. However, they are potent serotonergic agonists with no way to diminish the effect other than breakdown of active compound. These drugs have two problematic common side effects, namely, nausea and sexual dysfunction. They may paradoxically increase anxiety, irritability, and agitation, accentuate nausea, and disrupt sleep. There is a possible discontinuation syndrome, and clinically frequently loss of effects, or need for escalating dosage, occurs over time, and it is for these reasons particularly that we do not recommend the SSRIs to the CHIT patient. The serotonergic effects of all the current SSRIs appear nonspecific on supposedly all serotonin receptor subtypes. As such, the risk of paradoxic reactions is theoretically higher.

Fluoxetine (Prozac), with its extraordinarily long half-life (>400 hr, including the metabolite norfluoxetine), should be used with extreme caution. In fluoxetine particularly, there is controversy surrounding precipitation of suicidality, aggression, akathisia and tardive dyskinesia.

Paroxetine (Paxil) does not have an active metabolite but it inhibits the hepatic P-450 cytochrome enzyme system. It has a 1 day half-life. Start with doses of 20 mg per day initially and later 30 mg/day, built up as necessary to 50 mg/day.

Sertraline (Zoloft) has a minor, probably nonsignificant, active metabolite. We now know that it does effect the hepatic P-450 cytochrome enzyme system so there may be drug interactions. It has a slightly longer half-life than paroxetine—several days. Start with doses of 25 mg/day (half of 50-mg tablet) initially for 3 days and then 50 mg/day, built up as necessary to 100 mg/day.

More Uncommon Pharmacologic Options for the CHIT Patient

Physiologic Restabilization by Beta-Blockade. If numerous somatic (bodily) symptoms exist, this may be considered. Nadolol (Corgard) is the medication. Beta-blockers are useful in this instance for the somatic features of anxiety and agitation. They are not specifically FDA-approved for these indications. Nadolol is suggested as the only poorly lipid-soluble broad-spectrum (β_1 and β_2) beta-adrenergic blocker that can act peripherally, and because of its lack of intrinsic sympathomimetic activity, it can be dosed according to pulse.

The dose is similar to that of propranolol (Inderal).

The initial starting dose usually suggested is half of a 20 mg tablet t.i.d. (i.e., 10 mg t.i.d.). We suggest this be built up gradually by increasing by 10 mg every 3 days, as clinically necessary.

The drug should be administered as a t.i.d. dosage and is chosen over other beta-blockers because it is not very lipid soluble (avoiding central side effects), has both beta 1 and 2 effects, and has no intrinsic sympathomimetic activity, so that an initial titration of dose to a pulse of 66/min can be aimed at.

Important side effects relevant for the patient include:

1. Precipitation of asthma, diabetes, hypotension, cardiac failure, and peripheral vascular disease, leading to these conditions being contraindicated.
2. The awareness that too much is being taken if the pulse goes into the fifties.
3. Contact the treating physician if signs of cardiac failure such as pedal edema develop.

If the response to the nadolol is partial, we suggest changing to a lipid-soluble beta-blocker—to propranolol (Inderal)—and building up to a dose of about 480 mg/day or until side effects or till pulse is 60/min. The change around from nadolol can be milligram for milligram and direct substitution from 40 mg t.i.d. nadolol to 40 mg t.i.d. of propranolol. Thereafter maintain the dose for 1 week and increase by 20 mg t.i.d. more per week to 120 mg q.i.d. or pulse 60/min predosage or side effects such as dizziness (Neppe, 1989c).

Psychostimulants. Psychostimulants are occasionally worth considering in the CHIT, particularly in the context of residual focal nonepisodic phenomena and/or a history of paradoxic responses. These drugs should be used with caution based on potential dependence, misuse (also by others), tics, and possible tachyphylactic effects. One approach is to use these drugs in both attention deficit disorder and narcoleptic syndromes as provocative pharmacologic tests: Nonresponse without side effects indicates increase the dose; worsening indicates take patient off; improvement indicates maintain.

One preference is generally for the scheduled *methylphenidate (Ritalin),* which appears more effective than pemoline (Cylert) (which requires liver function tests 6-monthly) but requires b.i.d. or t.i.d. dosing; it should also be safer than dextroamphetamine sulfate (abuse potential, possible potential to a "model psychosis"/paranoid syndrome). Start with 10 mg q.d. and build up to 10 mg t.i.d. initially over 10 days. The patient should record responsiveness.

A second preference is for *pemoline (Cylert),* which requires liver function tests 6-monthly but is less highly scheduled, less likely to be abused and cause tics, and can be given daily, but it may be less effective than methylphenidate (Ritalin); it should also be safer than dextroamphetamine sulfate (abuse potential, possible potential to a "model psychosis"/paranoid syndrome). Start with 37.5 mg q.d. and build up to 75 mg q.d. initially over 10 days. The patient should record responsiveness.

Antipsychotic Use. There are many neurologic causes of psychosis (see Table 19.1), particularly seizure disorders and more so complex partial seizures (or temporal-lobe epilepsy). This may be a possible link to the rare onset of paranoid psychosis after brief traumatic brain injury.

In 1963, Slater, Beard, and Glithero (1963) pointed out that all of the symptoms that have been observed in schizophrenic patients can occur in patients with seizure disorders. Recent efforts using standardized diagnostic rating scales have shown that the positive symptoms of the psychotic state of patients with temporal lobe seizure disorders is almost identical to schizophrenics (Trimble & Perez, 1982). Seizure disorders present with a high incidence of behavioral disturbance, which may initially be interpreted as psychiatric in origin (Neppe & Tucker, 1994). The range of behavioral symptoms is listed in Table 19.2 and most patients have only one or two of these symptoms that remain consistent over the course of the illness (Neppe, 1989d).

Neuroleptics (antipsychotics; also called major tranquilizers) should be avoided in the head injured as there is a higher risk of tardive dyskinesia

(Neppe & Holden, 1989; Neppe, 1989d). Exceptions relate to the very occasional presence of or exacerbation of psychosis.

Perphenazine (Trilafon) medication has become our preferential drug in posttraumatic psychosis as part of the residual focal elements of the CHIT. Perphenazine is approved for use in psychotic conditions. Among the important side effects discussed is the long-term risk of tardive dyskinesia and related syndromes and its relevance to diagnosis, dosage, duration of treatment, smoking epidemiology, and the limited amounts of treatment.

Anticholinergic medication is sometimes prescribed to alleviate the extrapyramidal side effects of neuroleptic drugs. The patient should not routinely receive anticholinergic agents with the perphenazine, as this complicates pharmacokinetics, may accentuate psychosis, is usually unnecessary, and disputably increases the risk of tardive dyskinesia. Additionally, anticholinergics mask neuroleptic dosage somewhat. Also, additional potential side effects of dry mouth, dilated pupils with blurring of vision, constipation, confusion, memory impairment, and delirium may occur (Neppe & Ward, 1989). When there is a previous history of response to anticholinergics but with side effects of sedation, an anticholinergic that is relatively nonsedative, has low abuse potential, and that moreover has some muscle-relaxant effect, orphenadrine (Norflex), is recommended. A usual dose is 50 mg t.i.d. If not tolerated, lower doses can be tried. A maximum of 100 mg t.i.d. should be used. The most commonly used antiparkinsonian anticholinergic in the United States appears to be benztropine (Cogentin).

Special Replacement of Vitamins, Minerals, and Fatty Acids

This is speculative only.

Antioxidants. A recent area of some interest, theoretical speculation, and difficulty appreciating cause–effect relationships and consequent therapeutic efficacy is the use of antioxidant medications in instances of neuronal or neurologic diseases including pervasive developmental disorder, Landau–Kleffner syndrome, atypical epilepsies, multiple sclerosis, and mental retardation. These organic brain conditions may or may not prove to have endpoint biochemical similarities with CHIT. Antioxidants should be considered if the profile includes abnormal glutathione enzymes like glutathione peroxidase and transferase, and various trace elements like selenium plus a lipid peroxide index. These cannot be measured but speculatively may be abnormal in a CHIT with residual or postconcussional elements.

TABLE 19.3
Guidelines for Antioxidant Medications

RX Medication	Size	Dosing	Comments
Vitamin C	1,500 mg, long acting	1500 mg BID Or Daily	
Vitamin E as *d*-tocopherol	400 IU	400 iu BID	Use *d* isomer of tocopherol if possible
Selenized yeast	100 µg selenium	100 µg BID	Thought to be toxic beyond doses of 800 µg/day

The guidelines in Table 19.3 are thought appropriate at this time. Target symptoms to monitor at are energy, lethargy, concentration, daydreams, and communication.

Mineral, Vitamin, Omega Supplementation. Chromium picolinate at 200 to 400 µg daily, magnesium ion as chloride at 400 mg/day (with some calcium if necessary to avoid diarrhea), and zinc at 15 mg daily and the omega fatty acids are interesting mineral and vitamin or food supplements in this kind of patient. There is limited uncontrolled or anecdotal or lay literature suggesting this combination may assist potential toward hypoglycemia and may allow weight control (particularly chromium, based on its controversial effect in relation to glucose cell utilization, and possibly zinc), lower risk of heart attack (magnesium particularly), and diminished seizure risk (magnesium and secondarily chromium). Obviously, such supplementation is unnecessary in some, but as it is not easy to distinguish in any particular case, and the patient may wish to explore these possibilities, ensure that the best quality brands are bought and know that besides risks linked with the vehicles containing these medications (as with any vitamin or mineral or sometimes generic type medication), there may be unknown interactions occurring.

CONCLUSION

We are doing a full circle. Cesare Lombroso wrote in the last century about the constitutional psychopath (Lombroso, 1912). Sociologists and behaviorist psychologists claimed that there were no such constitutional givens and that all behavior was socially determined totally ignoring the organism. We have now returned to the stage where constitutional and biologic components have again become important and well demonstrated in our conceptualization of transient traumatic head injury.

ACKNOWLEDGMENT

We gratefully aknowledge the permission of the Pacific Neuropsychiatric Institute (www.pni.org) to publish the full version of this article plus Table 19.2.

REFERENCES

International League Against Epilepsy, Commission. (1981). Epilepsy International Congress, Kyoto, Japan.

Lombroso, C. (1912). *Crime, its causes and remedies*. Boston: Little, Brown.

McAllister, T. (1983). Pseudodementia. *American Journal of Psychiatry, 140*, 528.

McAllister, T. W. (1992). Neuropsychiatric sequelae of head injuries. *Psychiatric Clinics of North America, 15*(2), 395–415.

Neppe, V. M. (1982a). The new classification of epilepsy—An improvement? *South African Medical Journal, 61*(7), 219–220.

Neppe, V. M. (1982b). Olfactory hallucinations in the subjective paranormal experient. *Proceedings, Centenary SPR/Jubilee PA Convention, Cambridge, England, 2*, 1–17.

Neppe, V. M. (1983a). *The psychology of déjà vu: Have I been here before?* Johannesburg: Witwatersrand University Press.

Neppe, V. M. (1983b). The olfactory hallucination in the psychic. In W. G. Roll, J. Beloff, & R. A. White (Eds.), *Research in parapsychology 1982* (pp. 234–237). Metuchen, NJ: Scarecrow Press.

Neppe, V. M. (1983c). Temporal lobe symptomatology in subjective paranormal experients. *Journal of the American Society for Psychological Research, 77*, 1, 1–29.

Neppe, V. M. (1983d). Anomalies of smell in subjective paranormal experients. *Psychoenergetics—Journal of Psychophysical Systems, 5*, 1, 11–27.

Neppe, V. M. (1984a). The management of psychoses associated with complex partial seizures. In J. B. Carlile (Ed.), *Update on psychiatric management* (pp. 122–127). Durban: MASA.

Neppe V. M. (1984b). The relevance of the temporal lobe to anomalous subjective experience. In W. G. Roll, J. Beloff, & R. A. White (Eds.), *Research in parapsychology 1983* (pp. 7–10). Metuchen, NJ: Scarecrow Press.

Neppe, V. M. (1985a). Kindling and neuropsychological change: A model of dopaminergic involvement. In *Neuropsychology 2—Proceedings, Second South African Congress of Brain and Behaviour* (pp. 57–62). Pretoria, RSA: South African Brain and Behaviour Society.

Neppe, V. M. (1985b). The kindling phenomenon implications for animal and human behaviour. In *Neuropsychology 2—Proceedings, Second South African Congress of Brain and Behaviour* (pp. 47–51). Pretoria, RSA: South African Brain and Behaviour Society.

Neppe, V. M. (1985c). Non-responsive psychosis: Neuropsychological rehabilitation by antikindling agents. In *Neuropsychology 2—Proceedings, Second South African Congress of Brain and Behaviour* (pp. 52–56). Pretoria, RSA: South African Brain and Behaviour Society.

Neppe, V. M. (1988). Carbamazepine use in neuropsychiatry. *Journal of Clinical Psychiatry Suppl., 4*, 1–64.

Neppe, V. M. (1989a). The clinical neuropharmacology of buspirone. In V. M. Neppe (Ed.), *Innovative psychopharmacotherapy* (pp. 35–57). New York: Raven Press.

Neppe, V. M. (1989b). Beta-adrenergic blocking agents: Perspectives in psychiatry. In V. M. Neppe (Ed.), *Innovative psychopharmacotherapy* (pp. 1–31). New York: Raven Press.

Neppe, V. M. (1989c). Carbamazepine, limbic kindling and non-responsive psychosis. In V. M. Neppe (Ed.), *Innovative psychopharmacotherapy* (pp. 123–151). New York: Raven Press.

Neppe, V. M. (1989d). Psychopharmacological strategies in non-responsive psychotics. In V. M. Neppe (Ed.), *Innovative psychopharmacotherapy* (pp. 94–122). New York: Raven Press.

Neppe, V. M. (1990a). Buspirone: An anxioselective neuromodulator. In V. M. Neppe (Ed.), *Innovative psychopharmacotherapy* (pp. 35–57). New York: Raven Press.

Neppe, V. M. (1990b). Carbamazepine in the nonaffective psychotic and nonpsychotic dyscontrol. In H. Emrich, W. Schiwy, & T. Silverstone (Eds.), *Carbamazepine and ox-carbazepine in psychiatry: International clinical psychopharmacology* (pp. 43–54). London: Clinical Neuroscience.

Neppe, V. M. (1993). Serotonin 1A neuromodulators: Clinical implications for the elderly. In M. Bergener, R. H. Belmaker, & M. S. Tropper (Eds.), *Psychopharmacology for the elderly: Research and clinical implications* (pp. 222–238). New York: Springer.

Neppe, V. M. (1999). *Cry the beloved mind: A voyage of hope.* Seattle, WA: Brainquest Press.

Neppe, V. M., Bowman, B., & Sawchuk, K. S. L. J. (1991). Carbamazepine for atypical psychosis with episodic hostility. *Journal of Nervous Mental Disease, 179*(7), 339–340.

Neppe, V. M., & Holden, T. (1989). Innovations in schizophrenia management. In V. M. Neppe (Ed.), *Innovative psychopharmacotherapy* (pp. 58–93). New York: Raven Press.

Neppe, V. M., & Tucker, G. J. (1988a). Modern perspectives on epilepsy in relation to psychiatry: Classification and evaluation. *Hospital and Community Psychiatry, 39*(3), 263–271.

Neppe, V. M., & Tucker, G. J. (1988b). Modern perspectives on epilepsy in relation to psychiatry: Behavioral disturbances of epilepsy. *Hospital and Community Psychiatry, 39*(4), 389–396.

Neppe, V. M., & Tucker, G. J. (1989). Atypical, unusual and cultural psychoses. In H. I. Kaplan & B. J. Sadock (Eds.), *Comprehensive textbook of psychiatry* (5th ed., pp. 842–852). Baltimore, MD: Williams & Wilkins.

Neppe, V. M., & Tucker, G. J. (1992). Neuropsychiatric aspects of seizure disorders. In S. C. Yudofsky & R. E. Hales (Eds.), *Textbook of neuropsychiatry* (pp. 397–426). Washington, DC: American Psychiatric Press.

Neppe, V. M., & Tucker, G. J. (1994). Neuropsychiatric aspects of epilepsy and atypical spells. In S. C. Yudofsky & R. E. Hales (Eds.), *Synopsis of textbook of neuropsychiatry* (pp. 397–426). Washington, DC: American Psychiatric Press.

Neppe, V. M., Tucker, G. J., & Wilensky, A. J. (1988). Fundamentals of carbamazepine use in neuropsychiatry. *Journal of Clinical Psychiatry, 49*(4 suppl.), 4–6.

Neppe, V. M., & Ward, N. G. (1989). The management of neuroleptic-induced acute extrapyramidal syndromes. In V. M. Neppe (Ed.), *Innovative psychopharmacotherapy* (pp. 152–176). New York: Raven Press.

Robins, L. (1966). *Deviant children grow up.* Baltimore, MD: Williams & Wilkins.

Slater, E., Beard, A., & Glithero, E. (1963). The schizophrenia-like psychosis of epilepsy. *British Journal of Psychiatry, 109*, 95–105.

Thomas, A., & Chess, S. (1977). *Temperament and development.* New York: Brunner Mazel.

Trimble, M., & Perez, M. (1982). The phenomenology of the chronic psychosis of epilepsy. *Advances in Biological Psychiatry, 8*, 98–105.

Tucker, G. J., & Neppe, V. M. (1988). Neurology and psychiatry. *General Hospital Psychiatry, 10*(1), 24–33.

Tucker, G. J., & Neppe, V. M. (1991). Neurologic and neuropsychiatric assessment of brain injury. In H. O. Doerr & A. S. Carlin (Eds.), *Forensic neuropsychology: Legal and scientific basis* (pp. 70–85). New York: Guilford Press.

Tucker, G. J., & Neppe, V. M. (1994). Seizures, 1. In J. M. Silver, S. C. Yudofsky, & R. E. Hales (Eds.), *Neuropsychiatry of traumatic brain injury* (pp. 513–532). Washington, DC: American Psychiatric Press.

Tucker, G., & Pincus, J. (1980). Child, adolescent, and adult antisocial and dyssocial behavior. In A. Freedman, H. Kaplan, & B. Sadock (Eds.), *Comprehensive textbook of psychiatry III* (pp. 2816–2827). Baltimore, MD: Williams & Wilkins.
Tucker, G. J., Price, T., Johnson, V., & McAllister, T. (1986). Phenomenology of temporal lobe dysfunction: A link to atypical psychosis. *Journal of Nervous and Mental Disease, 174,* 348–356.

Emotion Recognition and Psychosocial Behavior in Closed Head Injury

Cynthia S. Kubu
London Health Sciences Centre, London, Ontario, Canada

Lezak (1989) argued that many patients who have sustained a significant head trauma seem to share a set of neuropsychological deficits that undermine their capacity for social competence in the broadest sense. This observation is often mirrored by family members of the head injured patient, who indicate that the psychosocial problems following closed head injury are among the most troubling sequelae.

Unfortunately, the research literature has tended to emphasize the cognitive consequences of head injuries, and relatively little emphasis has been placed on documenting and assessing sociobehavioral changes and their cognitive correlates (cf. Brooks, 1979, 1991; Levin, Benton, & Grossman, 1982; Levin, Eisenberg, & Benton, 1989; Oddy, Humphrey, & Uttley, 1978). One of the most basic aspects of appropriate psychosocial functioning is the ability to correctly perceive others' emotional state. Misperception of another's emotional state can lead to inappropriate responses in specific situations and potentially contribute to some of the sociobehavioral deficits found in patients with closed head injury.

The goals of this chapter are to briefly review the assessment of emotion recognition, particularly in patients with closed head injury; describe in some detail the Iowa Emotion Recognition Battery (Kubu, 1992); and discuss the relationship between performance on the Iowa Emotion Recognition Battery and various indices of psychosocial function in a group of patients with a history of remote closed head injury.

THE ASSESSMENT OF EMOTION RECOGNITION

The communication and recognition of emotion are multidetermined, dependent on a number of different modes or channels of communication (Borod, Koff, Lorch, & Nicholas, 1985). In natural settings, individuals use a variety of different nonverbal cues to communicate different emotional states, including vocal intonation and quality, facial expressions, postural cues, and eye contact (Hess, Kappas, & Scherer, 1988). In addition to nonverbal communication of emotion, the antecedent conditions and contextual information related to the expression of a specific emotion represent another channel that strongly influences the recognition of emotions (Scherer, 1986).

Benton (1967) suggested that a review of the relevant developmental literature may be particularly beneficial in the development of neuropsychological measures, for both theoretical and practical reasons. The developmental and cross-cultural data suggest that the recognition of emotion in various channels, particularly facial expressions and prosody, may represent largely innate, biologically determined abilities that are evident early in life and contribute greatly to adaptive behavior (Izard, 1971).

Children as young as 3 years of age can accurately recognize and label emotions, particularly positive emotions. Recognition and labeling improve with age, such that by approximately 10 to 11 years of age, most children's performance is correct using facial expression, prosodic, and contextual channels of emotion information. In general, both younger and older children are aware of multiple channels for obtaining emotion information; however, they tend not to use all of the information available to make a decision. Younger children tend to rely on facial expression and prosodic information, whereas older children' judgments are influenced more by contextual channels of emotion information. This discrepancy may reflect the acquisition of display rules in the middle school years, as older children realize that facial expressions may be easy to mask, and thus, more information may be obtained using contextual cues (Borke, 1971; Burns & Cavey, 1957; Gates, 1923; Gnepp, 1983; Gnepp & Hess, 1986; Gnepp, Klayman, & Trabasso, 1982; Izard, 1971; Reichenbach & Masters, 1983; Russell & Bullock, 1986; Saarni, 1979, 1984; Wiggers & van Lieshout, 1985; Zuckerman, Blanck, DePaulo, & Rosenthal, 1980).

Traditionally, neuropsychological studies of emotion recognition have primarily focused on groups of patients with unilateral lesions (e.g., Benowitz et al., 1983; Borod, Koff, Lorch, & Nicholas, 1986; Bowers, Bauer, Coslett, & Heilman, 1985; Bowers, Coslett, Bauer, Speedie, & Heilman, 1987; Cicone, Wapner, & Gardner, 1980; DeKosky, Heilman, Bowers, & Valenstein, 1980; Gardner, Ling, Flamm, & Silverman, 1975; Heilman, Bowers, & Valenstein, 1985; Heilman, Bowers, Speedie, & Coslett, 1983;

Heilman, Sholes, & Watson, 1975; Ross, 1981, 1988; Schlanger, Schlanger, & Gerstman, 1976; Tucker, Watson, & Heilman, 1977). This literature is limited by many factors, including small groups, lack of appropriate comparison groups, and dissimilar paradigms. In addition, potentially significant confounds were often not controlled (e.g., etiology, age, gender). Nonetheless, the bulk of the studies suggest that the right hemisphere is critical for the comprehension of affective nonverbal information in a number of different channels (i.e., facial expression, contextual, postural, prosodic). The role of the left hemisphere in affective comprehension appears to be much less significant and largely limited to affective verbal information. The literature also suggests that if there is a lateralization effect for emotion, it is clearly not as strong and invariant as that evident for language.

There are very few published reports assessing emotion recognition in closed head injury. In a sample of 15 patients with severe closed head injury (i.e., posttraumatic amnesia >24 hr), Jackson and Moffat (1987) found that the closed head injury patients were impaired relative to 15 normals on the recognition of emotional facial expressions and emotion postural cues. Similarly, Braun and colleagues (Braun, Baribeau, Ethier, Daigneault, & Proulx, 1989) found that 31 individuals with a severe head injury (i.e., duration of coma >5 days) were impaired relative to a group of normals on a task assessing recognition of emotional facial expressions. No differences were evident in the recognition of emotion based on verbal contextual statements. Unfortunately, both of these studies limited their subject selection to those with severe head injuries and only looked at recognition of emotion cues in facial expressions, postural cues, and verbal statements.

THE IOWA EMOTION RECOGNITION BATTERY

A study by Kubu et al. (1993) expanded on these earlier investigations and examined emotion recognition abilities in a larger group of patients with closed head injuries of varying degrees of severity using four different channels of emotion communication. Emotion recognition was assessed using the Iowa Emotion Recognition Battery.

The Iowa Emotion Recognition Battery focuses exclusively on the following channels of emotion communication: prosody, facial expression, visual contextual scenes, and verbal contextual statements. The same emotions are assessed using all four channels of expression and include happiness, surprise, anger, fear, and sadness (Ekman & Oster, 1979). For every channel of emotion expression the subject completes two tasks:

1. A matching task in which the subject identifies which of the four comparison items depicts the emotion portrayed in the target item (Cicone et al., 1980; DeKosky et al., 1980).

2. A verbal labeling task in which the subject identifies which of five emotion labels best describes the target items used in the matching tasks (Braun et al., 1989; DeKosky et al., 1980; Jackson & Moffat, 1987).

There are 25 items for every task with every emotion equally assessed.

All of the emotion stimuli were developed specifically for the Iowa Emotion Recognition Battery with the exception of the facial expressions stimuli. The Facial Expressions stimuli consist of black-and-white photographs of Ekman and Friesen's (1976) pictures of facial affect.

The prosody stimuli consist of an audiotape recording of 25 sentences stated in either happy, surprised, angry, sad, or frightened tones by an adult male or female. In order to evaluate the influence of prosodic information in as natural a manner as possible, only sentences whose content is emotionally neutral or could conceivably be stated in any of the affective tones were included (e.g., "Jane is working on the computer.").

The visual contextual stimuli consist of schematic line drawings of figures without facial expressions of approximately the same size in emotional scenes (e.g., trapped in a burning building, at a funeral). An arrow highlights the protagonist in every scene (i.e., the person whose feelings the subject was required to identify). See Fig. 20.1 for an example.

The verbal stimuli consist of a set of 25 statements that verbally describe the scenes depicted in the visual contextual task (e.g., "Joe was held up at gun point in the dark alley" or "Mary was trapped on the top floor of a burning building"). Boldface type highlights the protagonist in every sentence (or the person whose feelings the subject is to identify).

As stated earlier, matching and labeling tasks were designed for each mode of emotion expression. The labeling tasks assess the subject's ability to identify the most appropriate emotion label for the emotion depicted in the target stimuli for the matching tasks.

Unimodal matching tasks (i.e., matching tasks that utilized only one mode of emotion information) were designed for the facial expressions, visual contextual, and verbal contextual channels of emotion expression. The subject's task is to match the emotion depicted in the target stimulus with the item in the array that portrays the same emotion.

Due to concerns regarding demands on working memory, the prosody matching task was not designed as a unimodal matching task. Thus, during the prosody matching task the subjects listen to an audiotape of target sentences stated in either angry, sad, frightened, happy, or surprised tones. The subject's task is to identify which of four possible facial expressions corresponds to the emotion depicted in the prosodic cue.

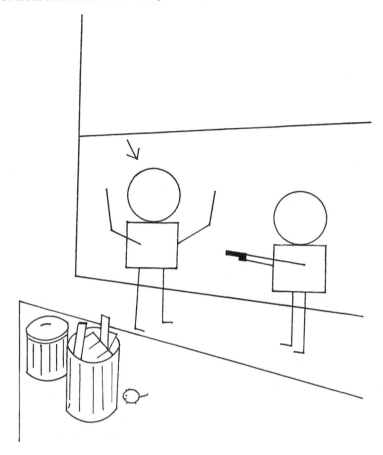

FIG. 20.1. Visual contextual example.

All of the emotion tasks are scored in the same way, with 1 point allotted for every correct response. Five summary scores were also derived:

1. Facial Expressions Total = Facial Expressions Matching Task + Facial Expression Labeling Task.
2. Visual Contextual Total = Visual Contextual Matching Task + Visual Contextual Labeling Task.
3. Verbal Contextual Total = Verbal Contextual Matching Task + Verbal Contextual Labeling Task.
4. Prosody Total = Prosody Matching Task + Prosody Labeling Task.
5. Emotion Recognition Total = sum of all of the emotion recognition tasks.

Closed Head Injury and the Iowa Emotion Recognition Battery

Kubu et al. (1993) demonstrated, in a sample of 40 men with a remote history of closed head injury, relative deficits on six out of eight of the Iowa Emotion Recognition Battery tasks (Table 20.1). The closed head injury subjects were 40 men between the ages of 25 and 55 years with a remote history of closed head injury (i.e., ≥2 years postinjury) who denied a history of premorbid psychiatric hospitalization or drug or alcohol abuse. Control subjects included 40 men with no reported neurological history. A comparison of the mean group scores on the Iowa Emotion Recognition Battery revealed that the clinical subjects' performance was significantly less than that of the control subjects for all measures except for the Facial Expressions Matching and Labeling Tasks. A significance level of $p < .01$ was chosen due to the large number of comparisons.

Equally important were the individual failure rate data. Failure was defined as a score falling below the 10th percentile of the normal control group. Using this definition of failure on the Iowa Emotion Recognition Battery, the failure rate in the clinical group ranged from 15% (Verbal Contextual Labeling Task) to 55% (Prosody Matching Task, Visual Contextual Labeling Task), with 36 or 90% of the closed head injury subjects failing at least one measure. The mean number of measures failed for the head injured group was 5 (Table 20.2).

The effect of level of severity was also assessed. Severity of head injury was defined by the duration of loss of consciousness. Loss of consciousness was measured in 5-min intervals and ranged from 5 min or less to 90 days. The majority of patients reported a mild head injury (i.e., loss

TABLE 20.1
Group Means on The Iowa Emotion Recognition Battery

Measure	Normal	CHI	t	p
Matching tasks				
Facial Expressions	21.85	20.39	−2.03	.023
Visual Contextual	19.27	15.44	−3.11	.001
Verbal Contextual	22.79	19.41	−4.05	.001
Prosody	20.27	16.13	−5.11	.001
Labeling tasks				
Facial Expression	21.85	20.72	−2.06	.021
Visual Contextual	23.10	20.89	−4.37	.001
Verbal Contextual	23.41	22.31	−2.93	.002
Prosody	24.12	21.72	−5.10	.001
ERB, total	176.54	156.32	−5.70	.001

Note. CHI, closed head injury group; ERB, total, Emotion Recognition total summary score (maximum score = 200).

TABLE 20.2
Percentage of Closed Head Injury Patients Who Fail the
Iowa Emotion Recognition Recognition Tasks

	10th %ile	Number Who Fail	Percent Who Fail
Matching tasks			
Facial Expressions	18	8	20
Visual Contextual	15	17	42.5
Verbal Contextual	19	12	30
Prosody	18	22	55
Labeling tasks			
Facial Expressions	18	7	17.5
Visual Contextual	22	22	55
Verbal Contextual	21	6	15
Prosody	23	21	52.5
ERB total	162	24	60

Note. The 10th percentile values were derived using the scores of the comparison sample (i.e., $n = 40$).

of consciousness of 5 min or less). In an attempt to control for the skewed distribution of severity scores, a logarithmic transformation of the data was done. None of the relationships between the transformed scores and performance on the emotion recognition tasks were significant. Nor were significant differences evident when the patients were divided into groups based on severity (mild = LOC <5 min; moderate = LOC 5 min to 24 hr; and severe = LOC >24 hr). Separate z tests (Fleiss, 1981) revealed that failure rates on the Emotion Recognition Total Summary Score did not differ significantly among the three groups at the alpha = .01 level. However, significant differences were evident between the mild and severe groups at a less conservative alpha level of .05 ($z = 1.715$, z critical = 1.645) (Table 20.3).

EMOTION RECOGNITION AND PSYCHOSOCIAL FUNCTIONING

The relationship between emotion recognition and psychosocial functioning was assessed in the same group of patients described in Kubu et al. (1993). The primary measure of psychosocial status was the Iowa Collateral Head Injury Interview (Varney, 1991). The relationship between current employment status and performance on the Iowa Emotion Recognition Battery was also assessed.

The Iowa Collateral Head Injury Interview is a standard collateral interview whose items were culled from the literature describing the

TABLE 20.3
Percentage of Mild, Moderate, and Severe Closed Head
Injury Patients Who Fail the Emotion Recognition Tasks

Measure	Mild (n = 25), % Who Fail	Moderate (n = 5), % Who Fail	Severe (n = 10), % Who Fail
Matching tasks			
Facial Expressions	20	20	50
Visual Contextual	48	40	50
Verbal Contextual	32	40	50
Prosody	52	80	90
Labeling tasks			
Facial Expressions	16	20	40
Visual Contextual	68	80	90
Verbal Contextual	28	40	30
Prosody	68	40	90
ERB, total	52	40	90

psychosocial, emotional, and executive cognitive deficits typically found in patients with frontal-lobe dysfunction, including that due to closed head injury (e.g., Damasio, 1985; Lezak, 1982; Stuss & Benson, 1984, 1986).

Every subject identified a collateral (e.g., spouse, family member), who was contacted and interviewed either in person or on the telephone. The score on the Iowa Collateral Head Injury Interview reflects the collateral's endorsement of a symptom's' presence as well as the collateral's evaluation of the severity of the present symptom (e.g., mild vs. severe). Thus, a high score indicates both a greater number and greater severity of symptoms typically found in patients with frontal system dysfunction. The closed head injury subjects' collaterals were instructed to only endorse a symptom's presence if it represented a significant change in the subject's behavior since the head injury. The present study represents the first time the interview has been administered to collaterals of a neurologically intact group.

Significant differences were evident between the head injured patients and the comparison subjects on the Iowa Collateral Head Injury Interview, with the clinical subjects' collaterals endorsing significantly more symptoms than the comparison subjects' collaterals (closed head injury group mean = 26.9, SD = 7.8; comparison group mean = 2.4, SD = 4.3, t = 17.23, $p < .01$). Furthermore, performances on the Emotion Recognition Summary Scores were negatively correlated with score on the Iowa Collateral Head Injury Interview for four of the summary scores (Table 20.4). These data suggest that performance on the Emotion Recognition Battery is related to psychosocial functioning as assessed by the Iowa Collateral Head Injury Interview.

TABLE 20.4

Correlations Between Iowa Collateral Head Injury
Interview and the Emotion Recognition Summary
Scores in Clinical and Comparison Subjects

Summary Score	r
Facial Expressions	−.26
Visual Contextual	−.45*
Verbal Contextual	−.46*
Prosody	−.53*
Total	−.55*

*$p < .01$.

TABLE 20.5

Employment Status and Emotion Recognition in Closed Head Injury

	Employed (n = 11)	Unemployed (n = 29)	Total (n = 40)
Portion who pass	.64 (7)	.31 (9)	.40 (16)
Portion who fail	.36 (4)	.69 (20)	.60 (24)

Note. Number of individuals given in parentheses.

Many of the clinical subjects were unemployed ($n = 29$). Examination of the percentage of subjects who failed the emotion recognition measures based on employment status indicated that, in general, a greater percentage of those CHI subjects who were unemployed tended to obtain a score below the 10th percentile for the Emotion Recognition Total Score than those clinical subjects who were employed. However, these differences were not significant ($z = 1.544$). (Table 20.5).

DISCUSSION

Impairment in the ability to recognize emotion cues communicated via various channels have independently been demonstrateed by two groups in patients with a history of severe closed head injury (CHI) (Braun et al., 1989; Jackson & Moffat, 1987). Kubu et al. (1993) demonstrated that this phenomenon is not limited to those with severe head injuries, but can be found in patients with mild and moderate head injury as well. Relative deficits involving multiple channels of emotion recognition including prosodic, visual contextual, and verbal contextual channels were evident. Furthermore, when only the severe head injured subjects were compared to the normal subjects on the Iowa Emotion Recognition Battery, significant differences on tasks assessing Facial Expressions were evident as well (Facial Expression Matching Task: $t = -2.722$, $p < .01$; Facial Expressions Labeling Task: $t = -2.628$, $p < .01$). This is consistent with the previous findings documented by Jackson and Moffat (1987) and Braun et al. (1989).

Furthermore, it is important to note that significant impairments in the ability of CHI subjects to recognize emotion cues are evident when one examines individual failure rates on the Iowa Emotion Recognition Battery as well as group means. Ninety percent of the CHI subjects (36/40) failed at least one of the emotion recognition measures, and the mean number of measures failed was 5.

Contrary to expectations, the available data do not support a significant relationship between severity of closed head injury and performance on emotion recognition tasks. Unfortunately, the Jackson and Moffat (1987) and Braun et al. (1989) studies limited subject selection to those with severe head injuries. Thus, this question could not be addressed. The Kubu et al. (1993) study was hampered in its ability to detect true group differences, if they were present, by the uneven distribution of severity. Inspection of the percentage of patients in each severity group who failed the emotion recognition tasks suggests a trend in which patients with more severe head injuries tended to fail the tasks more often than those with less severe injuries (see Table 20.3). This is consistent with other reports in the literature that demonstrated deficits in emotion recognition in severely injured patients (Braun et al., 1989; Jackson & Moffat, 1987).

It seems intuitively reasonable to believe, as Lezak (1989) argued, that greater emotional dysfunction is related to severity of injury. In contrast, Levin (1987) noted that clinical ratings of emotional dysfunction were just as prominent following minor closed head injuries as more severe injuries. Within this context, it is important to note that significant difficulties in emotion recognition were evident in patients who reported minor head injuries; thus this phenomenon is not limited to those with severe head injuries.

Although employment status was not related to performance on the Iowa Emotion Recognition Battery, the data suggested a trend in the correct direction supporting the relationship between the ability to correctly perceive emotion cues and be gainfully employed. It seems reasonable to believe that the ability to correctly perceive and interpret emotion information would be important in obtaining a job, particularly during an interview, and in maintaining a job.

Finally, the findings indicate that performance on the Iowa Emotion Recognition Battery is related to score on the Iowa Collateral Head Injury Interview. This suggests that impairments in the ability to recognize others' emotion cues might contribute to the posttraumatic psychosocial changes and interpersonal difficulties noted by the patients' collaterals.

In closing, it is important to note that the CHI patients, many of whom had only "mild" head injuries, manifested difficulties on emotion recognition tasks that the comparison subjects found to be trivial. In the real world, it is much more difficult to assess others' emotional state. Decisions must be made quickly and multiple pieces of information, often contradictory, must be noted, assessed, and integrated very quickly. The presence of difficulties on the basic tasks that comprise the Iowa Emotion Recognition Battery suggest that emotion recognition deficits in this population may be even more profound in their everyday life. Furthermore, the data support a relationship between poor psychosocial functioning and impairments in emotion recognition.

Lezak (1989) argued that the psychosocial deficits that characterize patients with closed head injury reflect a combination of executive cognitive deficits and emotional disorders. Executive cognitive disorders have been notoriously difficult to assess within the typical neuropsychological examination by their very nature. As soon as the structure of a neuropsychological examination is imposed, many of the executive cognitive demands have been minimized.

Emotional behavioral changes in closed head injury have been examined using standard psychiatric and personality measures (Prigatano, 1992). The use of such measures in a neurologically impaired group is inappropriate without an adequate normative sample. Others have employed structured interviews specifically designed to assess personality changes following neurological injury (e.g., Varney, 1991). These measures provide descriptive information and are useful in that regard. However, cautions regarding the use of personal and collateral interviews have been previously issued and must be noted (Prigatano, 1992). What is lacking in this area are tightly controlled experimental studies that examine all aspects of emotion behavior, including physiological, perceptual, somatic, and subjective experiential. Research in this area is challenging. However, these research endeavors are critically important to help scientifically document and ultimately explain the profound personality changes that can result from even "mild" closed head injury.

ACKNOWLEDGMENTS

This study was funded in part with funds from the University of Iowa, Student Grants Committee, and the Veterans' Administration. Special thanks to Tori Hansen, Derek Campbell, and Kris Franzen for their help in data collection and Drs. N. Varney and R. Roberts for their support.

REFERENCES

Benowitz, L. I., Bear, D. M., Rosenthal, R., Mesulam, M. M., Zaidel, E., & Sperry, R. W. (1983). Hemispheric specialization in nonverbal communication. *Cortex, 19*, 5–11.

Benton, A. L. (1967). Problems of test construction in the field of aphasia. Reprinted in L. Costa & O. Spreen (Eds.), *Studies in neuropsychology: Selected papers of Arthur Benton* (pp. 297–318). New York: Oxford.

Borke, H. (1971). Interpersonal perception of young children: Egocentrism or empathy? *Developmental Psychology, 5*, 263–269.

Borod, J. C., Koff, E., Lorch, M. P., & Nicholas, M. (1985). Channels of emotional expression in patients with unilateral brain damage. *Archives of Neurology, 42*, 345–348.

Borod, J. C., Koff, E., Lorch, M. P., & Nicholas, M. (1986). The expression and perception of facial emotion in brain-damaged patients. *Neuropsychologia, 24*, 169–180.

Bowers, D., Bauer, R. M., Coslett, H. B., & Heilman, K. M. (1985). Processing of faces by patients with unilateral hemisphere lesions. I. Dissociation between judgments of facial affect and facial identity. *Brain and Cognition, 4*, 258–272.

Bowers, D., Coslett, H. B., Bauer, R. M., Speedie, L. J., & Heilman, K. M. (1987). Comprehension of emotional prosody following unilateral hemispheric lesions: Processing defect versus distraction defect. *Neuropsychologia, 25*, 317–328.

Braun, C., Baribeau, J., Ethier, M., Daigneault, S., & Proulx, R. (1989). Processing of pragmatic and facial affective information by patients with closed-head injuries. *Brain Injury, 3*, 5–17.

Brooks, N. (1979). Psychological consequences of blunt head injury. *International Rehabilitation Medicine, 1*, 160–165.

Brooks, N. (1991). The head-injured family. *Journal of Clinical and Experimental Neuropsychology, 13*, 155–188.

Burns, N., & Cavey, L. (1957). Age differences in empathic ability among children. *Canadian Journal of Psychology, 11*, 227–230.

Cicone, M., Wapner, W., & Gardner, H. (1980). Sensitivity to emotional expressions and situations in organic patients. *Cortex, 16*, 145–158.

Damasio, A. R. (1985). The frontal lobes. In K. Heilman & E. Valenstein (Eds.), *Clinical neuropsychology* (pp. 339–375). New York: Oxford University Press.

DeKosky, S. T., Heilman, K. M., Bowers, D., & Valenstein, E. (1980). Recognition and discrimination of emotional faces and pictures. *Brain and Language, 9*, 206–214.

Ekman, P., & Friesen, W. V. (1976). *Pictures of facial affect*. Palo Alto, CA: Consulting Psychologist Press.

Ekman, P., & Oster, H. (1979). Facial expressions of emotion. *Annual Review of Psychology, 30*, 527–554.

Fleiss, J. L. (1981). *Statistical methods for rates and proportions*. New York: Wiley.

Gardner, H., Ling, P. K., Flamm, L., & Silverman, J. (1975). Comprehension and appreciation of humorous material following brain damage. *Brain, 98*, 399–412.

Gates, G. S. (1923). An experimental study of the growth of social perception. *Journal of Educational Psychology, 14*, 449–461.

Gnepp, J. (1983). Childrens' social sensitivity: Inferring emotions from conflicting cues. *Developmental Psychology, 22*, 1805–1814.

Gnepp, J., & Hess, D. L. R. (1986). Childrens' understanding of verbal and facial display rules. *Developmental Psychology, 22*, 103–108.

Gnepp, J., Klayman, J., & Trabasso, T. (1982). A hierarchy of information sources for inferring emotional reactions. *Journal of Experimental Child Psychology, 33*, 96–101.

Heilman, K. M., Bowers, D., Speedie, L., & Coslett, H. B. (1981). Comprehension of affective and nonaffective prosody. *Neurology, 34*, 917–921.

Heilman, K. M., Bowers, D., & Valenstein, E. (1985). Emotional disorders associated with neurological diseases. In K. Heilman & E. Valenstein (Eds.), *Clinical neuropsychology* (2nd ed., pp. 377–402). New York: Oxford Press.

Heilman, K. M., Sholes, R., & Watson, R. T. (1975). Auditory affective agnosia. Disturbed comprehension of affective speech. *Journal of Neurology, Neurosurgery and Psychiatry, 38*, 69–72.

Hess, V., Kappas, A., & Scherer, K. R. (1988). Multichannel communication of emotion: Synthetic signal production. In K. R. Scherer (Ed.), *Facets of emotion: Recent research* (pp. 161–182). Hillsdale, NJ: Lawrence Erlbaum Associates.

Izard, C. E. (1971). *The face of emotion*. NY: Meredith.

Jackson, H. F., & Moffat, N. J. (1987). Impaired emotional recognition following severe head injury. *Cortex, 23*, 293–300.

Kubu, C. S. (1992). *An investigation of emotion recognition in individuals with closed head injury*. Unpublished dissertation thesis, University of Iowa, Iowa City.

Kubu, C. S., Casey, R. J., Hanson, T. V., Campbell, D., Roberts, R., & Varney, N. R. (1993). An investigation of emotion recognition in patients with closed-head injury. *Journal of Clinical and Experimental Neuropsychology, 15*, 59.

Levin, H. S. (1987). Neurobehavioral sequelae of head injury. In P. R. Cooper (Ed.), *Head injury* (2nd ed., pp. 442–463). Baltimore, MD: Williams & Wilkins.

Levin, H. S., Benton, A. L., & Grossman, R. G. (1982). *Neurobehavioral consequences of closed head injury*. New York: Oxford University Press.

Levin, H. S., Eisenberg, H. M., & Benton, A. L. (1989). *Mild head injury*. New York: Oxford University Press.

Lezak, M. (1982). The problem of assessing executive functions. *International Journal of Psychology, 17*, 281–297.

Lezak, M. (1989). Assessment of psychosocial dysfunction resulting from head trauma. In M. Lezak (Ed.), *Assessment of the behavioral consequences of head trauma* (pp. 113–143). New York: Alan R. Liss.

Oddy, M., Humphrey, M., & Uttley, D. (1978). Subjective impairment and social recovery after closed head injury. *Journal of Neurology, Neurosurgery, and Psychiatry, 41*, 611–616.

Prigatano, G. P. (1992). Personality disturbances associated with traumatic brain injury. *Journal of Consulting and Clinical Psychology, 60*(3), 360–368.

Reichenbach, L., & Masters, J. C. (1983). Childrens' use of expressive and contextual cues in judgments of emotion. *Child Development, 54*, 993–1004.

Ross, E. D. (1981). The aprosodias. Functional-anatomic organization of the affective components of language in the right hemisphere. *Archives of Neurology, 38*, 561–569.

Ross, E. D. (1988). Language-related functions of the right cerebral hemisphere. In F. C. Rose, R. Whurr, & M. A. Wyke (Eds.), *Aphasia* (pp. 188–209). London: Whurr.

Russell, J. A., & Bullock, M. (1986). On the dimensions preschoolers use to interpret facial expressions of emotion. *Developmental Psychology, 22*, 97–102.

Saarni, C. (1979). Children's understanding of display rules for expressive behavior. *Developmental Psychology, 15*, 424–429.

Saarni, C. (1984). An observational study of childrens' attempts to monitor their expressive behavior. *Child Development, 55*, 1504–1513.

Scherer, K. R. (1986). Studying emotion empirically: Issues and a paradigm for research. In K. R. Scherer, H. G. Wallbott, & A. B. Summerfield (Eds.), *Experiencing emotion: A cross-cultural study* (pp. 3–28). New York: Cambridge University Press.

Schlanger, B. B., Schlanger, P., & Gerstman, L. J. (1976). The perception of emotionally toned sentences by right-hemisphere damaged and aphasic subjects. *Brain and Language, 3*, 396–403.

Stuss, D. T., & Benson, D. F. (1984). Neuropsychological studies of the frontal lobes. *Psychological Bulletin, 95*, 3–28.

Stuss, D. T., & Benson, D. F. (1986). *The frontal lobes*. New York: Raven Press.

Tucker, D. M., Watson, R. T., & Heilman, K. M. (1977). Discrimination and evocation of affectively intoned speech in patients with right parietal disease. *Neurology, 27,* 947–950.

Varney, N. R. (1991). Appendix. Iowa Collateral Head Injury Interview. *Neuropsychology, 5,* 223–225.

Wiggers, M., & van Lieshout, C. F. (1985). Development of recognition of emotions: Childrens' reliance on situational and facial expressive cues. *Developmental Psychology, 21,* 338–349.

Zuckerman, M., Blanck, P., DePaulo, B. M., & Rosenthal, R. (1980). Developmental changes in decoding discrepant and nondiscrepant nonverbal cues. *Developmental Psychology, 165,* 220–228.

The Problem of Comorbidity in Spouses

Kathleen Chwalisz
Southern Illinois University

> *While I have thought about a temporary separation when things are very stressful, I have an emotional conflict with myself because I feel as if I would be running away from, rather than dealing with our problems. I also know that if I were to physically leave my home for even a day or two, my spouse would not agree to a reconciliation, as in his present state of mind my leaving would be an irrevocable act. There is also the fact that I still love this man. Sometimes, very rarely, there are fleeting glimpses of the person he was and that makes me somewhat hopeful that perhaps some day there will be a partial return of his previous personality.*
>
> *In the past six months my physical health has been worse than I can ever remember—migraines, colds (3 times) and the flu—all of which seem harder to recuperate from. I have spent more on insurance co-pays due to Dr. visits than I have in the last few years. I find that I am exhausted physically and mentally by evening—sometimes by late afternoon and though [sic] I have no recollection of having been unable to sleep, the same feelings are present in the morning.*

This woman's spouse was in a motorcycle accident 9 months prior to her writing this in an essay about her situation (Chwalisz & Stark-Wroblewski, 1996). She reported that her husband was diagnosed with a "permanent frontal lobe injury," although the injury was mild enough for him to return to work. This caregiver is most disturbed by her husband's "inability to show any emotion beside anger." She receives assistance through counseling, a traumatic brain injury (TBI) support group, and friends. She takes Prozac for depression.

In many ways, she is typical of spouse caregivers of people with brain injuries. She copes with a variety of undesirable personality changes in her spouse—wondering if the person she married will ever return. She is at times painfully aware of the gradual disintegration of her physical and mental health, as she struggles to manage the endless demands of living, with neither the division of labor nor the support that was once a part of their marriage. In addition to managing the household and caring for her spouse, she is the primary source of emotional support for their five children. Sometimes she may wonder how much longer she can go on like this, but what else she could she do? He is not likely to change, and society wouldn't accept her leaving him.

Costs of caregiving such as these are often so severe that spouse caregivers have come to be referred to as hidden patients (Fengler & Goodrich, 1979). Because the majority of head injuries occur to young men, parents are frequently the caregivers, drawing more attention of professionals and contributing to the phenomenon of spouses as over-looked victims (Zeigler, 1987). The well-being of spouses of persons with brain injuries has received relatively little attention from health and mental health professionals and researchers alike, whereas most would agree that caregiver well-being is critical to the functioning of the head injured patient in the community. Caregiver breakdown can cause delays in rehabilitation and adjustment of the patient (Livingston, 1987). Although not previously addressed, it should be noted that caregiver breakdown creates two additional drains on the health care system. Not only are there expenses for treatment of caregivers' physical and mental health difficulties, but highly distressed caregivers are more likely to institutionalize the patient (Morycz, 1985).

CAREGIVERS OF PERSONS WITH MILD HEAD INJURIES

The majority of research on spouse caregivers of persons with brain injuries has been focused on caregivers of persons who have survived severe injuries (see Brooks, 1991, for a review). Many studies have included mild injuries along with severe or moderately severe injuries (e.g., Kreutzer, Serio, & Berquist, 1994; Livingston, Brooks, & Bond, 1985; Oddy, Humphrey, & Uttley, 1978), but little, if any, research has been directed specifically to studying caregivers of persons with mild head injuries. Therefore, we have information about how caregivers of persons with mild head injuries compare with those who are responding to more severe injuries, but we have virtually no information specifically describing caregivers of people with mild injuries.

Measures of the severity of the injury such as length of coma and posttraumatic amnesia (PTA) are not related to spouse outcome in a simple linear fashion (Livingston & Brooks, 1988). In a comparison of caregivers of 41 survivors of mild injuries and 57 survivors of severe injuries, there were significant differences at 3 months post-injury in anxiety-based insomnia and social dysfunction but no differences in somatic complaints and depression (Livingston, 1987). Perhaps these two groups of caregivers experience at least a threshold level of stress, sufficient to influence physical and mental health problems, and caregivers of more severely injured persons experience additional problems impacting social functioning and anxiety. Milder injuries (PTA <14 days) have been associated with low, medium, or high perceived burden, whereas PTA beyond 14 days was correlated with increasingly higher perceived burden (Brooks, Campsie, Symington, Beattie, & McKinlay, 1987). Severity of the injury was not related to caregivers' ratings of needs (Kreutzer et al., 1994) or marital satisfaction (Peters, Stambrook, Moore, & Esses, 1990). I also found no significant differences between spouse caregivers of persons who sustained mild versus severe injuries in terms on perceived stress, mental health status, physical health status, and coping strategies used (Chwalisz, 1992a). This finding should be judged with caution, however, because severity was not determined in this study by patient medical data but rather by variables such as perceived severity of the injury, patients' ability to return to work, and the need for care assistance.

Relatives of persons with brain injuries are particularly concerned with the nonspecific symptoms associated with brain injury such as tiredness, impatience, loss of temper, and emotional lability (Livingston & Brooks, 1988), and these symptoms are also often present in patients who have sustained mild injuries (Rutherford, Merrett, & McDonald, 1977; Wrightson & Gronwall, 1981). Lezak (1978) noted that "even mild irritability or a just noticeable diminution in drive can have stressful repercussions on family patterns geared to the patient's premorbid personality" (p. 593). Relatives of persons with minor and severe injuries have been found to report similar symptoms, but a significant difference in the magnitude of those complaints has been found (Livingston et al., 1985).

One might even suggest that caregivers of persons with mild injuries have a more difficult time coping, because the changes associated with mild injuries are not as apparent. Changes associated with mild head injury tend to be observed more in the personality realm than in the realm of physical or cognitive disability, which is much more apparent to persons who observe the patient for only brief periods of time. "Without day-to-day experience of the patient's irresponsibility, impulsivity, or foolishness, or of the onerous duties, vigilance, and sacrifices undertaken by the caretaker, they can easily misperceive the caretaker as being too protective or restrictive, too neglectful or uncaring" (Lezak, 1978, p. 593). Lezak (1988) noted that persons with brain injuries can often exhibit a chameleon-like character, controlling aberrant behavior for short periods of time or in structured situations, appearing normal to friends, relatives, and even professionals. Family members tend to react to the patient in terms of the person they remember rather than the person in front of them (Lezak, 1986), or family members or friends may distort perceptions of the patient due to denial or hope for recovery (Roueche & Fordyce, 1983). Therefore spouses may receive less support, and even opposition, from others. A number of researchers have described this phenomenon (e.g., Kreutzer et al., 1994; Lezak, 1978). One caregiver described it this way: "It is a terrible feeling to know that there is something different about your spouse and have doctors, friends, and family not believe you. I lived in hell thinking I was losing my mind" (Chwalisz & Stark-Wroblewski, 1996).

NEGATIVE REPERCUSSIONS FOR THE CAREGIVER

A number of negative mental health consequences have been reported among spouses of persons with brain injuries. Mood disorders, particularly depression, have been reported (e.g., Chwalisz, 1992a; Lezak, 1978; Livingston et al., 1985; Oddy et al., 1978). Anxiety has also been reported at significant levels (e.g., Livingston et al., 1985; Livingston, 1987). Panting and Merry (1972) reported that 60% of their sample of caregivers experienced problems significant enough to warrant psychotropic medication, which had not been needed prior to the injury. In contrast, 23 of 135 (17%) participants in a previous study of mine reported taking psychotropic medication (Chwalisz, 1992a), primarily antidepressants. These mental health difficulties also do not appear to diminish over time (Oddy et al., 1978).

Caregiving also has negative effects on spouses' physical health status. Twenty-five percent of relatives of brain-injured persons reported an illness within the first year postinjury (Oddy et al., 1978), including migraine headaches, asthma, and duodenal ulcers—illnesses that are often considered to have psychosomatic correlates (e.g., stress). An increased incidence of duodenal ulcer and heart attack was found in another sample of spouse caregivers (Bond, Brooks, & McKinlay, 1979). The most frequent health problems reported in my research included high blood pressure, stomach problems/ulcers, headaches, migraine headaches, back problems, exhaustion, heart problems/heart attack, and TMJ (temporomandibular joint) syndrome (Chwalisz, 1992a). Again, many of the health problems reported by spouse caregivers appear to have stress-related components. In addition to the physical outcomes associated with the stress of caregiving, spouses and dependent children may have the added physical risk that they may be abused by the patient (Lezak, 1978).

The generally unknown nature of head injury and accompanying societal response adds significantly to the difficulties experienced by spouse caregivers. The spouse is not permitted to mourn the loss of the patient, because the familiar body remains. Society neither recognizes the spouse's grief nor provides support and comfort that surrounds those bereaved by death (Lezak, 1978). Poor marital functioning has also been reported by spouses of persons with brain injuries (e.g., Livingston et al., 1985; Peters et al., 1990). However, these spouses cannot divorce with dignity or in good conscience, and marriages are often maintained through bonds of guilt and fear of disapproval (Lezak, 1978).

THE PHENOMENON OF CAREGIVER BURDEN

Efforts to assist spouse caregivers of persons with brain injuries have been impeded by the absence of a solid understanding of the caregiver burden phenomenon. Although much solid research has been conducted on spouse caregivers of persons with brain injuries, it has been limited by a lack of consensus regarding the definition of burden and how it should be measured and operationalized (Chwalisz, 1992b). If we examine the various conceptualizations of burden among caregivers of persons with brain injuries, we can see a number of trends that point us in the direction of a definition of burden.

A number of studies have focused on delineating the various negative consequences experienced by caregivers, which has been summarized earlier in this chapter. Some researchers, however, have equated those negative consequences with caregiver burden. For example, Oddy et al. (1978) used the Wakefield (depression) Scale as an indicator of spouse stress and used the terms *depression* and *stress* interchangeably. Caregiver outcomes vary considerably, even in response to similar circumstances. Therefore, outcome does not appear to be an adequate indicator of burden (Chwalisz, 1992b).

Other studies have examined burden as a psychological construct and have conceptualized burden as either *objective* or *subjective* (Hoenig & Hamilton, 1969). *Objective burden* includes observable changes in the patient as well as environmental changes such as financial strain, changing roles, and so forth. A number of studies have been directed toward using objective burden to predict spouses' subjective experience or outcomes. As previously noted, there is no simple linear relationship between objective severity of the injury and the caregiver's experience (Livingston & Brooks, 1988). Cognitive and physical impairments associated with brain injury were also not consistent predictors (Brooks et al., 1987). The emotional and characterological changes associated with brain injury have been found to be consistent predictors of spouse experiences and negative outcomes (e.g., Brooks, Campsie, Symington, Beatty, & McKinlay, 1986; Thomsen, 1974). The fact that emotional impairment is associated with burden and physical impairment is not suggests that some other variable that is only affected by the emotional changes is mediating the relationship between the patient's condition and the spouse's experience of that condition (Chwalisz, 1992b).

Subjective burden is defined as the caregiver's negative reaction resulting from the presence of objective burden (Hoenig & Hamilton, 1969). Because spouse outcomes and objective aspects of the injury do not adequately represent the caregiver phenomenon, burden should be conceptualized as this negative subjective experience (Chwalisz, 1992b). Indeed, measures of that more subjective experience have consistently predicted a variety of physical and mental health outcomes among spouses of persons with brain injuries (e.g., Livingston, 1985; Livingston & Brooks, 1988; Oddy et al., 1978). With the assumption that caregiver burden is a subjective cognitive or emotional process, our efforts should be directed to understanding the nature of that subjective experience.

THE BURDEN EXPERIENCE

Muriel Lezak's writings represent the most thorough efforts to date regarding the subjective experience of spouses of persons with brain injuries. In 1978, she described five areas of characterological alteration associated with brain injury (e.g., impaired social perceptiveness, emotional alterations) and the subsequent effects on family members. She described spouses as feeling trapped, isolated, and abandoned by extended family, who are inclined to be critical of the caregiver. A recent empirical study validated many of these observations, particularly feelings of being misunderstood, unsupported, and isolated (Kreutzer et al., 1994). Lezak (1978) also noted that spouses of persons with brain injuries cannot divorce with dignity nor mourn the loss of their spouse. Muir and Haffey (1984) described this grieving process as "mobile mourning," in which the tentative nature of the patient's prognosis leaves family members uncertain with regard to the extent to which they have permission to grieve the loss of the patient's former level of functioning.

In 1986, Lezak turned her attention to the importance of family expectations and their impact on reactions to the head injured patient, and she suggested that the stress associated with the patients altered behavior tends to be compounded by family members' unrealistically optimistic expectations. She described six different stages of family members' perceptions of the patient and associated reactions. The stages range from perceiving the patient as a little difficult (due to fatigue, weakness, etc.), expecting full recovery, and feeling happy the person is alive within 3 months of the injury, to perceiving the patient as a difficult childlike dependent, expecting little or no change, and becoming emotionally if not physically disengaged by 18 to 24 months postinjury.

Lezak's writings in this area laid the foundation for understanding the caregiver burden experience among spouses of persons with brain injuries. However, these insights have been based on clinical observations, and little, if any, research has been directed toward validating them. Furthermore, it is not clear if issues deemed relevant by professionals are those most important to caregivers.

When my research team analyzed spouse caregivers' essays about their experiences using qualitative research methods, some familiar ideas were revisited but other important ideas emerged (Chwalisz & Stark-Wroblewski, 1996). These essays were provided spontaneously by caregivers who had participated in a rather lengthy quantitative study of burden among spouses of persons with brain injuries, suggesting that the more traditional standardized measures had not sufficiently captured their experience. These ideas might also be considered to be those things particularly salient to these caregivers.

The individual ideas contained in the essays were categorized and clustered into themes (see Chwalisz & Stark-Wroblewski, 1996, for a description of the method). The different themes found among the essays might easily be identified as different aspects of objective and subjective burden. Furthermore, some of the themes reflect familiar ideas from previous research, and others represent new areas for exploration.

A number of objective aspects of the caregiving situation emerged from the spouses' essays. Familiar ideas contained in the objective themes included:

1. Changes in the patient (e.g., personality changes, intellectual and occupational losses, and wishful thinking about the return of the old spouse).
2. Changes in the caregiver and his or her life (e.g., physical and mental health consequences, changes in lifestyle, loss of life goals or dreams).
3. Changes in the marital relationship (e.g., loss of affection, sexual difficulties, thoughts of divorce).
4. The enigmatic nature of brain injury (e.g., every brain injury is different, difficulties predicting changes).

5. Others don't understand (e.g., lack of awareness and understanding from others, unsupportive and inappropriate reactions to the caregiver).
6. Coping strategies used by caregivers (e.g., keeping busy, journals, seeking professional assistance, social withdrawal).
7. Sources of support and assistance (e.g., family, friends, coworkers, professionals).

Several objective themes represent previously unexplored ideas:

1. My situation is different from and/or easier than others (i.e., making positive social comparisons with other caregivers).
2. Situational factors influencing survey responses (i.e., divorce, death of care-receiver do not relieve the stresses of the spouse).
3. Desire to be helpful to the researchers and other caregivers (i.e., healing aspects of helping others in a similar situation).
4. Problems with/advice for professionals (e.g., professionals' insensitive behavior or lack of information).
5. Miscellaneous stressors ancillary to the injury (i.e., brain injuries do not occur in a vacuum).
6. Personal resources helpful for the caregiver role (i.e., acknowledging one's skills as a caregiver).

This last theme was also observed in a recent study of a support group intervention with caregivers, who reported that having an opportunity to share caregiving successes was an important aspect of the group (Chwalisz, Wiersma, Cook, & Stark-Wroblewski, 1996).

The most informative aspect of our qualitative research, however, was the findings regarding subjective burden among spouse caregivers. A number of clusters of ideas were clearly distinct from the objective areas described above but not distinguishable from each other. These ideas suggest a multifaceted picture of subjective burden (Chwalisz & Stark-Wroblewski, 1996).

The core of burden appears to a be sense of *how terrible it is to have a loved one sustain a brain injury*, which was expressed directly by a number of caregivers (e.g., "you never really get used to it—because it's so different from being normal"). Another theme reflected the *wide range of emotional reactions experienced*, which one caregiver described as being on an emotional rollercoaster—with a lifetime pass. These caregivers also expressed ideas that illustrated *how overloaded and overworked they are* (e.g., "have had too many things to cope with") and as a result *feeling hopeless, exhausted, and at the end of one's rope* (e.g., "I just want this to be over," "I can't get to feeling better"). This hopelessness might be the key to the high frequency of depression among caregivers.

Caregivers also described *difficulties with trying to help the care-receiver cope* (e.g., "I also tried 'too hard' to solve his problems") and *having to support family and make decisions alone* (e.g., "feel like I have to do it all—can't depend on husband"). This loss of consortium appears to be a key variable distinguishing spouse from parent caregivers (e.g., Brooks, 1991; Thomsen, 1974; Zeigler, 1987). Finally, these caregivers were also troubled by *guilt or blame-related attributions about the cause of the injury* (e.g., "I initially devoted myself to his care, then became overwhelmed with guilt since I was driving when the accident occurred").

Our qualitative research suggests that subjective caregiver burden is a complex phenomenon incorporating physical (e.g., exhaustion), cognitive (e.g., guilt-related attributions, loss of consortium), and, most importantly, emotional components (e.g., emotional rollercoaster, hopelessness). Consequently, there may be a wide variety of environmental and psychological variables that impact caregiver burden. Therefore, it seems logical to conceptualize caregiver burden among spouses of persons with brain injuries as a complex process. Research and intervention efforts may then be directed toward aspects of the process or the process as a whole.

MODELS OF THE BURDEN PROCESS

A few attempts have been made to examine burden as a more complex process among caregivers of persons with brain injuries. The Perceived Stress Model of Caregiver Burden (PSB; Chwalisz, 1996) will be used to illustrate how such models might be developed, tested, and used. Then other current models are presented.

The Perceived Stress Model

The PSB grew out of the notions that the most predictive aspects of the caregiving situation come from subjective burden, which was discussed earlier in this chapter, and that subjective experience might just be a special case of stress. Particularly, perceived stress, or the perception that the situation exceeds one's available resources with which to manage it (Lazarus & Folkman, 1984), was determined to be the stress conceptualization most relevant to caregiver burden (Chwalisz, 1992a, 1992b). In fact, the Perceived Stress Scale (Cohen, Kamarck, & Marmelstein, 1983) was found to be a better predictor of spouse physical and mental health status than a scale containing the best items from traditional caregiver burden measures (Chwalisz & Kisler, 1995). The PSB was developed by testing an atheoretical model, representing all relationships among the variables in question that have been previously identified in caregiver literature, against a theoretical model in which perceived stress was hypothesized to be central to all of the relationships among the variables (Chwalisz, 1996). A few changes were made to the theoretical model based on empirical and theoretical considerations to create the PSB, and that model was found to be a good representation of the data.

Given perceived stress as the conceptualization of caregiver burden, other constructs are called into play from the stress literature in order to understand the relationships between the injury, the subjective experience of the spouse, and the physical and mental health consequences for the spouse. The PSB is presented in Fig. 21.1. Particularly, coping and social support become important constructs in relation to caregiver burden. The literature on burden among spouses of persons with brain injuries has, to some extent, examined coping and social support among spouse caregivers.

A breakdown in *coping* has been associated with various negative outcomes for spouse caregivers of persons with brain injuries (Livingston, 1987). A number of different coping strategies have been identified (Mauss-Clum & Ryan, 1981). The strategy most often examined among spouse caregivers is denial (e.g., Bond, 1983; Ridley, 1989; Romano, 1974). The examination of coping among spouses of persons with brain injuries, however, has suffered from a lack of theoretically sound measurement.

In the PSB model, coping is conceptualized in transactional terms (Lazarus & Folkman, 1984). First, coping abilities and previous coping experience are expected to affect the caregiver's appraisals surrounding the injury (i.e., whether the changes associated with the injury exceed the

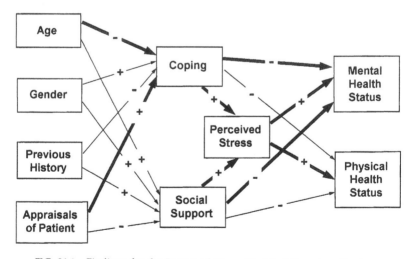

FIG. 21.1. Findings for the Perceived Stress Model of Caregiver Burden.

caregiver's resources). Caring for a person with a brain injury is a situation with which few individuals have had previous experience, so the presence of coping skill at the time of the injury may be critical to how the injury is perceived (Chwalisz, 1992b). Second, and more traditionally, coping is viewed as a response to a situation that is perceived as stressful, which mediates the relationship between the situation and negative stress-related outcomes.

Social support has not typically been measured among spouse caregivers of persons with brain injuries. Spouses of persons with brain injuries have been described as persons "in social limbo" or victims of a social handicap (Lezak, 1978; Rosenbaum & Najenson, 1976). A number of studies mentioned previously have described the lack of support caregivers often experience from friends and family after the injury. Like coping, social support is conceptualized in the PSB to have effects on both perceived stress and caregiver outcomes. That is, previously existing social support will impact on whether the caregiver perceives the injury as stressful, and subsequent mobilization of social support will impact on whether or not the caregiver suffers negative physical and mental health consequences.

Several other predictors of caregiver outcomes, which had been identified in previous research on spouses of persons with brain injuries, were included in the PSB. *Age* has consistently been associated with experienced burden. Particularly, younger spouses have been found to experience more subjective burden and reported more psychological distress (e.g., Barusch & Spaid, 1989; Fitting & Rabins, 1985). *Gender* has been associated with subjective burden, spouse outcomes, coping, and social support. Men and women report different needs and differential use of support groups (Kreutzer et al., 1994). Women have been found to report more subjective burden (e.g., Pruchno & Resch, 1989). Women used more avoidant coping strategies, whereas men used more problem-focused strategies and rated their coping as more effective (Barusch & Spaid, 1989). Men also tend to make more use of formal and informal support (Pruchno & Resch, 1989). *Previous history* of physical or mental health problems has been identified as a major predictor of caregiver outcomes (Livingston, 1987), but this variable has not typically been reported in the caregiver literature. *Appraisals of the patient* were also included in the PSB. Oddy et al. (1978) suggested that it is the perceptions of changes rather than the patient's actual level of disability that determines spouse stress. Unrealistic perceptions of the patient and expectations for recovery have been suggested as a determinant of caregiver status postinjury (Lezak, 1986)

The relationships found to be significant in the PSB model are indicated by bold lines in Fig. 21.1 (Chwalisz, 1996), and the direction of the relationship is indicated by a plus or minus sign. Indeed, perceived stress was significantly associated with spouse physical and mental health status. Coping and social support were significant predictors of mental health status, but not physical health status. There is some question regarding the adequacy of the physical health measure used in the test of the model, so this relationship should not be dismissed as of yet (Chwalisz, 1996). Coping and social support also had the hypothesized influence on perceived stress. That is, levels of coping and social support influenced the extent to which caregivers perceived their situations to be stressful. There were few findings for age, gender, previous history, and appraisals of the patient, suggesting that these variables may not be as important when other psychological constructs are considered in the burden process.

The findings for coping are somewhat counterintuitive and worth noting. Higher scores on coping were associated with more perceived stress and poorer mental health status. This appears to be a measurement artifact. The coping scale used in the test of the PSB model, the Revised Ways of Coping Checklist (WCC; Folkman & Lazarus, 1985), taps the frequency with which various coping strategies are used, but it does not measure how effective those strategies were. It is likely that individuals who are highly distressed may engage in a number of different coping strategies, and then engage in even more strategies if the initially chosen strategies are not effective. Furthermore, when I examined coping in terms of problem-focused (i.e., efforts to change something about the situation) versus emotion-focused strategies (e.g., distraction, denial, emotional expression), emotion-focused efforts were significantly related to poorer mental health status and problem-focused efforts were related to better mental health (although the relationship was not statistically significant).

It would be premature, however, to discard the nonsignificant relationships suggested by the model, because these findings are based on a single sample of caregivers. Clearly the model, which has theoretical support, should be tested with other groups of caregivers. Furthermore, there may be other variables that are relevant to the stress outcome relationship that have not been included in the model, and these relationships should also be explored.

Other Models

Graffi and Minnes (1989) applied the Double ABCX model of family adaptation (McCubbin & Patterson, 1983) to families of persons with brain injuries. In this model, the stressor event (A), the family's crisis-meeting resources (B), and the family's perception or definition of the stressor event (C) interact to determine the likelihood of family crisis (X), which is defined as a disruption in family functioning and calls for changes in the patterns of behavior in the family. Then additional postcrisis factors continue to affect the family. Additional stressors (aA) can pile up and affect the family's adjustment to the crisis. The psychological, social, material, and interpersonal characteristics of the family (bB) that are currently available may be developed or strengthened in response to the crisis. The cC factor is the family's postcrisis perspective on the crisis situation. The coping responses of the family determine the family's outcome, which can range from bonadaptation (e.g., maintenance or strengthening of the family unit or its members) to maladaptation (e.g., continuous conflict, imbalance among family members).

When applied to the traumatic brain injury event (Graffi & Minnes, 1989), how the model operates is more apparent. The characteristics of the person with the injury (A; e.g., personality changes, patient complaints) interact with the caregiver's or family's resources (B; e.g., financial, educational, health, and psychological) and the caregiver perceptions (C; e.g., anger, denial, mobile mourning). The aA (e.g., patient's changing characteristics), bB (e.g., changes in the personal, familial, and social resources), and cC (e.g., improvement in caregiver's perceptions) factors allow for consideration of the caregiver's response to the situation over time.

A number of *developmental stage models* have been developed regarding family members' adaptation to head injury (see Rape, Bush, & Slavin, 1992, for a review and critique). These models were developed to trace family members' reactions to brain injury over time postinjury. The developmental stage models describe various reactions to a family member's brain injury (Rape et al., 1992): (a) an initial shock response (Spanbock, 1987; Henry, Knippa, & Golden, 1985), (b) emotional relief, denial, and unrealistic expectations (Groveman & Brown, 1985; Henry et al., 1985; Lezak, 1986; Spanbock, 1987), (c) acknowledgement of permanent deficits and emotional turmoil (Groveman & Brown, 1985; Henry et al., 1985; Lezak, 1986; Spanbock, 1987), (d) bargaining (Groveman & Brown, 1985), (e) mourning or working through (Groveman & Brown, 1985; Lezak, 1986; Spanbock, 1987), and (f) acceptance and restructuring (Groveman & Brown, 1985; Henry et al., 1985; Lezak, 1986; Spanbock, 1987). Although these models are clinically compelling, they lack empirical support. Furthermore, they assume that families' adaptation progresses in a linear fashion, and they lack a principle that would explain why some families cope better than others (Rape et al., 1992). These authors suggest that the developmental-stage models would be more effective in explaining and predicting family adaptation if they were integrated with Minuchin's family systems theory, although such an integration has yet to be implemented and tested.

Implications and Future Directions for Models

Developing models of the burden process among spouses of persons with brain injuries certainly appears to be the most logical future direction for researchers and professionals interested in assisting caregivers. In fact, it is surprising that I was unable to find more models in the literature. In addition, many of the current models are purely theoretical and based on clinical observations rather than data provided by caregivers. In terms of the empirical literature, we have a great deal of descriptive information regarding objective burden, subjective burden, and outcome. My model-building research, however, suggests that if you consider all of those variables as part of a more complex process, some of the previously identified relationships do not appear to be as important (Chwalisz, 1996).

One particularly important aspect of developing models of caregiver burden is their relative strength in directing interventions with caregivers. Models allow for the prediction of caregivers who are at risk for difficulties, and they suggest mechanisms through which those difficulties can be averted. For example, if family members are indeed found to experience an acknowledgement of permanent deficits and accompanying emotional turmoil at 3 to 9 months post injury (Lezak, 1986), then individual counseling services geared toward those issues can be offered to the caregiver during that time frame. Intervention efforts have already been designed based on the PSB model, in which caregivers are encouraged in a support-group setting to identify their resources (to impact perceived stress) and engage in problem-focused coping efforts rather than emotion-focused coping (Chwalisz et al., 1996).

CONCLUSIONS

Comorbidity among spouses of persons with brain injuries is a serious problem, and one that may be to a larger extent preventable. Furthermore, the distinction between spouses of persons with mild versus severe injuries appears to be a somewhat arbitrary distinction, which continues to be supported by research that includes caregivers of persons with mild injuries merely as a comparison group. Such comparisons have revealed that severity of the injury alone does not predict spouse burden or outcome. In fact, caregivers of persons with mild and severe injuries have exhibited quite similar levels of depression, although there have been differences in terms of other indicators such as psychosocial disturbance. It might be suggested that spouses of persons with mild injuries may have a more difficult situation due to changes that are less readily observed. Clearly, efforts should be directed toward studying the unique experiences of caregivers of persons with mild injuries.

Spouses are typically high functioning prior to the injury and appear to remain so for at least the first 6 to 9 months post injury. This suggests that spouse caregivers are prime candidates for prevention-focused interventions; however, these efforts have been slow in coming. The various models of the caregiver burden process appear to be the most promising direction in improving our understanding of the caregiver experience and mechanisms through which we might develop and implement interventions with caregivers.

REFERENCES

Barusch, A. S., & Spaid, W. H. (1989). Gender differences in caregiving: Why do wives report greater burden? *Gerontologist, 29,* 667–676.

Bond, M. R. (1983). Effects on the family system. In M. Rosenthal, E. Griffith, M. R. Bond, & D. D. Miller (Eds.), *Rehabilitation of the head injured adult* (pp. 187–214). Philadelphia: F. A. Davis.

Bond, M. R., Brooks, D., & McKinlay, W. (1979). Burdens imposed on the relatives of those with severe brain damage due to injury. *Acta Neurochirurgica, 28*(1), S124–S125.

Brooks, D. N. (1991). The head-injured family. *Journal of Clinical and Experimental Neuropsychology, 13*(1), 155–188.

Brooks, N., Campsie, L., Symington, C., Beattie, A., & McKinlay, W. (1986). The five-year outcome of severe blunt head injury: A relative's view. *Journal of Neurology, Neurosurgery, and Psychiatry, 49,* 764–770.

Brooks, N., Campsie, L., Symington, C., Beattie, A., & McKinlay, W. (1987). The effects of severe head injury on patient and relative within seven years of injury. *Journal of Head Trauma Rehabilitation, 2*(3), 1–13.

Chwalisz, K. (1992a). *The perceived stress model of caregiver burden: Evidence from the spouses of head injured persons.* Unpublished doctoral dissertation, University of Iowa, Iowa City.

Chwalisz, K. (1992b). Perceived stress and caregiver burden after brain injury: A theoretical integration. *Rehabilitation Psychology, 37*(3), 189–203.

Chwalisz, K. (1996). The perceived stress model of caregiver burden: Evidence from spouses of persons with brain injuries. *Rehabilitation Psychology, 41*(2), 91–114.

Chwalisz, K., & Kisler, V. (1995). Perceived stress: A better measure of caregiver burden. *Measurement and Evaluation in Counseling and Development, 28,* 88–98.

Chwalisz, K., & Stark-Wroblewski, K. (1996). The subjective experiences of spouse caregivers of persons with brain injuries: A qualitative analysis. *Applied Neuropsychology, 3,* 28–40.

Chwalisz, K., Wiersma, N. S., Cook, C. A., & Stark-Wroblewski, K. S. (1996, August). *Critical events in a support group for caregivers of persons with brain injuries.* Paper presented at the annual convention of the American Psychological Association, Toronto.

Cohen, S., Kamarck, T., & Marmelstein, R. (1983). A global measure of perceived stress. *Journal of Health and Social Behavior, 24,* 385–396.

Fengler, A. P., & Goodrich, N. (1979). Wives of elderly disabled men: The hidden patients. *Gerontologist, 26,* 175–183.

Fitting, M., & Rabins, P. (1985). Men and women: Do they care differently? *Generations, Fall,* 23–26.

Folkman, S., & Lazarus, R. S. (1985). If it changes it must be a process: Study of emotion and coping during three stages of a college examination. *Journal of Personality and Social Psychology, 48*(1), 150–170.

Graffi, S., & Minnes, P. (1989). Stress and coping in caregivers of persons with traumatic head injuries. *Journal of Applied Social Sciences, 13*(2), 293–316.

Groveman, A., & Brown, E. (1985). Family therapy with closed head injured patients: Utilizing Kubler-Ross' model. *Family Systems Medicine, 3,* 440–446.

Henry, P., Knippa, J., & Golden, C. (1985). *Family Systems Medicine, 3,* 427–439.

Hoenig, G. J., & Hamilton, M. W. (1969). *Desegregation of the mentally ill.* London: Routledge and Kegan Paul.

Kreutzer, J. S., Serio, C. D., & Berquist, S. (1994). Family needs after brain injury: A quantitative analysis. *Journal of Head Trauma Rehabilitation, 9*(3), 104–115.

Lazarus, R. S., & Folkman, S. (1984). *Stress, appraisal, and coping.* New York: Springer.

Lezak, M. D. (1978). Living with the characterologically altered brain injured patient. *Journal of Clinical Psychiatry, 39*(7), 592–598.

Lezak, M. D. (1986). Psychological implications of traumatic brain damage for the patient's family. *Rehabilitation Psychology, 31*(4), 241–250.

Lezak, M. D. (1988). Brain damage is a family affair. *Journal of Clinical and Experimental Neuropsychology, 10*(1), 111–123.

Livingston, M. G. (1985). Families who care. *British Medical Journal, 291*, 919–920.

Livingston, M. G. (1987). Head injury: The relatives' response. *Brain Injury, 1*(1), 33–39.

Livingston, M. G., & Brooks, D. N. (1988). The burden on families of the brain injured: A review. *Journal of Head Trauma Rehabilitation, 3*(4), 6–15.

Livingston, M. G., Brooks, D. N., & Bond, M. R. (1985). Three months after severe head injury: Psychiatric and social impact on relatives. *Journal of Neurology, Neurosurgery, and Psychiatry, 48*, 870–875.

Mauss-Clum, N., & Ryan, M. (1981). Brain injury and the family. *Journal of Neurosurgical Nursing, 13*, 165–169.

McCubbin, H. I., & Patterson, J. M. (1983). The family stress process: The double ACBX model of adjustment and adaptation. *Marriage and Family Review, 6*(1–2), 7–37.

Morycz, R. K. (1985). Caregiver strain and the desire to institutionalize the patient. *Research on Aging, 7*(3), 329–361.

Muir, C. A., & Haffey, W. J. (1984). Psychological and neuropsychological interventions with the mobile mourning process. In B. A. Edelstein, & E. T. Courture (Eds.), *Behavioral assessment and rehabilitation of the traumatically brain damaged* (pp. 247–271). New York: Plenum Press.

Oddy, M., Humphrey, M., & Uttley, D. (1978). Stresses upon the relatives of head-injured patients. *British Journal of Psychiatry, 133*, 507–513.

Panting, A., & Merry, D. (1972). The long-term rehabilitation of severe head injuries with particular reference to the need for social and medical support for the patient's family. *Rehabilitation, 38*, 33–37.

Peters, L. C., Stambrook, M., Moore, A. D., & Esses, L. (1990). Psychosocial sequelae of closed head injury: Effects on the marital relationship. *Brain Injury, 4*(1), 39–47.

Pruchno, R. A., & Resch, N. L. (1989). Husbands and wives as caregivers: Antecedents of depression and burden. *Gerontologist, 29*, 159–165.

Rape, R. N., Bush, J. P., & Slavin, L. A. (1992). Toward a conceptualization of the family's adaptation to a member's head injury: A critique of developmental stage models. *Rehabilitation Psychology, 37*(1), 3–22.

Ridley, B. (1989). Family response to head injury: Denial . . . or hope for the future? *Social Science and Medicine, 29*(4), 555–561.

Romano, M. D. (1974). Family response to traumatic head injury. *Scandanavian Journal of Rehabilitation Medicine, 6*, 1–4.

Rosenbaum, M., & Najenson, T. (1976). Changes in life patterns and symptoms of low mood as reported by wives of severely brain-injured soldiers. *Journal of Consulting and Clinical Psychology, 44*(6), 881–888.

Roueche, J. R., & Fordyce, D. J. (1983). Perceptions of deficits following brain injury and their impact on psychosocial adjustment. *Cognitive Rehabilitation, 1*, 4–7.

Rutherford, W. H., Merrett, J. D., & McDonald, J. R. (1977). Sequelae of concussion caused by minor head injuries. *Lancet, i*, 1–4.

Spanbock, P. (1987). Understanding head injury from a family's perspective. *Cognitive Rehabilitation, 5,* 12–14.

Thomsen, I. V. (1974). The patient with severe head injury and his family. *Scandinavian Journal of Rehabilitation Medicine, 6,* 180–183.

Wrightson, P., & Gronwall, D. (1981). Time off work and symptoms after minor head injury. *Injury, 12,* 445–454.

Zeigler, E. A. (1987). Spouses of persons who are brain injured: Overlooked victims. *Journal of Rehabilitation, 53,* 50–53.

Therapy for Spouses of Head Injured Patients

Cathie T. Siders
Washington, DC

The changes in traumatically head injured persons extract an enormous cost from spouse caregivers. The resulting characterological defects, emotional upheavals, and behavioral changes in the head injured person disrupt usual family interactions and wreak havoc for the spouse (Chwalisz, this volume, chap. 21; Lezak, 1978, 1986; Varney, this volume, chap. 8). If the head injured person survives the injury, life does not resume as it was for either spouse. Usually, spouse caregivers endure a chronically high level of stress for several years, resulting in problems requiring psychological and medical treatment (Chwalisz, 1992; Oddy, Humphrey, & Uttley, 1978).

In general, the therapist's work with spouse caregivers is to help them develop appropriate expectations for their spouses (Lezak, 1986) and to turn the focus of treatment to their own health. The therapist should be alert to particular experiences that are common to spouse caregivers of traumatically brain injured (TBI) patients, and also to barriers to the therapy that may help them survive the devastating changes to their lives and their marriages.

THREATS TO THE WELL-BEING OF THE SPOUSE CAREGIVER

From clinical experience with women whose husbands suffered traumatic brain injury, I have observed factors that may worsen spouse caregivers' distress and/or keep them from appropriate individual psychological treatment.

Failure of Health Care Professionals to Recognize
the Spouse's Need for Individual Psychotherapy

It is appropriate for the initial treatment to focus on the TBI patient. However, sometimes the focus remains there, missing or ignoring the psychosocial, financial, and role adjustments the spouse must make. Fengler and Goodrich (1979) recognized this phenomenon in the wives of disabled men and referred to the untreated spouse caregiver as the "hidden patient."

Occasionally, TBI patients and their spouses are referred for marital therapy, a treatment experience often doomed to failure. A number of my clients had been referred for marital therapy before they were referred to me. The therapists or counselors appeared to work from a more classic relational orientation without sufficient recognition that many of the current marital problems were associated with the irreversible brain–behavior correlates of the head injury. Knowledge of the psychological sequelae of head trauma is essential. The TBI patient may suffer from impaired self-control, difficulties in modulating cognitive activities, and difficulties in modulating emotional reactions (Lezak, 1986). For example, the TBI patient may suffer changes that result in a childlike dependence, an absence of empathy, and the onset of impolitic speech (Varney, this volume, chap. 8).

Taking a traditional marital therapy approach to these types of problems may reinforce the spouse caregiver's denial about the seriousness or irreversible nature of the TBI patient's condition. The therapist's approach may add to the guilt and shame already experienced by the spouse caregiver. For the beleaguered spouse caregiver, the misplaced focus makes it easy to become soured on the mental health care system. A traditional marital therapy approach may drive feelings underground, making the spouse caregiver extremely reluctant to pursue individual therapy later.

The Difficulty of Grieving for Someone Who Is Not Dead

Spouse caregivers have suffered the death of a relationship, but continue to be married. Grieving the loss of the previous relationship and the TBI partner's former level of functioning flies in the face of societal expectations (Chwalisz, this volume, chap. 21; Lezak, 1986) and appears contrary to the process of a healthy adaptation to loss. Worden (1991) described the following four basic tasks of grieving that, once completed, enable such an adaptation: (a) to accept the reality of the loss, (b) to work through the pain of grief, (c) to adjust to an environment in which the deceased is missing, and (d) to emotionally relocate the deceased and move on with life.

When the victim survives, the very nature of head trauma presents obstacles to the spouse caregiver's grieving for the lost relationship. The spouse caregiver's partner is not deceased, but the marital relationship is permanently altered. Moving on with life becomes immensely complex. As the therapist, I found it helpful to think about integrating the concepts *mobile mourning* (Muir & Haffey, 1984) and *socially negated loss* (Lazare, 1979) into the conversations with the spouse caregivers. These concepts begin to put words to their current experience and begin to explain the challenges to the grieving process. Muir and Haffey (1984) coined the phrase *mobile mourning* to describe the process as one in which the tentative nature of the patient's prognosis leaves spouses in a quandary, that is, uncertain about the extent to which they have permission to grieve the loss of the patient's former level of functioning. This is particularly relevant to head injury in that all psychosocial and mental changes secondary to the trauma may not be manifest for weeks or months.

With the brain injured person alive, but irreparably changed, the spouse caregiver may experience what Lazare (1979) described as *socially negated loss*. The spouse caregiver may grapple with the loss of the previous relationship and all that this means, while family members and friends act as if the loss did not happen. Worden (1991) suggests that this is one social condition that portends a complicated grief reaction.

The opportunity for the phenomenon of socially negated loss is partially attributable to the variable nature of recovery from head injury. Family and friends not involved in the daily care of the TBI patient may be reacting to the patient's recovery of more immediately apparent motor and sensory capabilities. However, they do not see the absence of recovery of psychosocial and mental functions, especially the nuances of these capabilities that are essential to adult relationships. The TBI patient frequently lacks insight about his or her own diminished capacities (Lezak, 1986), compounding the possibility for a spouse caregiver's socially negated loss.

Family and friends may not be able or willing to acknowledge that the brain injury has significantly damaged the person they care about. As Lezak observed, family members respond to the person they remember, not the person in front of them (Lezak, 1978).

In some situations, extended family members behave in ways that make the situation more difficult for the spouse caregivers. The behaviors range from the nonproductive to the somewhat bizarre. For example, one of my clients endured accusations from her husband's family, who believed he had fully recovered from an auto accident that left him with frontal and temporal-lobe damage. My client's report of her husband's behavioral violence and severe memory deficits were met with the accusation that "it was all in her head." In this case, the TBI patient's mother and brother refused to see anything less than full recovery.

Another client reported an incident that occurred while her head injured husband was home for the weekend from a rehabilitation facility. He had sustained frontal-, temporal-, and parietal-lobe damage, resulting in severe memory problems, left hemispatial neglect, a severe decline in attentional abilities, and a defective temporal orientation. My client discovered her sister-in-law and her head injured husband viewing a videotape about sexual touch and massage. The sister-in-law, seeing that her brother's marital relationship had suffered since the accident, thought that learning these new techniques would help the marriage.

The actions of family or friends in these situations, however well intentioned, may deny grave realities for the spouse caregiver. The partners of TBI patient find themselves trapped in socially awkward and angering situations with their loss unacknowledged. Individual therapy for spouse caregivers can help them engage in the socially unacceptable behavior of mourning for a living person, assisting with the constructive disengagement from the past (Lezak, 1986).

The Emotional and Physical Exhaustion of Being Given All the Adult Roles and Responsibilities in the Family

The spouse caregiver's exhaustion is impressive. The spouse caregiver becomes head of household, negotiator with the insurance company, the sole decision maker, coordinator of the spouse's medical appointments, the only functioning parent, the financial manager, and the translator of the TBI patient's condition to children, family, and friends. Sometimes the spouse caregiver becomes the daily organizer and memory for the injured person. Sometimes the spouse caregiver becomes the protector of the children, shielding them from the TBI patient's violence or accidents associated with memory loss.

Initially, there is considerable self-imposed pressure to do it all. Occasionally, the extended family pressures the spouse caregiver to manage the new situation while pretending life hasn't changed. Spouse caregivers report sleep disruptions because of the increased demands, their own stress in response to the head injury, and their children's increased stress.

Children feel and reflect the changes imposed on the family as a result of the parent's head injury. My clients reported an increased frequency of physical ailments, disruptive behavior, anxieties, and school problems in their children. The children's sleep patterns were especially disrupted after intense arguments or violence between their parents. One client reported a problem that occurred whenever her husband discontinued his seizure medication. He would awaken the four children, age 8 and younger, in the middle of the night and harangue them about their mother. His tirades were marked by intense anger and peppered with profanity. All four children suffered stomach upset, an increase in crying episodes, sleep disturbance, an increase in respiratory illnesses, and seemed generally more anxious after their father's injury. Eventually, my client sought a divorce and legal protection from the violence of her head injured husband.

For the spouse caregiver, it is emotionally and physically exhausting to adjust to the increase in demands and loss of the adult relationship. It is emotionally exhausting to come to terms with the fact that the injured person cannot be satisfied or give satisfaction in any adult sense (Lezak, 1986).

Isolation

The spouse caregiver may be geographically isolated, as were several of my clients who lived in rural areas. This quickly became an issue in winter months when they were the only adult able to safely drive or when the distances to medical offices and other necessary services just became too much.

Most often the isolation is social. Spouse caregivers experience a dramatic increase in the demands on their time. They tend to the partner's health care needs, respond to newly acquired roles, and, if there are children in the family, respond to their reactions to the impact of the head injury. Spouse caregivers frequently lose contact with their previously established social network; there is no time for the usual activities. Friends and family begin to stay away from the TBI patient because of inappropriate verbal behaviors or an inability to modulate emotional responses. One client reported that her husband made extremely inappropriate sexual remarks to their adolescent children. This injury-related behavior occurred in front of friends and extended family, resulting in the children's bewilderment and their caution about who was present when they were with their father. Another client reported the decline in visits from friends in the months following her husband's accident. Their friends could not tolerate her husband's unpredictable, seemingly unprovoked verbal rage responses.

Spouse caregivers may develop affective or anxiety disorders in the months following their partner's head injury. The therapist should be alert to increasing isolation or withdrawal associated with long periods of high and uninterrupted stress.

THE WORK OF THE THERAPIST

Therapists need to be prepared to see considerable variation in the presenting picture of the spouse caregivers who come for treatment. The case-by-case differences depend on: (a) the nature of the TBI patient's injuries, (b) the resulting psychosocial and physical deficits, (c) the state of the marriage before the traumatic event, (d) the spouse caregiver's premorbid history, and (e) the length of time between the traumatic injury and the initial visit with the spouse caregiver. The work with spouse caregivers is multidimensional, requiring some knowledge of brain injury sequelae or a professional connection with a neuropsychologist who can be consulted about the behavioral and cognitive effects of the trauma. Therapists will be engaged in most or all of the following activities during treatment with a spouse caregiver.

Listening and Validating

These facets of therapy seem so fundamental that they need not be mentioned. However, spouse caregivers desperately need someone to speak to without editing their thoughts and feelings. The therapist may be the only person who's heard the unedited description of current life. Spouse caregivers make attempts to talk with friends or extended family about the condition of the TBI patient and the devastation to their own lives. These attempts are frequently met with reluctance or refusal to listen. The spouse caregivers may carry so much guilt, shame, anger, and/or fear that it seems unspeakable to friends and family.

The therapist must listen carefully without assuming that the issues the therapist has identified as most relevant are the ones most relevant to this particular spouse caregiver. It is important to validate feelings and communicate the naturalness of their reactions.

Translating and Consulting

The therapist will likely serve as translator and carrier of information, especially if other professionals are involved with the case. With appropriate releases secured, the therapist may consult with a neuropsychologist, a neurologist, or a lawyer. Consultation with a neuropsychologist brings valuable information to therapy by translating the brain–behavior correlates of the injuries into what this means for daily living and the state of the marital relationship. The spouse caregiver is one of the best sources of information regarding the TBI patient. The therapist may assist the spouse caregiver in conversations with the neurologist regarding changing symptom pictures and nonadherance with prescribed medication. If a legal action is in process because of the injury, the therapist may be called on to describe to the legal team the impact on the spouse caregiver. If the children develop a need for health care services, the therapist is postitioned to make the referral and describe the family's current circumstances. All of this is not to suggest that spouse caregivers should not communicate for themselves. Rather, spouse caregivers appreciate this assistance because of their own exhaustion and worry or because they have little experience conversing with physicians, psychologists, and lawyers. The therapist carries crucial information and understanding that facilitates the spouse caregiver's treatment.

Educating the Client About the Difficulty of Grieving

Speaking directly about the loss that the spouse caregiver has endured sometimes comes as a surprise. The freedom to acknowledge the loss of relationship in the safety and privacy of therapy begins to move the client forward. With an awareness for the timing, the therapist may acquaint the client with the concepts of mobile mourning (Muir & Haffey, 1984) and socially negated loss (Lazare, 1979). This helps by putting words to the spouse caregiver's experience and begins to address the tangle of mourning for someone who is living.

Depending on the client, bibliotherapy can be useful. Understandable readings about the impact of head trauma on the family and about grieving are most appropriate. These provide a framework for the process of grieving, assisting the client in what Lezak calls the eventual constructive disengagement from the past (Lezak, 1986).

Reducing Isolation

This work of the therapist generally involves connecting the spouse caregiver with resources. In a head injury support group, the client can speak privately with other spouse caregivers. There is much to be learned from spouse caregivers who are farther out in time from the injury event. Often spouse caregivers struggle with moral and spiritual issues about the marriage. One client was terribly conflicted about having more children and her own health. Her physician had diagnosed a serious medical condition, recommending that she not risk another pregnancy. Her head injured husband was pressuring her to have another child, which would have made four. On my recommendation, the client spoke with a priest outside her home parish. Their conversations helped with eventual decisions about this issue.

Spouse caregivers need time away from the demands of their many roles. The therapist must be creative and pragmatic when generating ideas for respite opportunities. For example, I encouraged one client to retain her babysitter an extra hour on the day of therapy. The client spent the extra hour with an old friend. Another client occasionally stayed overnight with extended family members, allowing her to relax in a supportive environment while they did much of the child care.

Diagnosing

A thorough psychological assessment is necessary with spouse caregivers. Depression and a spectrum of anxiety disorders are commonly observed in these cases, requiring referral for medication. Spouse caregivers often feel that they're "going crazy." They need to understand that they're not crazy, but that the situation is "crazy making." Treating this requires patience on the part of the therapist and the client because the spouse caregiver's situation typically does not get better or easier for several years.

CONCLUSION

I challenge the neuropsychologist to look beyond spouse caregivers as rich sources of information about the TBI patient (Varney, this volume, chap. 8). The head injury has damaged their lives too, inflicting changes they would not have chosen voluntarily. Knowing the extent of the TBI patient's injuries, the neuropsychologist is uniquely positioned to understand the spouse caregiver's psychological risks. A timely recommendation for individual therapy can begin the essential working through of this very complex tangle of circumstances.

It takes time for spouse caregivers to work through turbulent feelings about the partner's head injury and what this means for themselves and their families. The therapist turns the focus of treatment toward the spouse caregiver, identifying the unrecognizable and unacknowledged losses that the spouse caregiver suffers. A knowledgeable therapist can help the forgotten victim so that head injury does not claim two lives instead of one.

REFERENCES

Chwalisz, K. (1992). *The perceived stress model of caregiver burden: Evidence from the spouses of head injured persons.* Unpublished doctoral dissertation, University of Iowa, Iowa City.

Fengler, A. P., & Goodrich, N. (1979). Wives of elderly disabled men: The hidden patients. *Gerontologist, 26,* 175–183.

Lazare, A. (1979). Unresolved grief. In A. Lazare (Ed.), *Outpatient psychiatry: Diagnosis and treatment* (pp. 498–512). Baltimore, MD: Williams & Wilkins.

Lezak, M. D. (1978). Living with the characterologically altered brain injured patient. *Journal of Clinical Psychiatry, 39,* 592–598.

Lezak, M. D. (1986). Psychological implications of traumatic brain damage for the patient's family. *Rehabilitation Psychology, 31*(4), 241–250.

Muir, C., & Haffey, W. (1984). Psychological and neuropsychological interventions with the mobile mourning process. In B. Eldelstein & E. Courture (Eds.), *Behavioral assessment and rehabilitation of the traumatically brain damaged* (pp. 201–227). New York: Plenum Press.

Oddy, M., Humphrey, M., & Uttley, D. (1978). Stresses upon the relatives of head-injured patients. *British Journal of Psychiatry, 133,* 507–513.

Worden, W. (1991). *Grief counseling and grief therapy: A handbook for the mental health practitioner.* New York: Springer.

23

Mild Traumatic Brain Injury in Children and Adolescents

Mary Ann Roberts
University of Iowa

> *It is imperative that an increasing understanding on the part of pediatricians, school teachers, and other individuals likely to come into contact with children who have had head injuries be obtained so that children at risk for these difficulties can be seen, appreciated, and appropriately evaluated.*
> —Boll, 1983, p. 79

> *It would be unfortunate if this led to a casual dismissal of the testimony of parents or teachers of a child who has sustained an apparently trivial injury. The overall findings do not exclude the possibility that as a consequence of "mild" head injury, some children have in fact suffered behavioral disability that only becomes evident as they are confronted by increasing intellectual, academic, and social demands with advancing age.*
> —Benton, 1995, p. 288

PREVALENCE ESTIMATES AND DEFINITION

Significant numbers of individuals sustain a mild traumatic brain injury (TBI) at some point during their childhood or adolescence. Approximately 30% of the students in one survey (Segalowitz & Brown, 1991) of more than 600 high school students reported having experienced a history of head injury, with half of these adolescents reporting an associated period of loss of consciousness. The diagnosis of concussion, which may include brief or transient disruption of neurologic function, headache, nausea, or vomiting, has also been reported with considerable frequency in another

493

survey of adolescents and young adults (Roberts et al., 1990) and has been associated with persistent neurobehavioral dysfunction even years after the mild injury occurred (Klonoff, Clark, & Klonoff, 1995; Lundar & Nesvold, 1985; Roberts, Verduyn, Manshadi, & Hines, 1996; Wrightson, McGinn, & Gronwald, 1995). In one report of hospital admissions, approximately 90% of those pediatric patients admitted to a hospital for evaluation and treatment of TBI were considered mild or minor (Kraus, Fife, Cox, Ramstein, & Conroy, 1986). However, incidence figures based on hospital admissions alone, are lower than the actual rate of occurrence as they do not include those pediatric patients who are treated in the emergency room and released or examined by their local physician. The numbers begin to reach epidemic proportions as surveys (Alves & Jane, 1985; Boll, 1983; Jennett, 1989) report that as many as 20% of injuries sustained by school age children go unwitnessed by adults, whereas anywhere from 20% to 40% of mild TBI cases are never reported, and no medical attention is sought. Conservative estimates, based only on those admitted to the hospital, suggest that as many as 158 per 100,000 children and adolescents sustain a mild brain injury annually (Segalowitz & Brown, 1991). Although persistent and troublesome sequelae of mild TBI may occur in only a small proportion of these cases, research and clinical attention to this problem is critical because the incidence of mild TBI in the pediatric population is so great (Beers, 1992). Any reduction in morbidity would represent a vast savings to health costs and human suffering (Harrington, Malec, Cicerone, & Katz, 1993).

Boys are more likely than girls to experience a mild TBI in a ratio of approximately 2 to 1 (Segalowitz & Brown, 1991), with the ratio becoming more lopsided, growing to 4 boys for each girl when considering those who have experienced three or more mild TBIs (Bijur & Haslum, 1995). Relatively low velocity injuries such as falls experienced during play or sporting activities are the most common source of mild TBI in children and adolescents (Greenspan & MacKenzie, 1994; Segalowitz & Brown, 1991). One case known to the author is fairly typical, that of a 17-year-old male who experienced a concussion or "bell-ringer" in a pick-up football game with friends. When the game was over, he was unable to identify his car while standing in front of it. This young man experienced persistent sequelae described as staring spells, emotional outbursts, and memory problems. Whiplash injuries, in which a mild TBI may be sustained with no evidence of blunt trauma to the head, also occur and often involve greater forces of acceleration-deceleration and rotation (e.g., Roberts, Manshadi, Bushnell, & Hines, 1995; Varney & Varney, 1995; Yarnell & Rossie, 1988). Highest risk periods include weekend evenings during the spring and summer months (Boll, 1983). Roughly half of the mild TBIs sustained in one sample (Stewart-Scott & Douglas, 1998) of children and adolescents occurred during summer vacation from school. Coupled with the fact that physical disability is generally not associated with mild TBI, it is not surprising that a mild TBI seldom comes to the attention of the child's teacher (Gulbrandsen, 1984). Nonetheless, as documented later, mild TBI in children and adolescents is not always benign and may be of considerable educational significance.

Definition of mild TBI varies somewhat from study to study; however, there is general consensus with regard to the extreme or upper limit of most parameters, and thus, the cutoff between mild and moderate-to-severe TBI is relatively clear. The Glasgow Coma Scale is commonly employed, with ratings of 13 to 15 usually required at the time the child comes to medical attention, ratings that imply no more than minor alterations in verbal and motor responsiveness. The Abbreviated Injury Scale (Plant & Gifford, 1976) has also been employed in some research (e.g., Asarnow et al., 1995), but classification of an injury on this 1 to 6 rating includes both head and other physical (e.g., orthopedic) injuries. Loss of consciousness does not necessarily occur in mild TBI, but when it does it is brief, usually 30 min or less. Posttraumatic amnesia (i.e., failure to be age-appropriately oriented to person, place, and time, and poor recall of recent events) may also be included in rating brain injury severity and is generally limited to 24 hr or less for the categorization of a TBI as mild. Posttraumatic amnesia in children can now be evaluated with greater accuracy and reliability thanks to the efforts of Ewing-Cobbs and colleagues (Ewing-Cobbs, Levin, Fletcher, Miner, & Eisenberg, 1990), who developed and normed the Children's Orientation and Amnesia Test. Acute postconcussive symptoms may include headache, dizziness, transitory alterations in vision such as diplopia, brief loss of vision, or "seeing stars," as well as nausea and/or vomiting. Any required neurosurgical intervention, such as evacuation of a hematoma, is typically an exclusionary criterion for grading a TBI as mild, even in the absence of loss of consciousness (e.g., Levin et al., 1987).

Although the cutoff between mild and moderate-to-severe TBI is fairly clear, there is less agreement with regard to the definition of lower boundary limits for mild TBI. Some investigators (e.g., Asarnow et al., 1995) consider two or more acute symptoms such as headache and seeing stars as evidence of mild TBI, while others may contest this opinion, contending that such symptoms were insufficient evidence that any degree of brain injury had occurred. The American Congress of Rehabilitation Medicine (1993), however, has proposed that "any alteration in mental state at the time of the accident" (p. 86) is sufficient evidence that a mild TBI has occurred. Further, it should be pointed out that the qualifier *mild* applies to the neurologic disruption acutely at the time of the trauma and not necessarily to the extent of sequelae experienced.

THE CURRENT BOX SCORE

The multifaceted work of the Houston (e.g., Levin, Ewing-Cobbs & Eisenberg, 1995) and Seattle (e.g., Fay et al., 1993, 1994) research groups has demonstrated that, for pediatric mild TBI as a whole, attention, memory, and information-processing complaints registered acutely at the time of injury are essentially resolved by 3-month to 1-year follow-up. Comparing a large sample ($n = 247$) of children who had sustained mild TBIs with a control group of 280 children who had sustained trauma to regions of the body other than the head, Farmer (Farmer, Singer, Mellits, Hall, & Charney, 1987) also reported acute but transient emotional, behavioral, and physical complaints, including irritability, clingy behavior, sleep disturbance, and headache. Only headaches were more frequently experienced by the head-injured group when compared with the other injury group. The failure to identify persistent, severe, and disabling consequences of pediatric mild TBI as a whole is truly "gratifying" (p. 288), as was concluded by Benton (1995).

Epidemiologic studies of children who have sustained single (Bijur, Haslum, & Golding, 1990) and multiple (Bijur, Haslum, & Golding, 1996) mild TBIs have also been negative with respect to long-term sequelae when various statistical controls have been applied. As a group, Bijur concluded that children with a history of mild head injury were "statistically indistinguishable" from controls on all outcomes measured including global cognitive development, as well as reading and math achievement scores. One finding was significant at 5 years post-injury, and this was the teacher rating of hyperactivity. This finding remained significant even after partialing out variance attributable to demographic factors and the mother rating of the child's preinjury level of hyperactivity. Although the authors essentially dismissed the teacher data and concluded that there are no long-lasting behavioral effects of mild TBI in children, a vast body of research in developmental hyperactivity (e.g., Loney & Milich, 1982) has documented that teacher ratings are often more sensitive to the symptoms of attention deficit hyperactivity disorder (ADHD) than are informants in other settings, such as parents in the less structured home environment.

Bijur (Bijur et al., 1996) also studied groups of children who had sustained two ($n = 278$) and three ($n = 51$) mild head injuries, comparing them to a group of controls who had sustained injury to body regions other than the head. Once again, on global measures such as overall cognitive functioning or math and reading achievement scores, the authors concluded that multiple mild head injuries do not increase the risk of cognitive sequelae. Also, the authors failed to find an increased risk of posttraumatic behavioral sequelae (e.g., hyperactivity) following multiple mild injury

(Bijur & Haslum, 1995) once demographic factors had been statistically adjusted.

The issue of statistically controlling for premorbid risk factors, a common practice in epidemiological research, was addressed by Satz and colleagues (Satz et al., 1997) in their comprehensive and influential review of mild TBI in children and adolescents. The method investigators employ to accommodate for preinjury risk factors will dictate the generalizability of their findings. Although certain demographics (e.g., socioeconomic status [SES], gender) may put a child at greater risk of developing attention deficit hyperactivity disorder, these may be the very same factors that put a child at greater risk of acquiring a traumatic brain injury (Jacquess & Finney, 1994). Statistically disentangling these risk factors or excluding children with a history of multiple injury from studies of mild TBI may be ill-advised and result in atypical samples. Rather, it is proposed that the impact of each vulnerability (e.g., demographics, premorbid behavior problems, history of one or more mild TBIs) and their interactions be examined as they contribute to the child's current neurobehavioral status.

Traditional measures of neuroanatomy (i.e., computed tomography [CT]; magnetic resonance imaging [MRI]) and electroencephalography (EEG) often fail to document anatomic or electrophysiologic abnormalities in spite of a well-documented history of mild TBI and clear neurobehavioral deficits to corroborate the patient's subjective complaints (Bigler & Snyder, 1995). In one pediatric study (Levin et al., 1995), 3 of 10 mildly injured patients exhibited selected neuropsychological deficits, whereas none of the 10 manifested abnormal signal on MRI. Investigators also report that a normal neurological or mental status exam may be recorded even though the individual experiences persistent neurobehavioral sequelae (e.g., Roberts et al., 1995) or subsequently demonstrates other evidence of a potentially serious intracranial lesion (Snoek, Minderhoud, & Wilmink, 1984; Stein, Spettell, Young, & Ross, 1993).

Although seldom reported in children and adolescents, findings from the adult literature suggest that metabolic neuroimaging may be more promising in identifying posttraumatic neurologic abnormalities. In three separate series of adult cases (Jacobs, Put, Ingels, & Bossuyt, 1994; Kant, Smith-Seemiller, Isaac, & Duffy, 1997; Varney et al., 1995) neuroSPECT (single-photon emission computed tomography) using Tc-HMPAO proved to be more sensitive than CT or MRI in detecting cerebral abnormalities in those who experienced persistent postconcussion symptoms. A pediatric case report (Roberts et al., 1995) suggested similar findings for positron emission tomography (PET). In this case study, PET proved to have greater sensitivity than EEG in corroborating memory deficits and epilepsy spectrum disorder in an 11-year-old who sustained a mild TBI from a whiplash injury 4 years earlier.

Beers's (1992) comprehensive and thoughtful review concluded that there is sufficient evidence to document cognitive impairments persisting for periods as long as 6 months, as well as educational difficulties lasting as long as 5 years in a small but significant number of pediatric mild TBI cases. Further, Beers postulated that cognitive deficits are more likely to persist beyond the typical 3-month recovery period when the task is more complex or less well established in the child's repertoire (i.e., recently learned skills), a theme common to the goals of the educational curriculum. Empirical support is provided in a study of pediatric mild TBI reported by Gulbrandsen (1984). The mild TBI group performed at levels below a carefully matched control group on 29 of 32 variables. Statistical analyses identified the "concussion factor" as contributing significantly in 7 of the 29 comparisons, with the magnitude of difference between TBI and control groups increasing as a function of task complexity. Others (Bassett & Slater, 1990; Donders, 1993) documented that recall of verbal information after a delay, a critical skill in the academic environment, may be particularly susceptible to deterioration following pediatric mild TBI. Also, Andrews and colleagues (Andrews, Rose, & Johnson, 1998) presented evidence in a pediatric sample to suggest that persistent social, emotional, and behavioral deficits are "triggered by even mild TBI" (p. 137).

Finally, research is beginning to accumulate to document that deficits may persist for years following mild TBI in children and adolescents. Although Wrightson and colleagues (Wrightson et al., 1995) failed to identify acute cognitive deficits following mild TBI in a group of pre-schoolers, they did find emerging deficits on a visual closure task at 6 months and 1 year postinjury and, ultimately, significantly greater likelihood of reading deficits in this group at 6½ years of age. In the longest follow-up study available (Klonoff et al., 1995), 31% of adult subjects reported cognitive deficits including educational lag, as well as memory and concentration difficulties, 23 years after sustaining brain injury as a child, with 89% of these cases having been mild injuries. Although the TBI group had a higher than average unemployment rate, an even more striking finding in the Klonoff follow-up study is a fourfold increase in unemployment rate for those TBI subjects who continued to experience sequelae.

WHOM WE ASK, WHAT WE ASK, AND WHEN WE ASK IT

As reported earlier, research findings and opinions regarding the extent and duration of sequelae following pediatric mild TBI are inconsistent and run the gamut from no deficits (e.g., Bijur et al., 1990, 1996; Fay et al., 1993; Levin et al., 1995) to persistent and disabling consequences (e.g.,

Beers, 1992; Klonoff et al., 1995). Although slight differences in the definition of mild TBI may account for some of the variability in conclusions, other factors, such as *subject ascertainment*, are likely to contribute more. Investigators who recruit potential subjects from consecutive emergency room admissions are likely to identify a much lower base rate of residual sequelae in pediatric mild TBI than those investigators who report on patients from rehabilitation clinics where referrals are often made following incomplete recovery from injury. Investigation results, and ultimately conclusions as to the effects of mild TBI, will hang in the balance, as the experiences of the "Miserable Minority" (Ruff, Levin, & Marshall, 1986) may be too few in number to show up as statistically significant. It is of note, however, that even those investigators (e.g., Benton, 1995; Fay et al., 1993; Kaufmann, Fletcher, Levin, Miner & Ewing-Cobbs, 1993) who have concluded that pediatric mild TBI as a whole produces no long-lasting, disabling deficits still acknowledge that there may well be individual children who fail to recover.

The *dependent variables* selected for evaluation of deficit also contribute to inconsistency in findings across studies. A number of traditional neuropsychological assessment measures that may be critical in the evaluation of developmental learning disorders may fail to tap the "subtle" or elusive deficits (e.g., rate of processing) that may be disabling in the educational setting following mild TBI (Silver & Oakland, 1997). For example, research examining the effects of pediatric mild TBI on cognitive processing will come to very different conclusions if the dependent variable of study is the WISC–III or academic achievement scores (e.g., Fay et al., 1993; Rutter, Chadwick & Shaffer, 1983), as opposed to the Dichotic Word Listening Test (Roberts et al., 1994).

Finally, *timing of the assessment* postinjury and *age* of the child also contribute to variability in study outcomes of mild TBI. If, as some researchers (Roberts et al., 1996; Wrightson et al., 1995) have proposed, there is a delay of a year of more in the expression of certain deficits (e.g., first grade reading achievement, symptoms of epilepsy spectrum disorder; see Roberts, chap. 11, this volume) following pediatric mild TBI, the study that ends at 1 year postinjury may never see the problems incurred. Investigators who have published longer term follow-up studies have discounted the relationship between the delayed onset of deficits and previous mild TBI as implausible (e.g., Polissar et al., 1994). Also, some effects may be age dependent in their expression. For example, children who sustain a mild TBI during early elementary years may not exhibit posttraumatic executive dysfunction until adolescence, when the demand for such skills becomes ascendant. From a slightly different approach, Levin and colleagues (Levin et al., 1988) presented convincing evidence that neurobehavioral skills that are in a rapid stage of development (e.g., aspects of memory in children vs. adolescents) in the child at the time of assessment are also likely to reflect a greater degree of impairment than previously established skills.

As Satz and colleagues (Satz et al., 1997) pointed out, methodology, appropriate statistical procedures, and adequate control groups are important in reporting the box score on pediatric mild TBI. However, *whom* an investigator chooses to study, *what* neurobehavioral variables are selected for study, and *when* the research protocol is administered will have a profound impact on the conclusions drawn regarding pediatric mild TBI.

As researchers are just beginning to understand the importance of these parameters and their interactions on the outcome of pediatric mild TBI, it may be premature to draw conclusions about all individual cases based on the current box score. With recent (e.g., Roberts & Furuseth, 1997) and anticipated advances in developing new assessment methods that possess greater applicability to educational and behavioral functioning in children, we may well come to the position that pediatric mild TBI does have persistent disabling consequences for some children. Intense research efforts should then be focused on identification of the "Miserable Minority," as Ruff (Ruff et al., 1986) labeled this group, enumeration of the risk factors that characterize these individuals, and the development of effective intervention strategies that address their needs.

WHAT ABOUT THE "MISERABLE MINORITY"

Individual children and adolescents who sustain mild TBI may experience persistent sequelae in one or more of the following areas including neuropsychological, academic, behavioral, or emotional domains, deficits that will have an impact on the student's performance in the educational setting. A survey of rehabilitation professionals (Harrington et al., 1993) revealed that mild TBI patients are typically followed clinically for 6 to 18 months postinjury, with estimates as high as 25% of these individuals who continue to exhibit at least partial functional disability. Winogren, Knights, and Bawden (1984) reported that 6% to 18% of their pediatric sample continued to show impairment at 1-year follow-up, and Ylvisaker and colleagues (Ylvisaker, Feeney, & Mullins, 1995) observed that sequelae may persist indefinitely in rare cases. The percentage of cases that are considered to be "outliers" by some and the "miserable minority" by others varies across studies ranging from lows of 7% to 10% (Levin & Eisenberg, 1979) for selected neuropsychological measures to highs of 37% (Horowitz et al., 1983) to 40% (Chadwick, Rutter, Brown, Shaffer, & Traub, 1981) for poor scholastic progress and reading backwardness, rates that far surpass what would be explained by chance statistical variation alone.

At 1- and 2-year follow-up assessments, Klonoff and colleagues (Klonoff et al., 1995) reported that 40% of their pediatric subjects (average age at injury was 8.32 years) continued to experience physical, emotional, and cognitive symptoms, including the following most frequently reported problems: personality change, memory problems, concentration and learning problems, headaches, irritability, dizzy spells, visual and auditory defects, and a decline in school achievement. By follow-up year 5, 23.7% continued to exhibit neurobehavioral deficits that paralleled years 1 and 2, including personality change, headaches, learning problems, mood changes, and memory and concentration difficulties. As argued earlier, these persistent postconcussional symptoms will only be identified if specifically examined. Studies of pediatric mild TBI that survey behavioral and emotional sequelae by administering a parent rating scale encompassing stable dimensions of developmental psychopathology (Achenbach, 1991) may fail to identify the mood changes and emotional variability with which these children and adolescents continue to struggle. Simply because these emotional and behavioral complaints fail to match the templates of traditional externalizing and internalizing psychopathology does not negate their existence. Rather, it is incumbent upon us to take a broader perspective, investigate the natural course of these symptoms in the children and adolescents who fail to recover, and attempt to find the "best fit" templates to explain these symptoms with an eye toward postulating an underlying mechanism. The available literature on adult mild TBI does suggest some potential avenues of research implicating fronto-temporal dysfunction.

Posttraumatic anosmia in adults has been associated with executive dysfunction and persistent vocational disability in spite of medical clearance to return to work (Martzke, Swan, & Varney, 1991; Varney, 1988). Roberts (Roberts & Simcox, 1996) extended this work to children and adolescents. Samples of carefully matched mildly and severely brain-injured children, recruited from consecutive emergency room referrals, were examined as part of a larger retrospective study of neurobehavioral deficits following pediatric TBI. Sense of smell was evaluated in these two TBI groups by obtaining self-report and parent-report data through interviewing subjects and their parents separately, and formal assessment of olfactory function was also undertaken. In the mild TBI group, none of the children or adolescents and only one of the parents acknowledged awareness of reduced olfactory accuracy. Nonetheless, 45% of the sample exhibited an impaired sense of smell when presented with common liquid fragrances to identify. These investigators then went on to examine the relationship between olfactory accuracy and daily behavioral manifestations of executive dysfunction. Employing ratings on the Pediatric Inventory of Neurobehavioral Symptoms (PINS, Roberts, 1992; Roberts & Furuseth, 1997), a recently developed parent rating scale of executive dysfunction, Roberts found that subjects with impaired sense of smell were almost three times as likely to exhibit executive dysfunction as those TBI subjects with intact sense of smell. Given the interconnections of the olfactory nerve and frontal lobe structures, the postulated mechanism is abrasion or shearing of the inferior surface of the frontal lobes following mechanical trauma.

The persistent memory problems, headaches, irritability, and visual and auditory symptoms described by Klonoff (Klonoff et al., 1995) have also been studied from a broader neurobehavioral perspective. Clinical research (e.g., Tierney & Fogel, 1995) and survey studies (Ardila, Nino, Pulido, Rivera, & Vanegas, 1993; Roberts et al., 1990) have identified similar episodic neuropsychiatric sequelae in adults following mild TBI. Employing a semistructured child and parent interview format with a group of children and adolescents referred for neurobehavioral evaluation following failure to recover from mild TBI, Roberts and colleagues (Roberts et al., 1996) found that greater than two-thirds of their sample reported clinically significant episodic symptoms, including staring spells, temper outbursts, memory gaps, episodic tinnitus, and severe headaches. Thirty-five percent of this mild TBI sample failed a dichotic word listening task, and poorer performance on the dichotic task was associated with an increased number of reported episodic symptoms. In 92% of the cases, a moderate to substantial improvement was observed in response to anticonvulsant medications traditionally prescribed to treat partial complex seizures. The manifestation of posttraumatic episodic symptoms has been conceptualized elsewhere as epilepsy spectrum disorder (Roberts et al., 1992; see also Roberts, chap. 11, this volume). The postulated mechanism is "kindled" subclinical electrophysiological dysfunction (Moshé, Sperber, & Albala, 1991), which evolves as a functional lesion. Kindling may also provide a parsimonious explanation for the apparent delay in symptom onset of some patients with epilepsy spectrum disorder (Roberts et al., 1995).

Roberts and colleagues (Roberts et al., 1995) presented a detailed pediatric case study, with corroborating positron emission tomography (PET) scan findings, that exemplifies the clinical presentation of epilepsy spectrum disorder following a mild TBI. Staring spells with gradually increasing frequency were observed by the child's teacher over a 2-year period following history of a whiplash injury in a motor vehicle accident at 7 years of age. This girl began to experience depressive episodes as well, for which traditional psychiatric treatment was sought. This treatment included 2 years of counseling as well as prescription of psychotropic medications, neither of which were successful. By this time the accident had occurred 4 years previously, and any injury had been all but forgotten. Furthermore, in children, where the rate of future accomplishment is not precisely predictable and the etiology of developmental psychopathology often unknown, neurobehavioral deficits that occur following mild TBI may easily be misattributed to developmental factors or considered to be idiopathic. In spite of multimodal treatment, the patient's symptoms continued to persist, and further diagnostic workup was initiated. Neuropsychological evaluation revealed verbal and visual memory deficits in the context of high average intellect. Ambulatory electroencephalographs (EEGs) were interpreted to be abnormal and epileptiform, in spite of repeat standard EEGs that were read as normal. And finally, a PET scan documented bilaterally diminished glucose metabolism in the mesial temporal areas. When compared with the presentation of classic partial complex seizures, this patient is typical of others described clinically (Verduyn, Hilt, Roberts, & Roberts, 1992), in that a greater array of symptoms occur in nonstereotyped sequences, and classic motor automatisms are generally not reported.

Presumed fronto-temporal dysfunction following pediatric mild TBI may become manifest in executive dysfunction and/or episodic symptoms as described earlier. Clinical awareness of these symptoms depends on asking the right questions. However, justification for including such targeted questions in a neurobehavioral evaluation battery presupposes that investigative research has identified these dimensions as relevant areas of inquiry. It is here that subject ascertainment becomes the pivotal point of argument. Tables 23.1 and 23.2 present a comparison of prevalence estimates for executive-episodic dysfunction depending on whether the pediatric subjects were consecutive emergency room patients (Roberts & Simcox, 1996) or clinical referrals to a rehabilitation service following incomplete recovery from mild TBI (Roberts & Furuseth, 1997). A consecutively obtained orthopedic sample matched to the consecutive mild TBI cases is provided for comparison. With regard to the orthopedic sample, two observations may be made. Prevalence of executive dysfunction in the orthopedic group was comparable to normative base rates and established cutoff at the 90th percentile (Roberts & Furuseth, 1997). Second, none of the parents of the orthopedic subjects reported observation of clinically significant episodic symptoms in their children. Several observations regarding the mild TBI samples may also be made. Examination of Tables 23.1 and 23.2 indicates that the "miserable minority" in the research setting becomes the "miserable majority" in the clinical or rehabilitation setting. It is imperative that executive-episodic symptoms be monitored by primary care clinicians who evaluate and treat pediatric patients who have experienced mild TBI. It is unlikely that these patients will be referred for persistent orthopedic complaints or questions of intellectual decline. Rather, many parents and teachers will report behavior and personality changes or what has also been labeled *persistent postconcussional symptoms*, which fail to fit traditional criteria of attention deficit hyperactivity disorder. As Benton (1995) and Ylvisaker (Ylvisaker et al., 1995) commented,

TABLE 23.1

Percentage of Samples With and Without Executive Dysfunction on the
Pediatric Inventory of Neurobehavioral Symptoms (PINS)

	With Executive Dysfunction	Without Executive Dysfunction
Consecutive mild TBI referrals[a]	35%	65%
Clinical mild TBI referrals[b]	67%	33%
Consecutive orthopedic referrals[c]	12%	88%

Note. Executive dysfunction defined as scoring at or above the 90th percentile (Roberts & Furuseth, 1997) on one or more of the three PINS executive function dimensions (i.e., Mental Inertia, Social Inappropriateness, Disconnection of Affect and Behavior).

[a] $n = 20$. Sample from Roberts and Simcox (1996).
[b] $n = 25$. Sample from Roberts and Furuseth (1997).
[c] $n = 24$. Subject sample ascertainment as described in Roberts and Simcox (1996) after additional 4 subjects had been recruited.

TABLE 23.2

Percentage of Samples With and Without Episodic Symptoms

	With Episodic Symptoms	Without Episodic Symptoms
Consecutive mild TBI referrals[a]	12%	88%
Clinical mild TBI referrals[b]	92%	8%
Consecutive orthopedic referrals[a]	0%	100%

Note. To be scored as having episodic symptoms, parent interview indicated that the child experienced two or more of the four most prevalent symptoms based on phenomenologic description provided by Roberts et al. (1996): episodic tinnitus, headaches/cephalic pain, staring spells, and uncharacteristic/unprovoked temper outbursts.

[a] $n = 24$. Subject sample ascertainment from Roberts and Simcox (1996) after additional 4 subjects had been recruited.
[b] $n = 25$. Subject sample ascertainment from Roberts and Furuseth (1997).

these patients may not be identified as having behavior problems until several years postinjury, when increasing demands are placed on the executive system. Data presented in Table 23.2 suggests that the presence of episodic symptoms in clinical samples is exceedingly high. Clinical interview for these symptoms is also of paramount importance.

ASSESSMENT AND INTERVENTION STRATEGIES FOR THE EDUCATIONAL SETTING

Initial school reentry may be fraught with unexpected difficulties for the student following mild TBI. A student who is experiencing acute sequelae is, in most cases, returning to the same academic and social demands as prior to the injury and will not immediately be enrolled in formal academic support services. Depending on when and how the accident happened, school personnel and friends may be unaware that an injury had even occurred, and thus, informal classroom accommodations may not be forthcoming either, and peers may fail to "cut their friend some slack." In the absence of physical or orthopedic injuries, deficits attributable to mild TBI may not be apparent to school personnel who do not have daily contact with the student. Given that the injury incurred was reported to be mild, even those individuals who are aware of the trauma may fail to understand the magnitude of the student's struggles. Cognitive, behavior, and emotional changes may be misattributed to other factors. Memory deficits may be attributed to poor motivation, staring spells may be viewed as an attention problem, and emotional outbursts may be misinterpreted as a disciplinary problem. And the student him-/herself may be unable to account for recent onset memory deficits, word-finding problems, and periodic confusion, further exacerbating the frustration encountered.

Even those students with a history of mild TBI who have undergone cognitive evaluation prior to return to school may not fare much better, as traditional measures of intelligence and academic achievement often fail to pinpoint the deficits that may be experienced (Levin et al., 1995). Implementation of neurobehavioral screening protocols prior to school reentry following mild TBI has been proposed (Farmer & Peterson, 1995; Shurtleff, Massagli, Hays, Ross, & Sprunk-Greenfield, 1995), with selected aspects of screening measures that may be administered by available school personnel (e.g., school nurse, psychologist, speech/language pathologist). These efforts represent an excellent initial step. However, by and large, translation of these deficits into curriculum adaptations remains to be done. Table 23.3 provides a checklist of commonly observed deficits following mild TBI. Teachers may use this reference to identify aspects of the student's classroom performance that have been disrupted. Table 23.4 provides a parallel checklist of classroom accommodations that may be helpful on a temporary or permanent basis for some students following mild TBI. Persistent or serious concerns should always be brought to the attention of the student's parents/guardians, with consideration of referral for further professional evaluation.

Beginning in about fourth grade, one of the most common complaints the student perceives is inefficiency of retrieving information that has been recently read. Although continuing to be a fluent oral reader, the student with mild TBI often "forgets" what was read by the time he or she reaches the bottom of the page. A retrieval deficit is postulated to be the underlying mechanism accounting for the student's poor recall, as examination via a multiple-choice format often results in a return to preinjury levels of performance. Using single-case methodology and a

TABLE 23.3
Potential Problem Areas for the Student
Returning to School Following Mild TBI

Inefficient Processing

Lectures go too fast for the student to keep up with note-taking.

The student fails to catch on as quickly as classmates when a new concept is presented.

The student requires more in-class time to finish assignments or tests than classmates require.

Newly presented information appears to be confusing.

The student appears to be overwhelmed by bigger projects or longer term assignments and doesn't know where to begin.

Assignment book, notebooks, and backpack are disorganized.

Changes in the daily schedule or classroom routine are upsetting (e.g., classmates are excited about a field trip while this student becomes distressed).

The student has difficulty "switching gears" within an assignment (e.g., on a page of mixed addition and subtraction problems, the student is unable to flexibly switch from one to the other math process).

The student seems unable to perform two or more components of a task at one time (e.g., solving word problems in math, the student has difficulty reading the problem, identifying the correct math process, and doing the calculations).

Memory Difficulties

The student has difficulty retrieving previously learned math facts.

Responses on history, science, or social studies tests lack detail.

The student may read a passage fluently but cannot accurately answer comprehension questions even immediately after.

Episodic Difficulties

The student has brief staring spells.

The student exhibits uncharacteristic or unexplained emotional outbursts.

The student complains of headaches.

The student complains of sensitivity or irritability in noisy environments (e.g., gym or cafeteria).

Emotional/Behavioral Difficulties

The student becomes frustrated or confused by "too much going on at once."

The student becomes distressed by word-finding difficulties or taking a longer time to process information.

The student is experiencing difficulties with maintaining friendships or the give-and-take of conversation with peers.

crossover design, Franzen and colleagues (Franzen, Roberts, Schmits, Verduyn, & Manshadi, 1996) described the successful application of an elaborative encoding technique (Robinson, 1970) to assist two boys who had sustained mild-to-moderate traumatic brain injury from a blow to the head. The PQRST technique employed by these researchers is often known to special education resource teachers in their work with learning-disabled students. Although additional research to enhance the generalizability of this technique to daily classroom assignments is needed, the Franzen et al. (1996) study provides an initial example of the potential for cognitive remediation in pediatric mild traumatic brain injury.

TABLE 23.4
Potential Educational Accommodations to Address Difficulties
Experienced by the Student with a History of Mild TBI

Inefficient Processing

Provide an organized set of notes with key points highlighted.

Provide tutorials after school, during study halls, or other study time (For younger students do *not* use recess time to accomplish this).

Break down longer tasks or assignments into segments that may be finished in one day and review these mini-assignments with the student each day.

Avoid timed tests.

Reduce in-class assignments.

Eliminate repetition in assignments when possible (e.g., having the student complete 10 math problems accurately is preferable to assigning 30 problems of the same type).

Reduce homework assignments.

Provide a daily schedule that the student keeps with him or her. (Younger children may benefit from a picture schedule. It should be constructed in such a way that schedule changes can easily be incorporated.)

Memory Difficulties

Allow use of a calculator or manipulatives (for younger children) to decrease demands on retrieval for math facts.

Provide a fact sheet for history, social studies, science essay exams that include names, dates, events, etc., to reduce the demands on memory.

Avoid fill-in-the-blank questions on exams. Give multiple-choice questions instead.

Teach a strategy to help the student organize or encode information that is read (e.g., PQRST of Robinson, 1970) or written (e.g., story mapping).

Episodic Difficulties

Record the frequency of these events. Also, where possible, provide a narrative description of antecedents, behavior, and consequences to be given to the student's parents/guardian for review by the primary care physician. This information will facilitate a focused consultation evaluation, if needed.

Reduce background noise for the student when possible (e.g., eating lunch in a room that is quieter than the typical school cafeteria, perhaps allowing the student to invite a friend)

Following a staring spell, reorienting the student to the task at hand.

Providing a checklist of the steps to be accomplished, the daily schedule, etc.

Emotional/Behavioral Difficulties

When the student is frustrated, try to find a way to help the student calm down (e.g., give extra time to respond, take a few deep breaths).

Give the student some "space" and return to the problem later.

Help the student identify when the environment is too stimulating or confusing (too noisy, too much movement) and what to do about it (e.g., alert cafeteria supervisor, student may ask to go to the library or empty classroom etc. to eat lunch).

Avoid having the student present/perform in front of class.

If full academic load becomes overwhelming, at least "temporarily drop" one class for which the curriculum may be broken down into self-contained units (e.g., may be able to drop the science unit on batteries/electrical circuits and return to science class at the start of the next unit). Batteries/electrical circuits unit may be made up in summer session (if necessary).

Monitor student's friendships, with referral to guidance counselor if needed.

A consultation by a physician who specializes in evaluating, treating, and following patients who have experienced TBI may also be of considerable benefit in successfully addressing the entire complement of deficits the child or adolescent experiences. Gualtieri (1988) reviewed several classes of medications that have been employed to provide symptomatic relief and improve the patient's functional level, including stimulant medications for attention and anticonvulsants for episodic aggressive and affective symptoms. Roberts (Roberts et al., 1995, 1996) provided descriptions of a series of cases in which anticonvulsant treatment was successful with children and adolescents who failed to recover from mild TBI.

CONCLUSION

Mild TBI occurs with considerable frequency in the pediatric population. Although the vast majority of children and adolescents who experience a mild TBI will return to preinjury levels of functioning in 3 to 12 months, a small but significant number will fail to recover. The "miserable minority" will only be identified with attention to research parameters of subject ascertainment, careful attention to the selection of dependent variables, and further exploration of developmental changes unique to the pediatric age group. The present chapter proposes that many children and adolescents who fail to recover following mild TBI display fronto-temporal dysfunction that may be manifest as executive-episodic disorders. Assessment and treatment recommendations for the educational setting are provided.

REFERENCES

Achenbach, T. M. (1991). *Manual for the Child Behavior Checklist/4-18 and 1991 Profile*. Burlington, VT: Department of Psychiatry, University of Vermont.
Alves, W. M., & Jane, J. A. (1985). Mild brain injury: Damage and outcome. In D. P. Becker & J. T. Povlishock (Eds.), *Central nervous system trauma status report* (pp. 255–270). Bethesda, MD: National Institutes of Health.
American Congress of Rehabilitation Medicine. (1993). Definition of mild traumatic brain injury. *Journal of Head Trauma Rehabilitation, 8*, 86–87.
Andrews, T. K., Rose, F. D., & Johnson, D. A. (1998). Social and behavioral effects of traumatic brain injury in children. *Brain Injury, 12*, 133–138.
Ardila, A., Nino, C. R., Pulido, E., Rivera, D. B., & Vanegas, C. J. (1993). Episodic psychic symptoms in the general population. *Epilepsia, 34*, 133–140.
Asarnow, R. F., Satz, P., Light, R., Zaucha, K., Lewis, R., & McCleary, C. (1995). The UCLA study of mild closed head injury in children and adolescents. In S. H. Broman & M. E. Michel (Eds.), *Traumatic head injury in children* (pp. 117–146). New York: Oxford University Press.

Bassett, S. S., & Slater, E. J. (1990). Neuropsychological function in adolescents sustaining mild closed head injury. *Journal of Pediatric Psychology, 15,* 225–236.

Beers, S. R. (1992). Cognitive effects of mild head injury in children and adolescents. *Neuropsychology Review, 3,* 281–320.

Benton, A. (1995). A summing up. In S. H. Broman & M. E. Michel (Eds.), *Traumatic head injury in children* (pp. 281–293). New York: Oxford University Press.

Bigler, E. D., & Snyder, J. L. (1995). Neuropsychological outcome and quantitative neuroimaging in mild head injury. *Archives of Clinical Neuropsychology, 10,* 159–174.

Bijur, P. E., & Haslum, M. (1995). Cognitive, behavioral, and motoric sequelae of mild head injury in a national birth cohort. In S. H. Broman & M. E. Michel (Eds.), *Traumatic head injury in children* (pp. 147–164). New York: Oxford University Press.

Bijur, P. E., Haslum, M., & Golding, J. (1990). Cognitive and behavioral sequelae of mild head injury in children. *Pediatrics, 85,* 337–344.

Bijur, P. E., Haslum, M., & Golding, J. (1996). Cognitive outcomes of multiple mild head injuries in children. *Devlopmental and Behavioral Pediatrics, 17,* 143–148.

Boll, T. J. (1983). Minor head injury in children—Out of sight but not out of mind. *Journal of Clinical Child Psychology, 12,* 74–80.

Chadwick, O., Rutter, M., Brown, G., Shaffer, D., & Traub, M. (1981). A prospective study of children with head injuries. II. Cognitive sequelae. *Psychological Medicine, 11,* 42–65.

Donders, J. (1993). Memory functioning after traumatic brain injury in children. *Brain Injury, 7,* 431–437.

Ewing-Cobbs, L., Levin, H. S., Fletcher, J. M., Miner, M. E., & Eisenberg, H. M. (1990). The Children's Orientation and Amnesia Test: Relationship to severity of acute head injury and to recovery of memory. *Neurosurgery, 27,* 683–691.

Farmer, J. E., & Peterson, L. (1995). Pediatric traumatic brain injury: Promoting successful school reentry. *School Psychology Review, 24,* 230–243.

Farmer, M. Y., Singer, H. S., Mellits, E. D., Hall, D., & Charney, E. (1987). Neurobehavioral sequelae of minor head injuries in children. *Pediatric Neuroscience, 13,* 304–308.

Fay, G. C., Jaffe, K. M., Polissar, N. L., Liao, S., Martin, K. M., Shurtleff, H. A., Rivara, J., & Winn, R. (1993). Mild pediatric traumatic brain injury: A cohort study. *Archives of Physical Medicine and Rehabilitation, 74,* 895–901.

Fay, G. C., Jaffe, K. M., Polissar, N. L., Liao, S., Rivara, J., & Martin, K. M. (1994). Outcome of pediatric traumatic brain injury at three years: A cohort study. *Archives of Physical Medicine and Rehabilitation, 75,* 733–741.

Franzen, K. M., Roberts, M. A., Schmits, D., Verduyn, W., & Manshadi, F. (1996). Cognitive remediation in pediatric traumatic brain injury. *Child Neuropsychology, 2,* 176–184.

Greenspan, A. I., & MacKenzie, E. J. (1994). Functional outcome after pediatric head injury. *Pediatrics, 94,* 425–432.

Gualtieri, C. T. (1988). Pharmacotherapy and the neurobehavioral sequelae of traumatic brain injury. *Brain Injury, 2,* 101–129.

Gulbrandsen, G. B. (1984). Neuropsychological sequelae of light head injuries in older children 6 months after trauma. *Journal of Clinical Neuropsychology, 6,* 257–268.

Harrington, D. E., Malec, J., Cicerone, K., & Katz, H. T. (1993). Current perceptions of rehabilitation professionals towards mild traumatic brain injury. *Archives of Physical Medicine and Rehabilitation, 74,* 579–586.

Horowitz, I., Costeff, H., Sadan, N., Abraham, E., Geyer, S., & Najenson, T. (1983). Childhood head injuries in Israel: Epidemiology and outcome. *International Rehabilitation Medicine, 4,* 32–36.

Jacobs, A., Put, E., Ingels, M., & Bossuyt, A. (1994). Prospective evaluation of technetium-99m-HMPAO SPECT in mild and moderate traumatic brain injury. *Journal of Nuclear Medicine, 35,* 942–946.

Jacquess, D. L., & Finney, J. W. (1994). Previous injuries and behavior problems predict children's injuries. *Journal of Pediatric Psychology, 19,* 79–89.

Jennett, B. (1989). Some international comparisons. In H. S. Levin, H. M. Eisenberg, & A. L. Benton (Eds.), *Mild head injury* (pp. 23–34). New York: Oxford University Press.

Kant, R., Smith-Seemiller, L., Isaac, G., & Duffy, J. (1997). Tc-HMPAO SPECT in persistent post-concussion syndrome after mild head injury: Comparison with MRI/CT. *Brain Injury, 11,* 115–124.

Kaufmann, P. M., Fletcher, J. M., Levin, H. S., Miner, M. E., & Ewing-Cobbs, L. (1993). Attentional disturbance after pediatric closed head injury. *Journal of Child Neurology, 8,* 348–353.

Klonoff, H., Clark, C., & Klonoff, P. S. (1995). Outcome of head injuries from childhood to adulthood: A twenty-three year follow-up study. In S. H. Broman & M. E. Michel (Eds.), *Traumatic head injury in children* (pp. 219–234). New York: Oxford University Press.

Kraus, J. F., Fife, D., Cox, P., Ramstein, K., & Conroy, C. (1986). Incidence, severity, and external causes of pediatric brain injury. *American Journal of Diseases of Children, 140,* 687–693.

Levin, H. S., & Eisenberg, H. M., (1979). Neuropsychological outcome of closed head injury in children and adolescents. *Child's Brain, 5,* 281–292.

Levin, H. S., Ewing-Cobbs, L., & Eisenberg, H. M. (1995). Neurobehavioral outcome of pediatric closed head injury. In S. H. Broman & M. E. Michel (Eds.), *Traumatic head injury in children* (pp. 70–116). New York: Oxford University Press.

Levin, H. S., High, W. M., Ewing-Cobbs, L. Fletcher, J. M., Eisenberg, H. M., Miner, M. E., & Goldstein, F. C. (1988). Memory functioning during the first year after closed head injury in children and adolescents. *Neurosurgery, 22,* 1043–1052.

Levin, H. S., Mattis, S., Ruff, R. M., Eisenberg, H. M., Marshall, L. F., Tabaddor, K., High, W. M., & Frankowski, R. F. (1987). Neurobehavioral outcome following minor head injury: A three center study. *Journal of Neurosurgery, 66,* 234–243.

Loney, J., & Milich, R. (1982). Hyperactivity, inattention, and aggression in clinical practice. In M. Wolraich & D. K. Routh (Eds.), *Advances in developmental and behavioral pediatrics* (Vol. 3., pp. 70–116). Greenwich, CT: JAI Press.

Lundar, T., & Nesvold, K. (1985). Pediatric head injuries caused by traffic accidents: A prospective study with 5-year follow-up. *Child's Nervous System, 1,* 24–28.

Martzke, J. S., Swan, C. S., & Varney, N. R. (1991). Post-traumatic anosmia and orbital frontal damage: Neuropsychological and neuropsychiatric correlates. *Neuropsychology, 5,* 213–225.

Moshé, S. L., Sperber, E. F., & Albala, B. J. (1991). Kindling as a model of epilepsy in developing animals. In F. Morrell (Ed.), *Kindling and synaptic plasticity* (pp. 177–194). Boston: Birkhäuser.

Plant, M., & Gifford, R. (1976). Trivial head trauma and its consequences in a perspective of regional health care. *Military Medicine, 141,* 244–247.

Polissar, N. L., Fay, G. C., Jaffe, K. M., Liao, S., Martin, K. M., Shurtleff, H. A., Rivara, J. B., & Winn, H. R. (1994). Mild pediatric traumatic brain injury: Adjusting significance levels for multiple comparisons. *Brain Injury, 8,* 249–264.

Roberts, M. A. (1992). *Pediatric Inventory of Neurobehavioral Symptoms.* Department of Pediatrics, University of Iowa, Iowa City.

Roberts, M. A., & Furuseth, A. (1997). Eliciting parental report following pediatric traumatic brain injury: Preliminary findings on the Pediatric Inventory of Neurobehavioral Symptoms. *Archives of Clinical Neuropsychology, 12,* 449–457.

Roberts, M. A., Manshadi, F. F., Bushnell, D. L., & Hines, M. E. (1995). Neurobehavioral dysfunction following mild traumatic brain injury in childhood: A case report with positive findings on positron emission tomography. *Brain Injury, 9,* 427–436.

Roberts, M. A., Persinger, M. A., Grote, C., Evertowski, L. M., Springer, J. A., Tuten, T., Moulden, D., Franzen, K. M., Roberts, R. J., & Baglio, C. S. (1994). The Dichotic Word Listening Test: Preliminary observations in American and Canadian samples. *Applied Neuropsychology, 1*, 45–56.

Roberts, M. A., & Simcox, A. F. (1996). Assessing olfaction following pediatric traumatic brain injury. *Applied Neuropsychology, 3*, 86–88.

Roberts, M. A., Verduyn, W. H., Manshadi, F. F., & Hines, M. E. (1996). Episodic symptoms in dysfunctioning children and adolescents following mild and severe traumatic brain injury. *Brain Injury, 10*, 739–747.

Roberts, R. J., Gorman, L. L., Lee, G. P., Hines, M. E., Richardson, E. D., Riggle, T. A., & Varney, N. R. (1992). The phenomenology of multiple partial seizure-like symptoms without stereotyped spells: An epilepsy spectrum disorder? *Epilepsy Research, 13*, 167–177.

Roberts, R. J., Varney, N. R., Hulbert, J. R., Paulsen, J. S., Richardson, E. D., Springer, J. A., Smith-Shepherd, J., Swan, C. S., Legrand, J. A., Harvey, J. H., Struchen, M. A., & Hines, M. E. (1990). The neuropathology of everyday life: The frequency of partial seizure symptoms among normals. *Neuropsychology, 4*, 65–86.

Robinson, F. P. (1970). *Effective study.* New York: Harper.

Ruff, R. M., Levin, H. S., & Marshall, L. F. (1986). Neurobehavioral methods of assessment and the study of outcome in minor head injury. *Journal of Head Trauma Rehabilitation, 1*, 43–52.

Rutter, M. Chadwick, O., & Shaffer, D. (1983). Head injury. In M. Rutter (Ed.), *Developmental neuropsychiatry* (pp. 83–111). New York: Guilford Press.

Satz, P., Zaucha, K., McCleary, C., Light, R., Asarnow, R., & Becker, D. (1997). Mild head injury in children and adolescents: A review of studies (1970–1995). *Psychological Bulletin, 122*, 107–131.

Segalowitz, S. J., & Brown, D. (1991). Mild head injury as a source of developmental disabilities. *Journal of Learning Disabilities, 24*, 551–559.

Shurtleff, H. A., Massagli, T. L., Hays, R. M., Ross, B., & Sprunk-Greenfield, H. (1995). Screening children and adolescents with mild to moderate traumatic brain injury to assist school reentry. *Journal of Head Trauma Rehabilitation, 10*, 64–79.

Silver, C. H., & Oakland, T. D. (1997). Helping students with mild traumatic brain injury: Collaborative roles within schools. In E. D. Bigler, E. Clark, & J. E. Farmer (Eds.), *Childhood traumatic brain injury* (pp. 239–258). Austin, TX: Pro-Ed.

Snoek, J. W., Minderhoud, J. M., & Wilmink, J. T. (1984). Delayed deterioration following mild head injury in children. *Brain, 107*, 15–36.

Stein, S. C., Spettell, C., Young, G., & Ross, S. E. (1993). Limitations of neurological assessment in mild head injury. *Brain Injury, 7*, 425–430.

Stewart-Scott, A. M., & Douglas, J. M. (1998). Educational outcome for secondary and postsecondary students following traumatic brain injury. *Brain Injury, 12*, 317–331.

Tierney, J. G., & Fogel, B. S. (1995). Neuropsychiatric sequelae of mild traumatic brain injury. In A. Stoudemire & B. S. Fogel (Eds.), *Medical-psychiatric practice* (Vol. 3, pp. 307–346). Washington, DC: American Psychiatric Press.

Varney, N. R. (1988). Prognostic significance of anosmia in patients with closed-head trauma. *Journal of Clinical and Experimental Neuropsychology, 10*, 250–254.

Varney, N. R., Bushnell, D. L., Nathan, M., Kahn, D., Roberts, R., Rezai, K., Walker, W., & Kirchner, P. (1995). NeuroSPECT correlates of disabling mild head injury: Preliminary findings. *Journal of Head Trauma Rehabilitation, 10*, 18–28.

Varney, N. R., & Varney, R. N. (1995). Brain injury without head injury. Some physics of automobile collisions with particular reference to brain injuries occurring without physical head trauma. *Applied Neuropsychology, 2*, 47–62.

Verduyn, W. H., Hilt, J., Roberts, M. A., & Roberts, R. J. (1992). Multiple partial seizure-like symptoms following "minor" closed head injury. *Brain Injury, 6*, 245–260.

Winogren, H., Knights, R., & Bawden, H. (1984). Neuropsychological deficits following head injury in children. *Journal of Clinical Neuropsychology, 6,* 269–286.

Wrightson, P., McGinn, V., & Gronwall, D. (1995). Mild head injury in preschool children: Evidence that it can be associated with a persisting cognitive defect. *Journal of Neurology, Neurosurgery, and Psychiatry, 59,* 375–380.

Yarnell, P. R., & Rossie, G. V. (1988). Minor whiplash head injury with major debilitation. *Brain Injury, 2,* 255–258.

Ylvisaker, M., Feeney, T., & Mullins, K. (1995). School reentry following mild traumatic brain injury. A proposed hospital-to-school protocol. *Journal of Head Trauma Rehabilitation, 10,* 42–49.

Author Index

Subject Index

A

Acceleration, *see also* Car accidents; Low-velocity impact, occupant kinematics
   calculation, 41–43, 45, 86–90
   in low-velocity impact, 49–58
   practical definition, 41
   in sports, 86–90
   translational and rotational, 58
ACCLAIMED, 176
Acetylcholinesterase inhibitors, 415
Activities of daily living (ADLs), 119, 423–426
Acute care, need for guidelines for, 21, 23–24
Adolescent assessment, 170, *see also* Children and adolescents
Affective disorders, 27, 228–229, 347–348, 354–355, 367–368, *see also* Depression
   Dartmouth data on, 358–361
   drug treatment for, 439–443
   manic syndromes, 352–354
   treatment, 361–368
Affective status, 359–360
Affective symptoms, 241–242
Alcohol use, 424
Alzheimer-type dementia (AD), 334
American Academy of Neurology (AAN), 21
   system for grading concussion in sports, 17, 18
American Congress of Rehabilitation Medicine
   Brain Injury Interdisciplinary Special Interest Group Mild Traumatic Brain Injury Committee

(ACRM-BI-ISIG), 16, 17, 19–21, 151–153, 315, 322
Amnesia, *see* Posttraumatic amnesia
Amytryptaline, 414
Anosmia, posttraumatic, 127
   in children and adolescents, 501–502
   functional imaging and, 123–126
   outcome and, 126
   mechanisms and assessment, 116–117
   neuropathological significance, 117–118
   psychosocial outcome and, 121–122
   tests of executive functioning and, 118–119
   vocational outcome and, 122–123
Anticholinergic medication, 445
Anticonvulsants, 231, 364, 430–437
Antidepressants, 359–360, 362–363, 414–417, 440, 442
Antiepileptic drugs, 230–235
Antioxidants, 445–446
Antipsychotic drugs, 444–445
Anxiety disorders, 428–429
Apolipoprotein ɜ (apo ɜ), 26
Arthritis, cervical, 395
Assessment, 22–23, 91, 152, 361–362, *see also* Diagnosis; specific symptoms and disorders and assessment instruments
   of children and adolescents, 170, 499, 504–508
   of CHIT, 158–161, 167, 190, 421–423
   discipline-specific approach to
      clinician-specific biases, 102–103
      discipline-specific schemas, 100–101
      lack of integration, 102

533